SUPPRESSING THE DISEASES
OF ANIMALS AND MAN

THEOBALD SMITH,
MICROBIOLOGIST

SUPPRESSING THE DISEASES OF ANIMALS AND MAN

THEOBALD SMITH, MICROBIOLOGIST

CLAUDE E. DOLMAN

AND

RICHARD J. WOLFE

Boston

Published by the Boston Medical Library in The Francis A. Countway Library of Medicine

Distributed by the Harvard University Press

2003

ISBN 0-674-01220-8

CONTENTS

ILLUSTRATIONS

Daniel E. Salmon (right), depicted in later life in a photograph from the Department of Agriculture's files.

Illustration 4.   *Above:* Lilian H. Egleston (left), photographed in 1887 at about age 30, a year before her marriage to Theobald Smith; a studio portrait of Theobald Smith (right), taken in Washington in the late 1880s or early 1890s.
Below: (left) Grandfather Egleston with the Smith children on the grounds of the Bussey Institution or Arnold Arboretum, Jamaica Plain, Massachusetts, about 1897; (right) the Smith children, Dorothea, Philip and Lilian 2, left to right, a number of years later.

Illustration 5.   *Above:* The Bussey Institution (left) in the Jamaica Plain section of West Roxbury, about 5 miles from Boston, where Theobald Smith carried on his research between 1895 and 1915; the Bussey mansion (right), known as Woodland Hill, where the Smith family lived during the same period. Grandfather Egleston appears above the front steps.
Below: (left) Theobald Smith viewing a mountain scene in 1903 while on a trip to Montana during the Anaconda suit; (right) Theobald Smith, Theodor Madsen and Svante Arrhenius (left to right) in the doorway of Madsen's Serum Institute, Copenhagen, 1904. The scene was recorded by Marshall Fabyan, Smith's traveling companion.

Illustration 6.   *Above:* Lilian Egleston Smith (left), January 1903; studio portrait of Simon Gage (right), taken in 1906.
Below: The Board of Scientific Directors of the Rockefeller Institute, ca. 1909. Left to right, Simon Flexner (standing), Mitchell Pruden, Emmet Holt (standing), William H. Welch, Theobald Smith (standing), Christian Herter and Herman Biggs.

Illustration 7.   Souvenir card, commemorating Theobald Smith's many contributions to microbiology. This was prepared by Dr. Marshal Fabyan and was given to every participant at the Complimentary Farewell Dinner on June 2, 1915 honoring Smith for his 25 years of service to Harvard prior to his resignation from the University in August following.

Illustration 8.   Scenes of the Smith's life at their Silver Lake, New Hampshire camp:
Above: Theobald Smith (left), late August or early September 1916; daughter Lilian (Lilian 2) with Theobald (right), same period.
Below: Theobald rowing Lilian's (now Mrs. Robert Foerster's) children, September 1929 (left); Theobald Smith and Carl TenBroeck, September 1927 (right).

Illustration 9.   *Above:* (left) Theobald Smith (third from left) in the academic procession at the time he was awarded an honorary D.Sc. degree by Yale University on June 20, 1917. Behind him (second from left, looking out at the reader) is I. J. Paderewski, the pianist and future Prime Minister of Poland, with whom he conversed and joked; (right) Theobald, Lilian 2 and Lilian 1, with daughter Lilian's two children. Taken at Larkfields on March 8, 1925.
Below: The Smith family prepared for a tour in their Stanley Steamer automobile, September 1918. Son Philip is at the steering wheel, with his father Theobald beside him, and daughter Lilian directly behind him, in front of Lilian 1 (left) and Dorothea (right). In the scene below appear Philip, Dorothea, Lilian 2, Theobald and Lilian 1 after alighting.

Illustration 10.   *Above:* Lilian Smith in the Garden at Larkfields, the director's house of the Rockefeller Institute's Department of Animal Pathology in Princeton (left), June 1930; Theobald Smith (right), seated before a favorite tree at Silver Lake, early 1930s.
Below: The Smith's last residence, on Battle Road in Princeton, which they built in 1931–32 and occupied from September 1932.

Illustration 11.   *Above:* The Rockefeller Institute for Medical Research's Department of Animal Pathology, Princeton, New Jersey, pictured in its early years.
Below: The Board of Scientific Directors of the Rockefeller Institute, 1932. Left to right: Edric C. Smith, Secretary to the Board, James B. Conant; Eugene L. Opie, Francis G. Blake, Charles P. Stockard, Theobald Smith, and Simon Flexner (without glasses), and William Henry Welch. Courtesy of the American Philosophical Society.

Illustration 12.   *Above:* Theobald Smith pictured on his seventy-fifth birthday, July 31, 1934 (left); Lilian Egleston Smith before the fireplace of their Silver Lake camp, September 7, 1935 (right).
Center: Snapshot of Lilian and Theobald Smith at Silver Lake, summer of 1934.
Below: Philip Smith and his sister Lilian Foerster, October 1965 (left); Headstones of Vermont marble (right) erected in the Chorocua Churchyard following the reburial of Theobald and Lilian Smiths' ashes in the fall of 1967.

PREFACE

It is remarkable that nearly seventy years have elapsed from the end of Theobald Smith's life to the publication of a comprehensive biography of this preeminent pioneer microbiologist. Although Smith's important scientific achievements and discoveries were well appreciated during his lifetime, prompting deliberations about biographical recognition, Smith himself was reticent, preferring to leave his scientific work as adequate testimonial to his life.

In the mid 1950s, Theobald Smith's son, Philip, rekindled interest in a biography—proposing one that would appeal to readers uninitiated in scientific matters. At the same time, Malcolm Ferguson and Frederick Bang of the Johns Hopkins School of Public Health planned to collaborate on a formal biography. Philip eventually abandoned his plans, but Bang and Ferguson diligently archived a mass of reference material related to the life and work of Theobald Smith. Unfortunately, encumbered by other pressing engagements, their intentions eventually lost momentum and, by the early 1960s, they had to abandon their project and seek someone else to whom to pass the torch.

In 1964, while working in the Welch Library in Baltimore on essays on the history of microbiology, my father, Dr. Claude Dolman, met Mrs. Bang, who encouraged him to examine the material that her husband and Dr. Ferguson had collected. From the initial introductions, Dr. Dolman quickly assumed the mantle of biographer and he continued the industrious collection of Smith memorabilia that had characterized the efforts of Bang and Ferguson. Over a period of two years, he made visits to Boston, Princeton, the Rockefeller Institute in New York, the American Philosophical Society in Philadelphia, Baltimore, Washington, Cornell University in Ithaca, Albany, Bar Harbor, and Newfane, as well as to

Theobald's Children, Philip, Lilian and Dorothea. He became close friends with Philip, visiting him nine times at the latter's farm in Sherman, New York. Dr. Dolman returned home to Vancouver after each visit (the final one being in 1983) armed with ever more Smith memorabilia.

Following an auspicious beginning, writing progressed relatively slowly. Two complete revisions of the work were necessary to compress the text into a length that potential publishers might deem appropriate, and to achieve a quality and completeness that satisfied the author. Unfortunately, all this attention was focused on a work that was several chapters shy of completion. By the late 1980s, Dr. Dolman became progressively hampered by Parkinson's disease, and it was becoming apparent that the still incomplete biography might never come to fruition—a fate made more certain by his death in 1994. However, with the gracious help of Dr. Janet Robertson of the Department of Microbiology of the University of Alberta, one of my father's former students, we contacted Mr. Richard Wolfe, then Curator of Rare Books and Manuscripts at the Francis A. Countway Library in Boston, who had considerable experience in writing and editing medical history. Mr. Wolfe kindly undertook the final editing and completion of the book, as well as seeing to its ultimate publication. The completed book thus appears nearly fifty years after its initial conception, the product of several hands but hands united in a common goal!

Many acknowledgments are due. Mr. mother, Dr. Lore Dolman, provided inestimable financial, clerical and supportive help to my father over many decades until her death in 1988. Secretaries Cathy Liddle and Carrie Hirsch, both of whom endured numerous rewritings and editings in pre- word processor days, provided invaluable clerical assistance. Margeret Ettinger, granddaughter of Theobald Smith, has provided generous moral support, both to my father over the last few decades, and subsequently to his children as we pursued completion of the biography. Dr. Robertson was most gracious and helpful at a time when we were truly at a loss to see a way through to completion of the book. And a huge debt of thanks is due to Mr. Wolfe who has managed with efficiency and good grace to complete this lengthy task.

We hope that the reader will find the biography to be a fitting tribute to the life of a unique individual who made significant and fundamental contributions to the scientific knowledge of how microbiological organisms affect human and animal health.

John Dolman
Vancouver, British Columbia
January 2002

1

HERITAGE AND EARLY YEARS

"My parents, whose only interest in life was the welfare
of their children, were in straitened and humble circumstances.
No outstanding ancestry supplied a source of pride
or antidote to personal defects or failure."[1]

In the 1850s, swarms of German-speaking emigrants from Europe endured
the hardships and dangers of a long, dreary voyage to North America to escape the unrest caused by repeated eruptions and suppressions of the Union-
ist and Liberal movement in their homeland. Among those seeking the greater
security and opportunities of the New World were Philipp Schmitt and Theresia
Kexel, who had been married on July 16, 1854 at Limburg, a small city on the
River Lahn, a tributary of the Rhine. He was twenty-five and she two years
older.[2] Soon after their marriage they set out across the Atlantic from Antwerp.
In the fall of 1854 they landed at New York to find cholera rampant there. The
couple made their way to Albany, where a sister of Philipp had settled, and to
which some of his wife's relatives migrated later. Of the few possessions they
brought with them, one small relic is still treasured by their descendants—a
black wooden inkstand, intricately carved by Theresia's grandfather.

What little is known of the newcomers' background and antecedents is told in
a simple but moving account written thirty years later by their son, when he felt
the urge to make himself and his origins known to his future wife. Theobald, the
subject of this biography, informed his fiancée in 1886 that his mother's ancestors were a line of schoolmasters and that his mother had been born in a small
village in the Duchy of Nassau not far from Wiesbaden. His grandfather had died

young, leaving his grandmother with a large family. "The appearance of a step-father on the scene was coincident with the disappearance of her property. My grandmother, after much grief and suffering died soon afterward, leaving a large number of half-grown girls and one boy to take care of themselves. My mother and her sisters, orphaned and almost penniless, were forced to earn their living as servants in the near city of Limburg a/d Lahn."

Theobald's paternal grandfather was one of a number of brothers, sons of a well-to-do farmer in a large village in the same province. The expenses incurred in preparing one of the sons for the ministry virtually left the rest of the sons poor. His father was early apprenticed to a tailor in his native village, where at age fourteen he began his trade. "The privations of his childhood aggravated by an indolent father, had left a very deep impression upon his whole being which . . . has lasted a lifetime. He longed for a better education, but that was denied him." Upon reaching Limburg, he continued his trade, although he occasionally trampled afoot into distant cities, as was the custom with the journeyman tailor. "A strange peculiarity of his old province was its religious coloring . . . Some villages were Catholic in toto, others Lutheran or Reformed . . . Mother came from a Catholic village, father from a Protestant town, and of course they brought their respective beliefs with them . . . In the year 1854 they were married and came to this country. They tossed about on the ocean in a sailing vessel from Antwerp for eight long weeks."[3]

Where and how the Schmitts lived for the first year after arriving in Albany is untraceable. The Albany Directory for 1856 shows a Philip Smith, tailor, at 217 South Pearl Street. The 1857 and 1858 Directories list him at a nearby address, 177 Broad Street. There were many tailors and seamstresses in Albany, sustained by the special needs of senators and assemblymen for frock coats and their ladies for fashionable outfits. Competition was heavy, but Philipp was a skillful and industrious craftsman, and eventually had all the work he could handle. In October 1858, he bought a small property on Jay Street, then on the northwest edge of the city in almost open country. A row of three-story, red brick houses, simple but well-proportioned, lined both sides of the street. The Schmitt family lived for a decade in number 144 on the south side, about 100 yards east of the junction of Jay and Lark Streets.

The Schmitts had a daughter, Bertha, on March 14, 1856, and a son was born on July 31, 1859, the year his father became a naturalized citizen of the United States. When seven weeks old, the boy was baptized at the Church of the Holy Cross, then situated at Hamilton and Philip Streets, which cared for the spiritual needs of the German Catholic immigrant community through the Rev. Theodor Noethen, a well-educated but strictly orthodox parish priest. On the same occasion, Bertha Schmitt was baptized "sub conditione," indicating uncertainty whether the rite had been properly performed earlier. Her birthday is stated as May 14, 1856, two months in her favor.[4] The boy's date of birth is entered as July 30, 1859, only one day in error. An entry (in Latin) in the parish register for September 18, 1859 records the baptismal name as Theobald, the godparents being Jacob and Margaretha Theobald, who were next-door neighbors and recent immigrants from Germany. Jacob Theobald was listed sporadically in the Albany city Directories from 1854 to 1860, first as plain "Thieubalt," later as "Jacob Theobald" and "Jacob Theobilt," and his occupation as "varnisher."

For some years the godson adopted Jacob as his second name. The title-page of one of his 1875 diaries declares: "DIARY von Theobald Jakob Schmitt geboren Albany Juli den 31 im Jahre des Herren 1859."[5] Albany High School records usually listed him as Theobald J. Smith. The manuscript of his 1876 valedictory address and some school essays were signed likewise; on other documents he was T.J. Smith. The second initial was dropped soon afterwards, and he became plain Theobald Smith or T.S. Exactly when the name "Schmitt" turned into "Smith" is not clear. No formal steps were taken, but data collectors for city of Albany directories had been instructed to enter under SMITH all possible cognates, from Schmid and Schmitz to Smit and Smithe. Later Philipp's son brooded on this question:

> The ignorance of the Americans concerning German at that time was something quite unintelligible. They persisted in writing the name in what they presumed to be the translation. So I grew up in the second form. Names entered upon school records are indelible. They are carried in the form of certificates and diplomas from one institution to another until a name is stamped upon an individual as firmly as his nose upon his face. In latter years it seemed to me at times as if I were sailing under false colors without being able to take them down, yet when one feels so little Germanized as I do the deception becomes bearable and even seems justifiable in the acquisition of a new nationality.[6]

His parents spoke their native tongue, and sent both children to Professor Singer's Academy on Philip Street, a strict private school conducted in German, where they were still called Schmitt. Two married aunts and some cousins now lived in Albany. Visits were interchanged with them and with a limited circle of German-speaking friends.

In 1869, Theobald's father, who had been ailing, resolved to return to his home in Germany. Towards the end of April, the home on Jay Street was sold, and "one bright afternoon in May," Theobald remembered, "we steamed out of New York Bay."

What a glorious experience for a boy of ten! As soon as I could raise my head after four days of sea-sickness I moved about deck constantly, drank in every wave, every school of fishes, every sail. I will not dilate on the delightful time during the summer at the home of my parents. A city lad transplanted into the rural districts of an old country where every foot of ground is cultivated and so gains in beauty. We had left to stay in Germany. The summer rolled on and at last father was at his old trick again, trying to purchase a home. Nothing suited him. The slow pace in which everything moved, the diminished scale of income and living were beginning to be irksome. Autumn saw us again in Albany.[7]

Like Philipp Schmitt, a great many immigrants to the New World similarly assuaged their nostalgia for the Old. Theobald never forgot the tidiness and fertility of the fields, vineyards and gardens, nor the thrifty, ritualistic toil that made orderly harvesting possible. The visit reinforced his cultural inheritance. Given a book of selections from Schiller, he read them frequently from the age of twelve until manhood. "That calm, high ideal everywhere found in his works . . . had a powerful influence upon my ways of thinking for years after." In 1886 he still had "the dear old German volume much soiled and worn by my diligent use."[8] Later, his background yielded many practical advantages. He was able to correspond in German with overseas relatives and scientific colleagues; he savored and sifted German literature, both classical and bacteriological; and he reported some of his earlier work in that language. Certain Teutonic characteristics emerged— meticulous thoroughness, almost fanatical concern for detail, impatience with stupidity, and occasional authoritarian attitudes. Yet he was essentially American.

> A German in the strict sense I could never become. Most of those whom I have met never attracted me and their mode of life still less. [In the 1850s] there was a very strong, rather brutal feeling of a large class of "natives" towards the Germans. Germany at that time was still a *Teutoburger Wald*[9] to them, and the savages that emerged therefrom required corresponding treatment. These times have passed away. In fact . . . Germany is now the repository of our intellectual supplies. Should such a spirit ever again appear I should certainly be induced to forcibly readopt my parental name and stand by it.[10]

On returning to Albany, Philip Smith, tailor, lived for a while at 101 Lark Street. In April 1871 he bought a three-storied brick house at 54 Alexander Street, on the south side, between Clinton and Elizabeth Streets. The lot, of rather narrow frontage, was roughly 100 feet deep. On the ground floor were the tailoring workshop, parlor, kitchen and hall. The upper floors provided sleeping quarters for the family and occasional visitors, and also for lodgers. Behind the house was a garden about twenty-five by seventy feet, containing a few fruit trees, berry bushes, grape vines and a vegetable patch.[11]

Theobald served as general handyman, while his father attended to customers and made suits and overcoats for retail tailors, and his mother helped in the workshop, kept house, and managed the motley collection of lodgers. Theobald delivered clothes before school, bought fish and birdseed, skinned eels, glued chairs, varnished floors and doors, mended a skylight broken by March winds and hail, installed a lightning conductor, laid oilcloth on the stairs, and wall-papered the kitchen and hall. Occasionally he made neckties, either for himself or to give away. Ashes had to be carried out, rags picked clean, and new carpet fitted in the hall. In summer, he and his mother cleaned up the house and cellar. "Thus we white-washed, took up the carpets, threw over the beds, tumbled everything into the utmost confusion, for the more this is done, the more you are cleaning house."[12]

In early autumn Theobald filled the cellar with coal and in winter shovelled snow. In spring he might fence or pave part of the back yard with "flagging-stones," and each year he erected and took down the summer house. Regularly he tidied and swept the sidewalk. The gardening cycle, which began in April with compost dressing, ended in late fall when winter salad was lifted, evergreen trees bound up, and grapevines pruned and covered. He grew mainly vegetables, but flowers were planted too, competing with morning glory "about 2.75 ft high." Summer arrived suddenly in May, when digging and watering became frequent occupations. He kept a sharp eye on prices, once getting a plum tree for a dollar at the Madison Avenue nursery. The hired man "threw in" a currant bush, and the awkward load was lugged home by lamplight.[13]

The parents made ends meet with difficulty. Upkeep of the property was expensive: a wooden fence cost $77.50, painting of the front door and middle floor, $52.00. Nevertheless, through hard work and frugality, his father eventually owned 54 Alexander Street and left substantial bank savings. "One of his firm determinations in life was not to leave his children as he was left in childhood, and he certainly has done whatever was in his power to do."[14] Parental example made an indelible impression upon the son, whose deeply-rooted diligence and thrift were never discarded.[15] Theobald was kind and dutiful to his mother. On her forty-ninth birthday he bought her a shoulder shawl. When "pa reached his 47th year" a week before Christmas 1877, Theobald presented him with a pair of spectacles. He bought things occasionally for the household, when the price was right and he had the money. "This morn I found a barrel of Spitzenburgs $1.00 that exactly coincided with my opinions, & soon it was in our cellar."[16]

After the return from Germany, the boy was transferred from Singer's Academy to Public School No. 10, at 182 Washington Avenue. Even in late life he recalled with stern disfavor the two years of unhappy attendance at this school. His only recorded accomplishment there was to win "a pretty gold medal" for penmanship, just before he left in the summer of 1872. (His neat, clear handwriting changed remarkably little during his lifetime.)[17] Then, by a happy stroke of fortune, Theobald was admitted to the Albany Free Academy. He entered this school, known as "the High School," at the beginning of September, 1872, when just over thirteen years old, recalling in later life that "My four years at the High School were a most delightful period of my life."[18]

Albany became the permanent capital of New York State in 1797, nearly two centuries after Dutch traders built Fort Nassau, the first settlement in the area. Albanians traditionally upheld high standards of public education. In 1866, when the population numbered barely 65,000, a special committee named by the Board of Public Instruction recommended that the school system be enlarged and improved by the creation of a Free Academy. This was opposed by Mayor George H. Thacher and several members of the Common Council. However, in November 1867, General Charles P. Easton, President of the Albany Board of Public Instruction, secured for twelve hundred dollars annual rental a four-year lease on Van Vechten Hall. This three-storied building at 119 State Street, originally built in 1831 as terminal station of the old Mohawk and Hudson Railroad, which ran from Albany to Schenectady and carried the first passenger train in America,[19] had served as State Normal School, another pioneering venture, since 1844. A considerable sum was spent on adapting this building and purchasing furniture.

On September 7, 1868, the Albany Free Academy was launched, with ceremonies presided over by the chairman of the Board's Committee on the Free Academy, George W. Carpenter. It was staffed by Principal John E. Bradley and five men and women. By September 1870, the school's enrollment had doubled to about 280, and the Faculty increased by three men and four women. The predicted total student body for the school year beginning September 1872 was between 400 and 500, and the need for additional space became urgent. Besides, the ground level of the former railroad station was now used as a horse stable, which provoked Theobald to insert the following doggerel comment in his diary:

> And the odors, so fragrant,
> Wafted up from below,
> More "stable" than fickle were they;

> There may have been Horse Play indulged in above,
> There was Horse Work below every day."[20]

The Board of Public Instruction released plans for a new building, estimated to cost no more than $80,000. The Mayor addressed a printed pamphlet to the Common Council, headed "Mayor Thacher's Protest! Twenty Per Cent of Our Taxes for Public Instruction." He argued:

> We are under no obligation, either moral or civil, to tax ourselves for the purpose of conferring the higher and collegiate branches of learning in our public schools. What we are obligated to do is nothing more or less than to impart such an education as will enable the children of the state to perform, in an intelligent manner, all the ordinary duties of life.[21]

The Board fought back and the contest became very bitter. Libellous articles appeared in the public press. Looking back on those days a quarter-century later, the first Principal stated publicly: "From 1870 to 1874 the Free Academy encountered the fiercest opposition which has ever been arrayed against any educational institution within my knowledge."[22] The school's fate remained uncertain until 1874, when a popular petition was organized. A majority of votes favored the institution and ground was broken on Eagle Street between Steuben and Columbia Streets for a well-designed, much enlarged building.

John E. Bradley, a graduate of Williams College, was twenty-nine years old when he was appointed principal of the Free Academy, and also Professor of Mental and Moral Philosophy. Oscar D. Robinson of Dartmouth, an infantry captain during the Civil War, thirty-one years of age, was Professor of Latin and Greek, and eventually succeeded Bradley as principal. Both were educationists of demanding standards and outstanding organizing ability. They were assisted by Professors of English Literature, History, German, French, Mathematics and Natural Science. A professor of Music inspired those distinctive school songs—solos, duets, quartets, choruses, rounds and roundelays—which the first generation of Albany High School graduates enjoyed and never forgot. The staff and curriculum emphasized the conviction that a well-educated person should be both informed and able to convey knowledge. In the first examinations sponsored by the Board of Regents of New York State University, Albany High School placed foremost among comparable institutions in that state. Within a decade, this fledgling of a relatively small city won competitions open to the world.

Theobald attended the old school without missing a day during its last two years. A Certificate of Academic Scholarship, issued to Theobald J. Smith for passing an examination held at Albany High School in September 1873 became his earliest scrapbook trophy. All "Academies and Institutions of Learning" subject to visitation by the Regents of the University of the State of New York were authorized to receive him as an Academic Scholar without examination. Since from September 30 to December 19, 1873, he "received Free Instruction at the Institution known as Albany High School . . . to the amount of $15," he was entitled to further free instruction in "classics or the higher branches of English education, or both," at any school within the regents' jurisdiction. On November 1, 1874, he started a diary. Here he recorded in the spring of 1876: "The last week of school in the old building! The pleasant remembrances which cling around it are rather dusty & shabby, yet the building does not determine the knowledge diffused in it."[23] Three days later, he attended the "remarkably touching" final Public Rhetorical Exercises in Van Vechten Hall.

He enrolled as "Theobald J. Smith" in the English or First Division. The less patronized Classical Division demanded more Latin and Greek and less science and mathematics. He finished third in his First Year class, with a general average of 7.958—the maximum always being 8. His Junior Year average was 7.996. At the end of the year he noted: "The commencement ended at 6 P.M. I caught hold of a merit roll and felt very weak & shaky on seeing my name at the head of the list . . . My parents were exceedingly happy on seeing me head. Resolved—to go fishing tomorrow."[24]

His diary was sprinkled with comments on marks obtained. He noted 8s with quiet satisfaction. For example, on December 10, 1874: "très beau—received marks. 14 - 8s." Less than a full mark left him despondent and sometimes petulant. Thus, after a mathematics test, he wrote: "Horne [Charles A. Horne, Professor of Mathematics] & we had a quarrel about some 7s but he *caved* in."[25] Horne realized his pupil's talent for higher mathematics and took special pains to coach him outside school hours in spherical trigonometry and surveying.

The chemistry teacher, Charles H. Porter, M.D., gave a scrappy course with occasional demonstrations. Porter's chemistry and Prof. Cole's English literature periods were consecutive, so the diary for the first half of 1875 contained oddly cryptic conjunctions: "On Beowolf and Zinc," "On Chaucer, Iron &c," "On Decomposition of Gas & Theater," "Petroleum Review—Bunyan," "Wordsworth & Albuminoid Bodies." Theobald reached the finals of two spelling matches, but was stumped by "Lilliputian" and "dryad", losing in both instances to girls. His reactions to distinguished visiting lecturers were unpredictable but brief. For example, "Visit from Flack, Dr. LSD, AM, PD, BA. great talker."[26] Two renowned speakers—the gentle and high-minded poet-journalist, William Cullen Bryant, and the Congregationalist preacher and reformer, Henry Ward Beecher—were barely mentioned.

He enlivened his junior year by taking extra introductory courses—in Botany from an instructor in English, Miss Rebecca ("Becky") Hindman, and in Astronomy, offered by Prof. Horne. In his senior year, he began the study of Geology. These introductions to botany and geology were especially enjoyed. In his last high school year, he took extracurricular French lessons. Armed with a copy of Keetels's Grammar, Theobald inserted French words, phrases and occasionally long passages in his diary. During the last three months at the school, on Saturday afternoons, he enrolled in an unofficial course in drafting, which included shading and tinting. Thus he learned to draw pleasingly and accurately.

Theobald Smith's German was exceptionally good and literate, although the phraseology displayed colloquialisms and syntactical oddities. Apart from conversational opportunities with parents, relatives, and his old schoolmaster, he regularly read a German newspaper sponsored by the immigrant community in Albany. Moreover, he read in the State Library the great four-volume *German Grammar* by Jacob Grimm.[27] From the start, his diary carried occasional spontaneities in neat Gothic script. In his nineteenth year, there were numerous lengthy passages in German, which then diminished and ultimately vanished.

These educational diversions took less time than the English compositions to which many hours weekly were devoted throughout his high school years. The earliest of those preserved, entitled "Visit to a Castle," dealing with a family excursion during their 1869 visit to Germany, shows how clear and precise were Theobald's powers of observation when he was ten years old.[28] Another short manuscript of about the same date describes a visit to Seltzer Springs. Two longer compositions were also kept. The first, entitled "Historical Romance," and extending over twenty-three quarto pages, was assigned by Prof. Cole as a dissertation subject. Dated April 1875, it took two months to complete. Although the essay's central theme was that historical romance reached its culmination with the poems and novels of Sir Walter Scott, it ranged deftly from Homeric hexameters to the border ballads, from Robin Hood to Bishop Percy.

The other retained composition, completed six months later, was an exercise in science fiction. Entitled "A Journey to Mars," this curious tale exploited the idea that "The planet Mars, so near to us at present and the object of so much speculation and theory, is accessible to us since it is apparent that it is enveloped by an atmosphere, and from its indication appears to be inhabited." It concerned the adventures of three young students who, having discovered by laboratory experiment a gas infinitely lighter than hydrogen, which they named "Strinine," decided to use its lifting power for a voyage to Mars by space ship. The essay dealt with their construction of a cylindrical ship of aluminum. Their oxygen would come from heating potassium chlorate with an alcohol lamp, whose own needs for oxygen were met by a compressed supply. The upper and lower chambers communicated by means of a valve, whereby the two gases could be mixed together to make the machine heavier. "A substance to absorb the Carbonic Dioxide similar to lime was to be distributed in vessels around the room, and the water vapor was taken care of by means of Sulphuric acid." After provisions and equipment for a three-week journey had been put aboard, the fastenings were cut loose and the adventurers were whisked up rapidly through the air. They skirted the moon and, on reaching Mars, found a walled city with blond inhabitants eight feet tall. After exploring its equatorial continent and ice caps, the "astronauts," now in a warmer climate, descended and fell into a deep sleep, from which the dreaming narrator was shaken awake by his fellow students.[29]

Theobald Smith kept this essay in preference to compositions on numerous topics, many of them scientific, undertaken during his last two years at Albany High School. Perhaps it symbolized the assumption that progress depended upon the suitable application of sciences. The sixteen-year-old author produced some rousing descriptive passages, but in assessing the difficulties of the journey, and selecting appropriate equipment, he revealed very fragmentary knowledge; and in describing the Martian fauna and flora, his inventiveness showed mundane limitations. The inhabitants spoke a kind of Esperanto and their "head-dress was a hat similar to ours with a narrower brim."

Theobald was a moody youth. Shortly after the New Year Centennial celebrations, he complained: "No study, for my brain feels very bad. My head for a week seems bandaged & I am deeply depressed."[30] One Saturday was "Fooled away . . . without any beneficial result." Reading provided a year-round refuge from periodic disillusionment and emotional disequilibrium. He took advantage of the State Library's proximity to both school and home, often spending two or three evenings a week and parts of Saturday there. On winter nights he usually read by the kitchen stove, and in hot weather resorted to his summerhouse.

From age fifteen to seventeen Theobald favored romantic novels or poems and tales of travel. Enjoying Dickens as well as Scott, he recorded one evening "passed away with Scrooge." *A Christmas Carol* was followed by *Our Mutual Friend* and *Dombey and Son,* while Byron, Bronte and Wordsworth were sampled. Also read were Stanley's *How I found Livingstone* (1872); *Lalla Rookh,* a long metrical romance by Thomas Moore, whose oriental descriptions dazzled an earlier generation; Longfellow's verse-drama, *The Spanish Student,* and William H. Seward's *Travels Around the World* (1873). During his last school semester he tackled David Hume's *Political Discourses,* M.J. Schleiden's *Principles of Scientific Botany,* and Bishop Alonzo Potter's *Political Economy,* as well as informing himself on sleep, ventriloquism and electricity, phrenology and the Crusades.

Until Theobald Smith graduated from high school and began subscribing to *Scientific American,* his reading material hardly presaged an important scientific career. Then he noted exuberantly, early in 1877: "Reading Buckle's *History of [Civilization in] England,* a grand work . . . his truths are like thunderbolts, his language sublime."[31] When reviewing that period nearly a decade later, he admitted: "Another book among the many had a strong influence in directing my scientific tastes. I presume that for every growing mind the sweeping generalizations of such a book as Buckle's *History of Civilization* had a peculiar charm. Now, I fear, my attitude would be more skeptical."[32]

Buckle's ambition (thwarted by his early death in 1862) was to illustrate on a grandiose scale the laws governing human progress. Two introductory volumes developed several basic tenets, one being that mankind would advance through science. Another claim was that civilized progress depended on "skepticism," or the disposition to doubt and investigate, and declined with "credulity," or the tendency to protect, without scrutinizing, established beliefs and practices. Buckle rose quickly to literary and social fame after the first volume appeared; but his contribution to the prestige of science was overlooked in the controversies that arose about the more specific and disciplined doctrines of Darwin, Huxley, Lyell and their associates.

At the Academy, the Philologian Literary Society (Philologia) was organized as a friendly rival to the Philodoxian Literary Society (Philodoxia). Theobald joined the former in September 1874. He served briefly as Editor of the *Philologian Record* and became Corresponding Secretary in May 1875. Five months later, a new slate of officers listed T. J. Smith as Vice-President. "Ha-a-a," is the diary's only comment. Soon afterward, recording a declamation by Bishop "About the Sufferings of Negroes and their Emancipation," he noted, "I was in the chair and also in a puzzle sometimes."[33] On May 25, 1876, heading the list of newly elected executives was Theobald J. Smith ("myself") as President. He held this office for five months.

In sanctioning Philologia, Principal Bradley, who invented the name, stipulated that its meetings be open to the Faculty. Either he or a staff member suggested the topics for the programs and frequently attended. There were "topics by the peck." Theobald Smith spoke in debates, or read essays on matters as varied as "Albany as a Business Center," "The Influence of Wordsworth on Poetical Taste and Practice," "Chivalry," "Architecture," "Gunpowder," and "Tides." He tried (not always successfully) to avoid emotional involvement in social questions. For example, "Should Intemperance be arrested by legislative action? I took the negative and endeavored to show that the vice was too deeply rooted & could only be torn up by educating the intemperate to abhor the evil & abstain from it."[34] His private comments on meetings were apt to be especially disdainful during his presidency: "Is it of more advantage to study for a particular profession than to gain a general education—the arguments were farfetched & obscure & showed a remarkable ignorance of the subject—Initiated 4 members."[35]

The Society's affairs were conducted with high-toned formality. The Treasurer reminded members on printed letterhead that monthly dues (ten cents, soon raised to fifteen) were payable, and the Corresponding Secretary notified "Mr. Smith" or others that they were "appointed" to lecture or debate on a stated day. Upon one member's death, the Society printed a black-bordered *In Memoriam* tribute, and on the afternoon of the funeral "could be seen marching towards his house with crepe around the left arm."[36] They decorously enjoyed themselves when Faculty representatives responded to invitations. "A splendid time we had, speeches from our honorary & some active members, & on motion we went to Graham's Parlors to partake of some iced cream & cake & we went to Nelligar's & came a round of sodars."[37]

Nearly all thirty-five Philologians named in the diary during the period 1874–1876 had successful careers, as e.g., Congressman, rabbi, monsignor, schoolmaster-clergyman, architect and astronomer (Charles S. Wells, '77, gave his name to a comet). There were also five lawyers or attorneys, including Theobald's particular friend, George Addington, '78, who became a judge, four physicians, two university professors, and two engineers, one of whom, Henry Battin, '77, was another long-term friend. Seven prospered in business.

After graduation from High School, Theobald went only intermittently to meetings as an honorary member. In November 1876 he talked on "The Difference Between the Ancient & the Modern Civilization in Relation to the Arts & Sciences," and a few months later read an essay on "Africa." He attended the first debate between the Philodoxian and Philologian Societies in February 1877.[38] Although given the title Senior Editor, he soon resigned the office and before long ceased going to the meetings.

From the Society, Theobald reaped advantages in broadened horizons, heightened self-expression, opportunities for leadership, and commitment to orderly citizenship. In 1915, regretfully declining an invitation to the annual dinner meeting of the Old Philologians, he wrote: "I do not recall any single factor in my High School life to which I owe so much as the Philologian Society. Not only have the early friendships been strong and lasting but our earnest and persistent literary efforts have borne fruit in later years."[39]

Apart from meetings of the two Literary Societies, which reinforced the special encouragement given to elocution and public speaking at Albany High School, the Principal (a gifted orator) inaugurated a system of weekly exercises in rhetoric throughout the school year. Moreover, the customary Christmas and Spring Commencement rituals were supplemented by Public Rhetorical Exercises. In these strenuous "Publics" the Philologians and Philodoxians were fully represented. When not yet sixteen, Theobald was scheduled to take part in one of these "Publics." He confided to his diary: "Trembling all day about speaking which finally terminates with an 8."[40] For his declamation next day, he was awarded a prize—Tyndall's *Sound*.[41] On May 4, 1876, Theobald witnessed the new High School dedication ceremonies, involving numerous addresses from "honorable gentlemen," followed by "a grand soirée musicale . . . pa & ma there." Four days later, as the school occupied its new quarters, they mounted "the broad stairways & gaze upon the magnificence" to the strains of a solemn march.

At last the Annual Examination of his senior year arrived. "Today the grand affair took place, we recited moral Philosophy in the Chapel with 50 Clergymen & Commissioners as audience. I spoke eloquently on Reputation, the temptations to slander & Benevolent disposition of Caricature."[42] The following day "Bradley announced to me privately that I! ha! ha! must write & deliver the Valedictory." The news soon spread: "Joy among the Seniors . . . My brain seemed to contract & rise up at the trouble before it . . . After Bradley lugged me up to his house & gave me some previous vale- & vive-dictories I started for home."

He began to write. Bradley and Robinson read several drafts, and there were daily rehearsals with Miss Morgan, the Instructor in Rhetoric and Elocution. On the Sunday beforehand, having committed 1100-odd words to memory, he dressed up: "Today marks an epoch in my history—a long coat & an entirely new suit! White vest—black pants & neck tie."[43] At last, on June 30, 1876:

> The fearful day has dawned, when the Smith shall quiver & tremble, for today is the long wished for graduation day. The sun dawns bright & early & I go up to the Hall and back, got ready & went TO THE COMMENCEMENT. The time lies heavily upon me, the beginnings of my Valedictory flashes occasionally across my mind with a pang that tends to stop my heart . . . Is there no pit to receive me, no opening that shall be sealed after swallowing me? No, for the "Heroes"[44] is struck up, & I leave. Soon I am gesticulating violently & all is over. Then sheepskins are distributed & I feel happy.

In the four-page Valedictory manuscript—a conventionally phrased but grateful and sincere farewell—the injunctions to himself and his classmates were timely and prophetic for the years ahead: "Let us not suppose that the acquisition of knowledge ceases with our schooldays, for it is only begun."

> Some of us may go on still farther in the broad highway of knowledge, others will now begin the rugged path of life, but in whatever position we may be placed, into

whatever channel our energies may be directed, let us always endeavor to become useful to ourselves and to our fellow-men.

Remember that "Knowledge is power," that the educated man is honored and esteemed everywhere not for his material but for his mental riches. Let us be patient in all our labors, let us not expect distinction and success without earnest, diligent work and many disappointments, let us not despair at failures so common in life or be disheartened at petty obstacles, but let us press right on until perseverance will clear the road to success.[45]

After quietly celebrating over "Soda" with a few friends, Theobald "went to Bradley's there to spend a very pleasant evening in conversation & chatting. At 11 P.M. we left. Thus ended in A.H.S. 'MY GRADUATION DAY'."[46]

In the school's records, it was certified that "Theobald J. Smith has honorably completed the English and Mathematical Course of study in this Institution." Further, he was awarded the "highest expression of commendation . . . for his diligent application to study, thorough scholarship and exemplary deportment." He had achieved the remarkable overall average of 7.977, and was among fifteen on the 1875–76 Roll of Honor who "had not been absent or tardy during four years attendance." Ten years later he reflected: "My pride was transferred to my parents. It was for them that I rejoiced because I knew that their sacrifices would be best counterbalanced by such little things." After he left school, he helped to organize the Alumni Association and attended the first Annual Reunion. A century later, a small portrait of "T.J. Smith," taken two months before graduation, was still in the High School files.

Theobald recalled in his autobiographical letter to his finance that "After graduation I remained home a year, thinking what it were best to do."[47] Many of his classmates and fellow-Philologians found employment or planned to enter college; some had left Albany. "When I talked things over with father and mother, mother would finally say: 'Ach Kind, das musst Du am besten wissen.' They trusted me and that increased my responsibilities." As his parents could not afford to send him to college, he decided to mark time, living at home and earning what he could. He had "no friends to shove me into a comfortable place as bank clerk or book-keeper, from whence I might have become a staid business-man and never after emerged into the sunshine of a higher life. No advisers to point out for me the dangers of my own tastes, which were for more knowledge."[48] His seventeenth birthday provoked a gloomy soliloquy: "TODAY I AM 17 YEARS OLD . . . How quick does time fly & how do we arrive at our maturity & then slowly decay. How gr'tly are we disappointed in our expected amusements . . . what is life taken all in all but a painful road of uneven hilly country." He sought refuge from uncertainty through known and innocent pursuits.

In the fall of 1875, Theobald had formed a "brotherly quartette" with three classmates—John Whish, William Shaver, and Howard Watson. (Whish became a newspaper correspondent, Shaver a lawyer, Watson a civil service clerk.) Occasional companions from the class ahead included John Montignani and Joseph Guardenier, another future lawyer and bank clerk, respectively, and Maurice Lewi, later a well-known podiatrist, who lived to be ninety-nine. They all complemented his closest friends, together with Henry Battin and George Addington, who were in classes one or two years behind. With these companions or alone, Theobald prospected the countryside from early spring until late autumn. Neither ringleader nor hanger-on, standing always a little apart, he was yet looked upon as chief "tramp." A few called him "Baldy" but the nickname was not encouraged. An earlier diary entry expressed romantically the thoughts of all in the group: "There is something quiet & entertaining about country scenery not found in cities, nowhere can we find that quiet joy and happiness more than by studying Nature, sunshiny Nature."[49]

The season usually began with a hike to Kenwood, a favorite landmark on the southern outskirts of Albany. Occasionally they took an early ferry across the Hudson, and strolled along the railroad tracks. From hereabouts, they gained a fine view of the spires and steeples of Troy and the landmarks of Albany—"the top of the capitol rose above all the rest. At our feet rolled the Hudson . . . covered with tugs."[50] Theobald's diary in 1875 records that berry picking was undertaken systematically. Black and red raspberries and early blueberries opened the season in mid-July, followed in August by blackberries and elderberries. In mid-September, grapes ripened and apple trees were ready for plundering. As an amateur botanist, Theobald always learned something about the wild flowers of the region from his rambles. As he went around the city and countryside on foot, weather conditions closely affected his whole life—apparel, activities and mood. Lives ended with special frequency in winter. Tuberculosis galloped off with young and old, diphtheria took its toll high and low. The former killed Arthur Murphy's mother—Arthur then was courting Bertha—and diphtheria attacked Shaver, one of the quartette, but he recovered.

Because water had always been an attraction for Theobald, "which I could not overcome,"[51] with friends he fished and dug for clams. In the late summer of 1875 Joe Gaurdenier acquired a boat he named *Tawasentha,* which added zest to many expeditions. During the summer of 1876, *Tawasentha* was transformed into a sailing vessel, and early in September, Gaurdenier and Whish sailed her down the Hudson to New York. Even without a boat available, the river held Theobald in thrall. From their "old brick homestead" he would wander the wharf, only a few hundred yards away, during the days, and sometimes even at night.

One of Theobald's anxious pleas, "Is there no boat for me?" was answered favorably at last. Henry Battin disclosed that he had a skiff, the *Rosalie,* that Theobald and other friends might borrow for fishing trips and visits to old haunts on the Hudson. Soon Theobald and George rowed down the creek to the deep waters by the Rock of Hope, "to test the piscatorial power of my newly purchased pole."[52] "Sails" could be improvised from a spread-eagled coat or shirt, or even a suitably shaped bush or tree. With favorable wind and tide, such makeshifts stuck in the bow would carry the boat upstream. Theobald's diary mentions several such exploits, e.g., they "rowed near to the Dead Creek & caught the rollers of the 'City of Hudson'. Then planting a tree in the bow as a sail we scooted up to State Street."[53]

Though always happy manning a rowboat, Theobald never learned to swim. He tried and failed twice, at sixteen and seventeen years, on the Hudson's other shore. Eventually he "bought an immense life preserver, $1.25, with which to learn swimming." Next day he managed about four yards, commenting "the buoyancy of those 'ere life preservers is remarkable."[54] His last recorded attempts were some six years later.

Theobald revealed in his autobiographical letter that "I might be a priest today, had I followed the advice of . . . the Rev Theo Noethen, a remarkably intelligent man." The Schmitt children were raised in their mother's faith. Theobald remembered distinctly his daily attendance at mass before school.

> Often in the morning cold of winter, when the church seemed to gather within its walls all the frost there was, I would sit with fingers so benumbed that the pages of my little prayer-book would scarcely turn at their bidding . . . Even as a boy of nine I felt what the life of a priest must be and refused to think of it.[55]

The boy's diary, which began auspiciously on All Saint's Day, November 1, 1874, for a year or two recorded the main feasts of the Church. On Christmas Day (an almost purely religious celebration in his family) he arose at five o'clock for early Mass and attended church twice more. He went regularly to Confession and never missed weekly Mass. Besides assisting the organist, he joined the choir and took part in Sunday School.

In his youth and young adulthood, Theobald held religion very seriously. He found some comfort in its offices, and was prepared to concede that a mystical union with God sustained the priesthood and some laymen. But when curiosity challenged faith, he was unwilling to curb the former through irrational support of the latter. By contrast, although Father Noethen "brought with him all the classic learning of Germany," he resented any deviation from Roman Catholic orthodoxy. He was affronted when his young parishioner went to services, attended singing school, and played the organ in a Protestant church; and worse,

Theobald began questioning religious rituals and authoritarianism, even finding Confession distasteful.

Early in 1875, Noethen denounced his young parishioner before the congregation: "The invective & vituperative sentence . . . was hurled at me; I'll not forget."[56] Smith shrank from completing the "sentence." He was not yet ready for a complete break, but the iron entered his soul. Next Sunday he avoided church. The following week he attended Mass at Holy Cross Church, but Vespers at St. Vincent de Paul. Soon afterward, interrupted at the organ by Father Noethen, he spent a penitential evening. Confession and Communion followed this encounter and the routine was resumed.

Just before his sixteenth birthday, Theobald furthered his repentance by launching a "Jubilee" tour of Albany churches. "Today I began my jubilee at 7.20 A.M. I went to mass & then visited successively the Cathedral, St. Mary's, St. Joseph's and St. Anne's."[57] Each of the fourteen "rounds" occupied a full morning. The whole tour, including visits to various Protestant edifices, required four months. He attended mass throughout this period and substituted at the organ whenever needed. However on Palm Sunday, two months after his denunciation in church, he "took down" a sermon—an act of rebellion, for critically analyzed sermons imply a search for doctrinal inconsistencies. However, the final severance was again deferred; during his last year at home he sporadically attended or played the organ at various churches.

Theobald noted in his diary on February 7, 1877 that "Music is my greatest pleasure . . . How beautiful is Schubert—how exquisitely melodious!"[58] Before Theobald was thirteen years old, he took weekly piano and organ lessons from Hermann Singer, his old schoolmaster, now retired. Fifteen dollars quarterly covered his own and Bertha's piano lessons. (Bertha learned to play the piano pleasingly but lacked her brother's talent.) At age sixteen, he occasionally substituted as church organist, and had one or two piano pupils. The "grand" at home was more than a parlor symbol. Singer tuned the instrument when necessary, but the boy could clean it and make minor repairs. He also learned to judge mechanical and tonal qualities, so that relatives and friends sought his advice before closing a purchase. He developed a light baritone voice and for some time attended singing school once or twice weekly under Singer's direction. A liking for opera music accounted for allusions in his diary to *Norma*, *La Muette*, *Freischütz*, and *Trovatore*. The "sublimity" of Meyerbeer's *Robert le Diable* impressed him.

Singer's piano lessons ended discordantly. He sent his daughters to the Smith home to collect five dollars, presumably against overdue fees. The pupil reacted angrily. The organ lessons seemed unaffected, perhaps because Theobald earned them by "pumping" and in other ways served as Singer's unpaid assistant. As organist and choir-master at Holy Cross Church, Singer was often at loggerheads with Father Noethen, which ended in the former's discharge. Since the new organist proved unreliable, Noethen allowed Theobald to continue practicing, and he played a complete service there at age sixteen. Despite arthritis and worsening health, singer became organist at Dr. Neef's Dutch Reformed church. When he was too ill to play, Theobald substituted for him. Singer died in April 1877 and was buried four days later under overcast skies. "Tears flow unbidden & the solemn candles appear double as they stand near his coffin," Theobald observed.[59] Singer left his wife and five small children pitifully poor. Several years later, Theobald contributed three dollars to his gravestone.

Between September '76 and the end of August '77, Theobald obtained $90 from organ-playing and $135 for 285 one-hour piano lessons. Sometimes he committed himself to three or four lessons on a single day, despite being "terribly bored." He apparently hoped to amortize all past outlays upon music, although the prospects of doing so were negligible. The debit side of his accounting listed $100 for "Int[erest]," and $50 for "music," plus $500 for the piano, and $280 paid to Singer for his lessons, a total of $930.

Theobald rehearsed every service with perfectionist zeal, and on Sundays might play the "King of the Instruments" all day. This was no hardship, especially when Joe Guardeneir joined him at the console and George Addington pumped: "Joseph Guard. & I had a pleasing time in playing the Organ . . . What invisible harmonies trembled through the emptying pipes . . . How exquisitely beautiful & sweet, but only we have heard & know the secret!"[60] Within a month of having replaced Signer as organist at the Dutch Reformed church, Theobald became choir master. When the summer vacation ended, he also took over his old teacher's singing school, which resumed twice-weekly meetings in Neef's church. Of the two sopranos, two altos, three tenors, and three basses, all but one were of German descent. The leading tenor, Jacob Goebel, became a fishing companion. In eighteen months he died "after a long & serious illness. God has released him from pain."[61]

1876 was the United States of America's centennial year. Theobald's diary jottings reveal that he witnessed its beginning celebration in Albany, which commenced on New Year's Eve in 1875 with a procession of militia regiments and color guards and bands of societies with torches and a brass cannon. And on July 4, similarly appropriate festivities took place, with a procession at least four miles in length. On October 29, having earned $20 for playing the organ at Neef's church for three months, Theobald purchased an excursion ticket and travelled alone to Philadelphia to view the National Centennial Exhibition. After touring the Philadelphia waterworks, where he observed numerous forcing pumps, and then crossing the Schuykill in a hind-paddle boat to view the animals in the Zoo, he spent five days at the Exhibition, inspecting the Machine Hall and the Art Gallery three times, paying special attention to Krupp's cannon, gas engines and patent governors, steam hammers and a large blast engine. Then, in company with his sister's fiance, Arthur Murphy, who had arrived unexpectedly, he explored government buildings. In these, they admired beautiful models of lighthouses, the patent reversible oar, minerals of quartz and its varieties, educational books, and the envelope maker. They also visited the Aquarium and Agricultural Hall, where they found the labor-saving farm machinery impressive.

Theobald visited Horticultural Hall alone, viewing tree ferns, sago palms, banana trees and numerous other exotic plants. (The first boat-load of Jamaican bananas had been sold in Boston in 1870, and the fruit, introduced as a novelty at the Centennial Exhibition, proved spectacularly popular.) On November 4, after a final inspection of the main buildings, he went to the "Glass house where they were pressing goblets & other glassware" before catching the afternoon train to New York and the overnight boat home. His arrival in Albany coincided with the national elections to determine President Grant's successor, with Democrat Samuel J. Tilden pitted against Republican Rutherford B. Hayes. Tilden received more popular and electoral votes than his opponent; but because of irregular returns from three Southern states, Congress created an Electoral Commission in January 1877 of eight Republicans and seven Democrats which in March declared Hays the winner, corroborating Theobald's comment in his diary on Election Day: "Today is the great national holiday . . . noted . . . for the number of frauds that the American people will perpetrate, not only in buying & selling votes, but in stuffing the ballot box."[62] He had personally viewed such chicanery himself.

As the fall of '76 approached, Theobald improved his earnings by intermittently balancing the books and collecting debts for N.J. Dell, owner of the main tailor shop in Albany. ("I took the high chair at Dell's & kept his books," he remarked in his diary.)[63] Periodically he went every morning, including occasional whole Saturdays, to keep books, collect and pay accounts, and mail checks. Some weeks later he recorded, "Today I wear my new coat, which is a present from Mr. Dell. It costs thirty dollars, and is a very heavy coat. I like it."[64] Late in February 1877, he visited West Troy (upstream on the west bank) for the first time, seeing the Theological Seminary as well as some of Dell's debtors. Then, after interviewing a delinquent creditor on the far side of the river, he and a companion crossed the ice below Albany. Before they reached the shore, the ice cracked, but they found a solid bottom and made it to the bank.

On St. Patrick's Day the ardor of "former inhabitants of Erin," normally inflamed by the "solace of the cup" offered by ale and lager beer saloons, was damped by a cold wind and three inches of snow. Theobald coupled his longing for spring with loyal wishes for his employer: "The sun will soon have reached the *vernal* equinox . . . but let it open the hearts & pockets of Dell's customers that they may be clad in newer & more stylish rigs."[65]

In the spring of 1877, at age twenty-one, Bertha began preparations for a June wedding to Arthur Murphy, a carpenter, prompting Theobald to comment: "I bless the union & hope for continual happiness and bliss to the pair . . . when I go there will be emptiness in the house of Smith."[66] Theobald was fond of his sister and knew he would miss her teasing and taunting, her outgoing ways. On the wedding eve he noted: "Kneading & baking for the morrow, that the marriage-table may be well spread. A day detrimental to the good appearance of paper-collars."[67] The couple planned a week's honeymoon in New York, after which they would live at 258 Lark Street, "where no Lark was ever found or heard." Theobald often visited there for a chat with Bertha after giving piano lessons to his cousin Lena. As a special treat he would take some of his best raspberries and currants. In turn he was invited to their occasional evening parties.

In late June Theobald was "On the well-known stool again, counting Dell's money & balancing a/c's," making out checks, balancing accounts, and collecting bills. He enjoyed meticulously balancing accounts and in later life found many opportunities for practicing this skill. Nonetheless, Theobald yearned for further education, but he soon realized that his earnings from book-keeping and music would not cover college expenses. He kept in touch with Montignani, who had gone to Cornell University directly from the High School, and was intrigued with his friend's stereoscopic views of the University and its surroundings. Theobald's parents endorsed his ambition and offered modest support. Former teachers advised him about possibilities of lessening the financial load. After concluding that "my going to college would not be a great sacrifice to my parents provided I lived economically,"[68] he decided to register as freshman scholar at Cornell the coming fall, with civil engineering as first choice in career. In January, he mused in his diary:

> Waiting—still waiting for beautiful summer when the eelgrass glistens in the creek, when the wild flower lifts its head & is plucked by an analytic & botanic Smith in its freshest bloom, when the gates of Cornell open to bid him enter on a scientif-technical course, when he wanders in parallelopipedons & elliptical cycloids & epicycloids—tunnels & bridge construction, in safety valves & steam engines.[69]

Two months later, he was less confident about his choice of career: "Two questions press upon me. 1st, Religion—2nd, my future career. What shall I choose—do I not choose wrong—Will employment be at hand after graduation

& will it be pleasing? Shall I be a C.E. Civil Engineering Bach. of Architecture? Let us be decided in everything."[70]

Earnest preparations began for the June entrance examinations to Cornell. He browsed in book stores and picked up a second-hand Dalton's Physiology and Hooker's Natural History for $1.15. From Prof. Horne he bought Olney's Algebra & Geometry. He tackled English, German and French reading and grammar, along with mathematics, drawing, and a modicum of the sciences. He received a new catalogue from Cornell: "A mathematico-scientifico-physical course has been created & seems to meet my approval & wants exactly. So I am still on the fence, with pleasing landscapes on either side between which I can hardly choose."[71] He had several credits toward primary admission, but lacked Geography, Physiology, algebra, and Plane Geometry. Every candidate for university courses in Science or Mathematics had to pass a special examination in either French, German, or Solid Geometry and Trigonometry. His disdain for the easier foreign-language alternatives entailed additional work in mathematics and a frantic hunt for "Chauvenet," the needed text. A copy turned up just in time.

Montignani invited him to stay at Ithaca a whole week. Early on Saturday, June 16 1877, eel grass glistened in the creek as Theobald boarded the train. By the time he skirted Lake Cayuga and approached his destination, the setting sun lit up the University windows on the hill. Montignani met him at the depot, and "lugged me off to the boarding-house in the quiet Aurora Street, where I remained during my sojourn."[72]

"The jingling of many bells," an irreverent description of the "Cornell Chimes"—whose peal from an enlarged carillon still heralds each day—awakened Theobald. He spent Sunday writing home, listening to the Chapel sermon, and exploring the splendor of the neighboring gorge. The examinations were set for the next three days. First, Algebra and Plane Geometry, followed by Physiology and Geography, and finally, Solid Geometry and Plane Trigonometry. On the Tuesday evening, Montignani took him as guest to the initiation banquet of the Delta Upsilon fraternity house, situated with a fine view of the valley and opposite hills. Next day, after dinner, "'Monti' and I went to see the campus exercises of the graduating class, where . . . we heard the Ivy Speech, the Burying of the Hatchet, but did not wait to see the Calumet or Pipe of Peace."[73] (These ceremonies, apparently initiated in 1877, were dropped after a few years). Theobald attended the Commencement Exercises on the morning of June 21. "What was said was very good, but there was a lack of training, of elegance, to which a High School Scholar is unaccustomed." On Thursday he took the boat from Ithaca to Cayuga with "Monti" and other college lads. They changed trains at Syracuse and reached Albany in the late afternoon.

The old pattern of life was resumed without let-up. But no sooner was he informed of having passed the entrance requirements than preparations began for a competitive state scholarship. He studied hard up to the last moment throughout the first half of August. At ten o'clock on the 16th, "we were in the rooms of the Board to await with anxiety and suspense the disclosures of squire Cole. Only 2 scholarships on hand. Battin, the only one in the 3rd Assembly District received one gratis, while the rest, three in number, of which I was one, had to undergo the torture of an examination. Arithmetic in the morning, Grammar & Geography in the afternoon."[74] The suspense ended when the evening papers announced that Theobald had received the scholarship for the Second Assembly District. This news was confirmed promptly by the Office of the Board of Public Instruction:

> Dear Sir, I have the pleasure to inform you that you have been selected and appointed as a student from the second Assembly District of Albany County, for the year 1877 in the Cornell University. Please to call for your certificate, for you ought to be at the University as early as the 11th of Sept. inst. Yours faithfully, J.O. Cole.[75]

Choir practice and organ rehearsal came on the eve of his departure. "The last Sunday at church, I shall remember it as long as I live." Next morning, despite parental melancholy, he faced the future with resolution. "Now at last I must away from here. My parents are sad and I am unhappy. The suitcase is fetched and I rush away while Mother quietly weeps. So I wander to the Dell and say farewell to father—Watson waits in the railway station and we shake each other's hand and part."[76] After a tedious journey, he reached Ithaca in a rainstorm. An unsteady bus took him up the hill to the Delta Upsilon Society house, where he slept soundly in a guest room.

2

ABOVE CAYUGA'S WATERS:
UNDERGRADUATE LIFE
AT CORNELL

After the Civil War, American higher education was in a state of unsophisticated ambition. When Theobald Smith enrolled at Cornell University, that young institution—founded less than a decade before—had a slightly tarnished innocence, but its ambitions and enterprise were quite abundant. Ezra Cornell had been a farmer, carpenter and mechanic before making his fortune building telegraph systems. In September 1864, when a senator of the New York State legislature, he offered to donate his 300-acre hilltop farm "of first quality land . . . overlooking the village of Ithaca and Cayuga Lake" to erect suitable college buildings thereon, and to "make up an aggregate of three hundred thousand dollars," provided the Legislature would "place the college upon a firm and substantial basis" by guaranteeing an endowment of $30,000 per annum.

Early in 1865, Cornell increased his offer to $500,000. His fellow senator, Andrew Dickson White, a graduate of Yale and for seven years a professor of history at the University of Michigan, introduced into the State Senate a bill "to establish the Cornell University." Before the end of April, the University had its Charter in embryo and White had drawn up a Plan of Organization, while Cornell staked the location of the first buildings and indicated the future direction of campus growth. In November 1866, the University's Board of Trustees unanimously elected White as University President. In the fall of 1868, the doors opened to over 400 students.

The new University faced animosities, which arose from proclaimed nonsectarianism, the President's revolutionary views on education—he considered higher education in the United States "as stagnant as a Spanish convent"—, certain faculty appointments, and the founder's chronic shortages of cash to meet building commitments. Enrollments, revenues and prestige soon began to decline. During the six years from 1876 to 1882, total student registration fell from 561 to 384. Theobald Smith's own Class of 198 Freshmen shrank to eighty-nine seniors by 1881, of whom eighty-two graduated. The Trustees deferred expansion of classroom and laboratory facilities, kept faculty salaries low, and temporized about residential inadequacies and hazardous campus drainage.

White began one year's leave in October 1876, mainly for health reasons, Vice-President William C. Russel being appointed to act in his place. White's absence for all but seven months in a five-year period and the dissensions concerning Russel (whose religious liberalism forced his resignation in 1881) contributed to the low faculty morale of the period. However, many faculty members were young and zealous, eager to ignore local scandals. One of White's respected guidelines was that "the duty of acquaintance and social intercourse with students be impressed upon the faculty."[1]

When Theobald Smith enrolled in 1877, just before the ninth anniversary of Cornell University's inauguration, very few buildings were on the hill. Near the southwest corner stood Morrill Hall, a grey stone building; beyond it, to the north, was White Hall. Besides classrooms, each building contained dormitory accommodation for about sixty students; but despite a plenitude of natural running water, they lacked baths and had primitive toilet facilities. Below Morrill Hall, adjoining Cascadilla Creek, a four-story edifice (planned as a water-cure sanatorium) had been taken over and completed by the University as a residence for professors and students. Andrew White, who had himself lived in it, termed Cascadilla Place an "ill-ventilated, ill-smelling, uncomfortable, ill-looking almshouse." McGraw Hall, the gift of John McGraw of Ithaca, lumber merchant and Charter Trustee, housed the University Library and Museum, with a clock tower for a chime of nine bells, bestowed by his daughter, Jennie McGraw.[2] Another Trustee, Henry W. Sage, lumber merchant and partner of McGraw, had offered $250,000 for the instruction of women students "as broad and as thorough as that now offered to young men."

Sage College opened in 1875. Sage also endowed a nonsectarian chapel, styled in "upstate Gothic," to accommodate 500. East of the Halls was a wooden edifice, the "Chemistry Building," for the teaching of chemistry and physics (with a photographic laboratory in its attic). It soon housed Civil Engineering, as well as the lecture room and museum of Veterinary Science. To the north and at right angles to the line of the three Halls, a College of Mechanic Arts had been sponsored by another of the original Trustees, Hiram Sibley, a citizen of Rochester and first president of the Western Union Telegraph Company. An architecturally pompous mansion for the president, built at White's own expense—he had inherited wealth from his banker father—stood to the east upon a hillock. Just below, young elm trees, the gift of a farmer, bordered the makings of an avenue.

On the morning of September 13, 1877, Theobald made his way down the hill to Mrs. Crittenden's boarding house on Aurora Street, near its junction with Buffalo Street. Aurora continued northward, skirting the east shore of Cayuga Lake; South Hill mounted in the opposite direction, to be crossed by the Utica, Ithaca and Elmira Railroad. Buffalo Street began in the valley below West Hill, rose steeply some five hundred feet to the southwest corner of the campus, and ended near Cascadilla Place. Theobald enjoyed his daily climbs up Buffalo, but in heavy snow the early morning struggles were hard and sweaty. Winter's high winds made the street almost insurmountable, and toboggans could be an extra hazard. If ice formed, any means of descent became perilous.

Lodging in downtown boarding-houses was inexpensive. Theobald lived at Mrs. Crittenden's for all four academic years. As he shared a room with Henry W. Battin, his weekly outlays were probably under five dollars, meals included. The elastic academic program tended to encourage closer relations between fellow-boarders than among classmates. Thus Henry Battin became a long-cherished friend, whereas F. Cooper Curtice, Fred L. Kilborne, and Hermann M. Biggs, whose college courses (and future careers) impinged on Smith's own, were not mentioned in his contemporary diary.

On Sunday, Theobald wrote home and explored the nearby countryside. Next day, he mounted the slope to register. He took the "Boneyard Cut" through the village cemetery, "where lie the dead at an angle of 45° to the University Hill."[3] This route passed the "Villa Cornell"—a costly stone edifice, sometimes termed "Cornell's Folly" in the early days—to a cow path beyond. During and after heavy rains, this short-cut was unusable.

His scholarship exempted Theobald from tuition fees of $25 a term, or $75 per annum. He was spared further examination and granted sophomore status for French and German courses. Bachelor degrees were obtainable in various branches of engineering and science, in Arts and Literature, and even in Science *and* Letters. An independent program was also available, subject to faculty approval, which allowed a student to acquire knowledge likely to agree with his tastes, to encourage his aspirations, and to promote his work in life. The "elective system" introduced at Cornell—a distinction often claimed for Harvard, where President Charles W. Eliot merely carried the process further—was a logical outcome of White's dictum that "The usual imposition of a single fixed course is fatal to any true university spirit in this country; it cramps colleges and men."[4]

Meanwhile, it was foreseeable by 1877 that hard times might entail many unemployed engineers. The number of prospective graduates in engineering at Cornell University declined from ninety-four in 1872 to only ten seniors and four juniors by 1880–81. Theobald Smith decided to forego engineering. He longed to follow President White's doctrine of wide scholarship, but enrolled instead in mathematics.

Theobald's Course Book[5] shows a twenty-hour weekly program for the first year, with Rhetoric and Sophomore German and French absorbing ten of the hours. In the fall term he also took Physiology and Algebra (three and five hours weekly), Hygiene (six lectures), and Drill—the last two courses compulsory. The Hygiene lectures were given by Burt Green Wilder, Professor of Physiology, Comparative Anatomy, and Zoology.[6] President White admired Wilder's platform style, and believed his lectures on hygiene partly accounted for the excellent state of student health.[7] Much of Theobald Smith's admiration for Professor Wilder stemmed from their direct classroom contact. "It was a fortunate thing for us," he reminisced when honoring Wilder on his twenty-fifth anniversary at Cornell, "that your laboratories were so small and crowded, because all of your work was done in the presence of your pupils, and we could not very well escape the infection of your enthusiasm."[8]

The drill sessions were considered farcical. Theobald exchanged six periods of military training for an educational miscellany—duly entered in his *Course Book*—which comprised Trigonometry, Organic Chemistry, Faust, Physiology Laboratory (under Prof. Wilder), and Chemical Laboratory (Qualitative). In the first freshman term, he drilled on the Fairgrounds on Mondays, Wednesdays, and Fridays, weather permitting. The muskets distributed at the initial drill near the end of September were carried home in the rain. They often paraded without arms and had only token uniforms. "At present we carry no arms, but wear merely belts. We turn right at the command 'left' & left at the command 'right.' But we wheel in fours right & right about with a beauty & simultaneousness, which confounds our captain even."[9]

On weekdays, Theobald spent most spare hours in the library, reading journals on solid works, as well as *Le Cid, Wilhelm Tell,* and other classics for foreign language courses. The mathematical component of his curriculum was augmented in the winter term by five hours weekly in plane and spherical trigonometry, and in the following term by two-hour courses in harmonoid geometry and in trigonometry. The Associate Professor of Mathematics, Lucian

Augustus Wait, quickly discerned his pupil's mathematical talent, and they cooperated in translating from the French an already published "Essay on Imaginaries." That task was completed after several evening visits to Wait's house. Theobald had to negotiate the ditch-lined hill in complete darkness.

He passed "Honorably" (the highest level) in all subjects—a pattern sustained unbroken for the next two years. Despite this promising start, Theobald began to chafe at his specialty. "The course seemed too narrow to me. I was always afraid of getting a one-sided education."[10] In the winter term, despite a decision to compromise by taking both philosophy and mathematics, he continued to brood: "Mathematics disgusts me and philosophy beckons and Latin motions."[11] Three months later, he reflected: "The glitter of a B.Ph. is continually before. Shall I cram Latin for the next year & enter the course? Caesar does not seem to be so hard . . . I need a broader view, need air, & do not wish to be suffocated by the closeness of one subject."[12]

As soon as pre-Christmas examinations were over, the freshman longed to be home. "Here there is no more peace." The suitcase was packed, the umbrella readied for the trip. "How my heart jubileed and with what strides I rushed to the house. There I found Bertha and old Mrs. Kaufmann sitting by the stove. Mother came soon, then Father."[13] On Christmas Eve he went home, after lighting a fire at Bertha's house, but "did not receive any presents." Visiting the church of his youth he heard the High Mass. He called upon relatives, friends, and acquaintances. The second Annual Reunion of the Albany High School proved enjoyable. At Dell's, he did the accounts one day, and then helped to take the inventory. At Neef's church, he played the Sunday morning service and rehearsed the choir. Somehow the vacation did not quite come up to his expectations. With a slight sense of let-down, he returned to Ithaca on January 12. Then a letter came from home, followed by a parcel containing a dark brown spring overcoat. "It is nicely made. Oh, we do not know what good parents do for us until we miss their care over us."[14]

The Delta Upsilon Society, founded in 1834, was the last of seven fraternities established during Cornell University's first year. A chapter was started in an old house up the hill on Quarry Street. Montignani's departure in January to study law at Albany probably hastened Theobald's induction into the Society, for early in February he and Battin joined the eleven other active members. Theobald profited greatly in various ways from fellow-membership in Delta Upsilon with Wilder and several younger faculty scientists—William Russell Dudley ('74), Theodore B. Comstock ('74), Leland O. Howard ('77) and Simon Henry Gage ('77). In rambles with Prof. Dudley, he learned much botanical lore and tracked down unusual plants; up in McGraw Tower with J.H. Comstock and his pupil, L.O. Howard—both to attain renown as entomologists—he captured an enthusiasm for observing minute differences in species; in Gage he gained an admiring friend and life-long supporter.

The Society had outgrown its quarters, and Theobald was one of a six-member group who chose suitable fourth-floor rooms on State Street, to which they moved in mid-March. He soon presented the customary "autobiography" to the Society and during the spring term he contributed a paper on "The Jersey Centenarian" by Bret Hart (who had been born in Albany), led a discussion on "Drama," and, to the final gathering of his freshman year, spoke on "Toussaint L'Ouverture." The furnishings of the chapter included a piano, upon which Theobald soon became the habitual performer. More than half a century later, Gage recalled: "In the Society where we often met, he was of course the musician. I can see now his glowing young face playing the music for the Virginia Reel—the young men were having the time of their lives. It was a stag dance in the fraternity rooms, and in that group were Dr. Leland O. Howard, Professor J.H. Comstock, and many others who have been an honor to the University and to the country."[15]

One of the year's highlights was the banquet, celebrating a decade since the chapter was founded, which was attended in force by all faculty members of Delta Psi. Another was the formal call on General J.A. Garfield after he addressed the citizens of Ithaca as presidential candidate one evening in the fall of 1878. Next morning, the members were summoned to White's residence to be introduced to the "large-built man," with an "open frank countenance. He dwelt upon his college days" (at Williams College), when daily religious services were compulsory, and "snowy mornings at five saw them in the old Chapel."[16]

With Battin, Theobald shared many excursions to Fall Creek Gorge and Buttermilk Falls. On Easter Sunday, they climbed the South Hill to investigate Coy's Glen, returning with arbutus flowers; visited Lick Brook, three miles below Ithaca on the short-lived Geneva, Ithaca and Sayre Railroad; and tramped beyond Enfield, a village nestled in a glen over the western hills seven miles away, past dams and mills to the gorge. Theobald alone negotiated the bed for Cascadilla, at a time when up-stream mills had diverted most of the water, stone-hopping to get such trophies as columbine, Solomon's seal, wild honeysuckle and maidenhair. Once his group took shelter in a "glass house" near the lake. He carefully watched the workers blow the glowing molten glass, noting the rows of long hollow cylinders on the floor, the white-hot fire in the ovens, constantly replenished with coal, and barrels full of glass fragments in the building and yard. To climax the academic year, they planned a Decoration Day trip to Taughannock Falls, a 215-foot waterfall some ten miles north of Ithaca.[17] Heavy rain forced them to stay at home. The local celebrations were distastefully banal.

"The procession passed up the street, each man carrying a basket of flowers for the graves. In the evening the band aroused the town by wandering about followed by a horse-cart which had a monstrous bell attached to it. The streets being muddy, the whole procession walked on the sidewalk, lugging the horse-cart after."[18]

When in February the snow was deep enough for tobogganing through the graveyard, Theobald and Battin joined in the fun on a moonlit night, riding down with the boys. On one such occasion he met Lizzie C., an Ithaca High School girl. A week later, he escorted her to a party and danced until about 1 A.M. A few days later, while the "Stars twinkled clearly and the circle of the moon was surrounded by a red halo, we walked arm-in-arm to the show-place of joy. There I danced and had a good time with L., and time passed quickly and we had to get home, and so we left . . . Well that night I won't forget so soon. It was my first night spent under such circumstances. My feelings are soft, impressionable, and I hold them so tightly, hence my nature is more sensitive to such things, and woe to the after pains."[19]

One evening Theobald found that "Battin has gone out with my L. to some party and I am betrayed and deserted like yon Alceste of misanthropic renown, and am at home inwardly bemoaning my fate and bewailing the hour when L. first attracted me."[20] In remorse, Lizzie sent Theobald the first pansy in her garden. He decided to preserve it, labelled "from L;" but that entry was overwritten, "It is lost, gone forever, Mch. 6, 79." Until the end of the academic year, when the relationship ceased altogether, Theobald seldom saw her alone. He and Battin played whist with Lizzie and Kate Rhodes, her fellow-lodger, an Optional student at Cornell; explored the tunnel supplying the mill with water from Fall Creek; boated on the lake; and visited dairy-farming friends of Miss Rhodes. Toward the end of March, he left Ithaca again for Albany, this time by Ezra Cornell's rickety "Shoo-Fly Road."[21] Bertha was on the point of confinement. Within a week of his return to University, a letter announced that Bertha had a son. "God be praised, I know not what to say, for I am overjoyed."[22]

One hundred years ago, rail travel was far from relaxing. On his way home for his first long summer vacation, Theobald's train was delayed beyond Syracuse by engine trouble, and at Little Falls a woman was killed. Battin, who left Ithaca later, was met at the depot "with blackened dusty garments and an abject appearance." Familiar threads were picked up. Theobald gave organ lessons for fifty cents and piano lessons for twenty-five cents each; at home he painted the roof and the iron fence, laid a new floor in the cellar, and papered or whitewashed the walls. The garden's heavy demands included digging up the lawn so laboriously laid a few years before. He frequently visited Bertha to play with his three-months-old nephew, Artie. He had decided to change his course to philosophy, despite the extra work entailed in Latin and tackled one page daily of the *Gallic Wars* until Caesar became intelligible.

Theobald wandered around the city as of old, never tiring of the turmoil around the dock, where passengers and freight arrived from every quarter. Albany was growing in importance as a transportation hub and becoming heavily industrialized. Ore shipments collected on the Island, which now boasted a blast furnace. This industrialization was accompanied by ugliness. "My eyes," he noted, "accustomed to the green & varied landscape of Ithaca, rest with disgust upon the barren, clayey soil of Albany."[23] A boat ride down the Creek to the Normans Kill showed "The high tide had scattered here & there masses of debris on the water, bunches of water-grass & ivy, old bottles, cans, carcasses, and bubbles which gave the water an ugly appearance."[24] Nonetheless, life in the capital city had of course certain advantages: a fascinating waterfront, processions, boat races, fireworks, free concerts in the park—and good dentists. Having had a tooth and a half extracted, Theobald underwent "a very painful operation . . . two molars filled with Au . . . after an hour's work [for $4.50]."[25]

In mid-July Theobald rejoiced at Cornell's victory over Harvard in a freshman boat-race: "Hurrah! Cornell, I yell yell yell Cornell!!!"[26] He kept up with public affairs through the magazines in the "Y.M.A." rooms, and delved into Emerson and Herbert Spencer. The latter, with his "survival of the fittest" concept, then was considered in North America the leading interpreter of scientific advancement—the prophet of the inevitability of progress. Theobald noted that Spencer's *Education: Intellectual, Moral and Physical* (1862) "defends Science bravely against the assuming arrogance of the classics," and "conclusively shows how it is superior to the Languages in educating the mind." In short, science provided material benefits and was a necessary ingredient in all human affairs.[27]

In August, there were several memorable trips in the *Rosalie*—some with George Addington and finally, near the end of the month, a climactic one with Watson. They reached a sandy beach near Castleton, where they bathed, captured a floating barrel and ate lunch. "A schooner came by with a yawl behind, to which we clung and were towed up."

Watson suggested that we tie the rope of the yawl to the bow seat rather than hold it; so he did it. But this step almost cost us our lives, for no sooner was it tied than our boat was dragged broadsides and we could not pull her straight. We were both in the bow, and the water rose & rose and at last poured into the boat, & in a few seconds down it went & we sinking with it, the rope tied to the yawl snapped asunder & we were submerged in a moment. The boat turned bottom upwards &

rose, & we struggling & crying help! help! to the receding schooner snatched hold of it, & thus both lay helpless in deep water clinging to our only hope—the overturned boat. Our cries were heard aboard the schooner, & soon we saw the yawl loosened & two men in it coming towards us. We were saved. In a few minutes we were in the yawl wringing wet from head to foot, whilst the men were turning the boat over & gathering the stray articles floating about. We wrung our clothing, baled out the boat while we were being towed up, & soon had it in order, & left the schooner to row up, so as not to catch cold with our wet clothing.

Theobald recorded that the lock of the boat, his umbrella & napkin, Watson's cup & saucer & towel, had all dropped out. "But we were too glad to have escaped so luckily, and more & more the great danger in which we had been dawned upon me and continually occupied my mind . . . We reached home with wet clothing on our backs about 6.30 . . . All's well that ends well."[28] A chastened entry closed the month of August: "The dangerous adventure of yesterday still engages my thoughts. Its magnitude [and] possible results seem to grow in importance each moment."

My losses are:	umbrella	$2.00
	broken watch	1.00
		$3.00

Soon it was time to return to Cornell. At the boarding house, he and Battin had been assigned a pleasanter room, furnished with a new stove and a comfortable armchair. Mrs. Crittenden had put Theobald's bed in an alcove, with a "fiery mass of drapery hiding it from the vulgar eye." Theobald registered for "Philosophy Optional." The fall term program comprised eighteen hours weekly, with slightly less for winter and spring term. Five hours weekly were assigned each term to Analytical Geometry, Calculus, and Astronomy, respectively. Scientific interests led him to enroll in Geology, Organic Chemistry, and Vascular Cryptograms during the first trimester, Zoology in the second, and Entomology in the third, while Electricity and Magnetism were spread over the second and third trimesters. (In January 1879, Cornell made history by illuminating its campus with electric arc lights set up in the belfry of Sage Chapel.) Two hours of Italian and a one-hour essay every week completed the program.[29] The Latin requirements were postponable until his junior year. Meanwhile he could translate Cicero and Virgil privately.

Our sophomore was pleased at first with his new course. "My thoughts are philosophical to extremes, they delight in tracing the causes & effects of things which have happened, & to draw general conclusions."[30] His old love for geology was intensified by Theodore B. Comstock's enthusiasm. Burt Green Wilder's course in Zoology appealed to a mind seized by evolution. "All is evolution—plants, animals, mind, nature, knowledge, art, beauty—everything once was in a stage of rudimentary simplicity from which it has grown & developed into complexity."[31] Theobald likewise enjoyed studying insects, of which Wilder had donated a fine collection to the University, in the brilliant John Henry Comstock's custody. The University Entomological Museum was high up in McGraw Tower, where Comstock found it convenient to lodge, since he was also chimesmaster. Dudley's course in Vascular Cryptograms (implying a hidden mode of reproduction, a term rendered obsolete by improvements in microscopy) covered ferns, horsetails and club-mosses. Apart from the collection amassed for this course, Theobald had submitted a list of fifty-nine wild flowers gathered and classified during the spring term of 1878.[32]

Theobald was among those who welcomed President White back at the end of September 1878 from his extended leave, spent largely in European travel. Headed by a brass band, the students marched in columns of four with torches from Cascadilla to the President's house, where he made a long speech on the improved conditions in Europe. For a few months the University throbbed with new purpose, until it heard the news that White was to become American minister to Berlin, but would hold on to the Presidency.

At the outset of his sophomore year, Theobald became Secretary of Delta Upsilon for the customary stint of three months, and shared the presidential table. Within a few weeks, he presented a "Biography of Interest," and gave a short history of "The Colonization of N.Y., Penna, Mass." In March, he was elected Treasurer, and lectured on "The Moon." His friendship with Simon Henry Gage began early in 1879 following an enjoyable whist tournament. "Gage & myself as partners completely wiped out the others in a game and heartily rejoiced at the fact."[33] Theobald Smith, in a sixty-fifth birthday tribute to Gage, admitted that he "was largely responsible for turning me towards biology,"[34] and Wait told Gage affably some years later, in Smith's presence, that he held a grudge against him for converting a perfectly good mathematician into a biologist.

Whenever possible, Theobald practiced on church organs, but if necessary resorted to Mrs. Crittenden's harmonium, kept for singsongs and dances. He won the competition for the post of Sage Chapel organist, the runner-up being Hermann M. Biggs, a talented freshman who later gained fame in the public health field. The incumbent organist decided to stay on another year, thus postponing Theobald's assumption of this responsibility.

Sunday services at Sage Chapel were shared between eminent divines of various denominations and the local clergy. Theobald attended Chapel fairly regularly as a freshman, but never went twice on Sundays in his sophomore year. The Sage Chapel visiting preachers generally offered more to digest, but Theobald preferred to sample also some of the churches in Ithaca. He tried out the Congregational, Presbyterian, Episcopalian and Unitarian places of worship, more from curiosity and the hope of hearing good music than from spiritual hunger. None of these brought him satisfaction, though there was some appeal in the new Unitarian minister's definition of a Christian as a person who did a Christian's work, whatever his or her belief or creed. His churchgoing diminished as he grew more critical of the preachers' messages; and when spring came, church attendance very often gave way to the call of the outdoors. "The close, pent-up atmosphere of doctrines would not coincide or agree with my roaming, almost sacrilegious thoughts. The day of rude investigation is here & . . . all that is mystery must be unravelled."[35]

During vacations, visits to the church of his boyhood provoked acute nostalgia. On Christmas Day 1878, at Holy Cross Church, he enjoyed the singing, the organ playing and "the solemn ceremonial. My eye and my ears are used to it and for me they are always lovely." On his last day at home, as he rushed about to bid his friends farewell, "*vidi pater Noethen qui edixit me confiteri meos peccatus. Bon!*"[36] (I saw Father Noethen who declared that I should confess my sins. Good!) Father Noethen's decree was disobeyed. Three weeks after returning to Ithaca, Theobald received a painful letter from his sister. "The Rev. Noethen said openly in the pulpit that a certain person would not say Confession, and meant me. This offended me deeply and I feel the strength of the blow more and more."[37] There is no record of any threatened letter being sent and the spring vacation passed without allusion to priest or church. Soon after returning to college, Theobald observed "today the heaven is afflicted with light weeping . . . and—Father Noethen is dead."[38]

Before leaving home for his sophomore term, he penned a strange series of resolutions:

1. Be economical.
2. Take plenty of exercise & carefully build up your frame.
3. Never waste little spaces of time listlessly and aimlessly, but employ them to a good object.
4. Never sit by the window & look out vaguely, to be disturbed in your studies.
5. Study generally, no extra Mathematics.
6. Practice music on rainy indoor days.
7. Be not occupied with trivial frivolous matters during study hours, or in fact at any time.
8. Write at least two letters a week.
9. Frequently think of home and dear ones, & remember well the circumstances in which you are.

10. Do be contented every minute of your life. "Let not the sunlight on your path close" under whatever circumstances.
11. Do not worry over foolish things.
12. Cultivate friendship and good feeling everywhere.[39]

In a list of desirable qualities, few undergraduates would place thrift first and friendliness last. Theobald's high rating of exercise and physical buildup is also surprising. He had begun to fret about health and appearance. Recurrent gum-boils had yielded to radical dentistry, but now he worried about eyesight, head-aches and frequent colds. He was tough and wiry; otherwise he could not have shovelled coal and snow as a boy, nor enjoyed rowing and hiking as an adoles-cent, nor played "scrub" football at college—a rough Cornell specialty of that era. His height was recorded as 5'9–1/2" and weight as 132 pounds. He never weighed more.[40] "A little mental and bodily activity, a sound constitution and good living will soon fill out angular forms . . . The activity of mind which is un-doubtedly an heirloom with me can never cease save with death."[41]

"Les femmes are a powerful magnet to drag me into society," Theobald confided to his diary in February 1879.[42] The young women of Sage College were a doughty, spirited lot. One student went to Cornell in 1874 because "it has all the advantages of a university and a convent combined." Shortly after graduating, she married her instructor, John Henry Comstock.[43] Susanna Stuart Phelps, who enrolled in 1875, was the first woman to take laboratory work in Physics. She married Simon Henry Gage in 1881, raised a son, who attained a high position in the Corning Glass Company, and published her own researches in comparative neurology. Theobald's freshman class in 1877 included twenty-six women, about thirteen percent of the total. The student body was hotly di-vided about coeducation, but a small majority now favored it. By 1881, when the graduating class of eighty-nine included thirteen women, Theobald Smith was among forty-five seniors who declared themselves unconditionally "for;" four were "conditionally" in favor, e.g., "if coeds are pretty;" twenty-four were "against;" and six did not vote.

In the spring term of his sophomore year, Theobald gained entrée into Sage College. At a senior party, given by a student in his fraternity, Misses Alfreda Withington and Isabel Howland were met and they "spent the evening pleasantly with aid of cards, a penny, & shadowy figures on illumined sheets."[44] Several days later, Theobald and Battin were invited by Miss Howland to the Sage, where some of the "young folks amused themselves by dancing." Then they listened to the orators competing for the Woodford Prize.[45] He had "long desired to be-come acquainted with at least a few of the Misses of '81 & it has been realized."[46] After the spring examinations and a week's vacation at home, Theobald ceased curbing the impulse to revisit the Sage. He went with a friend, and they entertained the girls by playing a piano duet. He was emboldened to invite Isabel Howland to hear Llena di Murska,[47] the operatic soprano, at a concert in Ithaca early in June. "I am all awry today thinking continually of that lovely face . . . beside me." But he added unromantically: "Affection grows fungus-like in our hearts and perishes in the same manner."[48]

At the June examinations, all subjects taken during his sophomore year were passed "Honorably." By now he was well aware that he ought to pick a career and shape his studies towards it. He still felt more attracted to general culture than to a specialized or professional academic background. "But the world demands the latter & often turns a cold shoulder to the former. The development of our civilization has made specialists necessary. It has called in to being [a] hundred different vocations, and to choose among them is a hopeless task for one who has a kind regard towards all, and sees in all of them the gradual onward progress of the world."[49]

Theobald went home on June 17, 1879 in a train crowded with people going to Albany for a Grand Army Reunion. A few days later, he "spent a pleasant evening . . . calling on Miss Howland." Presumably she visited relatives in Albany for the Reunion celebrations. Following this brief encounter, Theobald considered how to get wealthy, something that never entered his head before. He had intended "to become a physician, but after my mind has roamed thro the whole list of occupations and professions it may return to the old idea of being a teacher or prof . . . Perhaps journalism is one most likely to respond to my multiplex likings."[50]

During the 1879 summer vacation, Theobald taught mathematics and German two or three hours daily for two months to the liberally paying R. S-. Delightful river excursions featured that long vacation. "The coolness & brightness of the late summer mornings, the fascinating appearance of the Hudson with its tugs & tows made me feel lifted above the plain of ordinary life."[51] On the 4th of July, he drove with Montignani, Addington and S-. in hired coach, complete with coachman, to Feura Bush, a village about ten miles beyond Kenwood. At last "the distant Helderbergs"[52] could be viewed from close quarters. When they visited the church, the "Dominie" invited them to play croquet in his garden with some young ladies of the neighborhood. His twentieth birthday passed without family celebration. However, it was an occasion for a more cheerful review of himself: "I am conscious of a tendency towards the improvement of my character . . . towards refinement of manners, partially due to social intercourse and partially to the ascendancy of reason . . . I am aware of a sharper intellect, a more searching and comprehending power of mind."[53]

In September 1879, Theobald began his last two undergraduate years, curtly noting in his diary that "I rolled back to Ithaca a sober Junior."[54] He passed the Latin examination and was accepted as a full-fledged B.Ph. candidate. Committed to four hours of Latin, two hours of English Literature, and one hour of Essays weekly throughout the year, he also took Roman History and Psychology in his first term, Moral Philosophy in the second, and Medieval History in the third term. He registered for a three-semester Physics course and enrolled in both Qualitative Analysis and Microscopy in the second term. In place of Military Drill, otherwise required in the first and third terms, he substituted Wilder's Physiology Laboratory course. The total load ranged from eighteen to twenty hours weekly.[55] He served conscientiously as President of the Junior Year, Class of '81. He also found time to practice "the Chapel organ 3 times a week with great delight to myself."[56]

Early in his junior year, he "dived deep into the mysteries of anatomy, overcame my dislike for death and blood and disease, and made up my mind that I was made for a physician."[57] Although no officially designated anatomy course was available until the senior year, Wilder and Gage encouraged extracurricular activities. Some pencil drawings of a cat's brain by Theobald are dated April 10, 1880.[58] Wilder later attested that "Theobald Smith . . . pursued with me the study of MEDICAL SCIENCE, from the 15th day of Sept. 1881 and that he is of good moral character."[59]

His closest instructor was the jovial Gage. Only eight years older than Theobald, he became his enduring confidant and adviser. Gage's textbook, *The Microscope,* first published in 1881, went through seventeen editions in sixty years. In 1893, in partnership with J.H. Comstock, Gage founded the famous Comstock Press. In later years, whenever Theobald's deep-seated conventionalisms welled up, it was easy to forget Gage's outbursts of enthusiasm for new bicycles and motor cars; his successful remarriage at nearly eighty-two after sincerely mourning his first wife; and (as a student) his triumphant retrieval of a circus camel for the Cornell collection of animal skeletons.[60]

After the second term passed, Theobald went home to recuperate from nitric acid and ammonia fumes, "of which I had inhaled a plentiful amt." After the short vacation, he and Battin moved again into more spacious but chilly quarters at Mrs. Crittenden's. He often had to wear an overcoat and hat indoors. In the laboratory, "the crack of bones resounds from various corners . . . We must pick to pieces the brain-case before we can get at the treasure within."[61]

For Theobald Smith's third summer vacation, Prof. Wilder had written a letter of introduction to an Albany practitioner, Dr. William Hailes, a graduate of Albany Medical College, ten years older than Theobald. Hailes had begun general practice in 1871 but soon specialized in surgery and later pioneered in X-ray diagnosis.[62] Theobald welcomed this summer holiday apprenticeship.

> For nearly three weeks I have worked in his private laboratory to my entire satisfaction thus far, and the 3–4 hrs daily spent in Histology. Laboratory work will I hope bring good fruit. Dr. Hailes is a young enthusiastic man, not overworking himself, and having his knowledge full blown without any hasty desire of increasing it; fond, perhaps a little too much, of praise and recognition of his abilities. We have become firm friends & he has not been tardy to help me in various ways.[63]

Hailes took a vacation and for several weeks left his pupil to his own devices. Theobald acknowledged the experience had been inestimably beneficial to him. By now he fully appreciated the growing emphasis on professional education. Before beginning the partial specialization of his senior year, he mused that life in society was comparable to a loom's complexities, in which each individual had his or her assigned movement. To ensure success, everyone "must calculate carefully and precisely what part of this huge machine he represents, and perform his work unflinchingly."[64] He still believed that harmonious human development was promoted best by a broad education, and he sometimes hankered after the limitless academic aspirations of his freshman year: "I should like to be a man of culture, an enjoyer of good literature, lover of nature and art, and of a peaceful religious disposition."[65] Instead, he must be content to have satisfied "profitably, enjoyably & uprightly" most of the intellectual cravings of his youth. "Thus far I have been able to gratify most of my desires, which thank Providence were of no vicious nature. My love for study has not yet died out, nor do I think it ever will."[66]

During that summer vacation, Gage had spent an afternoon at Albany with the Smith family and happily observed the parental pride in their son's accomplishments, especially the piano-playing.[67] The last systematic daily entry in Theobald's diary before it lapsed for a year and a half was a thoughtful tribute to those parents. He had "enjoyed the summer with every breath . . . Three months have passed by as in a dream and I stand before my last school year. In three days I shall travel away, again leaving my dear parents alone. I feel that I owe them everything and yet do not treat them as I should."[68]

Theobald's last year at Cornell was his busiest. He registered for a course load of from twenty to twenty-three hours weekly, enrolling in Veterinary Science and Chemistry (five and three hours weekly) throughout the year. The first term's two hours of Anatomy weekly were doubled in the third term, while a three-hour Physical Laboratory course fitted into the second. An appetite for cultural courses was still evident in his choice of Arts subjects—Ancient Oratory, American Law and American History, Dramatic Literature and Political Economy, the History of Philosophy and the Philosophy of History.[69]

The year had barely started when competition revived for the post of Sage Chapel organist. Theobald's main rival this time was a junior in Science and Letters, Elizabeth Van Pelt. "That afternoon I will never forget. Several professors (Wilder, White, Schaeffer, Fuertes) came as judges." (There was no professor of music at Cornell until 1907, but Latevan A. Fuertes, in charge of Civil Engineering, was a skilled flautist.) Through the stained-glass windows, "the sun shown so friendly . . . Miss Van Pelt played beautifully." The two competitors, adjudged of equal merit, were invited to share the appointment. They played the Chapel organ on alternate Sundays. On December 11, they gave a joint "soirée in the small chapel . . . It was triumph for both of us."[70] A pencilled outline of the program has survived.[71] Shortly before commencement, they produced another recital for an appreciative audience. "We closed with a duet . . . Thus my year at the Organ drew towards its close. I knew that the separation was to be a painful one, for I & my instrument had become acquainted & I loved it well."[72] Five years later, he recalled for Lilian Egleston how much he enjoyed "playing alone in the beautiful building as the sinking sun deepened the colors of the fine, stained windows."[73] He was not always alone. Long afterward, Gage related that "often when he was practicing I used to go to the chapel with him to hear some of the great music. The tones of these majestic pieces have never left me."[74]

In October 1880 a campus feud exploded. A majority of seniors, Theobald among them, elected George Lincoln Burr, a well-balanced and intelligent Arts student, as Class President. A minority elected a rival President. Burr's biographer stated that the minority "wanted to put on a graduation ball at a price which the others could not afford. Burr sided with the poorer boys."[75] The dispute was aired in the campus newspapers, and Theobald Smith was appointed to solve it. In his very first publication (a letter to the editor of the *Cornell Era*), he defined the alternatives as "economy and useless extravagance—an issue in which many a Cornell student is heartily interested."[76] His compromise plan involved the resignation of both Presidents, with nomination of a third party. Burr duly resigned, but the minority candidate intransigently refused to withdraw; whereupon Burr assumed the presidency and the controversy subsided.[77]

During the second term, Theobald competed for the Woodford Prize. His chosen subject, "The Ideals Destroyed by Science and Their Substitutes," provided a "torrent of ideas." But "It was a schoolboy production, and could be nothing else considering the distraction from any great subject caused by a variety of study and want of life experience."[78] James Stuart Ainslie, who was ordained a minister of the Congregational Church the following year, won the prize, his topic being "The Stoic and the Christian Type of Civilization."

Theobald's chagrin was mollified by publication of his effort (the second in print) in the March number of *The Cornell Review*.[79] The essay epitomized his current religious and philosophical outlook. By seeking to implant the ideal of Truth for its own sake in the heart of man, Science had loosened the bonds of political and religious despotism, and emancipated the individual.

Theobald's own limited social life expanded during his senior year. Fresh from a "sociable" at Sage College, he penned this diary entry:

> It is absolutely necessary either to dance or to stay at home, there can be no compromise between these two conclusions . . . A brilliantly lighted parlor with snow white cloth stretched upon the floor . . . the piano playing with vehemence the impulsive measures of the waltz, a number of flitting whirling couples gaily attired with trains to suit. Such was the spectacle to me standing in the doorway, deserted as I seemed to myself, awkward and stiff, not knowing what to do with myself, or the allotted hours.[80]

To avoid a recurrence of the situation, he formed a resolution: "Dancing— Tomorrow I shall begin!"[81] And later: "Weekly I have gone to whirl with my friends each in turn, & lastly with maidens . . . The dance has afforded me many agreeable hours; some of the most enjoyable of my life."[82]

During the short spring vacation, Theobald decided to try for a Johns Hopkins University fellowship. After returning to Cornell, he settled on a topic that should "win over" its Biological Department—"The Peritoneum of the Cat." He concentrated upon developing the project as a thesis, and in May submitted the final version to Baltimore, with letters of recommendation from Wilder and Gage.[83] He failed to win the fellowship but adopted the same subject for his Cornell graduation thesis.

His last springtime as an undergraduate was suffused with nostalgia: "The visit to the glass-house, the excursions on the lake." And there was an unforgettable excursion to Stratton Falls, south of Ithaca, with a dozen members of the Natural History Society. The group included the Van Pelt sisters, Misses Howland and Harriet Heyl, and Professors Dudley and W.R. Lazenby (Horticulture). They wandered for hours through the picturesque gorge, its moss-covered walls cascading or dripping water from innumerable crevices. "Oh, for another such day and such company."[84]

In May 1881, before the final examinations, Theobald began to collect testimonials. The Registrar, Rev. W.D. Wilson, certified him to be "a young man of excellent character & pleasing manners. He is one of the very best scholars in the class consisting of something like ninety members." Prof. Anthony wrote of Theobald's "excellent work in my department . . . Mr. Smith is a young man of marked ability and promise." The Acting President, William C. Russel, stated that his scholarship and industry in his Philosophy class had always been superior; he had shown high proficiency in all his studies; his conduct had been unexceptionable and his principles and character excellent; and he would graduate with honor next month. These handwritten documents (Cornell purchased its first typewriter in 1884) were preserved by Theobald Smith.[85]

The thirteenth Annual Commencement began at 9 A.M. on June 16, 1881 in the downtown Library Hall. Ezra Cornell had donated a fine library building in 1865 to the people of Ithaca and Tompkins County, which served for larger University functions until the campus Armory was built in 1883. The official Programme Exercises listed twenty-five items, besides presentation of prizes and conferring of degrees and certificates. Eight members of the graduating class made solemn speeches, beginning with a disquisition by Ainslie (Woodford Prize Orator) on "The Tendencies of our Time in Reference to Christianity," and ending with an oration by the Class President, George Lincoln Burr, on "Revolt and Revolution." Theobald's parents did not attend and he felt aloof from these formalities. He received a small prize of $5, with a scroll signed by William C. Russel as Acting President, "for merit and attainment in Veterinary Science."

The Class-Day Exercises had been held in the afternoon two days earlier, on June 14. The Prayer, the Roll Call, the Oration, the History, the Poem, the Essay, and the Class President's Address, were billed as "In the Valley" (Cornell Library Hall). The rest of the program took place "On the Hill," including the ceremonies of Planting the Ivy, followed by the Ivy Oration and the Prophecy, and the Presentation of the Class Pipe by the '81 to the '82 Custodian.[86] Theobald was a member of the Class Day committee which had approved the two-phase program "In the Valley" and "On the Hill." The claim[87] that there were "two rival class-day programs" in June 1881, due to "a war between fraternities and independents," is apparently incorrect. However, there was disharmony: "Class day came—but the division of the class had done enough to cool the interest usually taken in the occasion. The phrases of 'companionship,' 'brotherly love,' etc., were but a hollow mockery with the class of '81."[88]

The day of final departure arrived. As the boat moved up Cayuga Lake, Theobald kept his "eyes fastened upon the town and the tower of the University Building, surrounded by the light haze of a beautiful summer day . . . Thus Ithaca faded from View."[89] When disclosing his background and his scant family genealogy to his future wife some five years later, Theobald told her that "The four years spent there will forever remain an epoch in my history."[90]

3

MEDICAL SCHOOL TRAINING AND INITIAL WORK AT THE U.S. BUREAU OF ANIMAL INDUSTRY

Upon returning home to Albany, Theobald wrote to the New York Teacher's Agency and sought assistance from friends in getting summer work; but nothing turned up. "My only refuge from idleness as a last resort lay in medicine," he confided to his Diary, "So I worked steadily, studying the human skeleton & sundry kindred subjects . . . My time was spent partly at Dr. Hailes' office, partly at home."[1] At the end of August, he assisted Dr. Albert Van Derveer, who had an extensive practice besides being Professor of the Principles and Practice of Surgery at Albany Medical College. That fall, after a week's holiday in the Helderbergs, where he roamed and rowed and read George Eliot's *Felix Holt,* Theobald enrolled as a medical student.

The Albany Medical College (among the twenty oldest medical schools still extant in the United States) was organized in 1838, mainly through the efforts of Dr. Alden March, who remained president of the College's medical faculty, as well as Professor of surgery, until his death in 1869. His last registered pupil was Dr. William Hailes, who introduced Theobald Smith to the practice of medicine. Theobald's new mentor, Dr. Van Derveer, after postgraduate studies in Europe, occupied successive chairs in branches of anatomy and surgery and eventually became the college's dean and surgeon-in-chief. In 1873, the Medical

College amalgamated with the Albany Law School, the Dudley Observatory, and Union College of Albany, to form Union University.

Although Albany Medical College rated among the better "proprietary" medical schools that mushroomed in nineteenth-century North America, Abraham Flexner's 1910 report to the Carnegie Foundation on Medical Education in the United States and Canada classed it among schools that "belong to the past."[2] Allegedly, Flexner's visit was too cursory, entailing merely "a hasty glance here and there,"[3] and the faculty considered the report "unfriendly, unfair, incomplete and, indeed, distinctly hostile in its tone."[4] Nevertheless, the College instituted a drastic reorganization, and revolutionary improvements followed.

A few years later, in 1916, Maurice J. Lewi, Theobald's high school friend and fellow-Philologian, who had gone directly from Albany High School to the Medical College, recollected the old school's "dust-grimed library shelves, its creaky stairs, its foul-smelling dissecting room and its ramshackle cellar."[5] Several students and an occasional surgeon were generally at work in the dissecting room amidst the penetrating odor of preservative. Cadavers awaiting dissection were kept in the basement, "moored to the edge of the pool in which was some sort of 'brine' to preserve the bodies of the often unknown persons, picked up in various places . . . until graduation from the cellar to the upstairs dissecting room. There was always a reserve stock of four or five 'floaters'." Another alumnus remembered that "Some of the embryo medics broke into the building one night and appropriated one of the 'stiffs' from the pickle vat in the basement." Clothed and propped between two supporters at a favorite bar, he confronted and confounded the bartender and customers.[6]

The medical school course began early in October 1881. Theobald entered the dissecting room tense with excitement, but "the feeling of cutting up a human body was not a pleasant one for me."[7] He soon grew disgruntled for that and other reasons:

> The weeks sped in their monotonous round with their daily quantity of lectures, evening dissections, & Saturday clinics . . . but I was not happy. I felt not at home with my surroundings. I could not sympathize with the students there; the lectures were often grossly insufficient, the air was bad, and finally my own health was not good . . . My digestive apparatus was functionally deranged, & my imagination pictured all sorts of horrible maladies of which my present condition was the germ.[8]

The medical course closed for the summer on March 1, 1882. Of 170 students attending, almost one-third graduated. Theobald spent the rest of the month on anatomy, physiology, and music. One evening a week he read Horace, in a course organized by the Albany High School Society of the Alumni for the

Encouragement of Home Studies, with Oscar Robinson as Instructor. By the following winter, he had studied proficiently "thirty-eight Odes, two Epodes, three Satires, and two Epistles of Horace." His Diary for that period also recorded that "Prof. Martin of Johns Hopkins University, Baltimore offered me compensation of $125 for assistance in the Biol. Lab. for April and May."[9]

Theobald was much relieved at this chance to overlay the winter's deadening influence by work among strangers.[10] At the end of March 1882, he left by steamer for New York, whence the Pennsylvania Railroad took him to Baltimore. In the late afternoon, he "followed the well-known Donaldson up the stairs until I was ushered into the presence of Dr. Martin."

> The contrast between my imaginary portrait of him & the reality brought me to my senses again. His coat off & shirt sleeves rolled up, he was seated at a substantial table in his small room, manipulating a steel rule on paper. A short wooden pipe was in his mouth, and an empty bottle of some kind of beer stood near by. A plain blond face with large blue eyes & a delicate set of features to which may be added a light moustache of slight development, were turned toward me. He arose, welcoming me cordially, and introduced me to Dr. Sedgwick, his associate. The latter, a young man with a well-fed body-structure, full-blown cheeks, towards which tended a well-developed brown moustache, eyes shielded by spectacles, stood before me.[11]

Henry Newell Martin, trained in England under Thomas Huxley, William Sharpey and Michael Foster, though now aged only thirty-four, had developed his department into America's foremost center of teaching and research in physiology. Daniel Coit Gilman,[12] the first president of Johns Hopkins University, had offered him the Chair of biology only six years before. William Thompson Sedgwick was about four years older than Theobald. After graduating from Yale's Scientific School in 1877, he attended its School of Medicine for two years. Awarded a Biology fellowship at Johns Hopkins University in 1879, he was persuaded by Martin to forego medicine in favor of biological teaching and research. When Smith met him, the recently married Sedgwick had taken his Ph.D. and was a Associate in Biology.[13]

For Theobald, this temporary assistantship was "a period of continuous laboratory experience, of close application, not so much to mental effort as to observation and manual work."[14] Smith and his co-worker, F.S. Lee,[15] "hardened the chick embryos, prepared the cochleae of rats, colored the clays for Sedgwick's model of the still unhatched chick, and hung up the various charts of the respective lectures. For this simple work we were paid $62.50 a month each, and studied with zeal all the rest of the time." Theobald noted the department library's "book-lined walls, its tables concealed by periodicals from all quarters of the globe." Here, too, the research student "found the works dear to him beyond all else brought together within the compass of a dozen shelves, where he might sit & revel in the delights of his special line of study." The Peabody Library was especially admired—"Its large square room with five circumambient galleries all loaded with books, the whole filled with a mellow light from a large skylight overhead." Casts of famous statues reminded him of anatomy.[16]

Baltimore itself was pleasant with the neatness and quiet of its beautiful squares and parks contrasting favorably with "rusty old Albany." He secured accommodation at a boarding house run by Mrs. Osborne, a tall, graceful and kind-hearted landlady from Virginia, who had been through "the late rebellion and probably lost much." Around her table gathered an assortment of intelligent boarders, most of them graduate students. Arthur Henry Giles, son of a Methodist minister and a Latin graduate, was Theobald's companion on many a long walk and local expedition. Gerster and Kellogg took him to see *La Traviata* and *Faust*. Other boarders were Benjamin Lewis Hobson and William Scott Fleming, graduates in Greek; Edward Harrison Keiser, in Chemistry; de Witt Bristol Brace, in Mathematics; and Charles Albert Perkins, in Physics. Most of them took Ph.D. degrees and became well-known professors. Louis Alexander Witzenbacher, then an undergraduate, attained a judgeship.

Smith was introduced into this stimulating circle by "the diminutive Conn from the East,"[17] who worked for his Ph.D. in biology. Herbert William Conn (1859–1917) was a graduate of Boston University and grew to eminence in Bacteriology. According to H.J. Conn, also an outstanding bacteriologist, his father recalled "a tall, lanky young man" (later identified as Theobald Smith), who arrived at Johns Hopkins announcing that he wanted to study bacteriology. Receiving little encouragement, he went elsewhere.[18] However, Smith's diary conveys only the glad acceptance of a temporary assistantship in the spring of 1882. Half a century later, an autobiographical note alluded to his "spending a spring term at the Johns Hopkins in the biological department."[19] On a typed version of this *Curriculum Vitae,* Simon Flexner (at whose request it was prepared) penciled the suggestion that perhaps "Dr. Smith was influenced by the excitement attending the discovery" of Robert Koch's cultivation of the tubercle bacillus. There is no hint of any contemporary stir on that account, either in the Biological Laboratory or in Smith's own mind. In fact, Smith's concern with bacteria lay dormant until after his appointment by the U.S. Department of Agriculture at the end of 1883.

When Theobald left Baltimore for home, he was uncertain what the coming year would bring. In July he received two notices: "One from Prof. Martin that Johns Hopkins was not in need of my services next year—the other, an invitation from Prof. Gage to spend August at Ithaca in mounting skeletons. My sorry and disappointment at the first was only partially neutralized by the pleasant times augured by the second."[20]

Theobald spent a happy month quartered in a small room in Cascadilla Place. Daily he "sat in the Lab. below, boiling, scraping, drying, bleaching & mounting bones, and warding off too impetuous bands of picknickers who overran" his solitude. "A caravan of skeletons soon were gathered together. The mild but bloated frog, the large & small turtles, headed by two cats, comprised the work of the month. But our evenings on Cascadilla piazza were truly charming . . . our minds were borne on with irresistible mirth at our German Conversations in which we couched our simple wants . . . 'Am liebsten' was our host's endearing expression to Mrs. Gage, and it certainly deserved the credit of originality." (The Gages had been married about eight month before, on December 14, 1881.) Theobald wondered what to do next: "Go on with the Medical Lectures, for which I had a great aversion, or go to Ithaca where I might tutor & thus with Dr. Wilder's help push my way along financially. I had not yet heard from the West, where my name had been proposed as an instructor in Natural Science. After wasting several weeks in useless, inward debate . . . and receiving an adverse answer . . . from Oshkosh, I reentered the Medical School."[21]

He studied through the winter at home, where he fitted out a pleasant room over the kitchen. At the College he worked hard six days a week. On the seventh day, he sought relaxation (and $100 a year salary) by serving as organist and choirmaster at Trinity Church. "The Sundays mark this desert season like oases." He often saw Battin, who had returned from Dakota, where he had been a surveyor. Theobald and John Montignani spent Monday evenings perusing Cicero's *De Amicitia* "with a bevy of young ladies."

His graduating essay at the Medical College, entitled "Relations between Cell-activity in Health and in Disease," began with a quotation from Cicero.[22] Examinations took seven weary nights of scribbling on foolscap in the dark and dingy Chemical Lecture room, "now lighted with gas & filled with tobacco-smoke . . . New ideas were tortured into line . . . to do good service." Next morning, as he crossed the South Ferry Bridge to Greenbush in the warm sunlight, a buoyancy unknown for years swept over him. Finally, he heard that his "examination papers had won the prize—a pocket case of instruments, a pleasing triumph of close application."[23]

The fifty-first annual Commencement of the Albany Medical College was held in the Music Hall on Wednesday evening, March 7, 1883. The Graduating Class comprised fifty-one men. Theobald Smith was on the seven-man Executive Committee. Apart from the class prize, he received a parchment certifying (in Latin) that the college of Medicine of Albany University awarded him the diploma of Doctor of the Art of Medicine. The twenty signatories must have included every professor on the staff, among them A. Van Derveer, Chirurgery; William Hailes, Histology and Anatomical Pathology; and (surprisingly) S.O. Vanderpoel, Bacteriology and Pathology. The new graduates afterward repaired to the Alumni dinner,[24] where Theobald endured "poor speeches from unpracticed medical men . . . My mind was made up to return to Ithaca, at least for a time—to rest."[25] The "unsatisfactory state of the practice of medicine, the lack of accurate scientific knowledge concerning diseased conditions, and the means employed to cure them, led me to return to the laboratory as perhaps the most congenial and promising avenue towards a better understanding of pathological processes, their causation, and the means to their prevention."[26]

At the beginning of April, Theobald returned to Ithaca to continue mounting skeletons. His room, now facing the gorge, was furnished only with a little table and a single cot-bed, an armchair, a small bureau, and his trunk. "The bleakness of my room drove me into Prof. Gage's, where we usually had delightful times together," reading Andersen's fairy tales in German. "The cold drove me to bed & prevented my studying, thus giving me the long-needed rest & sleep."[27] He found time for many enjoyable tramps with Prof. Dudley.

His laboratory was in the McGraw Hall tower, which also housed the University Museum of Natural History. There he "mounted skeletons . . . and learned to become interested in Comparative Anatomy."[28] The *Cornell Review* praised his fine preparations and urged retention of his services, referring to Vertebrate Zoology as "a subject in which few persons have acquired the delicacy of manipulation which Dr. Smith possesses."[29] A campus newspaper announced that within the last month three former students of Profs. Wilder and Gage had graduated first in their class at different medical schools—Theobald Smith at Albany, Hermann Biggs at Bellevue, and Miss Potter at Buffalo.

In August, Theobald took a summer vacation of three weeks at home. He bathed in the Hudson and went on a walking tour through the Catskills with Joe Guardenier. Then he "doffed my wide-brimmed straw hat, & my blue flannel shirt, & prepared for Ithaca."[30] He now had two small rooms on the lower floor of Cascadilla. He papered a dado around the bedroom walls, put up pictures and curtains, laid a carpet and distributed his own furniture, all purchased in Albany. For the two weeks before the university opened, Prof. Wait entrusted him with some pupils at his private Cascadilla School, to whom Theobald taught Physiology, Geography, and German.

Soon, nearly 500 students returned to campus, many "thwarted by Entrance examinations." Fourteen of these were assigned to Theobald for elementary algebra three times a week. To others, he taught plane geometry. He also assembled the skeletons of a sloth and a camel. "The former soon climbed a branch under my treatment, while the latter required more time & labor to make him stand in his natural manner. Of both I am quite proud."[31] Neat records of completed specimens were kept as annotated sketches, meticulously headed with their dates of preparation. He mounted during summer and fall nine animals, including salamanders, a sloth and a large cat. A human skeleton required forty-five hours of work; a gorilla, whose sternum had to be cut out of heavy leather, took eighty hours to mount; the circus camel (which Gage had retrieved) had its bones already cleaned and assembled, but needed some "sternal cartilages prepared with tow & glue, with thin cloth wound around outside"—a total of 120 hours. Finally, in November, he prepared 648 microscopic sections of *Amphioxus,* and miscellaneous specimens for future classes, and devoted fifty-seven hours to mounting an alligator "cleaned with Mr. Kilborne's assistance." The evenings were spent usually with the Gages, the new task being to translate Claus' *Lehrbuch der Zoologie.*

In 1868, President White recruited James Law, a professor at the Veterinary College of Edinburgh, allegedly because Ezra Cornell had expressly requested a "horse-doctor."[32] The new professor did his utmost to elevate veterinary studies to parity with other sciences at Cornell University, which awarded the first Bachelor of Veterinary Science Degree in America in 1871. In the following year, Daniel E. Salmon also graduated with that degree. In 1876, Cornell University conferred the first American honorary doctorate of Veterinary Medicine upon Salmon, who seven years later became Chief of the Veterinary Division of the United States Department of Agriculture. After establishing a pathological laboratory in his Division, Salmon sought help from his former professor Burt Wilder in locating a well-trained assistant who could investigate animal diseases. Wilder passed the letter on to Gage (then Assistant Professor of Physiology and Lecturer on Microscopical Technology), who had known Salmon as a fellow-student. Gage wrote thus on October 12, 1883:

Dear Dr. Salmon, Professor Wilder showed me your letter of the 9th concerning an assistant. I know that Dr. Wilder is going to give you the name of Dr. Theobald Smith, B.Ph., M.D.

He is everything that you designate as desirable in the highest degree and a great deal more. He reads and speaks German like an educated native, and his ability to do careful work is, it seems to me, as great as that of any one I ever met. Perhaps if I tell you that we are writing a paper together it will show you that my expressed opinion is a genuine one.

I most sincerely regret to have him leave us, but of course feel glad to think of him doing better for himself. If you secure him, I can assure you that whatever he undertakes to do for you will be done ably, neatly and conscientiously—I am very Respectfully, Simon H. Gage.[33]

If Wilder's letter was equally complimentary, the prompt offer of a government position in Washington is no more surprising than Theobald's acceptance of it. The appointment was clinched in a handwritten letter from the Veterinary Division, U.S. Department of Agriculture, dated October 25, 1883:

> Sir, You are hereby appointed Assistant in the Veterinary Division of this Department at a salary of twelve hundred dollars per annum. Report for instruction to Dr. D. E. Salmon, Chief of the Veterinary Division, December 1, 1883. Very respectfully, E.A. Cameron, Acting Commissioner.[34]

The *Albany Medical Annals* announced that Dr. Theobald Smith ('83) had received an appointment "at an advanced salary" in the United States Agriculture Department. The *Cornell Sun* evidently thought the salary would be well earned:

> Another Cornellian has been captured by the U.S. Agricultural Department . . . Dr. D.E. Salmon . . . has been making experiments in the Veterinary Division upon the diseases of animals supposed to be due to microscopic organisms, and he later asked Professor Wilder to name some advanced student who would assist him in these difficult and important investigations. Professors Comstock and Gage . . . concurred in recommending Dr. Theobald Smith so emphatically that . . . compensation was fixed at $1200 a year instead of the $900 at first offered . . . His departure will be a great loss to the anatomical department.[35]

Theobald Smith "left Ithaca on Nov. 10th & staid at home to rest & prepare for Washington."[36] A few friends saw him off as he left on Thanksgiving Day for the nation's capital.

Charles E. Salmon was a freshman at Cornell University during its inaugural year. Prof. James Law advised him to take some science courses before starting veterinary studies, and to complete his final period of professional training in France. Salmon spent six months at the famous Alfort Veterinary School in Paris, where he learned about Pasteur's doctrines and bacteriological methods before returning to Cornell in the fall of 1872. He passed the examinations for the Bachelor of Veterinary Science degree, married an Ithaca girl, and took up practice in Newark, New Jersey, transferring to Asheville, North Carolina, three years later. In 1878, Commissioner William G. Le Duc hired Salmon for two months to investigate swine diseases, especially hog cholera, which caused huge losses and jeopardized the export trade in pork. Next year, Salmon was appointed a temporary inspector by New York State to assist James Law in overcoming bovine contagious pleuropneumonia. The federal government rehired him in 1880 to investigate Texas cattle fever as well as swine diseases.

Salmon's zeal and self-confidence were impressive. He supplemented his field inquiries by laboratory data procured largely with improvised equipment. He also wrote reports and scientific articles assiduously. He was appointed to the United States Department of Agriculture in July 1881, and when Congress approved the establishment of a Veterinary Division within this Department, Salmon was called to Washington as its Chief, effective May 1, 1883. The Department of Agriculture had been established by an Act of Congress, signed by President Abraham Lincoln in 1862. Thus, the Congress had responded slowly to pressures to create a Veterinary Division within the Department, despite serious livestock losses, which according to Horace Capron, Commissioner of Agriculture, in 1864 had amounted to not less than $50,000 and demanded the prompt attention of the Department.

Salmon set up his office and a pathological laboratory on the top floor of the Department of Agriculture Building, at the southwest corner of Thirteenth and B Streets. To facilitate observation and investigation of livestock diseases under natural environmental conditions, a seven-acre tract of rolling land was leased on Benning Road, just outside the northeast city boundary. With a few added structures, this served for several years as the Department's Experiment Station.[37] Salmon found it impossible to do significant laboratory work himself while administering the Division, and appealed to his former professors for an assistant. As described, they strongly recommended Theobald Smith, who arrived in Washington at the end of November 1883, ready for duty on December 1.

Smith found lodgings at 917 New York Avenue, within easy walking distance of the Agriculture Building. The Barnards, close friends of the Wilders, were on the second floor, which also had sufficient room for Theobald. William S. Barnard, Ph.D., was an entomologist with the U.S. Department of Agriculture. His wife worked in Salmon's office. In late August 1884, Smith wrote to Gage: "Please come to Washington if you are not all disposed. There is plenty of room for two here."[38]

At the outset, Smith was favorably impressed with his new situation. Salmon's enthusiasm for the "germ theory of disease" was genuine, and he was convinced that the newer knowledge of bacteriology, properly applied, could eliminate many of the animal plagues which jeopardized the country's health and prosperity; but a dictatorial, dogmatic and disputatious approach made Salmon unpopular with professional organizations. Theobald Smith, nine years younger than Salmon, and quite unversed in bacteriology, welcomed the doctrines and willingly adopted the techniques imparted by his chief. Salmon augmented the meager facilities of the new Division by providing a satisfactory microscope, adequate basic apparatus, and a fair sampling of relevant literature mostly in French and German. Theobald's ability to interpret the current reports of Koch and his co-workers at the Imperial Department of Health proved particularly advantageous. Communications from Koch's laboratory (*Mittheilungen aus dem Kaiserlichen Gesundheitsamt*) began in 1881. Besides, as Theobald wrote to Gage, he tried "to make abstracts at home from our best foreign monographs for my own use."[39]

Several animal diseases demanded investigation, mostly hog cholera, contagious pleuropneumonia, foot-and-mouth disease, glanders, and Texas cattle fever. As a total embargo on American cattle to Britain was threatened, while several European countries already prohibited entry of American salted and smoked meats because of hog cholera and trichinosis, it was generally agreed that elimination of such epizootics required national direction. The economic arguments were reinforced by compassionate and public health considerations, for long-distance domestic and foreign transport of animals subjected them to severe overcrowding, which was liable to affect the wholesomeness and safety of the meat.

In May 1884, the Congress narrowly passed, and President Arthur approved, an Act establishing the U.S. Bureau of Animal Industry, "to prevent the exportation of diseased cattle, and to provide means for the suppression and extirpation of pleuropneumonia and other contagious diseases among domestic animals." The Chief of the Bureau had to be a "competent veterinary surgeon," and the maximum staff should be twenty persons. Effective July 1, 1884, D.E. Salmon became Chief of the new Bureau under Commissioner Loring, at a salary of $3,000. Theobald Smith was also transferred to the Bureau and listed as Assistant in Laboratory, with William H. Rose as Superintendent, Experiment Station, each at $1,600 annual salary. A clerk, a messenger, and a laborer completed the salaried personnel of the Bureau. Two agents and several assistant veterinarians were on daily allowances.

The Bureau's extensive regulatory powers and the cooperative attitude of most state legislatures yielded early dividends. By 1887, pleuropneumonia was complete eradicated from Illinois, Ohio, Missouri and Kentucky; and on September 26, 1892, Secretary of Agriculture Jeremiah M. Rusk officially proclaimed the United States "free from the disease known as contagious pleuropneumonia." Much of this accomplishment, which entailed a total national government outlay of around one and a half million dollars, was due to Salmon's leadership as Chief of the bureau, and to his advisor, Dr. James Law. Salmon was often away pursuing the eradication policy, leaving Theobald Smith in charge of the laboratory quarters, which were very far from ideal.

Early in 1885, Smith apologized to Gage for tardily reporting the presence of tubercle bacilli in a slide-specimen kept in his table drawer instead of under a "bell-glass" or in a bottle. The roaches had eaten all the film off the cover glass. In

July the weather was so warm that "my culture media melt, which is fatal . . . While languishing in a stifling atmosphere at 90 - 95° with a hot blast billowing in thro my window and ice-water at my side, I will *try* to collect my leaking senses."[40] The desired alterations were long delayed. On his return from two weeks vacation, everything was as he had left it: "Even the roof of my laboratory was untouched, although I had expected to see a skylight there on my return."[41]

The period was notable for a great leap forward in medical microbiology, resulting largely from adoption of Robert Koch's criteria for specific pathogenicity, and his solid-media techniques for isolating bacterial pathogens. When Smith arrived in Washington, the recent discoveries of the tubercle bacillus by Koch (1882), of the bacterial cause of *roget de porc* or swine erysipelas by Pasteur and Thuillier (1882), and of the glanders bacillus by Löffler and Schütz (1883) were accepted by most bacteriologists. However, few American universities had adequate microscopes for revealing these parasites. Even Gage—eventually one of the country's best-known authorities on microscopy—was reminded by Smith, who had sent him a section of pathological material containing tubercle bacilli, "You will be unable to demonstrate them well unless you use Dr. Law's microscope with the Abbe ill minus the diaphragm." He was referring to a new light condenser, and immersion objectives, which had been evolved by Ernst Abbe and were manufactured by Carl Zeiss.[42]

Theobald Smith had learned a good deal about section-cutting and microscopic theory from his work with Gage at Cornell in the fall of 1883. They had co-authored two short papers on serial microscopic sections, the first of which appeared in November 1883, the other, describing a section flattener, in February 1884.[43] Gage demonstrated the flattener at the seventh annual meeting of the American Society of Microscopists, held at Rochester, New York, August 19–22, 1884. The junior author commented: "I am happy to know that people take notice of it: all due to your efforts too. If it depended on me I might write a public review denouncing it myself, because I had something to do with it. I have a mania of always putting a bushel basket over any light that might accidentally come from my unsnuffed candle."[44]

Knowledge of German and French literature, and personal experience, soon gave Theobald Smith enough material for several lectures and scientific articles. Following Koch's amplified report on tuberculosis (1884), he discussed the significance of tubercle bacilli in human sputum in the July 1884 issue of the *Albany Medical Annals*. Smith's review marked the beginning of his life-long concern to adapt "new facts to the amelioration or eradication of that fearful disease which more than decimates the race."[45] He concluded that the presence of *B. tu-*

berculosis in sputum signified pulmonary tuberculosis; that failure to find the parasite did not always rule out the disease; and that there was no correlation between numbers of bacilli present in the sputum and the severity of the disease.

The next issue of the *Annals* contained a detailed description by Smith of Koch's methods of demonstrating tubercle bacilli in sputum, citing Koch's newest report, which incorporated the staining modifications of Paul Ehrlich and his cousin Carl Weigert.[46] Smith felt that an already available English version should counter the drift of Americans to Koch's laboratory. On hearing that a Cornell undergraduate "had been sent abroad by the University to study Koch's methods in Germany," he inquired of Gage whether it was "true that the institution could perpetrate such a piece of folly and stupidity? His methods are fully published and quite simple."[47]

In a third article in the *Annals,* entitled "Pathogenic Bacteria and Wandering Cells,"[48] the relevant German and French literature from Cohnheim to Metchnikoff was appraised. This article initiated Theobald Smith's enduring concern with immunological problems, and foreshadowed two of his favorite themes: first, the intimate relationship between general biology and pathology, illustrated by Metchnikoff's researches that "the amoeba slowly flowing around its food particle is the prototype of the amoebiform leucocyte enveloping the death-bringing "parasite," and, secondly, the limited applicability of observations made on a small selection of diseases.

The fourth paper in the series, a translation of a monograph by Pierre Mégnin on gapeworm affecting peasantries in France, was published by the U.S. Department of Agriculture toward the end of 1884 in a special report on *Contagious Diseases of Domesticated Animals for 1883–84.*[49] It alerted Theobald to the wide range in size and complexity of disease-provoking parasites in poultry. He himself briefly investigated gape disease of fowls in 1885.

In the spring of 1885, Smith thought of translating Ferdinand Hueppe's monograph on the techniques of bacteriological investigation from the German;[50] but by the time Gage recommended him to the publisher's representative, the work had been assigned to Dr. Hermann Biggs, his organ-playing competitor at Cornell, now instructor at the Carnegie Laboratory of The Bellevue Hospital Medical College of New York. Bigg's translation was published in 1886.[51] Theobald Smith covered his chagrin by claiming the time could be "better spent in writing special chapters on the same subject for the forthcoming report of the Bureau."[52]

In 1884, Gage invited Theobald to attend the annual meeting of the American Association for the Advancement of Science at Philadelphia, beginning September 3, of which he and Wilder were fellows. Smith declined because he had to visit Albany the following month for his parents' return from a visit to Germany. However, he told his friend Gage, who would be in attendance, "If R. Hitchcock reads something about Dr. Salmon's methods and shows any slides, don't fail to gaze upon them, they are my preparations."[53] Romyn Hitchcock, a former science student at Cornell, now attached to the Smithsonian Institution, described and demonstrated a new culture-tube, invented by Salmon,[54] before the Histology and Microscopy Section of the meeting. The three-part glass apparatus was used for "the study of microscopic fungi in liquid media." The abstract named Theobald Smith, laboratory assistant to Salmon, as sole author.[55] It reported that in a room where dust is carefully managed, a short exposure to the air is not dangerous. The utensils, unless thoroughly sterilized, are the chief carriers of a miscellaneous contamination." Although the tube, flamed before use, allowed uncontaminated subculture from a pure culture, it was too complex and cumbersome to gain acceptance.

In April 1885, Theobald Smith presented a paper on Koch's methods in bacteriology before the Biological Society of Washington, which had elected him to active membership fourteen months before. Using the platinum loop, he reported, pure cultures could be obtained from the intestinal or respiratory tract by inoculating sterile nutrient gelatin from a broth culture of the sample to be tested. Samples of drinking-water likewise could be analyzed bacteriologically. The mixture solidified when poured on previously sterilized, cold glass plates. After keeping the plates for forty-eight hours under a bell-jar—the Petri dish was not yet available—minute "colonies" were examined under low-power microscopy for colonial form and gelatin-liquefying capacity.[56]

Also demonstrated were Koch's blood-serum and potato media—agar was introduced by Koch only in 1885—and various decoctions and infusions of lean meat, and also sterilized milk, used in the Bureau's laboratory. At the same meeting, Hitchcock showed microscopic preparations of Koch's "comma bacillus of cholera." The *National Republican* newspaper of April 23, 1885 printed two columns on Theobald Smith's "most interesting account of the cultivation . . . outside the body" of disease-producing bacteria. Smith's presentation appeared in abstract, under the joint authorship of Salmon and Smith, in the *American Monthly Microscopical Journal*.[57] Theobald had a low opinion of the Biological Society: "The Society languishes and, I think, ought to die."[58] Yet he presented twenty-one papers before it during the next nine years and was on the Society's council for over four years, beginning in January 1891.

Despite such co-authorship, there was no true collaboration with Salmon. Smith wrote to Gage: "I am going to send you . . . a photograph of my lab. I say 'my' because nobody else works in it. Dr. Salmon is too busy at his work; in fact, since I have come, the entire experimental work is left in my charge."[59] In another letter, he deplored having "degenerated to a scientific philistine . . . My daily labor has so absorbed my entire attention that I often feel like a packhorse destined to carry the same bundle over the same road for ever."[60] In mid-January 1885, Gage visited him, subsequently sending a note of thanks. Smith responded that he had been very busy lately, "preparing an index for the forthcoming *First Annual Report* of the Bureau, besides having to attend to everything else about the laboratory. Dr. Salmon went West again for a month or so."[61]

"In 1886 I appealed to the Columbian—now George Washington—medical faculty to let me give a voluntary course of lectures in hygiene and sanitation," Theobald Smith wrote in 1931 in the autobiographical sketch he prepared for John D. Rockefeller, Jr. The course gradually developed laboratory exercises in bacteriology. On February 2, 1886, Dean A.F.A. King of the National Medical College of the Columbian University advised Smith:

> Dear Doctor, it gives me pleasure to inform you that you were yesterday elected by the Medical Faculty: "Lecturer on Bacteriology" in the Spring Course of this College. Please notify me of your acceptance, or otherwise, at an early day.[62]

The once-weekly, unpaid lectures would begin early in April and continue for two months. (Like all the other appointed "Lecturers," Smith was soon designated "Prof." on the College's printed time tables.) Gage offered to assist with illustrations, and sent a copy of his just published *Notes on Histological Methods.*[63] Smith responded that he would make use of the notes, but "I shall not need any figs. Bacteria are, fortunately, not very complex in structure . . . I wish you might come down and neutralize the feeling I have in lecturing to medical students. I take such a personal interest in the subject that many of the facts I consider as pearls."[64] In 1885, when Theobald Smith resigned, his successor at the Medical College was Walter Reed.

Thus, Theobald Smith joined the ranks of pioneer American instructors in bacteriology. Before 1886, less than a dozen other Americans officially recognized bacteria as entities, and bacteriology as a specialty *sui generis.* Some of them will be mentioned here. In the 1870's, Thomas J. Burrill (1839–1916), professor of botany at the Illinois Industrial University, introduced the study of bacterial into his course on rusts and mildews. By 1880 he had verified his belief that the "fire-blight" ravaging pear trees in the Midwest was of bacterial origin.[65] William Trelease (1857–1945), Theobald Smith's contemporary at Cornell and a fellow-member of Delta Upsilon fraternity, organized a course in bacteriology at the University of Wisconsin in 1881.[66] In 1878, George M. Sternberg (1838–1915) began to investigate the value of disinfectants in controlling infectious disease. Three years later, he found in his saliva an organism, eventually known as Friedlanders's pneumococcus, that caused fatal septicemia when injected subcutaneously into rabbits. During the period 1885–86, Sternberg studied the thermal death point of pathogenic bacteria.[67]

T. Mitchell Prudden (1849–1924), after undertaking postgraduate studies in pathology at German universities, especially Heidelberg, in 1878 became assistant pathologist at the College of Physicians and Surgeons of New York, where he also directed an alumni-founded laboratory—a partitioned alcove for research—and teaching in bacteriology.[68] Within a year of Koch's discovery of the tubercle bacillus, Prudden published two papers on the bacteriology of tuberculous lesions,[69] following which he and W.H. Welch took Koch's new one-month course at Berlin in July 1885. He and his assistant T.M. Cheeseman began formal instruction in bacteriology in 1885. Six years later, Prudden became professor of pathology at Columbia University. Many of his hygienic principles were transformed into metropolitan practicalities by a close friend and disciple, Hermann M. Biggs, who was appointed director of the New York City Health Department Laboratory. In the fall of 1885, Biggs had taught bacteriology at the new Carnegie Laboratory of the Bellevue Hospital Medical College. In 1901, Biggs was nominated a Director of the Rockefeller Institute, as were Prudden and Theobald Smith himself.[70]

Harold C. Ernst gave six lectures in medical bacteriology at Harvard in 1885, where he was Professor of Bacteriology for many years.[71] He founded and edited the *Journal of the Boston Society of Medical Sciences* and its successor, the *Journal of Medical Research*. William H. Welch (1850–1934), after studying at German universities in 1876–78, taught pathology at Bellevue Hospital Medical College in New York. When appointed in 1884 to direct the proposed Pathological Institute at Johns Hopkins University, Welch revisited Germany to familiarize himself with the latest techniques. In October 1886 he instituted formal instruction and research projects in pathology and bacteriology for medical graduates at Johns Hopkins and himself gave the course in bacteriology. In 1901, Welch became chairman of the Rockefeller Institute's Board of Directors.[72]

Salmon's position was politically vulnerable. The Commissioner of Agriculture, George B. Loring (whose appointment dated from July 1, 1881, the day before President James Garfield was shot), held office at the whim of Garfield's successor, President Chester Arthur. By the second half of 1884, another presidential campaign was in full swing. If Grover Cleveland, the Democratic candidate, proved victorious over James B. Blaine, the Republican party's nominee, a new Commissioner of Agriculture would be appointed, and Salmon might lose his job and the Bureau cease to exist. Theobald Smith was unenthusiastic about the Republican candidate. He confided to Gage, "If my conscience should prick me for voting for Blaine, I will ask father to vote for Cleveland to make up for it. How's that? My father being a republican, generally speaking."[73]

Cleveland won the presidency and Commissioner Norman J. Colman assumed control of the Department on April 3, 1885. However, he soon reassured his senior staff, including the Chief of the Bureau of Animal Industry. The temporary threat to the Bureau thus being removed, Smith took stock of his own situation. The laboratory suffered many serious handicaps, especially from uncontrollable heat and cold. His teaching obligations were an agreeable solace, but offered no relief to the "pack horse" routine. If his duties were to include devoting any time to solving the many problems that multiplied before him, some assistance must be provided. "I wish we might have another Cornell man to help me," he had written to Gage nearly a year earlier.[74] He could not have foreseen how soon *two* of his university contemporaries would become associated with him.

Fred Cooper Curtice and Fred Lucius Kilborne also had entered Cornell University in 1877. They roomed together and ran an eating club.[75] During their junior and senior years they were elected to high offices in the Natural History Society. Curtice graduated in 1881 in Natural History (B.S.) and Kilborne in Agriculture (B.Agr.), the same year Smith received the B.Ph. in Philosophy. As seniors, they took certain courses in common, such as Veterinary Science under Professor Law and the Anatomical Laboratory of Professor Wilder and Gage; but Theobald apparently saw little of them otherwise.

After leaving Cornell, Cooper Curtice proceeded to the short-lived Columbia Veterinary College in New York, from which he received his D.V.S. degree in 1883. He then joined the United States Geological Survey. After spending the summer of 1884 in Wisconsin, Curtice informed Smith that he would be posted to Washington in the fall; and before the beginning of November, he had settled in as fellow-lodger. They roomed together for over a year, talked of many things, and occasionally explored the countryside. Curtice was three years older, and socially assumed the airs of the dominant partner. In mid-November 1885, he embarked upon a three-year, part-time course at the National Medical College, which granted him an M.D. degree in 1888. He was appointed, as of August 1, 1886, laboratory assistant in the Bureau of Animal Industry, where he concerned himself mainly with parasites of domestic animals. From the outset, Curtice was too ambitious and undependable to serve as a helpful laboratory assistant.

Meanwhile, Theobald Smith's concept that higher education should be general in scope had undergone a marked change. During his undergraduate years, he had considered trying for his Ph.D. at Cornell, but it came to nought, since he balked at Greek being a required subject. Now he was of the opinion that "No college graduate can afford to study subjects for general culture. Study must have an object in view . . . My study would be directed to the Sciences bearing on problems of *Hygiene*."[76]

Fred L. Kilborne was born, bred and died in up-state New York. The Cornell '81 "Class Statistics"[77] listed his future occupation as "Agriculturist." After graduation, he remained as anatomical preparator in vertebrate zoology and microscopy and demonstrator in botany, physiology and zoology. He married in September 1881. When Smith temporarily returned to Cornell in April 1883 as preparator in comparative anatomy, Kilborne assisted him in cleaning the alligator's skeleton. Kilborne enrolled in the autumn of 1881 in Prof. Law's course in veterinary medicine. The following summer, he investigated the lymphatic distribution in the common bullhead, and a "Preliminary Note on the Lymphatics of the Common Bullhead, *Amiurus catus* (L.)," duly appeared under Kilborne's name in the *Proceedings* for the 1884 meeting of the American Association for the Advancement of Science, although he was never elected to membership in the Association. (Salmon became a fellow in 1885, and Smith a member in 1886 and a fellow in 1887.) In the summer of 1885, Cornell University conferred upon Kilborne one of its few B.V.S. degrees bestowed in those years. A letter followed from the Bureau of Animal Industry, dated July 9, 1885:

> Dear Sir:—Dr. Salmon wishes to know if you could put yourself in readiness within a short time to come here, if the position were offered to you at the first of next month. There is a possibility that present incumbent may desire to leave at that time. Please answer as soon as convenient. Yours truly Theobald Smith.[78]

The first superintendent of the Experiment Station, W.H. Rose, had resigned after about a year, as of August 1, 1885. Kilborne accepted the vacant position. He and his wife moved into the superintendent's brick dwelling at the Station. Smith considered Kilborne his assistant. However, on visits from the Station, Kilborne reported directly to Salmon and took orders from him, while Smith seldom knew even the gist of their discussions.

Smith had complaints about his "Cornell man:" "Kilborne speaks with pride of what 'we' discovered. He can't understand how it was possible for me to have worked in vain for over a year, and why at his advent the pigs suddenly 'gave in' unless his personality had something to do with it."[79] A graduate student who worked under Smith's direction on a thesis project was referred to as "by far more agreeable than Kilborne, for whom I can't say I have a great personal liking, though he is capable in his work . . . You know it hurts some people to rise too suddenly and at too great a bound."[80]

Relations with Salmon became more difficult after Kilborne's appointment. Yet, Smith assured Gage, "I like Dr. S. very much, for I observe daily how honest and upright he is in managing a large appropriation."[81] With regard to Kilborne, he later wrote Gage, "In the past, I suppose, assistants of no training or capacity were appointed. The chiefs had to suffer for their ignorance at first, and after they had learnt something, took charge of the results in the same way."[82] When Salmon gave a paper on hog cholera to a National Public Health Association meeting in Washington, his report included Smith's latest work, but failed to give him any credit. "I should prefer to have been mentioned in this Association, because I may in the future be thrown in with work done by members of this body, while I have no sympathy with Veterinary medicine as such, or with practical Agriculture in general." But other problems competed with this grievance. Theobald Smith closed: "I feel very much like writing about more personal matters, but I will reserve them for another letter."[83]

4

COURTSHIP, MARRIAGE AND
EARLY FAMILY LIFE

Soon after arriving in Washington, Theobald had retorted to Gage's advice to follow his own example and get a bicycle and a "sweetheart:" "I should think it might be glorious to ride with one's wife, but I haven't tried the sweetheart yet. Life is too busy and serious to think of such trifles, my friend."[1] However, he rowed on the Potomac and played tennis—a game which "improves my temper wonderfully and is a benefit in every way." Washington had no ice rink so he did not invest in skates, but there was sleighing, while in spring and summer he hiked, alone or with Curtice. Nor was there a lack of social life, as he informed Gage early in 1885. "Almost every house at this season becomes a ring of parties, receptions and dances, so that the young people get exercise enough in their own peculiar way."[2]

Music was still important to him. He wrote of "a day of salvation" when he could play an organ once weekly. "I have often wished to hear with you the organ recitals which are given at Sage Chapel now . . . I shall be able to play for you a final song without words from Mendelssohn when you come."[3] He purchased Salmon's piano, and learned "some pretty German love songs . . . I have found singing a great relief (I wonder whether my neighbours above, below, right and left have. I hesitate to ask them.) Playing was well enough, but it did not rest the mind. I would go on calculating experiments etc. ad libitum . . . But singing does not allow this. It absorbs the mind wholly."[4]

Theobald Smith had been elected to the Phi Beta Kappa fraternity, shortly after a Cornell chapter of this pioneer honor-society was organized in 1882.[5] He had requested Gage to purchase a medium-grade key from the local jeweller: "Do not hurry about it . . . You need not communicate the price to me. I do not care for the best, nor for the worst from which the 'gold' will rub off."[6] Next spring Dr. Wilder invited him to Nantucket for the summer,[7] and Theobald gave the pin to Wilders' daughter Mary. She wore it for a few months and then re-turned it. To Gage she surmised that Theobald was pledged to another and relayed her congratulations. Smith responded ruefully that if possible he would return her good wishes tied with red ribbon for safe keeping until the "still cloud-wrapped female form" had arrived. "You must tell her that I shall . . . 'pi-geon hole' her congratulations for the present."[8] Happily no feelings were hurt, and they all remained on friendly terms. Mary Wilder married in 1897, and Theobald sent her a wedding present.

Nathaniel Hillyer Egleston, a patriarchal Unitarian clergyman, had been Asso-ciate Professor of Rhetoric at Williams College in 1869-1870. Until he retired in 1883, he had a church in Williamstown, Massachusetts. His essays on village life covered many aspects of country living and rural betterment, particularly the preservation of woodlands.[9] Now attached to the Forestry Division as a sort of conservationist, his office was in the Agriculture Building, adjacent to Theobald's laboratory. The exact date and circumstances of Theobald's initial encounter with his daughter Lilian are uncertain. Their acquaintanceship dates by family tradition to a tree-planing ceremony on the departmental grounds, when the old man presided at the Arbor Day celebration on April 22, 1886[10] and invited Theobald to his small Georgetown house at 1744 N Street, where he lived with his wife and Lilian—the blue-eyed belle of Washington. Intelligent, fond of music, of sunny disposition and sound principles, Lilian was about two years older than Theobald. Her brothers, Melville and Howard, married and considerably her senior, resided with their families at Elizabeth, New Jersey, and New Rochelle, New York, respectively. Melville, a successful lawyer, had gradu-ated from Williams College in 1870. Howard left the College in 1872 without graduating, to become a businessman. Two sisters, one younger and one older than Lilian, had died at ten and seventeen years of age, the latter in 1878. Lilian was religious, dutiful, and devoted to her parents, and largely managed the household.

The close-knit Eglestons welcomed and often visited friends and relatives. Mrs. Egleston had a very proper background and fine taste in household furnish-ings. She was snobbish to a degree which Theobald found discomfiting. Her hus-band's New England ancestors were directly traceable to Bagot Egleston, born in 1590 in Exeter, in southwest England. An oil portrait of Nathaniel's mother, Emily Egleston (1832-1874), a good-looking young matron, remains in the pos-session of the Smith family. Lilian played the piano quite well and invited selected friends to weekly *soirées musicales* at home. The earliest known written communication between her and Theobald was an invitation, sent probably in the latter half of April 1886, on a calling card inscribed "Miss Egleston:"

> Dear Dr. Smith:—Do you think your friend, whose name I do not know, is free on Saturday evening? . . . I am trying to find out how many I can coax away from *other* pleasures, to come here Saturday evening . . . I want to be sure of . . . Dr. Smith and his friend . . . I hope you are not bound to be at the Smithsonian that very night. Sincerely yours, Lilian H.E.[11]

About two weeks later, a similar note mentioned a concert previously attended together. "I am not a free agent in these days, and have to get the doctor's permission before I indulge in any sort of dissipation . . . If the weather is fairly pleasant tomorrow, I shall be very glad to hear the Wagner Society again. Very sincerely your friend, Lilian H. Egleston."[12] Occasional fainting spells, then fashionable among young women, had brought Lilian under suspicion of suffering from a weak heart or incipient consumption. As two sisters had been lost, her doctor viewed the prospects soberly. However, she consented readily to accompany Theobald one Saturday evening to see *The Lady of Lyons*. "I am no longer afraid of stairs, nor of a moderate amount of walking, so I shall not wait to consult my good Dr. Bromwell."[13]

The earliest letter from Theobald kept by Lilian was headed "Laboratory, May 25, 1886." He was nearly twenty-seven. The Eglestons were about to move to a larger house, so he asked "Would you accord me the favor of a last musicale in your old home . . . It is not such a simple matter to give up what one looks forward to throughout the week." While the Eglestons settled into their new home at 1667 Congress Street, the month came to a climactic end for Theobald, for into the night of May 31 he composed a declaration of love.

> My dear Miss Egleston, Do you recall that evening last winter when I asked you to play the Midsummer Night's Dream with me and you said No? It was said so decisively that it haunted me . . . It foreshadowed to me even at that time the possibilities of another no! which might be the turning point of a life . . . You see what power one soul already had over another. This influence . . . has now reached a degree when silence is but another name for pain . . . What claims of love could I have upon one who has been to me, ever since I knew you more intimately, the ideal of womanhood?

He had hoped that two lives brought together by some higher law "would come into a possession of each other's inner life without any such crisis as I certainly believe this to be." If her affections had already "found their object," he asked only for sympathy. "And now my life shall cease moving for a time until word shall have come from you. Yours in hope, Theobald Smith." The message seemed inadequate, and he considered declaring his love face to face; instead, he sent a second draft with a covering note.[14]

Overnight, Lilian put together a reply to this "unexpected revelation." She responded:

> If I gave you a decisive answer today it would of necessity be the 'No' you so dreaded . . . How can you think you know me as a man should know the woman he wishes to make his wife? Do you think I know you well enough put my whole life in your keeping? From this new point of view it almost seems that I do not know you at all . . . If I should ask you to be patient longer, and if, after all, I should not learn to give you what you wish, it would mean only more pain for you, and bitterer self-blame for me. Yet that is all I have to offer in return for your royal gift—an absolute uncertainty of the future . . . Unless you prefer not to see me, will you let me talk with you for a few minutes . . . Forgive me if anything I have said seems unjust to you—I send this note with a very heavy heart. Lilian.[15]

Theobald replied from the Laboratory that same afternoon. He had acted as a child in assuming that her knowledge of him was adequate. "As regards my knowing you—that has been settled with me long ago and if there are any risks to be run I am willing to assume them. Man can learn to know women so much better than women can hope to know man from the very nature of things."[16] He accepted her offer to see him. She gave him a sprig of honeysuckle, but though he later considered that their engagement dated from then, within two weeks they were again in turmoil.

One evening, however, Lilian admitted in an emotional outburst that she cared for him. Her father overheard the agitation and entered the room. Next morning Theobald complained, "We were so cruelly interrupted, that I came away still unsettled and doubting."[17] But she had divulged her feelings to her parents and wrote that she needed time to weigh the significance of her awakened reactions to a comparative stranger.[18] In answer, from his parents' house in Albany, he sent her the closely-written fourteen-page autobiographical sketch,[19] which has been freely quoted in the first chapter. His letter included a statement that he felt the Unitarian faith (her father's) suited him best.[20] Her response was warm but brief. "My dear friend: Is this what you wish me to tell you?—that I am still your friend and that your old welcome waits you? I wrote you a letter, but after all, I think this is enough . . . and send you only the assurance that I am, Your friend, wie immer—Lilian H. Egleston."[21]

A long letter from Champaign, Illinois, where Theobald had gone to investigate a western swine epizootic, assured her the thousand miles between them "were no better Lethe than cross-town."[22] On his return, Theobald moved to a boarding house at 1207 Connecticut Avenue. In mid-August, before leaving for the annual meeting of the American Association for the Advancement of Science in Buffalo, where he presented two papers on swine plague,[23] he again urged Lilian to make up her mind about him. If she deemed it best, he might even bring himself, "after the horrible storm & stress period when such an idea was unendurable, to relinquish the faint claim which love may have given . . . It is possible that I could stand a broken heart much better than you."[24] Lilian still sought delay. She wrote that with his help she wanted to avoid false postures with her parents, who sincerely believed he ought to remain unfettered by any tie until his position "in this workaday world" was more assured. She enclosed a photograph of herself.[25]

On their next Sunday walk, he broke down and wept at the prospect of lengthy separation.[26] Another short trip to Illinois was necessary, while she planned to visit Williamstown, where her parents kept their old home as summer retreat, and also New Rochelle. During his absence in the West, Lilian suffered a "little collapse," for which Dr. Bromwell prescribed "brandy and a green anondyne."[27] Early in October, Lilian left a desolate Theobald behind in Washington, where he had recently taken a room at 1918 Sunderland Place, a small hotel. Thence he dispatched four long letters, in which weather and other news alternated with bursts of reproachful self-analysis and health-protective instructions. Nine days after her departure, no news had come from Lilian, so he issued an ultimatum: "There must be either a free exchange and expression of love, such as the heart longs and yearns for as its daily sustenance . . . or else complete silence."[28]

On the tenth day a letter arrived from Lilian, glorying in the gold and crimson beauties of the autumn hills around their old home. Williamstown already had chilly snow flurries, so she would not linger there; but she could not close down the house until the carpenters, painters and paperers were finished.[29] In his reply, Theobald apologized for his impatience. She need not write at length; he merely wanted reassurance that she was well and happy. The Gages were the proud parents of a two-week-old boy and he would spend a week with them at Ithaca, whence he would go to Albany, returning perhaps through New York. Three days later, in a letter which discussed their relationship, Theobald told Lilian that "It all depends upon how much you will trust me, to be a true man, who will live for you, not selfishly but desirous ever of your happiness."[30]

Lilian wanted to see him on his way back. "Cannot you convince yourself that it is your duty to let me have your company for a little?" Better than New York itself would be New Rochelle, where her brother and sister-in-law would welcome him.[31] He sensed a changed attitude. He answered from Ithaca that he would come to New Rochelle and catch the late night train for Washington.

Cornell had grown astoundingly. He had declined Dr. Wilder's invitation to lecture to 135 sophomores, but talked briefly to a special class under Gage. He also addressed some invited faculty members, including former President White. Gage proposed to spend two months of his summer vacation in Washington "studying microbes." The account of the Cornell visit was completed from Albany. His mother handed him without comment a letter from Lilian. "I had not the courage to tell her what that letter meant to me . . . She is so good that she would not even embarrass me by asking."[32]

Lilian commanded him to spend the next weekend at New Rochelle. "You are to come straight to us . . . because we want you, my brother, my sister and I. Celia says 'tell Dr. Smith I want him to come and make my table balance better' . . . Give us all the time you can. If you do come on Friday, can you be here for a seven o'clock dinner? A good train leaves N.Y. at nine minutes after five o'c.—the Norwalk Special—and it would not be too dark for me to meet you!"[33] He was easily persuaded to spend two nights and they had an idyllic weekend. The Sunday midnight train was caught in New York. From the Laboratory, he asked Lilian to relay his gratitude to Howard and Celia for their early Thanksgiving dinner. He hardly knew "where to take up my work, so utterly has it gone from me, thanks to my vacation and to you especially."[34]

Despite the general distractions of being in love, Theobald's laboratory work never lapsed. Back in Washington, he studied his cultures in detail by day, and at night prepared the findings for publication.[35] Lilian regretted that his scientific life eluded her. She tried to bridge the gap, but his attitude was discouraging.

> There is a life-work which is always waiting for me at any hour of the day. There is the thought of those infinitesimal beings, whose fearful actuality is a greater surprise to me each day that I am gleaning a few things which applied to man may solve some perplexing problems in the future. You may have life-problems to solve too, but they are such in which you cannot lose yourself.[36]

Soon after returning to Washington, Lilian resumed her soirées. Theobald's letters did not diminish in frequency, but he had grievances: "I am afraid that before my mind is free to entertain others with you, I shall want to see a little more of you myself . . . I am naturally sensitive and shrinking and have worried concerning the distance between myself and your parents."[37] He also worried about his sudden depressions and dreaded to disappoint her. "I do wish you would scold me for being so dull and really spoiling your evenings now and then. I would always like to bring you so much happiness and lightheartedness."[38] His first Christmas present to Lilian—Mrs. Browning's *Sonnets from the Portuguese*—seemed to please her.[39]

By the end of 1886, Theobald and Lilian considered themselves betrothed, with marriage postponed until his career was more settled. The younger Eglestons favored the match. Even her parents grew reconciled to Theobald as their future son-in-law, though her mother still ignored him. Early in May 1887, Lilian visited her brother Melville and his family at Elizabeth, and Theobald completed his teaching duties at the National Medical College before leaving for Ithaca to be one of Cornell's twenty-six Special Lecturers. The series, which began with Andrew Dickson White ("German History in Nineteenth Century") and Goldwin Smith ("English Constitutional History"), ended with Alexander Graham Bell on "Telephony" and Theobald Smith on "Pathogenic bacteria and their relation to hygiene." For his first lecture, "The microscope in the study of micro-organisms," his audience numbered sixty to seventy. Local newspapers described him as one of the few Americans who had "done much in determining, cultivating and mounting micro-organisms. His work at the Bureau of Animal Industry in Washington has received great praise."[40]

Larger audiences attended "The method of isolating and cultivating bacteria" and "The diagnosis of bacteria by cultivation and inoculation." Before the fourth lecture, on "Some chemical and biological phenomena of bacterial life," Theobald took several buggy drives with Gage, who on one expedition wore rubber waders and netted more than fifty Cayuga Lake lampreys. (Gage described the identification and breeding habits of two species at the next meeting of the A.A.A.S.) Many faculty members attended the final two lectures, in Sage College, on "The bacteria of cholera, typhoid fever and tuberculosis and their relation to our environment," and "The bacteria of wounds, with reference to antiseptic surgery." The task of recasting all the lectures, he informed Lilian, proved harder than expected.[41] She expressed concern: "What can we do to rest you, my dear one? . . . I wish I could make the conditions for you such that the strained, over-weary feeling need not come . . . It is hard to stand on the outside of your life as it were, and not be able to life a finger for you!"[42]

Theobald went to Albany for a brief rest. His parents had moved to a smaller house at 260 Lark Street, next door to the Murphys, from which they could visit their daughter and grandchildren through the garden. His mother, who by now realized his commitment, appreciated his photographs of Lilian "and wanted one very much." She regarded marriage "as a necessary step in my life."[43] When Lilian went to Williamstown, Theobald became custodian of the Egleston household at 1667 Congress Street, where he coped with Lilian's pet bird Bobbie, and Ida the maid. How often did one clean out the cage? Was the old seed thrown away, or the new simply added twice weekly? What was the proper allowance of hempseed?

At the laboratory, Curtice had surprised him by introducing his wife—"a very nice lady, very shy and quiet. There seems to be quite an epidemic of this trouble about here." Three Museum friends were being married soon. His own similar fate was rumored, he told Lilian: "The report has been spread among a few that I went north to be married . . . Dr. Kilborne tried to congratulate me thro' the telephone from our Station, but I stopped him in the act . . . I told Mr. Curtice that I was so sorry to disappoint peoples' anticipations."[44] According to Lilian, "announcements" were being launched by the servants and children—"They like you, you know." Melville had offered months ago to "give his 'darling sister the pleasantest Berkshire wedding possible'."[45] In Williamstown, Lilian enjoyed the company of girlhood playmates, such as Suzy Hopkins, daughter of Mark Hopkins, the famous educationist, long-time president (1836-1872) of Williams College. She returned to Washington late in October.

At the end of February 1888, Howard neglected a cold and was stricken with pneumonia. As Melville wrote of a "discouraging weakness of circulation," Theobald caught an early morning train to New Rochelle. Howard's mind was lucid and heart strong. Intermittent oxygen brought relief, but breathing was still difficult. Theobald sat up with him overnight. Next day there was definite improvement and the consulting physician thought he would recover.[46] Lilian poured forth relief and gratitude: Theobald had brought hope and comfort to all. His standing in the family was now secure. They decided to marry in May, probably on the seventeenth. "Mother & father . . . are both glad of our speedy wedding,"[47] he told his fiance. His parents wished them every happiness. Lilian had written to Theobald's mother, enclosing violets. Theresia Schmitt replied in beautiful German script, welcoming her "as daughter."

> Your picture has brought us closer together . . . It is our dearest wish to see Theobald married and having a companion who shares happiness and suffering with him. He always was a good son to us and will be a good husband . . . Marriage is beautiful when both understand each other, when each lives for the other . . . then everything petty stays away.[48]

Lilian wrote to Theobald, then in Ithaca, urging him to persuade his parents to attend the wedding, but he replied that they "would not undertake the trouble & fatigue of a Washington trip. Besides, they would not and could not feel at home as things are, so do not think about it any more." He asked what flowers she wished, so that he could order them, though he would have preferred to do this without help. "I might get red where white is needed, green where blue is in place, and pansies where lilies should be."[49]

In the spring of 1888, Cornell University reappointed Theobald as Special Lecturer on Pathogenic Bacteria in their Relation to Hygiene, but allotted him

only four lectures. They were entitled, "The Natural Agencies at Work in Destroying Bacteria, and the Use of Heat in Disinfection;" "Chemical Substances as
Disinfectants and Antiseptics, with Remarks on . . . Compulsory Disinfection;"
"The Results Obtained by Pasteur and Others in Protective Inoculation;" and
"Immunity: Theories Based upon Recent Biological Researches." Now handicapped by absent-mindedness, he wrote out his presentations. A newspaper report told that he was said to have settled "some of the most obscure and difficult
questions relating to animal diseases . . . Dr. Smith is an original investigator of
the highest character."[50] Theobald returned to Washington and Lilian on Thursday, May 10.[51]

Their honeymoon and subsequent housing plans were modest. For living
quarters he would "conclude a bargain" with the landlord of her parents' house.
His own father and mother had helped him financially to this end, as part of their
wedding gift. Theobald wondered whether Lilian preferred reaching the honeymoon destination, the Hygeia Hotel at Old Point Comfort, Virginia, partly by
train via Baltimore, or wholly by boat down the Potomac—provided he could
reserve a comfortable stateroom. She should specify one or two good books
which he could procure. "We may not wish to read much with the ocean and
each other by day and night always about, yet it is well to be provided."[52]

Her father officiated at the wedding. A newspaper clipping announced that
"Theobald Smith, M.D., of Washington, D.C., was united in marriage to Lilian
H. Egleston, of Georgetown Heights, D.C., on May 17th, at the home of the
bride." It added: "To Dr. Smith and his co-worker, Dr. D.E. Salmon, has been
awarded the honor of being first in a recent brilliant discovery."[53] This reference
was to the experimental immunity reported in September 1887 to the Ninth International Medical Congress in Washington.[54] After a brief honeymoon, Theobald and Lilian returned to 1667 Congress Street, Washington, he to resume
work with unabated energy, she to keep house for parents as well as husband.

From the beginning, Lilian strove to assure that he could pursue his work in
peace. She deplored her limited scientific knowledge, but did her best to help. In
the spring of 1889, during their first year of marriage, she attended several of his
lectures on bacteriology at the National Medical College. Her sense of literary
style equalled or surpassed his, and she drew the diagrams for some of his early
papers. There is little evidence of his patience or encouragement in these en-
deavors. Theobald had raised no apparent objection to her presence at his lectures, although some introductory reading in, e.g. botany, would have seemed to
him a fitting prerequisite. He would have unreservedly approved her copying out
his reference cards.

Domestic tensions mainly arose from their sharing house with the Rev. and
Mrs. Egleston. Though warmly attached to her husband and dedicated to his ca-

reer, Lilian's intense loyalty to parents and brothers complicated the first years of her married life. In the spring of 1890, after several weeks of house-hunting, Theobald leased a slightly larger place at 1257 O Street N.W., nearer to his work. Lilian's mother and father moved with them. The new household also lured her brothers and sisters-in-law, who might arrive with little or no warning for visits of hours or even several days. If the old couple occasionally set out for a longish stay with Melville's family at Elizabeth, they soon returned, because his wife Jeanie found the strain too much for her. In mid-1891, Theobald complained to Lilian, "I wish that . . . your parents be kept as much as possible from our affairs."[55]

Melville—a prosperous lawyer—advised Theobald on investments in land or securities, handling some of the transactions himself. However, Theobald held the purse strings, routinely paid the household bills, and recorded the monthly expenditures and income to the nearest cent. He was undeniably careful with his money and frugal in habits. But he was not mean—indeed, he could be generous. In June 1889, he subscribed $5.00 for the Johnstown flood victims in Philadelphia, and in the same month gave $25 to the Delta Upsilon Chapter House Fund."[56] His fraternity never appealed to him in vain. He loaned a substantial sum to his laboratory assistant, who later took up dentistry. After about a decade, the following entry appeared in his accounts: "By loss of money left J.R. Stewart some years ago. $1300."[57] Other needy associates, as well as his family, relatives and friends, received financial help traceable to him, albeit often given anonymously.

At the end of April 1890, Theobald took Lilian, now nearly six months pregnant, to Williamstown, where she could rest up in a boarding house for a few weeks and visit friends. He returned at once to Washington, briefly looking up his parents at Albany. Theobald and his wife exchanged affectionate "patchworky" accounts of their daily activities. She was grateful for the coddling, and he cheerfully reported that without that long pull up the Georgetown hill he could bicycle to work. He inserted this message on a scrap of paper: "Wanted: a wife to sew on one button on my trousers and to mend a rip in my underclothing—also to kiss me when I come & go."[58]

On his way to join Lilian at the end of May he stopped in Albany, where he "found sister Bertha sitting up but vomiting freely . . . At 10 P.M. great dyspnea, dies quietly at 2.30 A.M. Saturday morning."[59] Death was attributed to a ruptured tubal pregnancy.[60] To his wife he wrote from 260 Lark Street: "I am glad to realize that you are a strong woman and that . . . I can get comfort from you. You have borne much sorrow and bereavement . . . and it has made your life's equal in its ups and downs." After Bertha's funeral at the Cathedral, with burial in St. Agnes Cemetery, he went to Williamstown and took Lilian home. There, on August 28, after a difficult labor in Washington heat, a daughter was born. Lilian's convalescence was complicated by breast abscesses and took several weeks. Although they had talked much about a little boy whom they could call "Philip," both parents doted upon the small newcomer, Dorothea.

Lilian's other brother, Howard, was financially venturesome and currently overextended. He had a farm at Sag Harbor, near the eastern end of Long Island. In June 1891, Theobald took Lilian and the infant "Dolly" to Sag Harbor to escape the capital's summer heat, while Dolly gained color and strength. Lilian was to try to give Celia enough money to cover at least her expenses. Theobald proceeded to Albany the same afternoon, arriving there around midnight. He summarized the long day: "Helped Lilian unpack and visited Howard's farm on the beach. Lent him $200... Arr. Albany 11.25. Parents waiting for me, dear old people. How sad to be away from them so much."[61] Theobald extended to "our little bawa" the kind of didactic solicitude he had displayed always toward Lilian. Dolly would need care "for neither one of her parents has too much vigor to give her."[62] He advised Lilian to "be careful of sudden changes & draughts and blowing of wind on her head, keep it covered excepting on real hot days . . . Do not give her unboiled water . . . Do not remain at the house without protection when Howard & Celia are away. Keep dog around."[63]

He himself was not robust and was subject to frequent colds and other indispositions, such as dental abscesses, intestinal upsets and cystitis—all recorded punctiliously. He sometimes took his temperature at short intervals, as if he were testing for Texas fever or bovine tuberculosis. Very hot weather especially sapped his energies. In the summer of 1889 he complained, "Very tired and used up from winter's work. How to gain strength?" and "Feeling some slight weakness of cor. Palpitations occasional and slight. Probably continual overstrain, so I shall give up bicycling for a time."[64]

While Lilian was away for the summer, Theobald complained to her that the maid, after serving breakfast, had packed off for good; and both stairs were "robed in your mamma's old carpet." He did not know why she put it here, since they intended to replace it with something "respectable." "Please tell her that the stairs are public highways in our house, and cannot be macadamized without a board or town meeting first . . . You know I have a strong prejudice against old things . . . I am sorry, for she wants to do so much for us in one way and another."[65] Mrs. Egleston had departed for Sag Harbor, leaving the two men alone in the house. His father-in-law thought making their own breakfast more economical; "this morning he cooked the breakfast and I have been washing dishes ever since (10 A.M.)." Theobald told Lilian that her mother should "*insist on his going out* to his meals even on Sunday morning ... his usual fastidiousness seems to forsake him entirely on these occasions and he is obstinate enough to eat what he pleases without heeding my protestations."

They had dinner either at the Women's Exchange or Faber's. Theobald preferred "the W.E., which gives less and charges less." Her father had "an ineffaceable predilection for Faber's"—which had a saloon. Ignoring the side entrance, "your papa returns by way of the saloon with as much naiveté as if he were walking up the church aisle, looking right and left at the interesting things." Lilian herself did not escape chastisement. "That you should try to keep your whole family in order, and worry if you can't succeed—that time has gone by and you now have other duties."⁶⁶

Lilian responded softly to all provocative comments. "About the carpets, of course we can change when we come back . . . I know such changes try you, and I am sorry to have anything bother you now . . . how often I am thinking of you and wishing I could do something for your comfort."⁶⁷ Her devotion to Dolly— "the blessed little one"—was evident from the references to her in every letter. "The darling is so sweet and good! She grows more cunning and interesting every day."

In August 1891, shortly before the International Zoological Congress and the A.A.A.S. opened consecutive meetings in Washington, the Gages stayed at the half-vacant household on O Street. When Lilian heard of the prospect, she wrote Mrs. Gage a letter to await their arrival, regretting her personal inability to welcome them and the inevitable disorder in a house "so long given over to the picnicking of two deserted men." Yet her absence was necessary "for our precious little daughter's sake."⁶⁸ Theobald reported the visitors were enjoying the house despite the fearful heat. But he must tackle Lilian's father about morning prayers. "If people are not in the habit of worshipping in this way it is hardly fair to throw them out of their equanimity for a few days and certainly does no good . . . I shall have to come to an understanding about this matter because . . . to hold my own opinions and feelings and theories in the background in our family life has not been satisfactory to me."⁶⁹

Lilian, who had joined the Church of the Covenant early in 1891,⁷⁰ wrote that her first reaction had been to avoid alluding to "the vexed questions" in his letter, but silence might be misunderstood.

> I cannot pretend to think as you do about it, for I cannot agree with you and I hope I never shall. I shall acquiesce in your will in all these matters, dear, and I accept the fact that I shall never have what is to me the ideal home . . . To me, a prayerless home . . . where the children are not being trained under a sense of re-

sponsibility to the great Master, is not the true home, it lacks the strongest bond of all . . .

The penalty for two marrying whose lives have been utterly unlike is that they find it so hard to understand each other; and have need of much patience in their gradual readjustment . . . We were . . . so much farther apart on many questions than I dreamed when we were married, that I only wonder now that we did not make worse of it than we did, especially under the unfavorable conditions . . . It has been life utterly unsuited to your needs, but it has been our life . . . After all, my beloved, I am your loyal, loving wife, finding my best happiness in being so, and God has given us a most precious child to love and care for.[71]

Nonetheless, writing to Mrs. Gage two weeks later, Lilian reported, "We are very happy in our changed surroundings and in the quiet life by ourselves."[72]

In early September, Theobald fetched his wife and baby daughter home from Granby, Connecticut, where they had gone from Sag Harbor to stay with other relatives. Despite meddlesome parents and demanding family, Lilian maintained and expanded her own circle of friends, and settled matters of etiquette, such as the ceremonial proprieties of the christening of her infant daughter by grandfather Egleston, and the proper dress for an evening Presidential Reception at the Executive Mansion in 1892. Theobald occasionally attended her afternoon teas but made up for such ill-spent hours by extra efforts at weekends. Lilian saw to it that social calls of neighbors and friends were not neglected. Former Cornell friends, such as Henry Battin and Dr. Alfreda Withington, were welcomed at their home. In March 1891, Smith wrote to Gage: "Miss Withington, M.D. has been here looking over the ground for a place of practice and has paid us several visits."[73] But "a Mr. Leitz, microscope maker of Wetzlar,"[74] did not get beyond the laboratory.

Walking remained Theobald's favorite recreation. At weekends he roamed in the Rock Creek woods, either alone or with Lilian, particularly in the early spring, when they sought such harbingers as hepaticas, bloodroot, arbutus, anemones and bluets. They went to as many concerts as they could afford and regularly attended the Boston Symphony Orchestra's visiting performances. There was little time for general reading, but Theobald managed to tackle such diversities as Scott's *The Heart of Midlothian*, *The Life and Letters of William and Lucy Smith*, and Goethe's *Wahlverwandschaften*. To each other they read aloud Hawthorne's *The Marble Faun*, Mrs. Hymphrey Ward's *Robert Elsmere*, and R.D. Blackmore's *Lorna Doone*. Now and again Theobald exercised his handiness at household jobs, such as putting up a paper frieze in the sitting room and hanging curtains in the guest room. He stained the border of his room only a few Saturdays before recording "Staining *flagella* of bact. for first time successful."[75] By preference, as well as of necessity, their joys were simple, their celebrations modest. Apart from his compulsive thriftiness, Theobald's maximum salary from the B.A.I.—less than $2400—was hardly conducive to spending sprees.

Despite modest earnings, Theobald Smith accumulated a sizable nest-egg, mostly in high-class bonds, stocks and bank savings accounts. He invested occasionally in land lots or mortgages, and made short-term loans to friends. In his thirtieth year, he recorded payments received on such loans—an ex-Cornellian, "Mr. Decker paid $100 on his note;" "Dr. Wilder sent check for 117.10 on note of 385;" and a Department of Agriculture colleague "Mr. Fernow paid Int. 13.12 on note of 400 (6 mos)."[76] By the end of 1891, his capital amounted to more than $4,000 apart from a Georgetown lot, which he bought for $2,185.[77]

On August 21, 1893, a second daughter was born, named Lilian after her mother, who had a "hard time," necessitating rest for the customary month. They now moved with their immediate family unit "to the edge of town," as Lilian informed Mrs. Gage soon afterwards, while her parents made for a boarding house. "We have a pleasant house in which we are sure of plenty of fresh air and sunshine, and we have ground enough to give the children exercise without leaving home. It is a relief to get them away from town for we were never reconciled to bringing up children in a city block. Already they are better for the change."[78]

5

HOG CHOLERA AND
SWINE PLAGUE

Hog cholera first appeared in Ohio in 1833. In North America, between then and 1845, nine separate outbreaks were reported from six southern states. In the next decade, ninety-three hog cholera outbreaks occurred, chiefly in southern states and along the lengthening lines of communication to the Far West.[1] From 1856 to 1860, no fewer than 168 epizootics were recorded in twenty-two states,[2] and by 1887 the disease had invaded thirty-five states. Extensive cyclical epizootics occurred in 1887, 1896, 1913, and 1926.[3] Annual losses to hog farmers mounted to $25 million,[4] and they remained substantial until recent years. Even after discovery of the true hog-cholera virus in 1904, seventy years elapsed before national freedom from the infection was reached in the United States. Canada became free of the disease about two decades earlier.

In the British Isles, the first clear-cut outbreak of hog cholera occurred in Berkshire in 1862. A century later, the government instituted an ultimately successful eradication policy, costing an estimated $1 million per annum,[5] involving slaughter of infected herds, improved diagnostic tests, quarantine of all pigs near suspected outbreaks, and enforced garbage-cooking. Elsewhere, hog cholera remains a formidable problem.[6] Indeed, it was reported in 1975 that "The virus of Hog Cholera is still the cause of more swine deaths than any other infectious organism."[7]

In 1865, Dr. William Budd, an authority on typhoid fever in England, accurately described the gross pathology, notably the "button ulcers" of the pig's large intestine, and advocated early segregation and slaughter of sick animals and destruction of their feces.[8] William Osler, investigating an epizootic of "pig typhoid" near Quebec City in 1878, concluded that this was a specific disease, unrelated to typhoid in man.[9] In 1876, from London, Emanuel Klein reported histological changes in the intestines and lung, suggestive of infection.[10] He contended that the contagious agent was an air- and food-borne, motile, filamentous sporulating bacillus, and proposed that the disease be designated *pneumoenteritis contagiosa,* or "infectious pneumo-enteritis of the pig."

Klein confused the picture by listing various synonyms for this infection—"typhoid fever of the pig," "hog plague," "*mal rouge,*" "red soldier" and "malignant erysipelas."[11] The popular terms "red soldier" and "*mal rouge*" derived from the patches of reddened skin, spreading from around the ears, which developed in severe cases. Such inflammatory areas also typified "swine erysipelas," an entirely different disease, uncommon in Britain and practically non-existent in North America, but prevalent in France and Germany, where it was called *mal rouge des porcs* or *rouget,* and *Rothlauf,* respectively.

In 1878, the United States Congress appropriated $10,000 for research into swine diseases. Among nine men appointed "examiners" for one to three months that year were H.J. Detmers, veterinary professor at Illinois Industrial University and vice-president of the American Berkshire (Pig) Association, James Law of Cornell University, and Daniel E. Salmon. They agreed that epizootics abated in the late fall or early winter, and that the clinical and pathological evidence suggested a single generalized disorder communicable from sick to healthy hogs.[12] Detmers designated the disease "swine plague," peculiar to swine, and the causative agent "*Bacillus suis,*" appearing as single cocci, diplococci and rods of varying length in the blood and tissue fluid of autopsied pigs.[13] Law thought he had succeeded in transmitting the disease to a sheep, a rabbit, and a puppy, and recommended isolation of all domestic animal contacts of sick pigs.[14] Salmon concluded that sanitary regulations, properly framed and enforced—slaughtering the infected herd, deeply burying the carcasses, thoroughly disinfecting the habitation, and not allowing hogs there until after a succeeding winter—were the only means of checking the ravages of "swine plague."[15]

Late in 1882 (a year when more than 20,000 pigs died of *rouget* in the Rhone Valley), Louis Pasteur told a meeting of agriculturists that the loss of 900,000 pigs in 1879 in the United States was very probably due to *rouget*. In March 1882, his young assistant, Louis Thuillier, had discovered a new microbe, formed like a figure eight, in the blood and body fluids of dead pigs.[16] This diplococcus produced fatal *rouget* if inoculated in minute doses into pigs. Pasteur dismissed Klein's paper as "entirely mistaken about the nature and properties of the parasite," while praising Detmers, who had described the same diplococcus as Thuillier almost simultaneously in an American journal.[17] Subsequently Pasteur outlined successful field trials of vaccine prepared from a strain of the *rouget* organism attenuated by passage through rabbits.[18] In January 1884, Klein reported having isolated his motile bacillus in fluid nutrient media from diseased organs of swine, rabbits and mice recently dead of "swine fever." He chided Pasteur for having overlooked this organism, and for the paucity of information supporting the causal role of his dumbbell-shaped micrococcus, which he considered an accidental contaminant.[19]

Before he became Chief of the Bureau of Animal Industry, Salmon had worked on the microbial cause of hog cholera, often with specimens procured through Detmers. He concluded that a micrococcus was the pathogenic agent of swine plague—the designation which superseded hog cholera, at least in the Bureau for a few years. Salmon initially viewed the bacilli described by Klein and by Detmers as septic bacteria of atmospheric origin.[20] He insisted that the American disease was the same as *rouget* and backed the claims of Pasteur and Thuillier. In October 1884, Theobald Smith told Gage that "I have been at work on the microbe of Swine Plague for some time now & have developed a few new facts," adding, "Klein has no doubt failed and we should be happy 'to show him up' if the cold weather did not put a stop to our inoculation experiments."[21]

Early in November, Theobald informed Gage[22] that a special report would be issued soon by the B.A.I.—Salmon's *Contagious Diseases of Domesticated Animals,*[23] later telling him that "My work lies in the chapter with the beautiful title Swine-plague . . . I have made a substantial debut in the investigation of infectious diseases, and [in] much of the technique and philosophy connected with that most fatal but exquisitely interesting chapter of diseases."[24] However, the section on "The results of experiments and investigations of Pleuropneumonia, Ergotism, Southern Cattle Fever, and Swine Plague" showed Salmon as sole author. Theobald Smith's name appeared only as translator of P. Mégnin's article on gape disease of fowls—his first official contribution to B.A.I. literature. Much of this material, including a photo-micrograph of the "swine-plague micrococcus," was reprinted in the Bureau's *First Annual Report* (for 1884).[25] The article on swine plague again carried Salmon's name alone.

Smith spurned hasty publication: "I have a large quantity of material for our next report if I could only get the work done satisfactorily,"[26] he subsequently told Gage. The search was hampered by the mixed flora in fluid culture media. A special cold-box was constructed to prevent liquefaction of gelatine cultures in the hot summer temperature of the laboratory. Thereby he isolated a bacillus from the peritoneal or pericardial exudates of certain cases of swine plague.

Further investigation led to his presenting a paper on a non-pathogenic, motile, chromogeneous bacillus, which he called *Bacillus luteus suis,* at the A.A.A.S. meeting at Ann Arbor in August 1885. This appeared in the Association's *Proceedings* under the authorship of Salmon and Smith[27] and in more detail in the B.A.I.'s *Second Annual Report.* "I am still as far, apparently, from the true cause of that delectable swine plague to which swine are heir, as ever," he confessed to Gage in July 1885.[28] Early in November, however, he wrote:

> Dr. Salmon & I are trying to say something in the next report about the real microbe of swine plague. Dr. Salmon feels pretty sure about the microbe & thinks he had him years ago. As I have been going over the whole ground again I don't believe so at all. I don't wish to tell him so flatly as he is too good a man to have his feelings hurt *all at once.* But I tell you the worst thing that can befall a man is to have published and then either have to recant or to fail in after-confirmation. This *inter nos.* The great and apparently insurmountable difficulty in this disease is the presence within the body of other microbes besides the pathogenic one which gets through ulcerations of the intestine. This fact I pride myself in having first pointed out, but not in print alas![29]

Shortly afterward, two pigs with typical swine plague were brought to the Station. One of them was killed next day. Its spleen and liver yielded a pure culture of a motile, round-ended, bacillary pathogen, which formed small, non-liquefying colonies on nutrient gelatin. While investigating the ensuing epizootic, Smith differentiated this pathogen from associated organisms and identified it as the cause of swine plague. In twenty-five rapidly-fatal cases, the spleen often yielded the bacillus in pure culture. In more chronic cases, with advanced intestinal ulceration, a varied flora reached the blood and spleen. Mice, guinea-pigs, and a rabbit developed fatal bacteremia when inoculated with this organism. Several pigs inoculated subcutaneously with liquid cultures died, and two out of four pigs fed with cultures contracted the acute disease. Others died after ingesting the viscera of swine-plague fatalities, and from their spleen and blood the same bacterium was isolated.[30] Apparently Koch's postulates for specific pathogenicity were satisfied.

The bacterium was also lethal for pigeons, to which Smith resorted during a shortage of rabbits. He determined the lethal subcutaneous dose for a pigeon to be 0.75 cc. of a five to fourteen day liquid culture, and prepared a vaccine by heating suspensions of the new swine-plague bacillus at 58–60°C. for at least two hours. Four pigeons were inoculated at roughly weekly intervals with an average of three doses of vaccine. When challenged one week later with 0.75 cc. of live culture they remained well, whereas an unvaccinated pigeon died within twenty-four hours.

By contrast, a sample of Pasteur's attenuated *rouget* vaccine from Paris failed to protect pigs against swine plague, indicating that the epizootics in the Untied States were not *rouget*. Microscopic examination and cultural tests showed the vaccine's predominant microbic component to be a slender, non-motile, non-sporulating bacillus: "The microbe of Pasteur's vaccine was not a figure-of-eight form, as he himself described, but a bacillus not to be mistaken for a micrococcus . . . We no longer consider a micrococcus as the cause of all outbreaks of the disease known as swine plague."[31] Nearly a year later, Salmon divulged that he had published Theobald Smith's results on the swine-plague bacillus "almost in the exact language in which he wrote them," but had made "slight changes." Smith's original version had stated: "We no longer consider a micrococcus as the cause of swine plague."[32]

In 1885, Loeffler and Schütz in Koch's laboratory established the identity of *rouget* and *Rothlauf.* Loeffler implicated a slender bacillus, resembling Koch's mouse septicemia organism (1880), as the causal agent. (It is now designated *Erysipelothrix rhusipathiae*.) He confirmed that American hog cholera was a distinct entity. Schütz suspected that Pasteur's cultures were impure, despite the protection afforded by Pasteur's attenuated *rouget* vaccine against *Rothlauf.*[33] Six fatalities occurred among 119 pigs inoculated with the vaccine.[34]

The 1885 B.A.I. *Report* stressed the superfluousness of vaccination with Pasteur's product in the United States, and the risk of its introducing a new contagious disease. Moreover, it failed to protect against swine plague, as was borne out in November in Nebraska, where most of twenty-six pigs inoculated with Pasteur's vaccine died on subsequent exposure to hog cholera.[35] To all outward appearances, Salmon was sole author of the 1885 B.A.I. *Report,* which detailed the swine plague results, with only the following acknowledgment in his Letter of Transmittal: "I have been ably assisted in these investigations by Dr. Theobald Smith, whose untiring services have been indispensable and invaluable: also by Dr. F.L. Kilborne, who has had charge of the experiment station." Yet, besides planning and performing the experiments, Theobald Smith was author of at least those parts of the 1885 and other *Annual Reports* which covered this work. When his bibliography was being prepared many decades later, he wrote to Simon Flexner: "There are some 6 or 7 annual reports of the Bureau of Animal Industry from 1885 to 1890?, covering some 200 printed pages, which are signed officially by the Chief, D.E. Salmon . . . they were written in toto by me."[36]

Early in 1886, Smith thanked Gage and Wilder for their appreciative comments about his paper on *Bacillus luteus suis* in the A.A.A.S. *Proceedings.*[37] As regards swine plague, the past few months' work had "cleared up a question which was apparently in a hopelessly involved condition in Europe, and now that we have the germ—a mostly ugly and vigorous one at that—we intend to find or at least look for a vaccine." Then he unburdened himself:

> Dr. S. read a paper on Swine plague before the American Public Health Association concerning recent work. Though he knew that the work was entirely my own, done with methods not heretofore employed, without assistance excepting our men at the station in helping at postmortems, though the germ had never been seen by him before, and the incubus of the "micrococcus" haunted me in my previous work and had to be thrown overboard first, yet he did not even mention my name in that paper. At least I have not seen it in any report of the meeting or in the manuscript which he has asked me to read over.[38]
>
> I do not see the justice of the above. Pasteur readily accorded to Thuillier the credit of having found the germ of swine plague. [Smith here meant the germ of *rouget.*] Personally I don't desire such at all but simply would like to be associated in print with the work in some capacity . . . But we will see what the forthcoming report brings out.

And later that year, he told Lilian that "It certainly is the last joint paper we shall have together."[39]

On February 20, 1886, Smith reported in person his immunization experiments with pigeons to the Biological Society of Washington. Two days later the paper was separately printed, with Salmon as senior author, under the title, "On a New Method of Producing Immunity from Contagious Diseases."[40] This first account of heat-killed bacilli as an effective immunizing agent antedated the B.A.I. report. Gage prophesied, on his copy of that preprint: "This paper is of fundamental importance for the history of immunization."

The paper provoked "a rather blunt letter about priority" from James Law for the failure to mention his experiment of 1880, in which he had injected a pig with 1 drachm of fecal infusion, filtered and heated for one-half hour to 130°F. The pig remained healthy after being inoculated with virulent "swine plague virus" one and two weeks later.[41] Smith commented to Gage that Law had meant well in the report, "But the experiments! Oh my!" Law had merely stirred up "the mucus-covered feces, which only contained the real germ by accident, partially killing the germs, partially not."

> I know you will think I am very severe and probably sarcastic. But I can't help it. When a man thrusts a thing under my nose in a peremptory manner, as he does when he claims to have demonstrated a principle, and considers our work quite superfluous and unreasonable, I reserve the right to pass judgment on it . . . The

matter of honor or priority . . . does not enter here. It is what I should call scientific indignation.[42]

Theobald Smith had soon amplified his first experiment on immunization, and was again reporting the findings to Gage.

A second series of experiments on pigeons just concluded has resulted equally well. I vaccinated 6 and inoculated 9. Of the three non-vaccinated ones two were dead next day, the third did not get sick. This was a hybrid with carrier blood and quite different from the other pigeons which were all alike. Vaccinated pigeons all well. Even if the hybrid be considered, the success is still 2/3. I am waiting for guinea pigs now, which are exceedingly susceptible to the virus. Lately two were inoculated with what corresponds to a 1/2000 cc. culture liquid; both died on the 8th day.[43]

Additional experiments were carried out. Salmon presented these results, without mentioning Smith, to the A.A.A.S. meeting at Buffalo in mid-August. In two further papers, he postulated that the immunized host prevented growth of a specific microbe through some unsolved mechanism of "vital resistance."[44] At the same meeting, Salmon and Smith were listed as co-authors of a short paper on the morphology and physiology of the swine-plague bacterium.[45] Smith himself discussed bacterial variation, as illustrated by this bacterium. The abstract of this work appeared in the *Proceedings* in January 1887;[46] fuller details were given, ostensibly by Salmon, in the *Third Annual Report* of the B.A.I.[47] A Western strain of the bacillus differed from Eastern strains by not being fatal to guinea-pigs, failing to grow in liquid gelatin, and forming a membrane on liquids. Although Smith believed that bacteria could be divided into well-defined species, he was convinced, and was the first bacteriologist to stress, that small differences existed in many species of microorganisms—a phenomenon "so well established among higher forms of life"—and, further, that such variation might influence the severity of epidemics.

Early in September 1887, Smith read the report on the pigeon-immunization results, prefaced with a fresh introduction, to the Ninth International Medical Congress in Washington, D.C. "The paper was well received, as it might be," Theobald wrote to Lilian, "being perhaps the newest development in the great effort towards preventing contagious diseases in man and animals, which is being made everywhere."[48] Salmon's name, however, was listed as sole author of the paper on the official program, and he told Lilian:

I was annoyed this week by the persistence with which the daily papers announced a paper by Dr. Salmon alone. The error was due to the general programme in which his name was entered alone. It was probably due to the wording of his letter to the president of the Section, in which he may have said that I could read a paper for him . . . It will of course appear properly in the official proceedings . . . Never mind, dearest, I care nothing for the omission, but such things are apt to put me in a peculiar light among those who don't have any other source of information than this same supplement."

Salmon appeared as senior author in the *Transactions*. Also, he incorporated the above findings, as though his own, in the *Third Annual Report* (for 1886) of the B.A.I.[49] As a result, Salmon, rather than Theobald Smith, is customarily credited with pioneering the use of heat-killed bacteria for specific immunization, and as being the predecessor of Almroth Wright in England and Richard Pfeiffer in Germany, who ten years later inoculated man with heat-killed typhoid bacilli for protection.

During the first half of 1886, Theobald Smith determined the resistance of his new bacillus to desiccation and its susceptibility to heat and antiseptics. It survived in Potomac River water for at least four months. He emphasized that to destroy the bacteria "in nature," the strength of disinfectants must be increased. Mice and guinea pigs were susceptible to the bacilli. But the infectivity of the test-tube cultures for swine had waned. Only a small proportion of pigs injected subcutaneously developed the disease. Yet, feeding of viscera from animals dead of the disease induced nearly always very severe hog cholera, as did inoculating heart blood from naturally infected pigs. Smith attributed such anachronisms, as well as the cyclical virulence, to bacterial attenuation or altered host resistance.

Although the preliminary results of immunizing pigeons were confirmed in ten experiments involving over forty birds, an effective vaccine could not be developed for swine. Smith administered various subcutaneous dosages of either heat-killed or untreated cultures to about ninety pigs, but when challenged, most of the animals died, which led him to conclude that "The ordinary methods of attenuation . . . are inapplicable to this particular disease for the unattenuated virus itself is incapable of conferring immunity."[50] This perplexing result was ascribed to speedy destruction of the vaccine in the pig's connective tissue, aided perhaps by attenuation. Today the true explanation is clear. The pigs were challenged by being fed with infected viscera or by confinement in infected pens. Thus, they were exposed, unlike the pigeons, to the real cause of hog cholera, a virus, against which the bacillary antigen induced no protection.

Henceforward, Smith investigated and published independently. In June, from the spleen of a dead rabbit in a shipment, he had isolated a microbe which proved invariably fatal to rabbits, although only feebly pathogenic for guinea-pigs, mice, pigeons and fowls. He also studied fluctuations in bacterial virulence and host resistance in this organism, which was similar to the rabbit septicemia microbe described by Koch in 1878, and studied further by Gaffky. Smith alone was the author of this report.[51]

Pigs were dying in Illinois. Theobald Smith once wrote effusively to Gage: "The epidemics among the festive swine in the West ought to be investigated . . . You can't imagine what a storehouse of knowledge pigs are. Full of interesting parasites . . . and plenty of all-colored bacteria."[52] William Welch also praised pigs. According to two of his biographers, "He would descant on their wisdom and beauty, calling particular attention to their elegant feet. They could easily enslave the human race, he would say, but fortunately they were too intelligent to take the trouble."[53] In July 1887, Smith went to Champaign, Illinois, where preliminary tests were facilitated at the Illinois Industrial University[54] by Prof. Burrill. The postmortem findings in nearby epizootics—widespread hemorrhages, lung consolidation, congestion of lymphatics, liver cirrhosis, and lack of intestinal ulcers—were not characteristic of hog cholera. One animal yielded a non-motile, ovoid bacillus which proved fatal to mice, rabbits and pigs. In September, on another field trip to Illinois, Smith autopsied two pigs with consolidated lungs. He isolated a bacterium, identical in all respects to the above, from the spleen of one pig and from the heart blood of the second. Microscopically, the isolate resembled the microbe of rat septicemia. From one of the animals, whose large intestine was ulcerated, the "swine plague" bacillus also was obtained.

The discovery of the new pathogen was disclosed in the Bureau's *Third Annual Report* of 1886. "In prosecuting investigations in the West in order to determine whether . . . hog cholera existed there also . . . another microbe was found . . . There are really two diseases . . . we call the micrococcus disease swine-plague, and the bacterium disease hog-cholera." In the light of this recent observation, the nomenclature had to be revised. The North American epizootic disease with intestinal lesions was still popularly known as "hog cholera," and although since 1879 the Department of Agriculture had favored "swine plague," reversion to the old name seemed logical at this point. The new syndrome, initially designated "infectious pneumonia" of swine, was eventually called "swine plague," since in Germany a comparable infection localized to the lungs and due to a similar microbe had been described by Schütz and named *Schweineseuche* ("swine plague").[55] This switch in nomenclature inevitably caused much confusion.

The confusion became even more confounded when Salmon tried to gloss over differences between his original micrococcus and Smith's short, ovoid bacillus. In an article, "Two Different Germs Found in Hog Cholera," published in the *Breeder's Gazette* of November 11, 1886, he mentioned the non-motile, figure-of-eight organism, which was presumably "the same germ . . . described in my report of 1884." Again, in addressing the United States Veterinary Medical Association, Salmon contended that the new malady was "associated with and undoubtedly caused by a microbe which differs radically from that found in hog cholera." This organism, he believed, was probably identical with his previously-described micrococcus, which "on account of pressure of other work and lack of assistance was imperfectly studied."[56]

From 1880 to 1885, the Bureau's investigations of swine epizootics had helped to resolve doubts about hog cholera and swine erysipelas. Their separate identify, and the specificity of the swine erysipelas microbe had been accepted. But the *Third* and succeeding *Annual Reports* were puzzling and disconcerting, and Theobald Smith began to question some of the reassurances he had penned to Lilian, such as: "It is a blessed thing to be able to forget one's self in work. My western trip proved in this respect a good investment. I have found another microbe, which will give our report a little additional interest in the biological world."[57]

During 1887, epizootics showed no correspondence between symptomatology and bacteriologic findings; and outbreaks, or even single animals, yielded both the motile "hog-cholera" bacillus, and the new short ovoid, non-motile "swine-plague" bacillus. Smith speculated that the clinical and pathological fluctuations illustrated the waxing and waning virulence of the two bacteria. Initially, hog cholera seemed a more prevalent and virulent disease than swing plague, but later, the conditions appeared equally malignant. There were other complexities; for instance, the swine plague cultures of 1887 differed in certain respects from the 1886 strains isolated in Illinois. Again, swine plague cultures were harmless to pigs when given intra-tracheally or in a spray. This fact he attributed to the rapid attenuation of subcultures, and to the likelihood that such pneumotropic bacteria only gained foothold in tissues already affected by lungworm infestation, bronchitis, or bronchopneumonia.

While wresting with these uncertainties, Smith cultivated other interests. He published five papers on several concurrent research projects. Two concerned the bacteriology of drinking water, tapped into the laboratory from the Potomac; one discussed the technique of obtaining pure bacterial cultures; another, the pros and cons of fluid and solid nutrient media; and the fifth was on bacterial variation.[58] In the spring of 1887, his evening lectures to medical students at the Columbian University stressed the public health applications of bacteriology, reflecting increased concern for sanitation and hygiene. In May, he was Special Lecturer at Cornell University for two weeks. In November, he reported on a spirillum, isolated from the consolidated lungs of a cow with pleuropneumonia, which differed culturally from Koch's comma-bacillus, but closely resembled an organism recently described by Finkler and Prior.[59]

Smith took only four days of vacation that year, despite having gained valuable professional help in the spring when Veranus A. Moore was appointed to the laboratory staff just before receiving his B.Sc. degree from Cornell University. A loyal associate for over eight years before he succeeded Theobald Smith in the B.A.I., Moore subsequently had a distinguished career as Dean of the State Veterinary College at Cornell.[60]

In 1888, Smith renewed his efforts to immunize pigs against hog cholera. Enormous dosages of heat-killed cultures, up to eight weekly intraperitoneal injections of 100 cc. each, were ineffective. The combined *Fourth* and *Fifth Annual Report* for 1887–1888 recorded these attempts. It also contained an article on the etiology and diagnosis of glanders including a review of the literature and experimentation written by Smith but published without his name.[61]

After his May marriage, Smith continued to study further outbreaks of hog cholera and swine plague. The end of September 1888 found him in Camden, New Jersey, whence he wrote to his bride that he had gone "to make one or two careful examinations of the internal organs of pigs." He recalled having stayed at the same hotel in November 1885—about a month before discovering the hog-cholera bacillus. He and a Department veterinarian had driven "for many miles in a drizzling rain." The farmers gathered around while he manipulated his tubes and flamed his scalpels in a little alcohol lamp before each incision. "Very likely they thought me either something wonderful or else a quack of the deepest dye, for how could they see the numerous concealed links between such an examination and a final cure? . . . But what a light it sheds on human typhoid and lung diseases. There is much that I should wish to publish, but I cannot use the material as my own."

For nearly a year he had worked "all at sea, on Dr. S's old theory. Then the facts crowded upon me . . . so overwhelmingly that everything else vanished . . . In those days it would have given me a permanent reputation if I could have published as I wished. I should have sent a German article to Virchow's Archiv immediately and published abstracts elsewhere." However, he was never "crazed by any success of this kind."

> When one is in the current of some good, permanently valuable work, it is unfair to leave it or be indifferent to it for money's sake until the proper time comes. We have so much of the mercantile spirit around us, that just a little of the other seems good to me, just a little enthusiasm not born of $ and ¢."[62]

Early in November 1888, Theobald went for three weeks to investigate several outbreaks of swine disease reported from near Mason City, Iowa, and to address the annual meeting of the American Public Health Association at Milwaukee on pathogenic bacteria. With specimens from three affected herds, he

entrained for Red Wing, Minnesota, to set up cultures in a local doctor's laboratory. Two pigs from one herd showed intestinal ulcers without lung disease—a
novel finding, which he conveyed to Lilian: "As usual, pathological changes are in
part new and puzzling. When we have a variable animal organism and a variable
germ, it is difficult to realize the result in all cases. Nature is very sportive, even
in disease."[63] To Gage he wrote:

> I spent a week at Red Wing, Minn . . . There I started a little embryo bacteriol.
> laboratory for the Sec. State Bd. Health and gave him some instructions. Then I
> went into Northern Iowa, dissected about 10 pigs of various sizes and returned to
> Red Wing to study my plunder . . . At Milwaukee I became a member of the Am.
> Pub. Health Ass'n and read a paper which was well received.[64]

Smith also outlined his findings to William Welch of Baltimore, who had
made some preliminary observations on the causation of hog cholera and swine
plague, which were published in the initial number of the *Johns Hopkins Hospital
Bulletin*. Welch answered: "our experience here would indicate that hog cholera
and swine plague are frequently combined with each other, and this complicates
the study greatly." He invited Smith to visit his laboratory at any time.[65] That letter exchange began the life-long association between William Welch and Theobald Smith.

The failure to immunize pigs against hog cholera by vaccination with the alleged causal bacillus led to rigorous criticism at home and abroad of many B.A.I.
claims regarding swine epizootics. Salmon was obsessed with Brieger's doctrines
about bacterial ptomaines[66]—that the pathogenicity of bacteria was due to poisonous substances they secreted into animal tissues or culture fluids. In the *Annual Report* for 1888, Salmon contended that the amount of immunity gained depended on "the quantity of ptomaines produced by the specific microbes, i.e.,
upon their poisonous nature." If the tissue-destroying effect of bacillary thrombi
in the blood vessels overshadowed the ptomaine element, the problem became
complicated and attempts to immunize might fail. He claimed priority in the
production of immunity by inoculating chemical products of bacterial growth.

In an historical review, Ferdinand Hueppe confirmed the priority of Salmon
and Smith's report of February 1886.[67] But Chantemesse and Widal announced
that a "new era in bacteriology" was inaugurated in December 1887,[68] when
Roux and Chamberland recorded the immunization of guinea pigs against
Vibrion septique.[69] Salmon objected to Pasteurian attempts to "secure the credit of
his discovery," and referred to Duclaux's explanation of why American studies
on hog cholera were so little known in France. They were not only published in
official reports and therefore buried in ministerial archives, or "in the grand
mausoleums hostile to visitors that we name, in France, public libraries;" but the

author was liable to pour the "entire contents of his notes of researches" upon the confused reader's head.[70] Smith learned in time to be more selective in placing his reports for publication.

The European muddle over this disease intensified in 1888, when Selander, working under Gaffky in Koch's laboratory at the Reichsgesundheitsamt, considered an epizootic of *svinpest,* which spread from Sweden to Denmark, the counterpart of American hog cholera.[71] A culture brought to Washington in that year differed from the hog-cholera bacillus, especially in being non-virulent for rabbit and pig. Selander moved to Roux's laboratory at the Pasteur Institute, and there increased the virulence of the culture by serial passage in rabbits and pigeons. But antigenicity was not enhanced, nor could pigeons be immunized with heat-sterilized cultures.

Metchnikoff confirmed Selander's work, and also observed that the blood serum of rabbits vaccinated with his "hog-cholera bacilli" protected against infections, but lacked bactericidal or antitoxic power and had no attenuating effect upon the specific microbe. Not surprisingly, Metchnikoff claimed that phagocytosis played an important role in the resistance of these vaccinated rabbits.[72] He designated the organism *Coccobacillus suinum.* Theobald Smith requested a culture of this alleged hog cholera bacillus and identified it as a swine plague organism. Welch and Clement independently reported similar results with another culture from Selander.[73] Smith concluded: "There has evidently been some misconception in the mind of this, as well as other European investigators, as to what the hog cholera bacillus really is."[74]

In 1888, a fierce attack was launched upon Salmon and the B.A.I. by Frank Seaver Billings, a native of Massachusetts, who had graduated from the Imperial Veterinary Institute in 1878. Now, as Director of the Pathobiological Laboratory of the State University of Nebraska at Lincoln, he published a 400-page Bulletin on *Swine Plague,* subtitled "With Especial Reference to the Porcine Pests of the World. An Etiological, Patho-Anatomical, Prophylactic, and Critical Contribution to General Pathology and State Medicine."[75] In this diatribe, Billings demanded that the question "whether there are two porcine pests in this country . . . be settled by a competent commission of experts." Salmon was pilloried and relentlessly taunted for seeking "to pose as the original and only investigator on animal diseases in this country," and as suffering from a "swine plague-hog cholera psychosis." His hog-cholera germ was a "Washingtonian-Bureaucratic nondescript . . . erroneous, and . . . a forgery." The document was remarkable for its vilification of a Federal Institution and of the public servant directing it. "For ten long years he has been at work—at what? . . . Let him show what he has done that has been an iota of value either to his country, his profession, or science." Billings believed that there was a single American swine epizootic that should be termed "swine plague," as originally advocated by H.J. Detmers, now professor of veterinary medicine at Ohio State University, Columbus.

Billings had begun to investigate swine plague in 1886. The blood, spleen, and other organs of every case examined had yielded Detmers' 1879 microbe—a pleomorphic, "belted, ovoid organism, which colors at its pole ends," resembling the bacterium isolated in Germany by Schütz from hogs with *Schweineseuche*. Salmon's claim to have identified another bacterial disease in swine was "unqualifiedly false," Billings contended. Further, swine plague was not contagious but was due to invasion by a microbe from the regional soil. Billings had isolated a kindred microbe from the blood and viscera of animals with Texas cattle fever and held that similar "extra-organismal, belted germs" caused other septicemic diseases, such as fowl cholera, rabbit septicemia, the *Schweineseuche* and *Wildseuche* of the German literature, and even yellow fever. "Facts are eternal! Authority transient!" trumpeted Billings. "I care no more for authority, when the facts are against it, than for the whisperings of a summer breeze." Theobald Smith got off lightly. "As the master is, so must the assistant be;" but in this case, the assistant was considered a mere acolyte. Finally, Billings demanded the appointment of a Commission of Inquiry, stipulating the exclusion of anyone connected with the government, and suggesting "Welch, of Baltimore, and Shakespeare and Osler, of Philadelphia."[76]

On November 27, 1888, Commissioner of Agriculture Norman J. Colman invited Dr. E.O. Shakespeare of Philadelphia, Prof. W.H. Welch of Johns Hopkins University, and Prof. T.J. Burrill of the University of Illinois to serve on the "United States Board of Inquiry Concerning Epidemic Diseases Among Swine." Welch declined and was replaced by Prof. B. Meade Bolton of the University of South Carolina. The Board was enjoined to convene shortly at the Department of Agriculture in Washington to decide upon plans "without instructions or interference" from the Department, whose facilities would be placed nevertheless at its disposal.[77]

The Board was to determine four main points: 1. Were the diseases of swine investigated by the B.A.I. properly designated in the official Reports for 1885 to 1887; were they caused by the germs specified; and were these germs accurately described? 2. To what extent were the descriptions of those germs original? 3. Was the disease investigated by Billings identical with one of the diseases described by the B.A.I., or did it differ from both of them? Did the Nebraska investigations establish facts that materially differed from the B.A.I. conclusions regarding swine diseases in the United States? 4. To what extent was Dr. Detmers justified in asserting that Dr. Salmon's *Bacterium suis, discovered by him in 1885 as a substitute for his* micrococcus, has nothing whatever to do with swine plague; that it is a septic germ, readily kills rabbits, and causes septicemia, but has no connection with the disease in question? If Detmers had identified any microbe as an infectious agent, did it specifically differ from the two agents described in the B.A.I. reports? Suggestions for treating and preventing these diseases were requested, with April 1, 1889 set as deadline for submission of findings.

William Welch's unavailability was regrettable, for he had considerable personal experience in this field. Indeed, his initial article in the *Johns Hopkins Hospital Bulletin,*[78] and the expanded version later published with Clement as co-author, declared that Billings's so-called "swine-plague" bacillus was "identical to the hog-cholera bacillus." According to Simon Flexner, Welch turned to bacteriological studies in 1887, when the Hospital was still unfinished and his access to human disease limited. Hence, he "chose as a major problem hog cholera, then prevalent in Maryland. Whenever he received word that a fatal illness had broken out on some farm near Baltimore, he hurried to the scene."[79]

The Board of Inquiry met at Washington during Christmas week 1888 and elected Shakespeare chairman and Bolton secretary. After inspecting the Bureau of Animal Industry in Washington, members planned to visit Billings and Detmers and proposed also to investigate swine epizootics in several badly-infected areas. Soon after the deadline had been extended by two months, the Board's appropriation was exhausted. The members continued their inquiries without pay and produced three reports—a short version by Bolton in May 1889; the main report by Shakespeare and Burrill on August 1, 1889; and a supplement by Shakespeare, dated February 27, 1890.

The Commissioners upheld the B.A.I. position in all important respects, thus vindicating Smith's contentions. They concluded that in the United States there existed two widespread epizootic diseases of swine with similar clinical and pathological features due to different microorganisms. The causal role of the hog-cholera bacillus had been established. Furthermore, "the discovery of . . . 'swine plague,' and of the microbe to which it is due, must be considered original on the part of the Bureau authorities." Billing's pathogen was identical with the "hog-cholera bacillus." His failure to find the swine plague organism sponsored by the B.A.I. did not incontestably prove its non-existence in Nebraska. Detmers's microbe also was probably the Bureau's hog-cholera bacillus.

The Commissioners believed that treatment of existing cases was futile. Preventive measures (since disinfection could not be effected under prevailing conditions) comprised three alternatives: quarantine, extermination of infected hogs with their surroundings, and artificial immunization. Attempts to induce immunity by using live germs was objectionable, since this would multiply centers of infections and stunt the growth of inoculated pigs. However, recent experience had shown that "the chemical products of certain disease-producing germs in artificial cultures possess the same power to create immunity as do the living germs themselves." The Commissioners urged that thorough and rapid investigation of the "hog-cholera germ" be made "in this direction and without stint of money or hampering limitations of time." The board submitted its report to Secretary of Agriculture Jeremiah M. Rusk, appointed in March 1889 by the new Republican president, Benjamin Harrison. The outgoing President Cleveland had raised the Department's status, giving Commissioner Colman and his successors the rank of Secretary.

Meanwhile, Smith continued to supply the grist to his Chief's mill. On January 25, 1889, he recorded, "Finished 100 pages foolscap, typewritten for annual dept. report for 1888." The following December 17 found him "Beginning on annual report for the current year." Among several visitors, apart from Lilian's relatives, were "Prof. Conn of Wesleyan," and his old friend, Henry Battin. In March, he gave the Annual Commencement Address before the National Medical College at Albaugh's Opera House. Various scientific presentations to the Biological Society of Washington included a report in May on his first protozoological investigation—renal coccidiosis in the mouse.

In the summer of 1889, the Bureau of Animal Industry issued its monograph on *Hog Cholera: Its History, Nature, and Treatment, As Determined by the Inquiries and Investigations of the Bureau of Animal Industry*.[80] Although Salmon referred to himself as "the author" in the introductory sections (the only part he wrote), Theobald Smith had assembled five-sixths of the text and sixteen pages of pathological and bacteriological illustrations, from notes on experiments which he initially planned, carried out or supervised, and meticulously recorded. Smith indignantly exposed the masquerade to Gage: "Now take the hog cholera bulletin which was mailed to you. I wrote 170 pp. out of 200 pp."[81] The purpose of the book was to provide the intelligent farmer, as well as the veterinarian, with an objective account of what had been established, and what remained unsettled, about hog cholera. Some sections were taken from earlier B.A.I. reports, others were preprinted from the combined *Fourth* and *Fifth Annual Reports* of the B.A.I., released later than summer.[82] Yet this was no patchwork. Facts were systematically rearranged, subheadings put in proper sequence, and new paragraphs inserted where needed.

A section headed, "Injections of Sterilized Culture Liquid to Produce Immunity," included Smith's pioneer experiments on pigeons, prefaced by comments indicating at least partial accord with Brieger's ptomaine theory. But he was horrified by any suggestion that bacterial *bodies* had no part to play, as witness the shock registered in one of his letters to Gage: "I don't intend to have you speak contemptuously of our bacteria as '*bacteria juice*,' how awful!"[83]

New material appeared in a section headed "Relation of Hog Cholera to Public Health." Here Smith reflected that the transmissibility to man of such animal diseases as glanders, tuberculosis, anthrax, and rabies was recognized "before the specific bacterial organisms of these diseases had been discovered." He had foreseen in the B.A.I. Report for 1885 that the "swine plague" (hog cholera) bacillus might be pathogenic for man. Now he amplified the theme. Typhoid fever and hog cholera, though entirely distinct diseases, were closely related as to cause, manner of infection, and symptomatology. Hog cholera also sufficiently resembled epidemic dysentery in man to warrant considering the hog-cholera bacillus "capable of producing diphtheritic and ulcerative lesions of the large intestine." Fortunately, the risk of human disease was lessened by the rapid death of this bacillus at 140°F, well below the temperatures at which pork was boiled or roasted. Eventually, the hog cholera bacillus became recognized as a dangerous human pathogen, liable to be ingested in poorly cooked pork products and causing human infections with a higher mortality than typhoid fever.[84]

Smith reiterated with complete conviction that this microbe caused hog cholera. Over 500 cases of the disease had been necropsied by him in the past three years. About three-quarters of them had died at the Experiment Station. The same bacillus was isolated from the spleen of about 400 of these pigs. It was pathogenic for rabbits, mice, guinea-pigs and pigeons. The pathogenicity for swine had been difficult to establish, except through oral administration of pure cultures. He considered that this not only confirmed the true cause of the disease but also illustrated the route of infection. Even after ingesting up to 100 cc. of culture, some very sick pigs recovered, while others showed no disturbance. Yet Smith averred, "The experiments prove conclusively the causal relation between the bacilli of hog cholera and the disease so called." Billings was not mentioned in the Hog cholera monograph, which had gone to the printer before his volume appeared. He would be dealt with in a companion volume, soon to be issued, on Swine Plague.

The Gages acknowledged Theobald's grievances, but counseled caution. He reassured them. "I do not intend anything rash, and I shall certainly have a kind open talk with Dr. S. before I make up my mind what to do."[85] Then, as they still did not seem to understand the situation, he brought them up to date.

Suppose that you & Dr. Wilder had been working together and he was advanced to the Presidency of the Univ. His time is filled up with details of business, appointments, speeches, payrolls & interviews. He has not time for scientific work or thought of any kind (exc. photography). Suppose that for four years thereafter he assumed all your work still, signs your reports, gives you a bare mention in the preface with your subordinates, so that no one could tell which was which. Do you think that is right? Now suppose that your work becomes too broad and another man is appointed to take part of it. At first he gets help and ideas from you, which you had to dig out yourself in some way. Within 3 years he publishes his first work under his own name and a bulletin also is to follow in his name . . . Curtice gets credit even for work done for me in Texas fever last year and for work done out West on taeniae. Of course he should have it, but why should I not be indignant at the selfish, unprincipled method which aims to keep all bact. work as emanating from him [Salmon].

Smith's denunciations of favoritism involved his fellow-Cornellians—a particularly painful situation to Gage, who yearned to be proud of them all. "Take the Bureau report just now in printer's hands," Theobald continued his letter to Gage:

> I wrote a long article on Glanders, the result of experiment chiefly, and four articles on swine diseases, one concerning work I did in Iowa, covering in all pp. 50–168 of the report. Curtice has an article on tapeworms, pp. 167–184, signed by himself. Now what credit do I get? After a long preface: "In conclusion, it affords me pleasure to acknowl. the ability, energy & devotion to work shown by Dr. T.S. & Dr. Kilborne in conducting the experimental work, the details of which are given in this report." Who knows what the work is, what each has done, how much independence of research, & who reads the preface?

When Smith complained to Assistant Secretary Willets, he was again advised to have a talk with Salmon. A measure of "proprietorship" was eventually promised for his future contributions to official reports, but no complete resolution was achieved and resentment remained. Secretary Rusk's actions brought more hope for the future. He informed President Harrison that the present facilities of the Bureau of Animal Industry were "utterly inadequate . . . Some diseases are communicable to mankind and can not be investigated because the laboratories are not sufficiently isolated from the remainder of the buildings, where many persons are employed."[86] Pending appropriations for a new laboratory, the old should be renovated. "The change is very great," wrote Theobald to Lilian, "as you will see when you call on me again there." He had removed objectionable water closets, his own room now had some privacy, a former "forestry room" (once her father's office) was in the laboratory domain, and skylights had been installed.[87]

In the *Sixth* and *Seventh Annual Reports* of the Bureau of Animal Industry, Theobald Smith's name headed the sections on infectious diseases. Although his views on hog cholera and swine plague as separate infections were now widely accepted, effective means of artificial immunization against either disease remained elusive. Two outbreaks of "modified hog cholera" yielded unusual strains of the hog-cholera bacillus. Abnormally large bacterial cells and colonies were associated with diminished cultural virulence. A live vaccine prepared from this "*b*" form protected rabbits (but not pigs) against lethal dosages of the virulent "*a*" form.[88]

As of January 1, 1890, Emil Alexander von Schweinitz was appointed (in his own words) "to take charge of the chemical work of the Bureau of Animal Industry and investigate the chemical side of the disease of animals, especially hog cholera and swine plague."[89] A chemical laboratory was temporarily "crowded into a damp, illy ventilated, and wholly unsuitable basement"[90] of the Agriculture Building until space for it was partitioned off in the adjacent National Museum. Water, gas and steam were installed, and operations began on April 1, 1890. Within four months, von Schweinitz reported on hog-cholera ptomaines at the Indianapolis meeting of the A.A.A.S. According to Smith, the greater part of this work was done in his own laboratory, planned by him, and executed by Veranus Moore.[91] Schweinitz acknowledged that Moore did the bacteriological work and thanked Drs. Salmon and Smith for valuable advice. Brieger's methods of treating the culture liquids had yielded chemical preparations that rendered guinea pigs "immune from hog-cholera." A follow-up report claimed that single subcutaneous inoculations of the germ-free ptomaine "sucholotoxin," although lethal in large doses, conferred on guinea pigs complete immunity to hog cholera.[92]

Gage read a paper on Smith's behalf at the same A.A.A.S. meeting. An earlier description of the *a* and *b* varieties of hog cholera, now termed α and β, was amplified. In suggesting that bacillus a might link bacillus β to *Bacillus coli,* Smith did not wish to imply that *B. coli* could be "converted into the hog-cholera bacillus and thus be an ever-present source of hog-cholera germs. The change of saprophytic into parasitic or disease germs probably goes on as slowly as changes in higher organisms, and has nothing sensational about it." Groupings of organisms, he claimed, based on thorough biological knowledge, safeguarded against confounding dissimilar organisms and separating organisms which belonged together. "In bacteriology, as in older departments of research, it is the care we bestow upon apparently trifling, unattractive, and very troublesome minutiae which determine the result."[93] Such intermingled philosophical musings and dicta about the fundamentals of technique based on personal laboratory experience characterized many of Smith's publications.

Although the *New York Medical Journal,* which published Smith's paper on bacterial variation, was more widely read than the reports of the U.S. Department of Agriculture, its circulation among bacteriologists was meager. There was no English counterpart to the *Zeitschrift für Hygiene und Infektionskrankheiten,* founded by Koch in 1885, the *Annales de l'Institut Pasteur* (1886), and the *Centralblatt für Bakteriologie* (1887). Smith had submitted two previous papers to the *Centralblatt.*[94] In the next ten years a dozen of his articles appeared in that journal and in Koch's *Zeitschrift.* The *Journal of the Boston Society of Medical Sciences* (which became the *Journal of Medical Research*) and the *Journal of Experimental Medicine,* were launched about a decade later. Smith then found it convenient to contribute to these periodicals, but meanwhile often published in German journals.

Several of these publications involved him in controversy with P. Frosch, one of Koch's assistants. Early in 1890, Frosch reviewed American "swine plague."[95] Cultures sent by Billings to Koch's Institute, labelled "SP" (swine plague), had proved identical with the B.A.I. hog-cholera bacillus, and Frosch concluded that this was the causal organism of American swine epizootics. He wondered, however, why the mortality was much higher on feeding the tissues of swine infected with hog cholera than after inoculation of the bacillary cultures. Salmon's "swine-plague" cultures resembled *Schweineseuche* bacteria and certainly were not micrococci. Although they were pathogenic and different from hog-cholera bacilli, Frosch viewed them as secondary invaders rather than prime agents of a distinct disease. Thus, he disputed some of the assertions of both Billings and Salmon.

Theobald Smith now entered the fray, publishing two papers in German, one on the hog-cholera bacillus, and the other on American swine plague.[96] In the second article, he designated as H- and S-bacilli the causal organisms of hog cholera and swine plague, respectively. He reported that his assistant, Veranus Moore, had isolated S-bacilli of widely different virulence from the upper respiratory tract of swine and various domestic animals. Smith criticized Frosch for having dealt so lightly with Billings, who had initially denounced hog cholera and its causal bacterium as fictitious, and yet spurned the S-bacillus when Frosch and others identified the Nebraskan "swine-plague organism" as the H-bacillus. Yet, using much faultier methods than the B.A.I. and after unjustified vituperation, Billings had produced the same bacillus.

Frosch's reply was printed consecutively by the chief editor of the *Zeitschrift für Hygiene,* Robert Koch. Smith should not deplore the inadequacy of Billing's animal experiments, since his own positive results were quite scanty. The initial evidence, according to Frosch, pointed to a secondary role for the S-bacillus, which the findings of the last five years had confirmed. Salmon had increased the confusion by intruding himself into the literature. The situation had been clarified somewhat by the disclosure that Theobald Smith had sponsored both organisms.[97]

In March 1891, Smith was officially informed by Secretary of Agriculture Rusk that "You are hereby appointed Chief of the Division of Animal Pathology."[98] He was to report to the Chief of the Bureau for instructions as to duties. His salary, $2,250 since July 1, 1890, was to remain unchanged. Salmon advised him that "this Division will include the scientific investigations of disease as carried on in the bacteriological laboratory and the experiment station, and the study of animal parasites."[99] Nine staff members, including Moore, Kilborne and Cooper Curtice, were to be under his supervision and direction. Cooper Curtice thereupon resigned on April 8. While this promotion both defined his status and salved his pride, Theobald Smith felt no long-term commitment to Washington. He was thoroughly disenchanted about the "Bureau" which "might be considered a big overgrown Jerry with one foot deep in the mire of politics and the other vainly trying to plant itself in scientific ground."[100] Yet its administrative weaknesses were outweighed by the unrivalled research opportunities. He would stay on as long as his talents and ambitions found worthwhile outlets, or until a more promising job was offered.

In 1891, the Congress, prodded by Secretary Rusk, provided for a new B.A.I. laboratory. Theobald Smith supervised the detailed planning, the selection and installation of equipment, and the final move—the whole task lasting many months. During August, the laboratory transferred to a new brick building two blocks away. It was thirty-five feet wide and fifty feet deep, three-storied, with a basement for small experimental animals. The first floor, dealing with the parasitology of domestic animals, was in charge of Dr. C.W. Stiles; the second floor was for pathological and bacteriological work; and the third was chemistry's domain, under Dr. E.A. *de* (changed from *von*) Schweinitz. The Experiment Station, improved by adding a few wooden structures, remained separated from the laboratory, so that travel to and fro used much time and energy.[101] Salmon's office remained in the Department of Agriculture Building.

Between February and August 1891, Smith prepared and proof-read a report on swine plague. "Manuscript on Swine Plague pract. finished today: amount 200 t.p. [typed pages] of my own part."[102] On October 17, the *Special Report on the Cause and Prevention of Swine Plague* was published. The sub-heading was *Results of Experiments Conducted under the Direction of Dr. D.E. Salmon, Chief of the Bureau of Animal Industry*.[103] Smith had written almost the whole work (140 pages) and had prepared specimens for the twelve plates. He summarized practical preventive measures for swine-breeders, appropriate for a communicable disease. Some of his assertions were erroneous enough to have haunted him in later years. For instance, his claim that swine-plague bacteria "in pure culture can be made to produce by inoculation the disease itself in healthy animals," a fallacy reiterated in the *Annual Report* for 1891: "The proof that swine-plague bacteria do produce a fatal infectious disease is thus complete, and any further discussion of that part of the subject is useless."[104] He restated his 1887 postulate that this parasite acquired virulence when the host's resistance was lowered by parasites, malnutrition, or other factors. Further, it could live harmlessly in the air pas-

sages of one host species, and yet prove pathogenic to another. These proposi-
tions were "not yet fully demonstrated," but "in applying facts of science, it is often necessary to anticipate actual demonstration of a presumed truth, especially
when we are thereby put on the conservative side, and our attention aroused to
probable dangers of the future." Billings was disposed of in a five-page exposé.
His methods of cultivation were too inaccurate to determine which cultures
were pure so that the pleomorphic organisms described by him might represent
either or both of the Bureau's species.

Austin Peters of Boston, as Chairman of the Committee on Intelligence and
Education of the United States Veterinary Medical Association for the two years
1890–91, addressed the Annual Meeting at Washington in September 1891.[105]
He advocated higher standards of veterinary education, discussed the disappointing results of Koch's tuberculin, and summarized the anti-rabies activities
of the new Pasteur Institute of New York. Then he attacked the Bureau of Animal Industry, especially as regards "scientific investigation of swine diseases." He
had read the Bureau reports, the Billings monograph, and the Frosch-Smith articles in the German literature. Personal involvement in swine plague outbreaks
in Massachusetts had brought him into contact with Theobald Smith. Salmon
ought to be the scapegoat for the "chaos" surrounding the whole question, he
charged. His changes of nomenclature had started the confusion. If the B.A.I.'s
scientific labors were judged by its investigations of swine diseases, veterinarians
should feel "disgraced when we think of the opinions which must be held in
Koch's laboratory." Salmon had gained credit for Smith's researches, Peters asserted, as Frosch doubtless came to realize during his literary exchange with
Theobald Smith, adding, "It has been no secret to me . . . who was actually conducting these investigations in the Bureau of Animal Industry."

Peters wondered whether Frosch's "admiration for the honesty and generosity
of the pseudo-scientist whose work he supposed he was reviewing when he
wrote his first article[106] were equal to his . . . pity and contempt for the assistant,
who was obliged to give the credit for his hard work to his chief."[107] Billings was
not spared: "Personalities that so often pervade the writings of the investigator
employed by the State of Nevada . . . have done so much to detract from the dignity of his work." Finally, although "modern political methods are not to be tolerated in the conduction of scientific research," if the B.A.I. were to be a political
organization, its chief should "simply write the letter of transmittal of his annual
report to the Secretary of Agriculture, and have a few true scientists in its employ to work unhampered, and make their own reports."

Salmon was in Europe as Secretary Rusk's nominee at the International Congresses of Hygiene and Demography in London and of Agriculture in the Hague.
Upon his return, he sent an open letter to two periodicals, accusing Peters of

taking advantage of his absence. "This attack was the more cowardly since he also knew that Dr. Smith, who has charge of the investigations, was not a member of the Association, and was therefore not in a position to reply." (Theobald Smith became a member of the U.S. Veterinary Medical Association in September 1892.) In his own letters of transmittal of B.A.I. reports, and also in his statement in the *Breeder's Gazette* of November 11, 1886, Salmon had made known "the exact position and work of each one connected with the investigations."[108] Peters had set up straw men—"the well-known dodge of polemical writers"— and mercilessly criticized the Bureau, while praising Billings, who had discarded his swine-plague germ for the Bureau's hog-cholera microbe, whose existence he had denied up to 1889. Peters' view that swine plague was "one of those septic diseases due to filth" was too sweeping, based on experience limited to swill-feeding hogs in the Boston vicinity. "Condemning personalities, political methods and lack of honesty in others," his patently fallacious allegations laid Peters himself, according to Salmon, open to all these charges.

At the next annual meeting of the U.S. Veterinary Medical Association, Salmon again denounced this grievous affront: "The entire field of scientific investigation in this country can be explored without finding an example of such rank injustice or of such uncalled-for defamation."[109] He called Billings "a bungler as an investigator, and an ignoramus in bacteriology." Did the Association take no pride in the investigations of the Bureau, or did it propose to stigmatize them as a disgrace to the veterinary profession?

Contributing to the Association's indifference was Salmon's posture on veterinary education. That very meeting had endorsed three-year courses and had resolved to exclude graduates of two-years courses, after 1895, from membership in the Association. Yet Salmon and some B.A.I. associates subsequently sponsored a two-year course at a new National Veterinary College in Washington, an action that was censored by several professional organizations. In 1895, its Fundamental Faculty was headed by Salmon and included Moore and Kilborne. Theobald Smith gave four lectures and a quiz on bacteriology at the National Veterinary College in the fall of 1892, but otherwise kept entirely aloof.

In 1891, de Schweinitz reported that "albumoses" of swine plague cultures immunized guinea pigs and hogs, while similar attempts to protect pigs against hog cholera had little or no success.[110] In September 1892, he described the antigenic properties of the enzymes in hog cholera bacillary cultures.[111] Smith relayed his annoyance to Welch, who replied: "Of course I saw that Dr. S. does not bring forward the slightest proof that the enzymes or ferments produce immunity. He certainly had a good deal besides ferments in the material he injected." But Welch was anxious to dissuade his able and zealous new acquaintance, now bristling with indignation, from open warfare with his Chief. "I hope you will not fall out with the management," was his way of putting things. "I know that there is much about the work of the Bureau which must be annoying to you . . . Nevertheless, the Bureau has afforded you opportunity for excellent work."[112]

> You are responsible only for the work which is credited to you, although I know that there is much for which you have never received proper credit . . . The only reputation of real value for a scientific man is that which he earns among his peers . . . Be content to rest upon good scientific work and in the long run it must be recognized and the notoriety seeker must go to the wall.

By 1892, the hog cholera-swine plague problem was no longer Smith's main concern. In 1893, he edited and contributed to a miscellany of nine articles by himself and laboratory associates. The collection, "Conducted under the direction of Dr. D.E. Salmon, Chief of the Bureau of Animal Industry," and issued as B.A.I. *Bulletin No. 3,* included only three papers relating directly or indirectly to swine infections.[113] Veranus Moore described a non-motile form of the hog-cholera bacillus. In a separate paper he reported further observations on the bacterial flora, including swine-plague organisms, in the upper air passages of domesticated animals.

Smith himself reported the isolation of a pathogenic organism, closely resembling the hog-cholera bacillus, from the vagina of a mare which had aborted. His last recorded trip in quest of swine epizootics was early in May 1893, when he journeyed by rail and buggy with Veranus Moore to Brookville, Maryland, to investigate an outbreak of hog cholera on a farm.[114] However, with Moore's assistance, Theobald Smith continued to accumulate data on swine diseases, outbreaks of which continued in diversity, prevalence, and intractibility. In March he completed *Additional Investigations Concerning Swine Diseases.* Salmon transmitted to Secretary Morton these hitherto unpublished results of "my assistants in the laboratory," and it became *Bulletin No. 6* of the B.A.I.[115]

Smith recapitulated, or first recorded here in collaboration with V.A. Moore, important observations on the production of immunity against hog-cholera and swine-plague bacteria. Smith and Moore defined the general relationship between the virulence of the bacterial parasite, the degree of pre-existing immunity in the host, and the character of the resulting infectious disease: "The greater the immunity short of complete protection, the more prolonged and chronic the disease induced subsequently by inoculation." This generalization represented an early step in Theobald Smith's long pilgrimage toward clearer understanding of the host-parasite relationship. Independently of Ehrlich, he differentiated passive immunity and described its disadvantages. "The blood serum of animals protected against hog cholera and swine plague is almost as efficacious in producing immunity soon after treatment as the bacterial products obtained from cultures;" but the protective effects were transient, and it was often difficult to obtain the blood serum.

At the end of August 1894, Theobald Smith sent a copy of *Bulletin No. 6* to Welch, whose own results, based on twenty swine epizootics investigated, confirmed those of the B.A.I., although he believed that *B. cholerae suis* was the sole cause of hog cholera and the swine plague bacillus a secondary invader.[116] Welch thanked Smith: "You ought not be discontented with your work on swine diseases. Time will prove, has proven, its essential accuracy . . . You are ahead of us in nearly all our conclusions, but it is only fair that you should be, as you occupied the field first and have made it peculiarly your own."[117]

In *Bulletin No. 6,* earlier results were rearranged and amplified, along with new data and ideas. Smith outlined the bacteriologic and pathogenic properties of seven varieties of *Bacillus cholerae suis,* so-named for the first time. The six varieties, a to ?, all discovered by him, and Moore's non-motile ? variety, were compared with allied species unconnected with hog cholera outbreaks—including the bacillus isolated by himself in 1891 from a mare following abortion,[118] Gärtner's *Bacillus enteritidis* (1888), and Loeffler's *Bacillus typhi murium* (1890). The general characteristics of these organisms, which he termed the "hog-cholera group" of bacteria, were tabulated. The short, non-sporulating rods were all motile, except for variant ?; they failed to liquefy gelatin; and their fermentative reactions against specific carbohydrates had a constant pattern, "differentiating such group sharply from the colon group." They produced acid and gas from dextrose, but none from lactose or saccharose. Since their pathogenicity could be lost or changed on repeated subculture, Smith suggested that morphologically typical bacteria "which do not liquefy gelatin and whose fermentative properties are the same as those described for this group, should be ranged under it." Although the "hog-cholera group" (later expanded to *Salmonella* genus) eventually included many hundreds of species, Theobald Smith's 1894 proposal for their separate classification remains valid, with minor exceptions.

The duality of hog cholera and swine plague was supported by J. Lignières, who studied swine diseases in Argentina and at the Alfort Veterinary School. Lignières proposed the generic name *Pasteurella* for organisms causing hemorrhagic septicemias,[119] including *Schweineseuche*—the "swine plague" of Salmon and Smith.[120] This condition differed from Salmon's "hog-cholera," whose causal organism "could serve as prototype for the creation of another group, the *Salmonella.*" Lignières also suggested that diseases due to these genera should be termed pasteurelloses and salmonelloses, respectively (1901),[121] and this nomenclature was accepted by taxonomists.

Weedin (1927) recognized a *Salmonella* genus within the colon-typhoid group of bacteria, designating the type species *Salmnella cholerae suis* (Smith, Th., 1894).[122] Theobald Smith disdained protesting this eponymous tribute to Salmon, which Bergey's *Manual of Determinative Bacteriology* perpetuated. But his resentment smoldered. More than three decades after Lignières' proposal, he wrote to Gage: "Salmon's relation to the entire work of the Bureau from 1884 on was less than nominal. Although he had nothing to do with the discovery & first description of the hog cholera bacillus, an entire group of bacilli of which the hog chol. bacillus was the father so to speak, is now called Salmonella.[123]

After leaving the Bureau of Animal Industry, Smith never resumed intensive researches in swine infections, though he maintained a collection of cultures for many years. In 1899, he identified as a hog-cholera bacillus a non-motile organism sent him by Prof. Burrill from an infected herd. A report on this culture, verifying Moore's earlier isolation of the ? variant, was Smith's only further German publication in the hog cholera field.[124] In 1902, he confirmed the finding by Reed and Carroll[125] that Sanarelli's *Bacillus icteroides,* isolated from yellow fever cases in Uruguay and Brazil,[126] was the hog-cholera bacillus. In 1914–15, when one of the main objectives of the Rockefeller Institute's new department of animal pathology at Princeton was to combat hog cholera, Smith readily outlined a thorough program of laboratory researches into this disease.

In 1897, a devastating outbreak in the Iowa corn belt led the B.A.I. to send out there Marion Dorset, a young member of de Schweinitz's Biochemic Division. Since horse antiserum prepared against *B. cholerae suis* proved ineffective, Dorset became skeptical about the role of this bacillus. After closely studying the natural disease and its relation to the bacillus for some years, Dorset and colleagues in 1903 demonstrated the infectiviity of blood taken from a sick pig before bacilli were demonstrable in its blood or tissues. Moreover, bacteria-free filtrates of such serum proved infective for normal pigs, leading them to conclude that "An infectious disease among hogs . . . which cannot be distinguished clinically from hog cholera . . . may be reproduced by infecting with material which contains no hog cholera bacilli."[127]

Six years after Loeffler and Frosch had discovered that foot-and-mouth disease was due to a filterable virus,[128] Dorset (who had succeeded the recently deceased de Schweinitz) confirmed with his colleagues Bolton and McBryde the viral etiology of hog cholera.[129] When Smith's major experiments were repeated in the light of these findings, the potential pathogenicity of *B. cholerae suis* for pigs remained undisputed, but this bacillus became grouped with swine-plague organisms as a secondary invader of pigs infected with the hog cholera virus.

6

TEXAS (SOUTHERN)
CATTLE FEVER

Texas fever was probably introduced into the more southerly American colonies in the seventeenth century by cattle brought in from the Spanish West Indies and Mexico. The infection spread until a high degree of herd immunity prevailed in the south; but any breeding stock imported there was liable to be lost after a period of ten days to several weeks. James Mease, a physician of Philadelphia who wrote the earliest professional account in 1826 of what became known as Texas, or southern, cattle fever, observed in August 1796 that successive droves of cattle from South Carolina "so certainly disease all others with which they mix in their progress to the North that they are prohibited by the people of Virginia from passing through the state."[1] Several other border states also banned the transit of southern cattle.

Following the Civil War, after demands grew for a hardy breed to replenish the scarcity of livestock in the West and for cheap beef in the northeastern states, vast herds were driven from the South into Illinois and the expanding West, where no such laws existed. In the summer of 1868, a disastrous epizootic broke out in Illinois and Indiana following the importation of apparently healthy southern cattle. At least 15,000 native animals died. Early in August, dead animals turned up in Pittsburgh and in the stockyards and abattoirs supplying New York, and a public health hazard from the consumption of the butchered beeves was feared, especially as there was a concurrent increase of obstinate and fatal human diarrhea. *The Times* of London of August 28, 1868 reported that this new "Cattle plague . . . furnishes the principal topic of public interest." A subsequent investigation concluded that kindred diseases in Europe were associated with "ill-drained retentive soils in warm localities," and it was presumed that something in the Texas soil gave it a peculiar virulence.[2]

The Metropolitan Board of Health of New York, in cooperation with the Cattle Commissioners of New York State, sponsored a thorough inquiry. The U.S. Department of Agriculture also hired several investigators: Professor John Gamgee, an English veterinarian and expert on rinderpest, who happened to be in Chicago; John Shaw Billings, an authority on public health and later famous as a medical historian and founder of the Army Medical Library; and J.R. Dodge, Daniel E. Salmon and H.J. Detmers. Unsought and consistently inaccurate findings were also reported by Frank S. Billings (no relation to John S. Billings).

There was general agreement that any theory about the cause of Texas fever had to explain the following peculiarities: 1. The disease spread only during the warmer months. In winter the southern cattle were harmless. 2. The infection was not conveyed directly from southern to northern cattle, but *via* ground infected by north-bound migrants over which susceptible native animals later passed. 3. The incubation period ranged from ten to ninety days, with an average of four to six weeks. 4. Southern cattle lost their infectivity after several weeks on northern pastures, or after a prolonged drive. 5. Northern cattle with Texas fever apparently did not communicate the disease to other natives; sick mothers even failed to infect their calves. Nonetheless, its nature was perplexing, and its cause and transmission remained unknown, despite the several inquiries on the subject.

The *Gamgee Report* (1871). Gamgee accurately described the symptomatology of "splenic fever," comprising an enlarged spleen, high fever, hemoglobinuria ("red water"), marked anemia and weakness. Southern herds often carried a latent infection and "none but a trained expert, thermometer and scalpel in hand, can declare positively that any stock is in the enjoyment of perfect health." He emphasized the season incidence: "A few nipping frosts check its ravages." He scoffed at the "tick theory," which had "acquired quite a renown during the past summer; but a little thought should have satisfied anyone of the absurdity of the idea . . . There is not the slightest foundation for the view that the ticks disseminated the disease." A wood fence hardly restrained ticks, yet could effectively protect cattle from Texas fever. Besides, the malady might be absent from tick-infested regions, yet malignant in some localities where few or no ticks were apparent. Southern cattle fever was neither inoculable nor "propagated by the bites of insects." Gamgee postulated a toxic principle in the Texas soil, which permeated the wild grasses and water ingested by the regional cattle. Herds driven northward or westward excreted this agent, polluting the vegetation upon which non-immune cattle fed and thus contracted the disease. The cycle was broken when frosts killed the herbage. Gamgee, accompanied by the botanist H. W. Ravenal, was unable to find the source and nature of the toxic principle in Texas.[3]

The Dodge Report (1871). Dodge reviewed statistical and historical investigations into Texas cattle disease. He urged greater uniformity in the laws imposed by various states. In describing a Pennsylvania outbreak, he also dismissed the "tick theory."[4]

Salmon's Reports (1881–1883). Salmon's first report (1881) predicted that the agent must be a "living contagion," in view of the lengthy incubation period. He scorned the "tick theory" as "simply an evidence of the desire of the human mind to explain the origin of mysterious phenomena."

> The same principle is exhibited in the popular views regarding the pathogenic nature of *hollow-horn, hollow-tail, wolf-teeth, black-teeth, hooks,* etc., none of which have the least foundation in fact or reason. The tick theory scarcely explains a single one or the many peculiar phenomena of the disease . . . The *postmortem* examination plainly indicates the cause . . . to be an agent taken into the circulation, and causing the most important changes in the composition of the blood.[5]

For three years, beginning in November 1879, Salmon intermittently attempted to transmit Texas fever by injecting or drenching healthy animals with blood, bile, spleen pulp, urine, or fecal suspension from diseased cattle. He apparently succeeded with three out of five spleen-pulp inoculations. The victims showed micrococci in their spleen pulp, and a diplococcus culture was isolated from two such samples. Although no distinctive illness followed large inocula of the micrococci into six head of cattle, Salmon's 1883 report anticipated that "the diplococcus of the spleen is the true germ of the disease."[6] He also traced the northern boundary of the enzootic area, which followed roughly the 37th parallel of latitude. This line, extending about five miles westward annually, was plotted in his office, using data from farmers, livestock agents, and veterinarians. While the enzootic area corresponded with the habitat of the cattle tick, Salmon never suggested any such relationship until February 1893, ten years later, when he transmitted Smith and Kilborne's Texas fever *Bulletin No. 1* to the Secretary of Agriculture for publication.

Detmers's Reports (1881, 1885). In his first report (1881),[7] Detmers described the gross and microscopic postmortem lesions in Texas fever, as noted by him in 1880. He contended that the "pathogenic principle" was deposited in the saliva wherever southern cattle grazed, drank and slavered, rather than by feces or urine. Sections of the liver and spleen from infected animals showed a peculiar bacillus, similar to one present in infusions of decaying grasses from Texas hog-wallow land. Detmers likewise disparaged the "tick theory," despite numerous adherents among practical cattle men.[8]

Frank S. Billings (1888, 1892). Among other countrymen of Smith who championed a bacterial cause of Texas fever, the bellicose Frank S. Billings was the most obtrusive. In 1888, he claimed to have isolated the cultivable germ of southern cattle plague in Nebraska, and announced that "the sun of original investigation seems to be rising in the West."[9] According to him, tissues of affected cattle yielded an ovoid, pleomorphic, "belted" bacterium, which closely resembled his swine plague and yellow fever germs. The main source of infection with this bacillus was polluted grasses, whose infectivity was maintained from dried manure disseminated by cattle hooves.

In 1892, Billings published a further series of articles.[10] The first two parts continued his attacks upon Salmon, Smith, and the Swine Plague Commission. The last three installments alleged that Koch's postulates were "fulfilled in connection with the bacillus of the Southern Cattle Plague," and that cultures of this bacillus killed small laboratory animals as well as calves. Theobald Smith's final monograph on Texas fever (1893) dismissed all the findings of F.S. Billings in a single generalization: "In scientific research . . . it is incumbent upon the investigator to give . . . the details of his experiments, so that others may form an opinion . . . as to whether the work was properly done and the conclusions of inferences warranted." Any particular claim might be "safely left to the judgment of future workers in this field."[11]

Paul Paquin, at the Missouri Agricultural Experiment Station, found a germ resembling that of Billings in blood, bile and tissues from Texas fever fatalities, and also in samples of soil, water, fodder and excreta. His findings, with illustrations of this microorganism, appeared in a special bulletin from that Station in 1890.[12] Various microscopic particles interpreted by Paquin as protean forms of a single organism were viewed by Theobald Smith as merely blood, bile and liver debris.

About four years after the publication of Smith's monograph on Texas fever, a lengthy letter to the editor appeared in a livestock periodical. The author conceded, "Though I cannot possibly see the cause of any error in my own work, the tick-plasmodium theory of Dr. Smith must be accepted as correct, though it is still as incomprehensible to me as is the fact that my own work is erroneous." The letter came from Frank S. Billings, M.D., "Founder and Late Director of the Patho-Biological Laboratory, University of Nebraska," now of Grafton, Massachusetts.[13]

The New York State Cattle Commissioners' Report (1869). Before any of the foregoing reports appeared, Dr. R. Cresson Stiles, Deputy Registrar of the New York City Metropolitan Board of Health, described his postmortem findings of the cattle dying in the New York City area from Texas fever. Stiles reported his findings after examining specimens from the first animals to die of Texas cattle fever in a stockyard near Jersey City in the late summer of 1868, and they were subsequently published, together with the inquiry of the New York State Cattle Commissioners, in the state Agricultural Society's journal in 1869.[14] Dr. Stiles found that the kidneys "were deeply congested . . . and their glomeruli and tubuli uriniferi were filled with extravasated blood." The urine "was of a glutinous character, excessively albuminous . . . of a claret color, and contained a few casts." In the blood, "not a single red blood disk could be detected. The red disks had parted with their coloring matter and the serum was of a dark mahogany color."

In an amplified portion of the report, Stiles noted, "The red blood-corpuscles when examined immediately after removal from the body were shriveled and *crenated,* without artifial provocation." They looked "as if a circular piece had been punched out" . . . and "many of the discs appeared to have lost a portion of their substances. Some red cells disappeared like a light blown out." Unwittingly, Stiles had viewed the causal parasite. His critical observations, had he lived longer to pursue them, might have led to the earlier identification of the pathogenesis of the disease. Stiles developed a mental disorder in 1870, and died of pneumonia three years later.

The red cell abnormalities were attributed to the solvent action of bile from the invariably enlarged, congested, bile-injected, and fatty liver. Stiles dismissed the alternative hypothesis that an infective agent destroyed blood corpuscles, causing an accumulation of bile pigment in the blood, "beyond the capacity of the liver to remove it." In the bile of diseased cattle he observed micrococci, which developed into cryptococci in the laboratory. So he communicated with Prof. Ernst Hallier[15] of Jena, who believed that certain micrococci and cryptococci were "grades in the life of higher organisms." From a bile sample sent by Stiles from an infected beast, Hallier grew a previously unknown fungus, which he proposed to name *Coniothecium Stilesianum,* "in honor of the first discoverer." He urged Stiles to seek the natural habitat of this parasitical fungus among the cattle's plant food. J.S. Billings and Edward Curtis (1871) rejected the claims of Stiles and Hallier, and stressed the necessity of inoculating animals to determine the pathogenicity of a suspected microorganism.[16]

Although Theobald Smith informed Simon Gage on November 30, 1884 that "we shall soon attack the still unsolved mystery of Texas fever,"[17] he actually did not begin working on the disease until the beginning of September 1886, when two enlarged spleens from cows that had died in an outbreak at Hamilton, Virginia, arrived at the B.A.I. laboratory. One spleen yielded various bacterial cultures. The other, although bacteriologically sterile, showed "in or on many red

corpuscles . . . small round bodies, perhaps 1 μ in diameter, centrally or somewhat eccentrically situated." The bodies resembled micrococci in size and form;
unstained they appeared as "mere, transparent spaces in the corpuscles." Few
were found outside the red cells. This preliminary finding was not published until three years later, in December 1889, in *The Medical News*, where it was reported that "the disease must be due to a blood parasite."[18]

In September 1888, Cooper Curtice made field studies of an outbreak in
Carroll County, Maryland, which he described in the next *Annual Report* of the
B.A.I.[19] Although some animals were heavily tick-infested, he did not relate
these arthropods to the disease. Smith tried to cultivate bacteria from refriger-
ated blood, urine, spleen and kidney samples, since "in these days it is necessary
first to demonstrate the absence of bacteria before other results are credited."[20]
The condition of the blood elements was unsuitable for critical microscopy; but
Smith concluded from the histology of the liver, kidneys and spleen that the basic
disorder in Texas fever was destruction of the red blood cells, due either to absorption of a hemolytic agent, perhaps elaborated by intestinal bacteria, or
(more likely) to disintegration because of an intraglobular parasite.

If a blood parasite were involved, frequent microscopic studies of the blood
and absolutely fresh postmortem material would be essential. Hence, in 1888,
Smith proposed to Salmon that Texas fever should be produced at the Bureau's
Experiment Station. Smith's diary, after a five-year gap, bears witness that for almost four years, from February 5, 1889, when he began "Working on Texas
Fever notes and literature," until November 10, 1892, when the Texas Fever Report was completed, he dedicated himself to finding the causal agent and solving
the mechanism of transmission. Even on the day when Lilian underwent her first
difficult labor, with delivery by forceps, he was five hours at the laboratory, and
spent the following Sunday there "to make up for lost time."[21]

Late in June 1889, seven head of tick-infested cattle arrived in Washington
from North Carolina. They have been procured by Kilborne, on Salmon's authorization, and were held at the Experiment Station. Smith recorded in his diary
for Saturday, June 29: "Spent morning at Station examining the arrangements
for Texas cattle fever study." Four of the southern animals were segregated in an
enclosed pasture with thirteen native (northern) cattle. Of the latter, ten eventually died of Texas fever. They served for studies of the causal parasite.

Smith made blood counts for many hours daily at the Station—a tedious but
necessary task because mild or early infections were often detectable only
through a lowered red-cell count. During the first three weeks of August, feeling
"very tired and used up," he and Lilian took a seaside vacation, first at a small hotel on Nantucket Island close to the Wilder's summer home, and then at Sag
Harbor where they stayed with Howard and Celia Egleston at their farm. By the

time of their return, Texas fever was in full spate at the Station. The first animal died late in August. On Saturday, August 31, 1889, appeared this statement in Theobald's diary: "Quite hot—two postmortems of Texas fever at Station. Cause definitely established with microscope." The opposite page overflowed with a list of expenses incurred on his recent holiday. The total of $42.72 (for both of them) included haircut .35, hotel room 4.00, "not a/c for," 2.70.

A whole week was now devoted to weighing "arguments for and against the parasitic nature" of the intracellular bodies.[22] During the next month, he spent many hours at the laboratory studying the parasite microscopically and also at the Station examining cases before and after death. The cause of every fatality was verified at autopsy. Milder cases were revealed by frequent thermometry and by blood examinations for reduced cell counts and the presence of the characteristic parasite. In the evenings he perused the international literature on the formed elements of the blood.

By the end of October, nine additional animals succumbed. All of them revealed bodies which careful focusing showed to be definitely within the red blood cells. A single red cell might contain from one to four spherical, ovoid, or pear-shaped bodies, ranging in size from 0.5 to 2μ. When pyriform, they were generally in pairs. They were sparse in the circulating blood, presumably because of the filtering action of liver and spleen, which often contained large numbers of the parasite. He concluded that they might "belong to the group of sporozoa, some of which are pronounced cell parasites."

On a visit to Baltimore, Smith fascinated Welch with an account of the Texas fever parasite "over dinner at the Club." He was urged to unravel the mystery of its transmission.[23] At last, he reported his findings to the Annual Meeting of the American Public Health Association at the Brooklyn Institute on October 23, 1889.

> There is a continuous or paroxysmal destruction of red blood-corpuscles due to an intraglobular parasite, and the disease results mainly from the incapacity of the internal organs, primarily the liver, secondarily the spleen and kidneys, to transform and remove the waste products resulting from such destruction. In milder cases the protracted anaemia, which results from the loss of corpuscles, may become the chief cause of exhaustion and death.[24]

He cited R.C. Stiles as a preceding explorer, who assuredly "had before him the intra-globular bodies . . . At that stage of our knowledge it was entirely excusable for Dr. Stiles to pass these bodies by without further attention." He avoided discussing other former investigations of Texas fever, except to generalize that readily cultivable germs no doubt had "a *post-mortem* history . . . There seems to be nothing which literally breeds bacteria so rapidly as a dead body in midsummer." However, Smith mentioned in closing the work of Babes on epizootic hemoglobiunuria in Roumania, a disease having "many features in common with Texas fever, and many peculiar to itself."

In the summer of 1888, Victor Babes (1854–1926), a Roumanian bacteriologist, founder of the Institute of Pathology and Bacteriology in Bucharest, began to investigate hemoglobinuria of cattle, an enzootic disease prevalent in the Danubian marshlands of Roumania. As many as 50,000 oxen had succumbed in a single epizootic. At the end of October, the Académie des Sciences in Paris received his account of a bacterium which he considered the undoubted pathogenic agent. The microbe resembled the gonococcus, but its diplococcal elements were often linked at an angle by a filament. In the heart and great vessels the organisms might be "free, adhering to the red cells or even situated in their interior." The cocci were cultivable on nutrient media at body temperature. A variety of experimental animals remained well after being inoculated or fed either with disease products or with cultures of this microbe; but rabbits, treated likewise, developed a febrile, often mortal illness.[25]

A longer, illustrated report by Babes in German[26] stated that the hematococcus, which produced hemoglobinuria by penetrating and destroying the red blood cells, differed from previously known bacterial species. It had a saprophytic phase, during which it multiplied in puddles, thence reaching the bovine intestinal tract. Excessive stress, mucosal injury or digestive irregularities allowed the parasite to traverse the intestinal wall to adjacent lymph glands and eventually to the blood stream.

In his own preliminary report on the intraglobular parasite of Texas fever, Theobald Smith acknowledged the resemblances in Babes's description of the Roumanian cattle plague and its causal agent. However, he concluded that the two parasites were "quite different," since the Texas fever agent was not bacterial, was usually inside the red blood cells, and could not be cultivated on artificial media. Smith ended his first report on the protozoon of Texas fever with a clumsily worded but prophetic allusion to Babes's work: "Inasmuch as both his and our investigations must be regarded as just begun, the future will have to decide how near of kin these two diseases are."[27]

As winter approached, the Station cattle exposed to Texas fever were affected less severely. The animals no longer succumbed to an acute disease, "characterized by the sudden enormous destruction of corpuscles," whose waste products "clog up the liver, disintegrate the spleen, and lastly pass out unchanged through the kidneys, producing the 'red water'." Instead there was only moderate red-cell destruction, and the resulting anaemia gradually disappeared. Practically symptomless animals might carry the infection, although intraglobular parasites might not be found in their circulating blood. In such cases, the diagnosis of suspected Texas fever might be clinched by demonstrating the parasite in the spleen or liver tissue post-mortem, or by a low red-cell count during life. These conclusions appeared under Smith's name in a section headed "Investigations of Infectious Animal Diseases" in the Secretary of Agriculture's *Annual Report* for 1889.[28]

Kilborne's initial importation of the southern cattle was supplemented by another nine head in September 1889, and by further shipments from North Carolina and Texas in the summer of 1890. This reservoir of partially immune animals at the Station would ensure enough induced cases of Texas fever to confirm Smith's observations on the intraglobular parasite, as well as to facilitate solution of the interlinked problem of transmission. He wrote to Gage: "I have no doubt that I shall confirm my work this summer . . . If then I can have it go under my own name I shall consider myself fortunate."[29]

By the end of the summer of 1891, Theobald's observations on the potential extent of red-cell destruction covered sixty cases of Texas fever and many control animals. During these two summer seasons he determined that up to one million cells per c.mm., or about one-sixth the total number, might be destroyed in acute, fatal cases. The red cells generated to replace the destroyed cells showed abnormalities which might be related to or mistaken for the intraglobular parasite. Hence he investigated red cell morphology in sheep made severely anemic by venesection. In his published report,[30] Smith punctiliously acknowledged that Kilborne took the blood samples, while E.C. Schroeder, a veterinarian recently added to the Station staff, relieved him of many of the tiresome corpuscle counts. Smith concluded that whatever the cause of the severe anemia, embryonic red cells appeared in the circulation in a definite sequence: 1. Macrocytes (simple enlargement of the cells); 2. Macrocytes containing stainable granules, later diffusely staining macrocytes; 3. Hematoblasts (nucleated red cells). Such embryonic or transitional erythrocytes appeared early in mild cases of Texas fever, or after severe blood loss in otherwise healthy animals. He was invited to present these findings in 1891 to the Association of American Physicians.

Despite unbearably hot weather in Washington throughout the meeting (September 22–25), Smith rated his paper as "Quite successful." William Welch officially commented that "Dr. Smith's admirable contribution" illustrated the unity of comparative and human medicine.

> As Virchow long ago has said, the diseases of animals and those of man are of equal scientific interest, the only difference being in the dignity of the subject of the disease. Dr. Smith has not solicited discussion on the etiology of Texas fever, but

those familiar with the subject know that his discovery of a protozooid parasite in the red blood-corpuscles of the subjects of this disease, analogous to the malarial parasite, is of the highest importance.[31]

The Association elected him to membership. After the 1892 meeting, Welch wrote to him: "We have now got in the Association a number of good men interested in bacteriology and hygiene . . . I hope that you will publish under your own name a full monograph on Texas fever. I regard this as an extremely important contribution."[32]

In his final "full monograph," Smith detailed the morphology, intraglobular "movement," and tissue distribution of the parasite, and discussed the coccoid, amoeboid and pyriform shapes assumed by it during its developmental cycle. Comparisons with other erythrocytic parasites of man and animals led him to conclude that here was a new genus. He named it *Pyrosoma bigeminum, n.sp.,* from the Latin *pyrum,* pear, the *bigeminum* referring to "the peculiar character which this organism has of appearing in pairs within the red blood corpuscles."[33]

His observations on the parasite were incorporated in two sections, headed respectively, "History of the Microorganism in the Body of Cattle" and "Probable Action of the Microorganism in the Body of Susceptible Animals." Of these, the latter has stood the test of time; but the uncertainties of the other section persisted until most parasitologists conceded that the stainable "peripheral coccus-like bodies" associated with some red cells signified a double infection with *B. bigeminum* and *Anaplasma marginale.* Smith himself anticipated this possibility. In his view, these bodies probably represented a stage in the life cycle of *Pyrosoma bigeminum,* but admittedly "we have still the question before us whether they are stages of the Texas fever parasite or of another parasite transmitted with it."[34] Smith's generic term turned out to be invalid, for *Pyrosoma* was assigned already to an ascidian (*Ascidium:* a genus of molluscs, including the sea-squirts). W.H. Patton proposed in 1895 that *Piroplasma* be substituted for *Pyrosoma.*[35] This change was accepted widely, particularly in North America. But Victor Babes and his son Mircea, and their supporters, had other designs.

Babes's initial papers on hemoglobinuria of cattle termed the causal microbe a bacterium. In 1890, having read Theobald Smith's 1889 report, he modified his views: "This is a special organism, whose place in microbic classification is not well established."[36] In August 1892, he stated that his previously reported parasite was analogous to that causing "Texas fever, subsequently described by Theobald Smith." The microbe should be put in an intermediate group of "hematococci" of epizootic hemoglobinuria and of Texas fever, augmented by another of "these curious parasites" discovered by him to cause *Carceag,* a disease liable to attack sheep that migrated to the marshy areas of the lower Danube. Although the disease was similar to cattle fever, he could not cultivate this particular hematococcus.

Soon after Smith's Texas fever monograph appeared, an address by Babes to the Roumanian Academy included the following translated passage:

> Based on my research, Dr. Theobald Smith followed up the story of the Texas fever and established again that the sickness is produced by my parasite, but classifies it among the protozoa . . . By discovering the parasite, I have established not only the cause of the sickness of our animals, but also the phylogenetic tie—unknown until now—which exists between bacteria and protozoa. I have also given the impulse for the discovery of the cause of the most dreadful disease of animals in America.[37]

Smith's Texas fever discoveries were neither initiated by nor based on the writings of Babes. According to Smith's 1889 report, he observed the intraglobular parasite of Texas fever at his first scientific encounter with the disease in 1886, two years before Babes began his investigation of hemoglobinuria in Danubian cattle. But while the former kept aloof and had no champion among his associates, Babes' claims were energetically promoted. The veterinarian C. Starcovici, Assistant to the State Commission appointed to investigate hemoglobinuria, asserted in July 1893 that Babes had discovered the peculiar blood-cell parasite (or three closely related varieties thereof) responsible for epizootic hemoglobinuria, Texas fever, and *Carceag.* He advocated the name *"Babesia"* for this genus, to comprise Smith's *Pyrosoma bigeminum,* as well as the two other parasites which Babes had first described, *Babesia bovis* and *Babesia ovis.* Since their characteristics "differ so markedly from those of known protozoa, and resemble so much those of bacteria," it was proposed to place the Babesia in the "lowest grade of protozoa," immediately above the bacteria.[38]

Nationalistic and familial loyalties of Roumanian origin probably influenced the delegates to various committees on taxonomy, including protozoal nomenclature, in the second half of the twentieth century. Their recommendations helped to give the designations *Babesia* and "babesiosis" the sanction of increasing usage, so that these terms have largely supplanted *Piroplasma* and "piroplasmosis."[39] Consequently some credit may have been diverted from work of superior quality—though with less distortion of the truth than in the case of *Salmonella* and "salmonellosis."

Smith surmised that the "redwater" of cattle observed at the Cape of Good Hope over twenty years earlier, the Roumanian bovine hemoglobinuria of Babes, and possibly the "Tschichir" affecting Caucasian cattle, were all equivalents of Texas fever.[40] In 1897, Robert Koch found the coastal cattle in East Africa afflicted with a disease resembling Texas fever. He observed erythrocytic parasites and considered them young forms of *Piroplasma bigemina.* In 1903 he identified "Rhodesian redwater" in Bulawayo as "East Coast fever," but later agreed with Theiler[41] that a different piroplasmic species was involved. Koch's basic knowledge of Texas fever dated from personal contact with Smith when the latter visited Berlin in 1896, and also from the condensed account in German[42] which Theobald Smith summarized from the original monograph. Other domestic animals such as sheep, goats, swine, dogs, and cats, as well as various wild ruminants and rodents, are liable to babesiosis. The total of about twenty recognized *Babesia* species probably will increase. Nor should current taxonomy be regarded as final.

Despite the analogies which led Theobald Smith to refer to Texas fever as cattle malaria, human babesiosis was first recorded as such only in 1956 when *B. bovis* was found to be the cause of anemia, jaundice and hemoglobinuria in a splenectomized Jugoslav farmer. Since then a few other cases have been reported in patients without spleen, including a fatal case due to *B. divergens.*[43] Beginning in 1970, *B. microti,* a rodent piroplasm conveyed by the tick *Ixodes scapularis,* was responsible for outbreaks among previously healthy vacationers on Nantucket Island, some thirty miles south of Cape Cod, Massachusetts.[44]

Theobald Smith expressed no fears of infection in persons intimately exposed to the Texas fever parasite. Yet, a comment in his diary possibly signifies such a case in a close colleague. In December 1892, Smith and Schroeder went to Ames, Iowa, to visit Veranus Moore and Kilborne, who had been studying the mysterious "cornstalk disease" of cattle. They found "Dr. Moore very sick ex[amined] blood and found intra-glob. parasites." They departed after six days, leaving behind "Dr. Moore but little better."[45] Three years later, in 1895, Smith recorded having "for the first time" personally identified *Plasmodium vivax* in a blood film made near Boston; thus, Moore's intraglobular parasites may have been associated with an attack of acute babesiosis.

In 1893, soon after publication of the Texas fever monograph, Smith, Kilborne and Schroeder recorded further observations on the disease. Their article described persistence of the microparasite in the blood of a southern cow sheltered from all sources of Texas fever infection for more than three years after it had left the enzootic area. Small numbers of the parasite were observed also in the blood of a native animal which had been inoculated, with consequent Texas fever, nearly one year previously. This animal proved insusceptible to reinfection, foreshadowing the development of a simple method of preventive inoculation.[46]

Smith considered it essential to seek some method of prevention through immunization, even although since "a single attack of the disease itself does not afford complete protection it is not likely that any process or method of artificial inoculation will be successful in this respect." He urged further research on that type of non-sterile partial immunity often termed "premunity." Babesicidal drugs are now available for controlling the disease induced by inoculating infected blood in the "premunition" of young stock. Even more promising as a preventive measure is the active immunization of cattle by means of antigens prepared from *B. bovis* cultures, using similar methods to those adopted for *Plamodium falciparum*.[47]

For the transmission experiments, most of the B.A.I. farm was divided into several enclosed "fields." Theobald Smith consulted Kilborne about the size and purpose of these enclosures; but otherwise, with one exception, took the initiative in all aspects of the project. Smith was initially skeptical about the tick's role in Texas fever, although he never committed this opinion to print. He acknowledged that Kilborne "during the summer of 1889 . . . in arranging the various enclosures at the Experiment Station for the exposure of native cattle to the infection of Texas fever, conceived the happy idea of testing this popular theory of the relation of ticks to the disease."[48] Seven head of cattle, all tick-infested, reached Washington from North Carolina near the end of June. Four animals were segregated in a field with thirteen native (Northern) cattle, of which ten died of Texas fever. Four native animals, exposed in a separate field to three deticked southern cattle, remained healthy.

Through a second shipment of nine southern cattle in mid-September, the foregoing results were confirmed. Further, several thousand ticks collected around New Berne, North Carolina, were scattered by Kilborne over a hitherto unused enclosure. Three of four native cattle exposed thereto contracted Texas fever. Smith concluded from these 1889 experiments that "a field must be infected with ticks before Texas fever appeared among natives;" but the mode or vehicle of operation remained a mystery. Feeding a heifer with grass from an infected field did not pass on the infection. From 1890 to 1892, Smith devised experiments to illuminate this question.

He observed that under natural conditions the cattle tick (*Boophilus bovis*) failed to survive the winter, for native cattle pastured in a field infected the previous summer remained tick-free and healthy. The mortality rate in older, naturally-exposed cattle might reach 80 percent, while similarly-exposed calves had relatively mild attacks. Smith noted, besides, that all animals which succumbed had young ticks on them, and that the incubation period of fifteen to sixty-four days was shortest when young ticks appeared promptly on the cattle.

Crucial to elucidation of the problem was his discovery that adult female ticks laid eggs even if confined in bottles. Such eggs, kept warm in a covered glass dish with a little soil or moistened leaves, hatched larvae within three to four weeks.

When these larvae were attached to a host's hide, they developed normally, with a cycle of two molts and an intervening nymphal stage. Texas fever was produced thus in native cattle in late summer by laboratory-hatched larval ticks originating from North Carolina stock, and likewise even in mid-winter in a heated stable—thus illustrating that Texas fever was transmissible in any season provided the temperature was warm enough for the cattle tick to remain active.

The probability that young ticks transmitted the disease through the hide into the blood stream was strengthened by the following experiments. Heifers remained well after being fed with 2,000 live adult ticks, or several thousand young ticks and egg cases; or after pasturing on a field containing blood and spleen pulp from fatal cases of Texas fever. By contrast, the disease was transmitted to healthy cattle, with multiplication of the parasite in the new hosts, by small subcutaneous or intravenous inoculations of blood from a diseased animal. Inoculations into sheep, rabbits, guinea-pigs, and pigeons produced no ill effects. By the end of November 1890, Smith could state for the *Annual Report* of the B.A.I. that young ticks produced Texas fever. However, his knowledge of the parasite's life history was incomplete and baffling. He attempted unsuccessfully to infect cattle by intravenous injection of crushed young ticks from artificially-hatched lots of known activity.

In the summer of 1891, experiments were repeated and earlier findings confirmed. One native cow, exposed to southern animals but removed from the enclosure before young ticks appeared, remained unaffected. Two native animals, placed nearly three weeks apart in the same field, acquired the disease and died within a day of each other, illustrating that the infectivity of the field depended on the hatching of the young ticks twenty to twenty-five days after southern cattle had pastured on it. Finally, to verify his conviction that all tick-infested southern cattle were dangerous, whether sick or healthy, Smith demonstrated the presence of the microparasite in the circulating blood of apparently healthy southern cattle. Six native cattle each received intravenously 28 cc of blood drawn from one of three cows that left southern pastures up to seventy-four days before; all developed Texas fever.

Eventually, the field experiments extended over the four summers of 1889 to 1892. By then all crucial findings had been verified, discrepant results rectified, and residual doubts swept away. Every such experiment was supplemented by multiple laboratory tests, especially blood film microscopy, upon which specific evidence of infection depended. But the development and fate of the parasite in the tick remained elusive. Within a month of his discovery of the parasite in August 1889, Smith already considered ticks as possible vectors and began to investigate them microscopically. Even before delivering his paper on the protozoon, he recorded "looking on stray cases of h. chol. from Va. and Md. Also on Texas

fever, contents of ticks and healthy blood. Reading on blood platelets and formation of red blood corpuscles."[49] In July 1890, a diary entry read: "Probably discovery of Texas fever parasite in tick eggs this afternoon. Mrs. Egleston returns
fr. North. Finished reading Lorna Doone this week. Using hose on grass almost
every evening."[50]

About that time, the twenty-year old David Fairchild, who became a distinguished botanist, was quartered near Theobald Smith's laboratory under the
mansard roof. Almost half a century later, he wrote to the widowed Lilian
Smith:

> It was late! I was the only worker about the building except Theobald Smith, and I
> was surprised to have him walk into my laboratory and ask me if I wouldn't like to
> see the organism of Texas cattle fever in the blood of a tick. He was in the first ex-
> citing moments of his discovery and spoke brilliantly of it and its bearing upon the
> transmission of blood-infecting parasites. Of course I was thrilled! It was the first
> time that I had been in the presence—actual presence—of an epoch-making dis-
> covery.[51]

This experience influenced Fairchild's whole scientific life. He repeated the
story in his autobiography, contrasting Smith with the "fossils" represented by
other employees of the Department of Agriculture—though now the parasite
was said to have been discovered "in a drop of steer's blood . . . taken from a cattle tick."[52] That preliminary confidence was not fulfilled in Smith's later microscopic examination of "the contents of the bodies of ticks in various stages of
growth." The search was obscured by the many particles "resulting from the
breaking up of the ingested corpuscles. The very minute size of the microorganism renders its identification well-nigh impossible, and any attempt will be
fraught with great difficulties."[53]

In 1906, Koch attempted without success to follow the various developmental
phases of *Babesia bigemina* in the gut of replete cattle ticks. Dennis first demonstrated the sexual cycle of *B. bigemina* in *Boophilus bovis* in 1932. He contended
that because *B. bovis* was attached to a single host for life, its protozoal parasite
could be transferred only through the tick's offspring. "The extremely intimate
relationship of the digestive tract and the reproductive organs makes it almost a
foregone conclusion that any parasites leaving the gut . . . will . . . occupy the
ova."[54] According to Riek, parasites ingested early during engorgement appear
to be destroyed, whereas in replete female ticks the bovine blood may display
extracellular parasites and parasitized erythrocytes.[55] Fairchild's reference to being shown the parasite in a drop of steer's blood taken from a cattle tick may thus
be reconciled with Smith's later uncertainties about identifying the parasite
within the tick.

Early in May 1892, a diary entry signalled the beginning of Theobald Smith's monograph, *Investigations into . . . Texas, or Southern Cattle Fever*. At the beginning of June, he packed up his family, including "three trunks and a baby carriage [and] Ella the servant,"[56] and took a steamboat for Old Point, Virginia, where they settled into a small cottage on the shores of Hampton Roads. He wrote steadily every day. "If I were not so busy with the Texas fever report I would like to be a real out-door naturalist for a while."[57] After three weeks the Egleston parents arrived. He returned to Washington, "running about for an obstetrician for Aug."[58] before resuming work on the report at Hampton. They returned to an "extremely hot" Washington in mid-July. At the Station, the last batch of Texas fever experiments was launched. On August 21, their daughter Lilian was born. Theobald's activities were undiminished. He relaxed only on Sundays, when he took Dolly on cable-car excursions to Mount Pleasant, and once rode with her "on the new Rock Creek electric road" as far as Chevy Chase.[59]

During September and October, several hours daily and all his evenings were devoted to the Texas Fever report. At last it was completed and handed in— "638 pages quarto typewritten."[60] In his Letter of Submittal, dated November 15, 1892, Smith outlined the contributions of his colleagues. Kilborne carried out "the planning and arranging of the field experiments in general and those relating to the cattle ticks in particular." Schroeder was mostly responsible for the red blood cell estimations and later assisted with autopsies. Smith himself handled "that part of the work dealing with the intimate nature of the disease, its pathology and etiology, and the microscopical and bacteriological work involved in their elucidations."

Early in 1893, Theobald Smith began six weeks of proof-reading and completed a report on the etiology of Texas fever for the *Centralblatt für Bakteriologie*.[61] Toward the end of March the diary laconically declared: "Report on Texas Cattle Fever issued . . . beginning to be distributed."[62] The title page was headed "U.S. Department of Agriculture. Bureau of Animal Industry. Bulletin No. 1." Beneath this, Salmon had freely exercised his prerogatives. The "Investigations" were defined as "Made under the direction of Dr. D.E. Salmon, Chief of the Bureau of Animal Industry." The term "Texas Fever" in the main title was replaced by "Texas or Southern Cattle Fever," despite Smith's preference for the former, as explicitly indicated in his (unpublished) Letter of Submittal; and F.L. Kilborne appeared as coauthor. Curtice later volunteered that "Dr. Smith wrote the entire work . . . To my surprise (and I believe to Dr. Smith's) Dr. Kilborne was made co-author, an injustice to Dr. Smith that should not have been allowed."[63]

B.A.I. *Bulletin No. 1*, welcomed by Welch and hailed by Gage as "this monumental piece of work,"[64] was ascribed in due course by George W. Corner as "one of the classics of modern biology . . . clear in style, vivid in detail, telling a great story of successful research."[65] But very soon it was the focus of an unseemly scramble for credit. Salmon's Letter of Transmittal to the Secretary of Agriculture, dated February 6, 1893, emphasized his own antecedent observation that the infected cattle zone corresponded with the natural distribution of the tick. "This led to the experiments which demonstrated that ticks carried the infection."[66] Conveniently forgotten was his own previous contention that "the tick theory scarcely explains a single one of the many peculiar phenomena of the disease."[67]

Smith made no public protest at any time, but early in 1903 he requested Curtice for Kilborne's postal address. He wished to ascertain whether or not Salmon had ordered Kilborne to start work on Texas fever. Secretary of Agriculture James Wilson, in a recent lecture at Boston, had named "Salmon as the Texas fever discoverer and pointed out its influence on yellow fever, etc." Smith complained to Curtice that "Dr. Salmon is making efforts to establish his claim to the discovery of the tick as transmitter . . . In 15 or 20 years after the event Salmon will have swallowed up everything."[68] Curtice replied that Smith's monograph had given Kilborne "entirely too much credit for original work done." He cast doubts upon the dependability of Kilborne's account: "You must remember that K's interests are bound up with Doctor Salmon's, that both are Masons and that you will get a version from their standpoint."[69]

In Senator Wilson's audience was Austin Peters, a senior veterinarian, who became one of Theobald Smith's staunchest friends and supporters in Massachusetts. Peters expressed surprise at Wilson's reference to Salmon as discoverer of the tick-borne nature of Texas fever. Surely, he urged, "the scientist who did this work or the greater part of it, is Dr. Theobald Smith."[70] In reply, the Acting Secretary bluntly asserted that Kilborne had made the discovery, under his Chief's "specific directions."[71]

Thirty years later, in a long retrospective letter to Gage about the Texas fever work, Theobald Smith dismissed Salmon's and Kilborne's research contributions in two scornful paragraphs:

> Salmon wished to be executive & scientist at the same time, so he had his name put on the title page. His only contribution to the whole work was a "micrococcus" when he worked in North Carolina, and I still remember the disappointment that came over him when I first showed him the intraglobular parasite. That ended his connection with the whole 4 years of very trying work.
>
> When the cattle were first brot [sic] up from N. Carolina, Kilborne picked the ticks off the Southern animals & threw them into a field for exposure to the Northern animals . . . I asked Kilborne why he did this without consulting me. He

said that he had read in agric. papers that ticks were the cause . . . Kilborne was put on the title page as co-author on account of the first expt. That gave him ample credit . . . for he did nothing beyond this.[72]

During the decade that followed publication of *Bulletin No. 1,* Salmon repeatedly claimed that he had instructed Kilborne to start the cattle tick experiments.[73] Salmon argued that since these experiments were conducted despite Smith's objections to the tick theory, "to Dr. Kilborne" (acting on his orders) "should be given the credit of carrying out these investigations." However, according to Smith, when he started his investigations, although "Nothing was known of the nature of the disease . . . [in] the very first cases . . . the existence of blood parasites naturally suggested some ectoparasite to draw them out."

> Kilborne's tick expt. helped the work forward a year . . . Thereafter Kilborne had . . . [only] to buy cows & have the temp. taken. I doubt that he looked into a microscope. The entire work fell on me. The final expt of breeding & putting the young ticks on cattle I did myself . . . After it had been shown that disease failed without ticks, everything was still to be done . . . To say that a protozoon parasite passed from old to young ticks through the egg & then into the mouth parts required *some* proof before it could be accepted *at that time.*[74]

Smith agreed that Kilborne "was faithful to his work and did what he was told [but] he was not always careful, for we lost a whole year when ticks were washed from one field into another." While defective isolation arrangements could be tolerated, Smith was angered by the rumor that he had compiled *Bulletin No. 1* from notes handed him by Kilborne—"following 4 years of slavery at the microscope, at autopsy, at watching tick broods, at the long labor of preparing the report while others looked on over my shoulders . . . God save the mark."[75]

In March 1936, fifteen months after Theobald Smith had died, Kilborne recounted his own version of these events. Although long retired from veterinary practice, he now recollected clearly being in the chief's office in June 1889. His three pages of single-spaced typing were accompanied by a shaky handwritten note of reassurance to the reader: "My conversations with Dr. Salmon on starting the Expts. are as vivid in my mind as if it were last month, so that I can recall almost the exact words used." Salmon had said: "I wish you and Dr. Smith would start some experiments on Texas fever."

> I asked him, "Along what line would you suggest, Doctor." His reply was, "I do not know. You and Dr. Smith will have to work them out" . . . It is hardly fair to Dr. Smith to say that the experiments were planned over his protest. While he did not believe in the tick theory (who did) and thought I was giving too much

prominence to the tick, which I intended to do, we planned the experiments together . . . .

Dr. Smith . . . was then Bacteriologist and Microscopist, and to him belongs the credit of the discovery of the parasite in Texas fever patients. As Veterinarian and Director of the Veterinary Experiment Station of the B.A.I., the planning and carrying out of the experiments, the operations and autopsies fell on me. As the first tick experiments were planned by myself, I claim the credit of the discovery that the tick was the cause of or the carrier of the parasite of Texas fever."[76]

Kilborne had responded straightforwardly to a request from Hubert Schmidt of the Division of Veterinary Science, A. and M. (Agricultural and Mechanical) College of Texas. That institution had been invited to prepare an exhibit on Texas fever and the cattle tick for the Texas Centennial Celebrations in Dallas during the summer of 1936. Schmidt was Acting Chairman of the organizing committee for this exhibit, and sought to provoke Kilborne to some startling revelations, saying, "I am sure that you . . . deserve much more credit than Smith does."[77] No doubt the old man exaggerated his own part, but he did not denigrate Theobald Smith.

The official linking of Kilborne's name with the tick experiments may have spoiled Theobald Smith's Nobel Prize candidacy for these investigations. When his name was submitted for the 1925 Nobel Prize for Physiology and Medicine, the Committee admitted the "similarity to malaria" displayed by Texas fever; agreed that the specific agent was a protozoon identified by Smith more than ten years before Ross reported his findings from India; and considered it likely that these discoveries "had an encouraging effect on Manson, Ross and others." Yet no award was made to Smith. "The Nobel Committee examiner found that the work on Texas fever deserved a prize," one commentator has observed, but speculated that "the Committee objected, possibly because Kilbourne [sic] had not been included in the nomination."[78]

In 1901, Curtice claimed that he and Kilborne together planned the 1889 tick experiment, and that early in 1890 Salmon authorized him to test the effect of applying artificially-hatched ticks to native cattle,[79] leading him to conclude that "I should have had a larger credit for my part in it."[80] However, these crucial transmission experiments were carried out by Smith himself in 1890, possibly with Kilborne's assistance, while Curtice took summer leave to collect fossils for the Geological Survey. Curtice admitted[81] that his work on the "history of the tick" was initiated by Theobald Smith's observation (as early as October 1889) that adult female ticks would lay their eggs even when confined in glass receptacles. Smith passed the specimens on to Curtice, and they furnished the starting point of the latter's work on the life cycle of *Boophilus bovis*. After the larvae hatched, Curtice placed them on a stabled calf at the Station and observed their three-stage development to adult ticks, which he reported to the Biological Society of Washington on February 3, 1890. This paper was discussed by Prof. C.V. Riley (who had first described the cattle tick in 1868) and also by Theobald Smith.

In later years Curtice asserted that "Experiment No. 12"—proving the percutaneous infectivity of laboratory-hatched young ticks—stemmed from a proposal made by him during this discussion. "Drs. Kilborne and Curtice (Veterinarians) placed themselves as willing to investigate and Drs. Salmon and Smith as believing the quest an idle one."[82] That story is inaccurate. The meeting Curtice referred to was actually on November 30, 1889, when Salmon made "General Remarks on Texas Fever," followed by Smith on "The Microorganisms of Texas Fever." Both papers were discussed by Prof. Riley and Drs. Curtice, Salmon and Smith.[83] Smith and Kilborne knew already that cattle ticks must be present in a field for Texas fever to be transmitted, a fact of which Salmon surely was also aware. The proposition that Salmon and Smith vetoed the quest as irrelevant therefore seems absurd.

Curtice's report on the life cycle of the cattle tick appeared in July 1891, three months after he left the Bureau. He had inserted a paragraph about his proposal to place young ticks on Northern cattle. Although Salmon's sanction for these experiments had been obtained,[84] others carried them out since Curtice was away that summer. In 1903, Curtice complained to Smith: "I feel that Dr. Salmon did me out of my share, that which belonged to the tick work . . . it is one of the reasons that led up to my leaving the department of agriculture."[85] To that Smith replied:[86]

> I am voicing a unanimous opinion and precept among scientists that the one who first successfully demonstrates, especially by new methods, a new fact, is entitled to the credit of such discovery or demonstration. This is the case with malaria today. I worked on the mosquito theory since 1896 here in Mass[achusetts] but I should not think of claiming Ross's credit for 1898 . . . I regret that the report did not state that you had believed the transfer [of Texas fever] occurs through the bite of the young tick . . . But . . . the world would not pay attention . . . because where would the stimulus and credit for the active worker come from who felt his territory preempted but not occupied?

Smith emphasized that such questions demanded experimentation rather than mere discussion, "for the migration of the blood parasite from one cow to another through the young [ticks] could hardly have been conceived biologically until the proof forced it upon me. It took over 5 years for Europe to even believe the fact."

Within two years of resigning from the Bureau in April 1891, Curtice applied for Salmon's job, forecast to become vacant.[87] But Salmon weathered the storm created by establishment of the two-year National Veterinary College in Washington. Curtice set up private practice in Moravia, New York, and became a part-time inspector under the New York State Board of Health. He was reinstated in the Bureau of Animal Industry as Livestock Agent in September 1894 and remained there for two years. Subsequently he held a variety of positions, many connected with a tick eradication program, until his retirement in 1930.

In the earlier years, Theobald Smith wanted to be friendly and helpful to his former colleague and roommate. "I am trying to keep him from starting quarrels for his own sake," he wrote to Gage in 1894. "He has 5 little ones to support."[88] Two years later, Smith urged Gage to find a job for Curtice at Cornell. Many disappointments had "warped him a little, but I believe in proper environment that would wear off."[89] Ultimately, Smith grew resentful of Curtice's unreliability, and in his last assessment dismissed him as "a rolling stone [who] did nothing as a scientist after he left the B.A.I." Moreover, "he always had a bad tongue besides rationalizing while I was working." Smith's impatience increased with Curtice's obsession to secure more recognition for his involvement in the Texas fever researches. "He got all the credit belonging to him. The relation of the young tick to the disease he had nothing to do with. He put them on cattle to watch their development. I presume he may have produced disease, but he did not know how to diagnose mild attacks."[90]

By contrast, Curtice ascribed his resignation from the B.A.I. to an inherent incompatibility between himself and Smith, "whom I had learned to know had the artist's temperament." Writing some thirty years after that event, Curtice blamed it on "Dr. Salmon's reorganization—placing my Animal parasite work under the Supervision of Dr. Smith . . . I could live with him without friction as an equal but was unwilling to work under him . . . Besides it irked me to confine myself steadily to the details of his work."[91]

W.A. Hagan, a staff member of the New York State Veterinary College of Cornell University since 1916, and Dean of the College from 1932 to 1959, discussed the Texas fever issues several times with Kilborne, Curtice, Moore, and Smith himself. He expressed his views of the situation thus:

> I know perfectly well that the story told by Fred Kilbourne [sic] on the tick matter differs considerably from that told by Smith. I have talked with Kilbourne at various times, also with Cooper Curtice . . . V.A. Moore . . . as well as with Smith

himself. The composite that I get is that Smith was quite reluctant to believe the tick transmission story [at first] . . . Knowing all the men concerned rather well . . . I am sure that he [Smith] supplied the brains for the outfit . . . I feel quite confident that Smith has not received more credit than he deserves in the matter.[92]

More than "brains" were needed to unveil the Texas fever mysteries and also to cope with Salmon's machinations, Kilborne's artless casualness, and Curtice's paranoidal pretensions. The Texas fever monograph displayed the antitheses of those qualities—modest skepticism, painstaking methodology, carefully planned experiments, and full verification of all findings, its author's hallmarks. Assuredly, Smith deserved more credit than he received. But his attitude toward the veterinary profession had aroused antagonisms.

As Smith declared to Gage in 1886, he lacked sympathy with veterinary medicine or practical agriculture, and made no attempt to conceal his leanings toward human medicine and hygiene.[93] Nevertheless, in 1892 he joined veterinary colleagues in attending monthly dinners organized by the Department of Agriculture Club and became a member of the United States (later American) Veterinary Medical Association. He soon became chairman of the Committee on Diseases—a committee which he recommended should be abolished—and in 1897 was elected to honorary membership in the association. Yet he kept quiet about this affiliation.

Paul de Kruif, a former research worker at the Rockefeller Institute for Medical Research in New York, published an article in 1926 in *The Country Gentleman* entitled "Theobald Smith and the Texas-Fever Tick." This reappeared later that year as "Theobald Smith: Ticks and Texas Fever" in the best seller, *Microbe Hunters*.[94] The article was based on two interviews with Smith in 1925, who apparently underestimated de Kruif's bias toward sensationalism, and merely urged de Kruif to be "objective."[95] The Texas fever story was dressed up in a fashion that riled many veterinarians and some parasitologists.

In 1933, the American Veterinary Medical Association awarded gold medals to Cooper Curtice and Fred L. Kilborne, "In recognition for their outstanding accomplishment of demonstrating for the first time, in collaboration with Salmon and Smith, that a microbial disease can be transmitted exclusively by an insect carrier or host." This was a deliberate effort to recompense Kilborne and Curtice for their contributions and entailed a gross miscarriage of justice to Theobald Smith. Curtice attended the presentation ceremony in August 1933, but Kilborne was too unwell to go. In 1894, he had left the Bureau of Animal Industry and in 1900 set up his life-time business as a hardware merchant in Kellogsville, New York, where he became a Justice of the Peace and a leading citizen. According to his daughter, "The whole village was proud of that medal, and anyone who wanted to see it, was welcome to."[96]

Fortunately, Theobald Smith had powerful supporters. His Texas fever efforts culminated in an address before the Association of American Physicians at the end of May 1893. As soon as the proof-reading of *Bulletin No. 1* was completed in mid-February, he began to prepare for that meeting a tentative outline of the life cycle of the microparasite; a review of the special changes induced in the blood of the infected cattle; and a discussion of the immunological peculiarity whereby "animals from the enzootic territory may scatter the seeds of a fatal disease without becoming victims themselves." The modification of the disease, apparently due to progressive immunity, "has an important bearing on the interpretation of irregular malarial fevers."[97] Although he did not know how or in what form "the micro-parasite passes from the old to the young tick . . . the agency of parasites in transferring the microbes of protozoan diseases should henceforth receive more attention." At the end of the actual paper, as sole discussant, Welch remarked that "The etiology of Texas cattle fever has become . . . probably clearer than that of any other protozoan disease . . . Dr. Smith is to be congratulated upon such an important contribution to science."

William Osler, another of Smith's admirers who was also present at the meeting, deferred his tribute; but he would have agreed with the appraisal of his own biographer written many years later:

> The most notable contribution was made by Theobald Smith on "Texas Cattle Fever" . . . One wonders whether the great significance of the discovery, which was to be followed by a succession of others—the mosquito in malaria and yellow fever, the tsetse fly in sleeping sickness, the flea in plague, the louse in typhus—could then have been fully taken in by the majority of Theobald Smith's auditors.[98]

In 1895, Osler spoke on "The Practical Value of Laveran's Discoveries" before the Medical Society of the District of Columbia. He referred to "the really brilliant discovery by Theobald Smith of the parasite of Texas fever, also a haematozoon, connected in its life-history with the cattle-tick (Boophilus bovis). No more interesting problem in comparative pathology has been solved of late years."[99] Smith attended this meeting and wrote down Osler's comment in his diary—a fitting final tribute to his work for the Department of Agriculture. It was the first day of two weeks' terminal leave from the B.A.I. After leaving Washington, Smith ceased Texas fever research. The Bureau and other organizations continued experiments with control measures directed toward eradication of the cattle tick.[100] Stringent application of the arsenical dip, which was standardized in 1911 by the B.A.I., eventually brought the disease under control.

The Bureau of Animal Industry's *Bulletin No. 1* remains Smith's best known and most ambitious project. Nowadays rarely purchasable, even in tattered condition, its general reception initially was lukewarm, if not incredulous, and no doubt many mint copies went to waste. The significance was remarkable for the novelty of its conclusions respecting the nature of the causal agent and mode of transmission of Texas fever, as well as for the inspired imagination, boundless patience, and extremely thorough experimental evidence marshalled to support these claims.

7

MISCELLANEOUS RESEARCHES
AT THE B.A.I.—
LEAVING THE B.A.I.

The Tubercle Bacillus, Tuberculin, & Bovine Tuberculosis

The news of Koch's discovery of the tubercle bacillus reached North America on May 3, 1882 when the *New York Times* reproduced from *The Times* of London a letter headed "Tubercular Disease" by the physicist and amateur bacteriologist John Tyndall. Koch's accomplishment was soon verified independently by Mitchell Prudden, William Welch, Theobald Smith[1] and George Sternberg; while many Americans, including Prudden, Welch and Hermann Biggs went to Germany to study either with Koch or his disciples. Biggs returned from Germany to launch a pioneering anti-tuberculous campaign in New York City,[2] and Prudden taught E.L. Trudeau how to follow his own and his patients' bacteriological condition at the Saranac Lake Sanitarium.[3]

Smith could not afford to go abroad then, but used his knowledge of German to keep abreast of reports from Koch's laboratory. Intermittently, throughout his life, he investigated various aspects of the pathogenesis and control of tuberculosis. Decades later, a former fellow-passenger on a transatlantic crossing wrote percipiently of him in an obituary tribute that "his first and last biological love was the study of tuberculosis."[4] That love was not unrequited: it bore important fruits. But the intensity of Theobald Smith's attachment waxed and waned according to factors largely beyond his control. During his B.A.I. period (1884–

1895), the many problems of tuberculosis in man and animals were complicated for Smith by Salmon's priorities—often directed by political considerations—and by Koch's authoritarian but devious pronouncements on tubercle bacilli and tuberculin.

Perhaps Koch's gravest mistake, in terms of the confusion created in policies designed to control tuberculosis, was to proclaim in 1884 the "unity" of all forms of the disease, in man and animals, on the grounds that they "contain the same bacilli, yield similar cultures, and when inoculated produce identical results."[5] Koch considered bovine tuberculosis definitely liable to affect human health. But since primary intestinal tuberculosis was comparatively rare, and he was convinced that human infection usually occurred from inhalation of dried particles of phthisical sputum, he believed that eating flesh from a tuberculous carcass posed no great hazard. Although he cautioned, "It is certain that the milk of tubercular animals may give rise to infection," he minimized even the milk-borne risks. "As pearl-nodules do not commonly occur in the udder, the milk of cows with *perlsucht* will very often have no infective properties."

In September 1883, the Fourth International Veterinary Congress at Brussels adopted the following recommendations, which were relayed to United States Commissioner of Agriculture G.B. Loring by Prof. James Law, the Department's delegate to the Congress, who reported that "An appreciable part of the tuberculosis that affects man is obtained through his food."[6]

> The flesh and viscera of a tuberculous animal can only be utilized for human food when the disease if found in the cadaver in the incipient stage, when the lesions are confined to a very small portion of the body, when the lymphatic glands are still free from all morbid tubercular lesions, when the tuberculous formations have not yet undergone softening, when the flesh presents the characters of meat of first quality, and when the animal is in good state of nutrition at the time of slaughter.
>
> The milk of animals affected with tuberculosis or suspected of it should not be taken by man nor by certain animals. The sale of this milk should be severely interdicted.[7]

Theobald Smith joined the Department of Agriculture soon after the Brussels Congress passed its resolution. The Bureau of Animal Industry, created a few months later, endorsed the recommendations that every tuberculous animal should be inspected by a veterinarian, who would decide if the flesh were fit for human consumption. Otherwise the Bureau's early support was passive.

The Eighth International Medical Congress at Copenhagen (1884) accepted the contention of the leading Danish veterinary pathologist, B. Bang, that consumption of milk from cows with tuberculous mammitis was hazardous. After the Congress, dairy herds supplying Copenhagen were regularly inspected. In 1888, G. Sims Woodhead, an English bacteriologist and medical hygienist, with the veterinarian Prof. J. McFadyean, found thirty-seven instances of mammitis (using microscopic methods) among over 600 cows supplying Edinburgh dairies. Six of them yielded milk containing tubercle bacilli. In their udders, disseminated tuberculous tissue contained "almost inconceivable numbers" of the specific bacilli, some in milk ducts. In other words, bacillary excretion could be associated with changes neither visible to the naked eye nor palpable.[8]

The First International Congress on Tuberculosis, held at Paris in July 1888 under J.B.A. Chauveau's presidency, declared bovine tuberculosis a contagious animal disease. Rigid inspection of all dairies and dairy farms was advocated, with seizure and destruction of every tuberculous carcass, however small the lesions.[9] A Standing Committee, which drew up public "Instructions" for protection against tuberculosis, recognized the possible propagation of the disease through meat.[10] At the International Veterinary Congress held during the Paris Universal Exhibition in 1889,[11] with J.A. Villemin presiding, it was agreed that milk from any suspected cow should be boiled or altogether banned. A carcass might be consumed if foci of infection were few and readily removable. In Berlin, meat of dubious infectivity was rendered safe for the poor by being cooked under official supervision.

In the United Kingdom, a Departmental Committee, appointed in 1888, recommended that tuberculous animals should be slaughtered and the owner compensated, since neither the flesh nor the uncooked milk of such animals could be used safely as food.[12] In Scotland, where traffickers profited from feeding "the inhabitants of Glasgow and the west of Scotland on the abominable carrion,"[13] that city's Sanitary Department seized a sick bullock and cow, claiming the right to condemn the whole carcass, "if indubitable evidence were present of tubercle, however localized." The Sheriff found the carcasses unfit for human food and public health was declared the paramount issue.[14] But in Britain as a whole the Committee's recommendations were rejected, after dairymen and stock dealers protested to the Privy Council that the proposed "stamping-out" measures, so successful against rinderpest in 1865, would be too costly, and that difficulties in early detection made eradication impracticable.

Nevertheless, operating under the Public Health Act of 1885, medical health officers and inspectors of nuisances seized and destroyed diseased animals without compensation. Continued complaints led in July 1890 to the appointment of a Royal Commission on Tuberculosis to look into the possible effect of food derived from tuberculous animals on human health. The Report, submitted five years later, concluded that "the conditions conducing to human tuberculosis are the presence of active tuberculous matter in the animal food, and its consumption in a raw or insufficiently cooked state."[15] The Commission considered any discussion of procedures for reducing the infective risk from such sources as beyond its mandate.

In January 1890, Smith prepared a review, "Tuberculosis in Domesticated Animals," destined for the 1889 *Annual Report* of the B.A.I., which summarized the status of legislation on bovine tuberculosis in various European countries. His diary recorded that he had "Spent all week in writing up Tuberculosis article for annual."[16] Though these laws reflected the resolutions of the various preceding congresses, little had been enforced owing to medical and veterinary disputes over the dangers involved. The recommended preventive measures ranged from improved sanitation in the cowshed to slaughter of infected cattle, with burial or burning of their carcasses; but the consensus was that eradication, with compensation to the livestock owners, should not be enacted until diagnostic methods had improved and the incidence of the disease was better known.

When Theobald Smith was deficient in personal experience, as he was initially in the field of tuberculosis, he provisionally accepted Koch's dicta, some of which were incorrect or confusing. For example, he did not dispute (as yet) Koch's claims that the tubercle bacillus formed spores; and that bacillary cultures isolated from different animals had the same appearance and produced similar pathogenic effects upon experimental animals. He made clear, however, his own conviction that the flesh of tuberculous animals was potentially dangerous; that the milk of tuberculous cows was hazardous, especially for children; and that on these grounds alone the suppression of bovine tuberculosis would be beneficial to public health.[17]

The B.A.I.'s own data on the incidence of bovine tuberculosis were very limited. Among cattle slaughtered at Baltimore under its supervision, 2.5 to 3.5 percent proved tuberculous. However, Smith was able to cite studies carried out by Harold C. Ernst, Professor Bacteriology at the Harvard Medical School, with the assistance of Austin Peters, the official veterinarian of the Massachusetts Society for Promoting Agriculture. Tubercle bacilli were demonstrated in the milk of ten among thirty-six tuberculous cows with no recognizable disease of the udder. Of fourteen guinea-pigs each inoculated with milk from a different individual cow, six developed tuberculosis.

At the Seventh International Congress of Hygiene and Demography, held in London August 10-17, 1891 under Sir Joseph Lister's presidency, the Sections of "Bacteriology" and on "The Relation of Diseases of Animals to those Man" arranged a joint session on Tuberculosis. The keynote speaker, the physiologist J. Burdon Sanderson, minimized the risks from tuberculous meat, but urged that the sale of contaminated milk be stopped. There was general agreement on the need for more skilled inspectors to be maintained at abattoirs under close governmental scrutiny.[18] Salmon attended this meeting as delegate of the U.S. Department of Agriculture. Among some impressive museum exhibits was one from the Bureau of Animal Industry—assembled anonymously by Theobald Smith—comprising cultures of the organisms of hog cholera, hemorrhagic septicemia (swine plague), and other bacteria as well as microscopic specimens illustrating Texas fever.

In 1885, after five fruitful years at the Reichsgesundheitsamt (Imperial Health Department), during which his associates had identified the bacilli of swine erysipelas, glanders, diphtheria and typhoid fever, Koch accepted a newly established chair of hygiene, including directorship of a proposed Hygienic Institute, at the University of Berlin. In improvised quarters, he had to cope with a changing coterie of assistants, devotees and trainees, as well as local part-time clinicians and visitors from abroad. He grew unhappy and restless. Late in 1886, "very soon after the discovery of tubercle bacilli," Koch began a quest, largely secret, for a specific cure for tuberculosis: "I set about seeking for substances which could be used therapeutically against tuberculosis."[19] Having determined the negligible disinfectant value of various chemicals given internally, he investigated the growth products of tubercle bacilli.

Near the end of a plodding review of bacteriological research, presented in Berlin on August 16, 1890 to the Tenth International Medical Congress, Koch calmly announced a startling discovery. Recently, he had "hit upon"

> A substance which has the power of preventing the growth of tubercle bacilli, not only in a test tube, but in the body of an animal. Guinea pigs . . . exposed to the influence of this substance, cease to react to the inoculation of tuberculous virus . . . In guinea-pigs suffering from general tuberculosis even to a high degree, the morbid process can be brought completely to a standstill, without the body being in any way injuriously affected.[20]

Koch had departed from his "usual custom . . . [and] made a communication on a research which is not yet completed," in order to encourage further research in this direction. By mid-November 1890, Koch reported good results in clinical trials with this subcutaneously-injected "transparent brownish liquid." Despite its undisclosed origin and composition, the new product—first known as "Koch's lymph," later as "tuberculin"—aroused extraordinary enthusiasm. Thousands of consumptives flocked to Berlin, vainly hoping for prompt treatment. Pending establishment of a research institute promised by the Prussian government, Koch's son-in-law, Dr. E. Pfuhl, with a long-time friend, Dr. A. Libbertz of the Höchst pharmaceutical firm, hired a private house in which to manufacture the agent. Pfuhl and Libbertz also administered the injections, un-

der Koch's direction, to patients in private institutions; for Koch initially controlled no beds in Berlin's public hospitals.

   Tuberculous patients were sent there for treatment by Clinics, or by chiefs of
university-services, such as the Professor of Surgery, Ernst von Bergmann. Early
cases of lupus, and of bone or joint tuberculosis, had cleared up speedily.
Phthisical patients—the majority of those treated—"in the beginning can be
cured with certainty by this remedy." The therapeutic effects were ascribed to
the destruction of tuberculous tissue rather than to any lethal action upon tubercle bacilli. Statistical analyses and detailed descriptions were omitted.[21]

   English and American reports on clinical usage of the "lymph" were based on
small amounts obtained from Libbertz. The product was channelled mainly
through physicians known personally to Koch, such as John Shaw Billings in
Washington. Billings found much improvement, but no cures, in four cases of
lupus. Of eight cases of "incipient tuberculosis, two left the hospital . . . apparently well. Two were much improved, in two there has been little change, and
one is worse."[22]   E.L. Trudeau, who ran a Sanitarium in the Adirondacks, recalled later—while himself dying from intractable phthisis—"the intense excitement that pervaded the little colony of invalids at Saranac Lake when Koch's first
announcement of his specific was published in the daily press." Osler shared
with him "the first bottle of the priceless fluid he had just received from Germany. This small bulb, which was supposed to contain a fluid capable of giving
life to hopeless invalids, was gazed at with deep emotion by many."[23]   By contrast, a sample sent to Pasteur was banned from France, as "a medicinal agent of
unknown composition."[24]

   Evidence accumulated that the agent, far from being a remedy, often proved
toxic. A clamor mounted for the disclosure of the formula and mode of preparation. The German Cultus Minister, Gustav von Gossler, to whom Koch had
confided that the manufacturing process was time-consuming and complex, decided that in the public interest the secret remedy should be produced under
government supervision. In January 1891, Koch announced that his material
was "a glycerine extract of pure cultures of tubercle bacilli."[25] This revelation
satisfied nobody, especially because inadequate identification was coupled with
further vagueness about the postulated mode of action.

   In March 1891, the results of administering tuberculin by some sixty leading
physicians and surgeons in Prussia were officially reported. Of 1,769 cases followed through treatment, fifty-five had died, twenty-eight were classed as cured,
and the majority showed no improvement.[26] One editorial stated it was "absolutely impossible" to judge the merits of tuberculin. Von Gossler resigned. In
April the twentieth Surgical Congress in Berlin reported that in many appar-

ently cured cases relapses occurred.[27] Von Bergmann's presidential address dealt skeptically with the longer-term effectiveness of tuberculin. He was disillusioned especially by Koch's private admission that he had not autopsied his infected guinea-pigs after their tuberculin treatment, but had merely assumed their apparent improvement meant actual cure.[28]

Despite all these setbacks, Koch declared his prime task in the new institute would be to purify and identify tuberculin. In August 1892, his associate Paul Ehrlich, at the Seventh International Congress of Hygiene and Demography in London, reported encouraging results following tuberculin treatment of pulmonary tuberculosis patients at the Moabit Hospital in Berlin.[29] Ehrlich believed moreover that tuberculin injections had prevented recurrence of his own occupationally-acquired phthisis.

Two months after the London Congress, Koch disclosed the method of preparing his product. It was merely a filtrate of tubercle bacilli cultured for six to eight weeks in a glycerinated medium and then evaporated to one-tenth volume. The medium had been described before by Nocard and Roux, but this fact was unacknowledged.[30] While any bacteriological technician could handle the procedure, crucial details regarding standardization of the agent were missing from the outline.

Throughout these early trials of tuberculin as a therapeutic agent, Theobald Smith was so preoccupied with hog cholera and Texas fever controversies that he avoided embroilment in this new question. However, he could not escape helping to prepare for injection, by diluting with saline, one of the first samples of tuberculin to reach the United States. Early in December 1891, Smith recorded "Helped Dr. Magruder do the first bottle of Koch lymph, arrived here today." The next day he "Attended first injection of lymph at Garfield Hospital." Subsequent visits allowed him to observe the second injection and its effects.[31]

Francis E. Leupps, editor of *Kate Field's Washington*, a weekly magazine devoted to topical problems, asked Smith to submit "to an interview on the Koch lymph theory . . . Most of the articles in the daily press have been either too verbose or too careless to satisfy a class of readers to whom we especially minister."[32] The Smiths and Leupps were on friendly social terms. Within a month the magazine featured an article "By Grapevine Telephone" from Theobald Smith, which dealt succinctly with bacteriology in general, as well as Koch's "lymph." In reply to the question, "Where do you find the necessary apparatus, when there are so few laboratories of the sort in America?" Smith ascribed the dependence on Germany to insufficient local demand and lack of public interest in science. American scientific literature was not well known in Europe. "I am now at work upon a paper which I have to write in German in order to bring the facts it contains quickly before other investigators in similar lines. We may, in time, have a sufficiently strong body of workers here to be independent of transatlantic influence, but such a condition is as yet remote."

Professional appraisal of Koch's "lymph," Theobald Smith admitted, was severely handicapped by the secrecy surrounding its composition. Even the specificity of the remedy for tuberculosis was uncertain, and the extent of its efficacy must be determined experimentally. Dosages should be properly diluted and the patient's temperature carefully followed. Initial injections of any but minimal quantities might be dangerous. Finally, notwithstanding the incomplete knowledge of Koch's discovery, it had aroused interest in "bacteriology as a branch of medical science. The subject has been already, for the last half-dozen years, the most interesting and commanding one before the medical profession. Specialists are now searching for the microscopic agencies of every communicable disease."[33]

By now, the German literature in general was denouncing Koch's premature judgment in submitting tuberculin to clinical trial as a specific remedy for all kinds and degrees of tuberculosis. Theobald Smith took no part in any trials, but a few well-known North American physicians, including John S. Billings, remained convinced that tuberculin had important clinical value. If Koch cared to pay a short visit to the United States, Billings wrote, he would gladly offer him restful privacy. "I have a room in my house always ready for you, and you shall do as you like—see no one you do not wish to see—make no speeches that you do not wish to make, and not be troubled in any way so far as I can prevent it."[34]

Early in 1891, two severely tuberculous but mammitis-free cows arrived at the Experiment Station. Milk samples taken at intervals from each cow were inoculated into separate guinea-pigs. One of these, which received milk from an emaciated, dying animal, developed typical lesions. Smith deduced that "tuberculosis of this udder is necessary to an infection of the milk when the disease is not too far advanced," and contended optimistically that regular inspections of the herd should eliminate milk from cows with tuberculous udders. No "self-respecting owner" of a very emaciated cow would permit its milk to be used; and he held that suburban dairy farmers, whose herds seemed especially prone to tuberculosis, could be educated to familiarity with its common manifestations and with the hazards of milk from mastitic or emaciated cattle.[35]

Between August 1892 and March 1893, similar tests were conducted on four cows, two with advanced and two with moderate tuberculosis. All had normal udders. Milk samples from one badly infected animal conveyed tuberculosis to inoculated guinea-pigs. The data on the six cows were reported by Smith and Schroeder in B.A.I. *Bulletin No. 3*. Although they reiterated the importance of rigidly enforced inspection of dairy herds, their wording lacked full confidence. If "all animals showing any affection whatever of the udder, or any emaciation, could be at once removed from the herd and the milk condemned, perhaps most of the infected milk would be thereby excluded."[36] In other words, inspection alone could not guarantee safety.

At the close of 1890, W. Gutmann, of the old Hanseatic city of Dorpat, reported that Koch's tuberculin had diagnostic value in tuberculous cattle.[37] Extensive trials of tuberculin were inaugurated by B. Bang of Copenhagen, and by 1892 free tuberculin was provided in Denmark to cattle owners who undertook to separate reactors from healthy cattle.[38] Research on Koch's tuberculin began to alter direction, and in March 1892, Eber summarized reports on the new usage. Of 247 head of cattle injected therewith, 134 gave a febrile reaction. When slaughtered, 115 of these reactors proved tuberculous, whereas of the 113 nonreactors, 101 were free of the disease. The correspondence rate was therefore about 87.5 percent.[39] Leonard Pearson, head of the Pennsylvania State Livestock Sanitary Board, was the first to test cattle in North America with tuberculin. In March 1892, he tested a privately-owned herd of seventy-nine Jersey cattle and thirty positive reactors were slaughtered.[40]

The tuberculin-testing of cattle under Theobald Smith's supervision began at the end of August 1892, when a sick cow reached the Experiment Station with physical signs of tuberculosis. Its tuberculin reaction was positive and postmortem findings confirmatory. About three months later, a suspected bull, after repeatedly reacting to tuberculin, was sacrificed and found extensively infected. In the summer of 1893, again under B.A.I. auspices, Schroeder used the tuberculin test in further studies of milk from tuberculous cows. Among sixteen reactors, he identified only one, practically moribund but without evident mastitis, that yielded milk causing typical lesions when inoculated into guinea-pigs. However, he also found tubercle bacilli in one of nineteen samples of market milk, each from a different dairy supplying Washington, D.C.[41]

A larger-scale investigation involved a dairy herd of sixty head at the soldier's Home, near the northern outskirts of the capital. The previously mentioned bull had associated freely with the herd. Although only a few cows showed clinical disease, parallel tests with "tuberculinum Kochii" and a B.A.I.-prepared tuberculin revealed infection so widespread that all of the animals were slaughtered. At autopsy, only seven were free from tuberculosis. Kilborne and Schroeder reported these findings, supplemented by Smith's detailed post-mortem observations, in B.A.I. *Bulletin No. 7*.[42] This bulletin, a collection of papers relating to diagnosis and prevention of bovine tuberculosis edited by Smith, Kilborne and Schroeder, contained three articles by Theobald Smith, and was published late in 1894.[43]

By now, Theobald Smith was convinced that tuberculin-reactors in a dairy herd should be eliminated as a potential source of tuberculosis to other cows and to man. In 1893, the State of New York adopted a policy of slaughtering and autopsying tuberculin-reactors. In October, Smith went to Oneanta, New York, to meet Cooper Curtice, now a veterinary inspector for the New York State Department of Health. In a few days, together they slaughtered and autopsied forty-five reactors, most of which proved tuberculous.[44] One of Smith's articles[45] in *Bulletin No. 7* contained the pooled pathological data on 126 tuberculous cattle of the Oneanta region and the Soldier's Home herd. The same data appeared in his official 1893 Report.[46] That winter, in sub-zero weather, Smith twice visited Rochester, New York "to attend the slaughter of tuberculous cattle under the State Board of Health . . . Dr. Curtice examined 14 Jerseys yesterday in a barn and took the notes. Icicles on our beards and the tissues freezing to the knife in a second. Dr. Salmon came along to see the fun."[47] During the spring of 1894, Smith autopsied slaughtered herds at Rochester, Williamstown, Massachusetts, and Richmond, Virginia. Near Richmond, in April, he autopsied seven tuberculous animals in a ditch of an old Confederate earthworks, shovelling dirt on the carcasses from above.

Curtice lost his state inspectorship because of mounting protests against the slaughter. He was reappointed by the B.A.I. in September 1894 to work on tuberculosis in the District of Columbia. With Curtice assisting, Smith continued zealously to autopsy tuberculin-reactors in the District, finding an infection rate of 20 percent. All his post-mortem examinations were conducted with scrupulous care, as witness his report of a fetal vascular disturbance in two pregnant cows following the injection of tuberculin.[48]

When the Chief of the B.A.I. submitted his Report for 1893 to the Secretary of Agriculture, pleuropneumonia had been eradicated from the United States and the chief Texas fever riddles solved; but the incidence of bovine tuberculosis was increasing. Without minimizing the huge livestock losses caused by this disease, Salmon concluded that the B.A.I. should not launch an extensive control campaign until budgetary increases were forthcoming, although he believed that "Tuberculosis considered as a disease of the domesticated animals is . . . the most important of any with which we have to deal."[49] The U.S. Treasury was very depleted, and President Cleveland had inaugurated his second term by imposing many economies.

Late in 1893, A.W. Clement, Chairman of the Tuberculosis Committee of the United States Veterinary Medical Association, presented his Committee's Report. Noting the extraordinary accuracy of the tuberculin test, the Report advocated thorough testing of cattle, with removal of reactors from dairy herds. A veterinarian should examine all carcasses at the time of slaughter. The Bureau of

Animal Industry "should not be hampered by lack of facilities" for investigating animal diseases transmissible to man; and the Bureau's employees should be chosen "on account of their special fitness for the work and not for purely political reasons."

Furthermore, he alleged, despite Salmon's warning that bovine tuberculosis was undoubtedly contagious, and "spread from one State to another by the shipment of affected animals," the Bureau had not undertaken its control or eradication.[50] Salmon continued nevertheless to downplay the need for drastic action. He informed Secretary of Agriculture Sterling Morton that the Bureau's investigations revealed a lesser danger to public health from the milk of tuberculous cows than some authorities had maintained. The meat-borne hazard was even smaller. He believed that the Bureau's manufacture of tuberculin for distribution to State authorities would prove an inexpensive means of determining cooperatively and accurately the incidence of the disease.[51]

In November 1894, the Secretary in turn advised the President that the B.A.I.'s duty was to seek "scientific enlightenment . . . it is not believed that the Department of Agriculture is justified in much other than educational work." Individual States of the Union should undertake the necessary police work for preventing the spread of livestock diseases, leaving much "to the enlightened self-interest of the stock-owners themselves." The Department would purchase only sufficient animals "to intelligently prosecute its scientific work and for purposes of illustration, description, and definition."[52] Salmon echoed this opinion in his Letter of Transmittal for *Bulletin 7*. Farmers should decide "whether it would not be preferable to themselves free their herds from this plague, rather than wait the necessarily slow and unpleasant action of the constituted authorities."

Such irresolution contradicts the suggestion that "The vision of the eradication of bovine tuberculosis seems to have been the creation primarily of D.E. Salmon and his junior associate, Theobald Smith."[53] Smith espoused this aim much more aggressively than Salmon, and he emphasized that the paramount issue was the public health. The control of the disease "should not be left to the interested dairyman and cattle dealer, but should become a subject of surveillance by those who are appointed to watch over the public health . . . Whenever the history of a herd points to the existence of tuberculosis for many years, this herd should be slaughtered entire . . . The sale of the milk of tuberculous cows should be forbidden as directly inimical to public health."[54] This principle, outlined in an article by Theobald Smith in the Secretary of Agriculture's Report for 1893,[55] provoked resentment and alarm, and was not republished in the corresponding B.A.I. Report. Nor was Smith's reputation among dairy farmers enhanced by the content of two lectures he delivered to the Sanitary League of

Washington in June 1893 and in February 1894.[56] One of the main themes was that "All milk destined for the use of children should be sterilized."

Salmon was too parsimonious. His expenditure of less than $500,000 out of an appropriation of $850,000 for the fiscal year ending June 30, 1894 was considered niggardly by the Tuberculosis Commission of the Veterinary Congress of America at the 1893 Chicago Exposition. "We have no regular inspection of herds, nor a complete inspection of meat . . . It is only by an extensive examination with tuberculin . . . that reliable statistics can be obtained."[57] Salmon responded to the ensuing pressures by recommending an expanded program, to involve "a larger force and more rigorous operations . . . with twice as many men and better facilities for getting over the ground, several times as much work can be accomplished."[58]

Theobald Smith meanwhile decided to modify his approach to the bovine tuberculosis problem, a decision reflected in his Letter of Submittal for *Bulletin No. 7*, dated July 1894, which purported to deal with the disease "from an economic and a sanitary point of view."[59] One of Smith's contributions in this bulletin, "Studies in Bovine Tuberculosis with Special Reference to Prevention," contained a key statement, echoed in the Letter of Submittal: "If the disease can be restricted and repressed among cattle during life, the hygienic problem will take care of itself."[60] Then followed illustrated studies of the commoner forms of bovine tuberculosis (pulmonary, intestinal, and lymphatic) as well as those rarer forms, involving certain lymph glands of the head, neck and thorax—often overlooked sites of occult infection—based on his detailed records of post-mortems conducted on tuberculin-positive cattle.

Another of his contributions, "Some Practical Suggestions for the Suppression and Prevention of Tuberculosis," offered a mixture of simple injunctions, such as "Cattle should not be placed so that their heads are close together," with exhortations to the livestock owner to "understand precisely what to expect after the disease has entered his herd."[61] As treatment was unavailing, only the radical measure of segregation and slaughter of tuberculin-reactors would be effective in eliminating sources of infection. Smith's suggestions were republished, slightly modified, in the Department of Agriculture's Yearbook for 1894, immediately after an article on the pasteurization and sterilization of milk by the Bureau's versatile chemist, de Schweinitz.[62] Salmon reprinted de Schweinitz's article (without acknowledgment) as the *Bureau of Animal Industry Circular No. 1*, to illustrate how milk suspected of containing tubercle bacilli could be rendered safe. The same material was reproduced again by Secretary of Agriculture Morton in his report for 1894, this time credited to the Bureau's Chief.

Koch's doctrine of the contagiousness and unity of tubercle bacilli isolated from human and various mammalian sources presented this enigma to Theobald

Smith: Granted that without the tubercle bacillus, no tuberculosis can develop, yet if "more than three-fourths of all tuberculous cattle have been infected through the air of cow stables, why is not the air of stables equally dangerous to human beings frequenting them?"[63] Much later, in Denmark, Jensen found that where the incidence of tuberculosis was high in the livestock, the bovine type was more liable to be transmitted by inhalation to workers in infected sheds or barns.[64] But at that earlier time much of the anachronism remained unexplained, until Smith himself threw light upon it by demonstrating distinctive *human* and *bovine* types of tubercle bacilli, whose different pathogenicities for certain experimental animal species revealed the possibility that the two types might differ also in their infectivity for man.

In 1890, Trudeau had noted specific differences in cell morphology, growth on glycerol agar, and virulence for rabbits between two strains of tubercle bacilli isolated from human sources.[65] One culture came from a recent case of miliary tuberculosis, while the other originated in an old phthisical cavity, and had been subcultured repeatedly, sometimes at lengthy intervals. Trudeau was uncertain whether the dissimilarity was due to the distinctive host lesions that yielded the isolates. Smith initially attributed it to different rates of cultural adaptation to laboratory media. His more recent observations concerned a more complex kind of bacterial variation.

On April 30, 1896, Theobald Smith addressed the American Association of Physicians at their annual meeting in Washington on "Two Varieties of the Tubercle Bacillus from Mammals." One culture, of presumed human origin, was isolated in May 1894 from a mesenteric gland of a pet *Nasua* or coatimundi (a raccoon-like animal) that died from extensive tuberculosis after its owner succumbed to that disease. The other culture came in January 1895 from a retropharyngeal gland of a tuberculous bull. The bovine bacillus was shorter and straighter, and proved more difficult to grow in artificial media. Its culture was definitely more pathogenic than the *Nasua* (human) culture when injected into guinea pigs, rabbits and two heifers. Osler was present but took no part in the lively discussion. Smith closed his presentation by stating, "I believe I was the first to demonstrate the existence of varieties among pathogenic bacteria, as far back as 1886. The subject has been a favorite of mine ever since."[66] Two years before, he had written to Gage: "The changeability of bacteria has always been an interesting subject to me."[67]

Final notes on the animal inoculations were furnished by Drs. Moore and Schroeder to Smith after he left Washington. Smith's findings appeared under his name in the B.A.I.'s combined 1895/96 *Annual Report*, but this was not published until 1897. Before then, however, he had addressed the Association of American Physicians, whose *Transactions* first printed his pioneering report.

Water Bacteria and the Fermentation Tube

The first volume of the German Imperial Health Office journal (*Arbeiten aus dem Kaiserlichen Gesundheitsamte*, 1884) contained three articles on the significance of microbes in a water supply. Soon the German, French and English literature expressed an anxiety to establish biological control of municipal water supplies, and Smith cautioned that American cities should do likewise. He began to investigate the bacterial content of untreated Potomac water, which, along with more than 200 scattered wells, supplied the capital city. The river skirted the grounds of the Agriculture Building and was piped in for drinking and other purposes, such as media-making. The samples for bacteriological counts were collected from a constantly flowing faucet in the basement.

Smith first reported his analyses to the Biological Society of Washington early in 1886, followed during the next decade by a dozen articles about the bacteriology of water and water-borne diseases. In dry weather, the number of germs was 50-200, well within the arbitrary limit of 1000 per cc. set by Koch for drinking water. Between December and May, however, heavy rains washed soil and decaying vegetation into the Potomac, increasing the bacterial count twenty-fold and leading to marked turbidity. Since the typhoid incidence was usually low, Theobald concluded that a high bacterial count did not necessarily indicate the presence of harmful organisms, but pointed to possible danger.[68]

In October 1891, responding to editorial allegations in *The Medical News* that Washington water had caused intestinal disturbances in physicians attending a recent Congress, Smith declared Potomac water "much safer than that of most large cities of this continent."[69] He foretold, however, that sanitarians would demand sedimentation or sand filtration when population growth along the river banks caused contamination of the Potomac with sewage.[70] Berlin's water supply had been clarified and its bacterial count markedly reduced by the introduction of sand filtration. In the London area, after the Metropolitan Water Act (1852) was enforced, the Thames water supply had improved remarkably in quality and safety, while sand filtration, as the Franklands showed,[71] substantially reduced the incidence of water-borne epidemics.

In January 1891, at the request of Prof. Charles C. Brown of the School of Civil Engineering, Union College, Schenectady, and Lewis Balch, M.D., Secretary of the State Board of Health at Albany, Theobald Smith had begun to test water samples from the Hudson and Mohawk Rivers and several tributary creeks. During a short visit to Albany, he prepared plates and inoculated them with river samples "from various sources at Albany Med. College—Tucker's lab." He returned to Washington by overnight train, and worked on the cultures during the weekend and afterwards,[72] for one of Theobald's diary entries for

May 1891 reveals that he was "At lab. in morning [Sunday] working on some samples of water fr. Albany."

In late June, during his vacation, Smith stayed at Prof. Brown's house on the Union College campus for several days. He and one or two companions would set out in the early morning and take buggy, train, or a new-fangled electric trolley car to within walking distance of their point of embarkation. Samples were collected from a rowboat, though once a small sidewheel steamer was hired to accommodate the bulky galvanized-iron cans needed to surround the bottles of water with ice. Plates were inoculated in duplicate the same evening and colonies counted after two days of incubation at 37°C. Smith recorded taking twenty-two Mohawk samples, having "rowed above Schenectady and then down to dam," as well as from above and below the falls at Cohoes. On the Hudson a few days later, he "took twenty-six samples of water from State Dam to Van Wie's Point." The Norman's Kill was sampled with special thoroughness.[73] He assured Lilian, who was summering at Sag Harbor, "My work has done me much good and it has been equivalent to a vacation in many respects."[74]

Upon returning to Washington in mid-July, Smith further tested the isolated cultures and later sent Dr. Van Derveer a report on the Norman's Kill samples. On New Year's Day 1892, he completed a report on the Hudson and Mohawk investigations, which was submitted to Balch with Brown shown as senior author. Although typhoid bacilli were not detected in epidemiologically-suspected water, Smith knew that failure to find them was no proof of their absence. *Bacillus coli communis* (in modern nomenclature *Escherichia coli*, after Theodor Escherich, its discoverer) was often so numerous in rivers and streams polluted with human or animal excreta "as to render the appearance of typhoid bacilli in our tests practically impossible." A system for indicating the potential presence of pathogenic bacteria in water specimens was obviously needed.

The report's tables and maps illustrated the relationship between increased numbers of "sewage bacteria" and probable sources of pollution.[75] By contrast, tributaries flowing direct from the Adirondacks, or through thinly settled country, or from those few cities which adequately treated their sewage, served as diluents rather than pollutants. In fact, the survey provided estimates, at small cost, of the extent of pollution and the capacity for self-purification at various sites. The expenses incurred and "moneys paid for expert and temporary services" amounted to about $9,000. Payments were made to eight individuals, ranging from about $1,700 to C.C. Brown and $1,500 to W.G. Tucker, down to Theobald Smith's total of $160.07.

The Mohawk and Hudson Rivers were sampled again in 1892. At the start, Smith conducted only total bacterial counts, on the principle enunciated six years before: "The number of bacteria is a measure of organic contamination and the introduction of saprophytic bacteria into streams from polluted sources may be taken as a broad indication that pathogenic bacteria, whenever present, will gain entrance through the same channels."[76] This argument seemed too imprecise and even misleading when that summer's widely fluctuating counts were unconnected with the incidence of enteric disease. Smith persuaded Brown and the State Board of Health that the degree of water pollution was less fairly indicated by the total number than by "the number of bacteria which could be recognized as coming from suspicious sources."[77]

A more specific and quantitative index of fecal pollution involved the fermentation tube, whose new applications Smith had outlined early in 1890 in the *Centralblatt für Backteriologie*.[78] The method, applied to water samples taken from several miles of river in the Schenectady, Troy and Castleton triangle, was described separately by Smith in the Board's *Report* for 1892.[79] Theobald's own section was not completed until May 1893, though he had helped to compile the main report since the previous September. The bacteriological principles and standards of water safety control thus initiated have withstood the test of time. The Board acknowledged the aid so rendered, sometimes at much personal inconvenience, "but his interest in the cause is too great to allow him to refuse our requests."[80] For that year's work his ledger recorded one payment of $50 from Prof. Brown.

The new method depended on the fermentative properties of the *E. coli* group of intestinal bacteria, which produce carbon dioxide and hydrogen when incubated at 37°C in nutrient broth containing 2 percent of added glucose. Because of their normal habitat, the presence of these organisms in soil and water was presumptive evidence of fecal contamination by man or animals. The number of *E. coli* per cc. of the sample could be estimated by inoculating multiple fermentation tubes with measured amounts of a given water sample. Thus, the method was predicated on Theobald's belief that "Intestinal bacteria . . . furnish us a very good index of the pollution of water."[81]

Theobald Smith did not "invent" the fermentation tube, but adapted to bacteriological purposes Einhorn's saccharimeter (1885) for determining the presence of sugar in urine.[82] His own words succinctly described the form and usage of this V-shaped glass tube:

> One end is closed. The other is open, much shorter than the closed end, and enlarged into a bulb. A glass foot soldered to the angle permits the tube to stand upright. The closed branch and a portion of the bulb is filled with peptone bouillon containing two percent anhydrous dextrose and the tube sterilized by discontinuous steaming. When the fluid in these tubes is inoculated with certain species of bacteria, a fermentation is begun and the gas set free collects in the upper portion

of the closed branch . . . If a fermentation tube . . . be inoculated from a pure culture of *B. coli*, gas is always set free.[83]

The modified tube was first illustrated in Smith's article in the *Centralblatt* for
April 1890.[84] Further descriptions and details of its uses appeared in several of
his subsequent publications.

At the meeting of the American Public Health Association in Montreal in
1894, an attempt was made through the initiative of Wyatt G. Johnston of
McGill University's Department of Pathology to arrange collective investigations of current methods of bacteriological analysis of water. After fruitless efforts to settle the issues by correspondence, many prominent bacteriologists of
the United States and Canada assembled the following summer in New York.
Smith was nominated to an eight-man committee, chaired by William H. Welch,
to formulate techniques for the study and differentiation of bacterial species in
water supplies. The full report, submitted to the Philadelphia meeting of the Association in September 1897, and published early in 1898, won considerable
approval.[85]

In 1899, the Association again appointed a Committee to recommend procedures for additional kinds of analyses. Its report, presented to the Laboratory
Section of the Association in December 1904, appeared as a supplement to the
Journal of Infectious Diseases in May 1905.[86] This was the first of many editions of
Standard Methods of Water Analysis. Theobald Smith was cited as an adviser and
participant in comparative studies of bacterial species. His fermentation tube
methods gave way eventually to less cumbersome arrangements, but the principles and techniques which he initiated were a fundamental contribution to the
concept and performance of modern "presumptive tests" for coliform bacilli.

From the outset, Smith considered the fermentation tube a device for studying the physiological and chemical activities of bacteria, which supplemented
the morphological bases for recognition. It constituted "A simple procedure basic to many methods of differential isolation, for soil and water analysis, and for
the recognition of forms in . . . systematic bacteriology."[87] Bacteria displayed
"unmistakable activity." He defined the tube as an important expedient for differentiating various species and for providing "a fairly good conception of their
powers of fermentation."[88] The tube's major function was clearly to demonstrate production of gas (of determinable composition) in its closed limb; yet
Theobald Smith sought to broaden the applications, even in his earliest description.[89] Obligate aerobes could be readily distinguished from obligate anaerobes
by failing to grow in the long, closed limb, whereas motile facultative anaerobes
would spread turbidity to the top. In a dozen articles scattered over the next
fifteen years, beginning with several written in German for the *Centralblatt für*

Bakteriologie, Smith reported the results of more detailed inquiries into these various usages. For example, by adding litmus to the medium, he was able to note that alkalinization was often a delayed phenomenon that might mask initial acidification.[90]

The first of these papers recorded tests on three cultures of typhoid bacilli. They produced no gas when grown in peptone-broth containing 2 percent of glucose. This fortuitous observation led to Smith's development of a simple method of differentiating typhoid bacilli from other pathogens, such as the hog-cholera bacillus and from *B. coli*. Two years later, in March 1892, Smith amplified his observations on the different fermentative reactions of typhoid and colon bacilli, using three nutrient media containing respectively 2 percent glucose, lactose, or sucrose.[91] The coliforms produced acid and gas in glucose-broth and lactose-broth, whereas typhoid cultures produced no gas in any of the three sugar-containing media. Although typhoid cultures ferment neither lactose nor sucrose, the use of bouillon containing muscle-sugar (glucose) led Smith to claim wrongly that typhoid cultures produce acid, but no gas, in all three media. Subsequently he corrected the error and advised how the confusion could be avoided.[92]

These procedures left unresolved the problem of detecting pathogens in polluted water containing harmless intestinal bacteria. Smith was unable to isolate typhoid bacilli from epidemiologically-implicated or even artificially-infected water, and grew skeptical about positive reports by others. He did not believe that colon bacilli transformed into typhoid bacilli, despite obtaining "a number of intermediate stages from the water cultures which puzzle me very much."[93]

In 1887 the State Board of Health of Massachusetts established an Experiment Station at Lawrence. Following an extensive outbreak of water-borne typhoid, the city of Lawrence installed sand-filtration for its river water supply. George W. Fuller, bacteriologist at the Station, applied a modification of Smith's fermentation tube technique to the differentiation of true typhoid cultures from several strains of "pseudo-typhoid" bacilli isolated from the Merrimack River.[94] In a personal letter, Fuller assured Theobald Smith that his methods for distinguishing *B. coli communis* and *B. typhosus* had given "excellent satisfaction."[95]

Another paper tabulated the fermentative reaction of thirty-six isolates from water and other sources in media containing 1 percent dextrose, lactose or saccarose, along with such properties as motility, form of colony on gelatine and potato media, milk coagulation, and indol reaction. From their behavior pattern, Smith classified fifteen cultures as *B. coli* and five as *B. lactis aerogenes*. The remainder included "transitional forms," "pseudo-colon" and "pseudo-typhoid" bacilli, and *B. cloacae*. The surest fecal indicator remained *B. coli communis*. The related forms did not invalidate his presumptive test results. If any doubt arose, he recommended that plates be inoculated "to confirm the indications of B. coli."[96]

A paper in German showed that obligate anaerobes would not proliferate if sugar were absent, while certain species developed facultative anaerobiasis only when sugar was added to the medium. Smith speculated that the presence of fermentable carbohydrates in the intestinal tract and tissue fluids might be crucial to the proliferation therein of obligatory anaerobes.[97] This report was highly praised by Erwin F. Smith, phytopathologist in the Department of Agriculture, whose contributions to plant bacteriology were commemorated eponymously in the genus *Erwinia*. He termed it "unquestionably the most discriminating and important paper that has yet appeared on this subject."[98]

In February 1894, Smith addressed the Sanitary League of Washington on water and milk as channels of infection.[99] A detailed review of the lecture appeared in next day's *Evening Star*, and it was republished promptly by *Popular Health Magazine*. The League had been founded about one year previously by the redoubtable sanitarian John Shaw Billings, who had nominated Theobald Smith to membership, as well as D.E. Salmon, E.A. de Schweinitz, Erwin F. Smith, C.V. Riley and C.W. Stiles. A report prepared by Smith for the League's Committee on Water Supply was prematurely published. Billings protested to Smith for apparently attributing the capital's high enteric fever incidence to its water supply—the untreated Potomac river and private wells. Smith replied that the report had been drawn up merely "as a basis for discussion" and that its publication was contrary to his intention. His recent bacteriological findings had indicated that there were some good wells, and nowhere in the report had he brought Potomac water "in causal relation to enteric fever." But even if the river water were guiltless of typhoid, "we ought not to be compelled to drink the filth that is served to us in winter."[100]

When Theobald Smith received the 1926 George M. Kober Medal from the Association of American Physicians, the donor's citation mentioned his important contributions to the bacteriology of water. "Your investigations in distinguishing members of the colon, typhoid and paratyphoid groups on the basis of gas production, and a method of using the colon bacillus as an indicator of sewage pollution, have had a tremendous effect on the purification of public water supplies and the marvelous reduction of typhoid and other water-borne diseases."[101]

In safeguarding milk and water supplies, Smith's dogged thoroughness extended from the performance of laboratory tests to the elaboration of suitable control measures. Nor were his interests in sanitation confined to milk and water. For many years he advocated scientifically-based techniques covering several other conveyors and harborages of pathogenic bacteria, such as hospitals, farms, dairies, sewage and the house-fly. As long ago as 1888, he had published a pamphlet on the disinfection of sick rooms in hospitals and private dwellings, based on a recent ordinance of the city of Berlin.[102] On the whole, he endorsed Koch's tenet that the control of disease germs entailed their destruction outside the host—rather than the Pasteurian doctrine of protecting the prospective host by immunization. But Smith always carefully weighed the pros and cons in such issues. His conclusions carried the authority that stemmed from intimate knowledge and personal performance of the appropriate laboratory tests.

Leaving the B.A.I.—Regretfully, Not for Cornell

Several months before Cornell University reached its first quarter-century in 1892, some of Burt Wilder's colleagues and former students, headed by Gage, decided to commemorate simultaneously his twenty-five years of service to the University. They proposed to present him during the University's Quarter-Centennial Celebrations with a book of articles by selected former students. Smith was invited to contribute to this compilation. He soon discarded for lack of material his original plan to write about "the Cattle gregarine," a new sporozoon in the intestinal villi of cattle, which he eventually reported to the 1893 meeting of the A.A.A.S. at Madison, Wisconsin.[103] As an alternative topic—"The ideas are mine but Dr. Moore has carried out many of the expts, hence the article would be in both our names"—he proposed the following:

> 1. Given a certain disease germ, a variety of lesions may be produced in the same species of animal by inoculating different degrees of attenuation. 2. The same variety of diseases may be produced in the same species by inoculating the same degree of virulence into animals which have received different *degrees of immunity beforehand*. Hence we have the formula …

$$\frac{V}{D} = r \qquad \begin{aligned} v &= \text{(virulence)}, \\ r &= \text{(resistance)} \end{aligned}$$

> The idea is new (altho' there has been some beating about the bush lately in foreign journals) and we have some striking demonstrations . . . I have one other new piece unpublished which may suit if this does not, "on the peculiar modification of species in mixed cultures owing to mutual influence."[104]

Smith's pseudo-algebraic expression of certain "ideas" eventually found its way into *Bulletin No. 6*. His naiveté seems of the same order as was displayed by Ehrlich in his attempts to represent the degradation of diphtheria toxin by balanced chemical equations. The "other new piece" was presented at the August

1893 meeting of the A.A.A.S. at Madison, under the title "The Production of Races and Varieties of Bacteria in Mixed Cultures."[105] Eventually he settled for the fermentation tube.

The Gages invited the whole Smith family to stay with them during the Celebrations in October. Lilian regretfully declined, telling Susanna Gage that she could not leave the children. Her letter crossed with one from Gage, requesting Smith to make the presentation to Wilder. "Now my dear friend, we cannot take no for an answer. We have considered the matter most carefully and are unanimous in our choice. It will be an honor to you also. The President of the United States, the Governor of N.Y., Goldwin Smith etc will be here and take part."[106]

Smith agreed to play his part. "Will it be in good taste to read such an address, or even to hold a manuscript as a ready help to forgetfulness or as a stimulant for stage paralysis? If the address is to be offhand I shall have to complete it soon and begin to chew the cud of sweet memory promptly." He proposed to hand the book to Dr. Wilder during the "peroration" and to accompany the action with a concluding sentence. "I take it for granted that there is a "best form" of address and I ask these questions in order to get at it . . . Am I wrong in regarding this as the first *American Festchrift?*"[107]

Among the sixteen contributors to the volume were two women, whose husbands, Profs. J.H. Comstock and S.H. Gage, also participated. Others included David Starr Jordan, installed two years before as first president of Stanford University, L.O. Howard, H.M. Biggs, V.A. Moore, and Prof. W.R. Dudley, two of whom also chose bacteriological topics. Hermann Biggs presented "A Bacteriological Study of Acute Cerebral and Cerebro-spinal Leptomeningitis;" Veranus A. Moore wrote on the flagella of *B. cholerae suis*, *B. coli communis*, and *B. typhi*. Smith's article, titled "The Fermentation Tube, with Special Reference to Anaerobiasis and Gas Production among Bacteria,"[108] appeared in print before the 1892 *Report of the New York State Department of Health*,[109] and hence became the first and fullest exposition in English of the structure, mechanism, and functions of the fermentation tube. The limited circulation of the *Wilder quarter-Century Book, 1868-1893*, unfortunately impaired Smith's claim to priority.

Smith stayed with the Gages. After a General Reception and Reunion in the University Library on Friday evening, October 6, the ceremonies began early next morning with a twenty-five gun Salute, followed by one hour of the Chimes. A long series of addresses culminated in the presentation of the commemorative volumes to Professor Burt G. Wilder and to the University, following which all participants dined at the Gymnasium.[110] President J.A. Schurman had advised that five to seven minutes should suffice for the presentation addresses and three to five minutes for acceptance speeches.[111] Smith's address, reproduced in *The Cornell Era*, praised the constancy and range of Wilder's researches, especially commending his efforts to popularize the doctrine of evolution. "However insignificant your facilities, however crowded your quarters, however burdensome the instruction," he had delved into pure as well as medical biology. The message to the University was unmistakable:

> When this spirit and its fruits are absent, a university does not deserve the name . . . Original investigation may spasmodically show itself through private munificence or under government auspices, but the difficulty will always lie in the atmosphere, the environment. Those who devote themselves to the solution of problems whose virtues, like those of Emerson's weeks, have not yet been discovered, cannot hope to get light in an atmosphere befogged by false utilitarianism.[112]

Wilder gracefully thanked all the contributors, especially the two women. One of them (Anna Botsford Comstock) was an artist "highly accomplished in the drawing and engraving of natural history objects, a work demanding the difficult subordination of the artistic sense to the scientific conscience." The other (Susanna Phelps Gage) had written an article "second to none in fact, philosophy, or illustration," that gainsaid allegations about "the incompatibility of the feminine constitution with delicate manipulation, close observation, accurate delineation, clear description, logical reasoning, intellectual initiative, and persistent endeavor." Wilder's highest wish for the rest of his 3,261 former students was that they resemble the authors in not cultivating "the true and the beautiful at the expense of the good."[113] This experience deepened Theobald Smith's nostalgia for Cornell. His address was included in a book containing the Quarter-Centennial speeches published by the University.[114]

As Smith's reputation grew, extracurricular demands increased. He welcomed opportunities to spread the gospel about the importance of microbes. In that spirit, he addressed farmers on "Texas fever," and a church congregation on "Micro-organisms and Disease." He gave interviews to selected newspaper representatives and closely associated himself with the Sanitary League. In the summer of 1893 he won a gold medal and Diploma of Honorable Mention for "A large and instructive collection of bacteria, beautifully mounted and well displayed," at the World's Columbian Exposition at Chicago. (C.F. Dawson, V.A. Moore, and W.M. Sawyer assisted him in this endeavor.) New duties included those of examiner for the Civil Service Meat Inspector's Certificate, Chairman of the Civic Center Committee on Housing, member (by invitation) of the District of Columbia Medical Society, and President of the Association of Albany Medical College Alumni.

Although the mounting commitments increasingly interfered with Smith's work, his final researches under the Bureau of Animal Industry's auspices were particularly productive. Besides his pioneer reports on the diagnosis and control of bovine tuberculosis and on the microbiology of water, he began to investigate infectious enterohepatitis of turkeys. Several vacation weeks were spent in Rhode Island on the study of this disease, of which he had "found the cause and worked out the pathology roughly."[115] A preliminary report appeared in *Bulletin No. 8.*[116] He also investigated bronchopneumonia of calves, differentiating this disease from pleuropneumonia. Some of his findings appeared in the combined *12th and 13th Annual Reports* of the B.A.I., published in 1897,[117] well after his departure.

Two novel phenomena, each meriting a separate descriptive article, were first observed during that period. One was the liability to fatal (scorbutic) hemorrhages of guinea pigs fed a diet lacking greens (vitamin C)—mounted casually in a report on a different topic.[118] The other discovery involved post-mortem observations on two guinea-pigs inoculated intraperitoneally with cow's milk several weeks before. Smith's unpublished notes for 1894 concluded that the interstitial inflammatory changes in spleen, liver and kidneys were not due to tuberculosis or "pseudo-tuberculosis" but to an unknown infectious agent, "no longer recognizable in the tissues of the host . . . That the hypothetical infectious agent came from the milk is highly probable." He concluded, "No tuberculosis, but another peculiar disease present."[119]

In 1970, the late Dr. K.F. Meyer, Director Emeritus of the Hooper Foundation, University of California Medical School, San Francisco, described to the author a visit to Theobald Smith at the Harvard Medical School. (Smith's diary for February 18, 1913, noted: "Luncheon with Guernsey Club & discuss cattle abortion with K. Meyer.") According to Meyer, when brucellosis in cattle was discussed, Smith said that he had demonstrated this disease in 1892 by inoculating milk into guinea pigs. Unfalteringly, he reached for his working notebook of that year, which described the lesions. Meyer told the same story in his taped autobiography.[120] The discrepancy in dates represents only a slight aberration in Meyer's remarkably accurate memory.

For several years, Smith's letters to Gage had contained grumblings of dissatisfaction with his job, such as, "I have so many irons in the fire at the laboratory, I presume they multiply with our years."[121] Early complaints about the "pack-horse" role were replaced by thinly-veiled resentment at the complexity of his subject and the compulsive pressures to master it.

I envy you the summer's go-as-you-please. This is my Sabbatical year here, but only 20 days at a time . . . such [a] busy, pushing, expanding field . . . microbiology has become . . . My mind is like the sausage machine in our lab. for making culture media. It is constantly ejecting contents to make room for fresh material.[122]

Seven months later, this afflatus had given place to skepticism bordering on cynicism. "The Government is not a place for those who have ideas of their own to air. If one can draw his salary and get a little truly scientific work in without being detected at it he ought to be satisfied."[123]

Increasingly, Smith sought to compare the research opportunities and facilities for governmental and university employees. To Gage's contention that "the teacher has to put off the working out of ideas for months and perhaps longer," he responded: "I realize that hardship, but it is not less serious with an investigator, because he wishes to work out ten problems to the teacher's one, since he is constantly turning over the stones and sees more."[124] Assuming that Smith's self-analytical comment in September 1894 were an accurate appraisal—"the birds in the bush always draw me more than those in the hand"[125] — and that in those days many publications in sound journals indicated successful research, he should have been content with thirteen published items in 1893, and more than satisfied with the prospective eighteen for 1894. Gage knew that no university could offer so many birds in the bush, and discouraged any rash decision. When Smith wrote him (nearly two years after leaving the B.A.I.), "Too much research is weariness to the flesh,"[126] Gage replied: "Perhaps you are right that all research is tiresome! Teaching I know is. I would enjoy the chance of getting tired once on research work."[127]

As the disillusionment with his present position grew more bitter and persistent, Smith's yearning for a return to Ithaca intensified and in due course demanded recognition. Already as early as September 1890, he wrote to Gage, "I am quite homesick for the campus again."[128] Driven by growing disgust with the politico-bureaucratic web which entangled him, Theobald Smith accepted elective offices in alumni and fraternity associations of Cornell; attended local lectures by Cornell's president and prominent faculty members; gave special training to occasional students from that University; and at times toyed with the idea of joint researches on the campus with Gage.

As President of the Washington Alumni Association of Cornell University, he was toastmaster at the Annual Banquet early in 1892. D.E. Salmon toasted "Cornell's Progress," and several persons took their turn.[129] When he accompanied some twenty others to an organizational banquet of the Delta Upsilon Alumni Association of Washington, he was assigned to toast "The contagium of Delta U," with text from Alexander Pope: "Why has not a man a microscopic eye? For this plain reason: man is not a fly."[130] The following summer, he was notified by

Corresponding Secretary George L. Burr (Theobald's '81 classmate, now Cornell's Professor of Ancient and Medieval History) of his election as Third Vice-President of the Associate Alumni for 1893-94.[131]

In September 1896, a Veterinary College opened at Cornell University which was directed by Prof. James Law until his retirement in 1908. Gage had suggested to Smith four years earlier that he should appraise the possibility of an appointment. Smith expressed his concerns: "I am afraid Dr. Law would 'turn me down' as a member of the faculty. My views on tuberculosis are not quite as radical as his."[132] (Salmon publicly and Smith privately later heaped scorn on Law's suggestion that tuberculin secreted in the milk of tuberculous cows might slowly kill the children drinking it.)[133] Further, "The researches of the past fifteen years have wiped out the academic boundaries between different departments such as chemistry and biology, and no one can go far unless he makes use of both."

> If you want a bacteriologist simply to isolate the milk bacteria for the making of butter, etc . . . my acceptance would be a great step backward for me . . . Why could not the Univ. establish a chair in bacteriology and make the incumbent bacteriologist of the Expt. Station, to be called on for all work deemed necessary by the Station? The work on animal diseases would suit me very well.

Later he added that it seemed best "that the Univ. have a chair of general path. & bacteriol. combined, or of bact. and hygiene combined . . . Would the Station pay travelling expenses, so that the disease could be studied on the spot—an absolutely essential thing?" For salary he could hardly accept less than $2,500.[134]

When no concrete offer appeared, Smith ruefully surmised that he had not done enough "boosting" of himself and that his own situation was appraised as "such a sinecure that I would not leave and hence am not taken into consideration."[135] Subsequent events showed that Gage, Schurman, and Law strove to bring him to Cornell. But by the time the New York State Legislature unequivocally covered the budget for the College, Smith's allegiance was pledged elsewhere.

Early in July 1894, Theobald requested Gage's opinion on a tentative offer from Dr. Van Derveer of the Chair of Pathological Anatomy and Bacteriology in Albany Medical College at $2000 per annum, with opportunity to earn considerably more outside.[136] Gage's response is missing, but apparently a wait-and-see policy was recommended. Early in 1895, Smith reiterated to Gage his anxiety to leave his situation in Washington.

> I wish Cornell would hurry up so that I might know what is going to be done. Dr. Billings [J.S. Billings] asked me the other day if I wanted a better place and I un-

derstand Jordan [David Starr Jordan, Cornell '72, Stanford University's first Pres-
ident] is keeping an eye on me. Last summer I refused to consider an offer to the
Rush Med. College, Chicago. The difficulty will be to hold off long enough without making a false step.[137]

Then, early in the New Year, came a letter from a recent visitor, Henry
Pickering Walcott, Chief of the Massachusetts State Board of Health. He was a
graduate of Harvard, a long-time fellow of the Corporation, and twice served as
Acting President of the University. Could the Board make an offer that would
entice him to Boston?

> The present interest in serum therapy, the belief . . . that the control of the pro-
> tective material must . . . rest in the hands of the public authority, lead me to look
> for some one of the highest quality to take charge of the work. We also need
> equally good assistance in the many investigations as to the control of diseases
> which bacteriology has done so much to explain.[138]

Smith forwarded the letter to Gage, with a brief message: "If I go to Boston to
look over the ground I may stop over a few hours with you . . . If there is to be a
change, I want to keep it quiet as long as possible."[139] He felt it best to get out of
Washington soon; the Massachusetts Board of Health was "the most progressive
as well as properly conservative sanitary body in the country," and they offered a
salary of $3000.[140] A few days later, Dr. Van Derveer wrote of a gift of $20,000
to build a bacteriological laboratory, evidently expecting him to come. "What
can I do?"[141]

This time, Theobald Smith soon made up his mind. At the end of January, during a hurried visit to Boston, he saw Dr. Walcott in the morning at the State
House and lunched with Prof. Sedgwick at the Massachusetts Institute of Technology. That afternoon he went to Cambridge with Walcott, at whose house he
stayed overnight. Returning to Washington via Albany and Ithaca, he found all
well with his parents, and at Cornell looked up Gage, President Schurman and
Law.[142] Schurman requested ideas about the Veterinary School's future organization, particularly as regards bacteriology and pathology. In Smith's view, "the
pivotal point is the choice of a faculty which will work together, whose fields
overlap as little as possible, and yet supplement each other."[143] He complained to
Gage, who had suggested he should travel to Europe, that before venturing
official suggestions it would have been preferable for him to have seen Berlin's
similar school.

He conveyed this desire to Walcott, who promised on February 18 to "con-
trive to secure the visit to Europe." Payment of the salary would be divided be-

tween the State and the Bussey Institute of Harvard College. The Board would provide "a sufficient laboratory with such accessories as shall, from time to time, be found to be necessary." Duties were not to be limited to the question of serum therapy. "You are to investigate the epidemic and contagious diseases, and to consider measures for their restriction and, if possible, prevention . . . diseases of animals are to be taken into account." Smith agreed to these terms before the end of February.

Around the middle of March, Theobald Smith verbally informed Sterling Morton and Salmon that he had accepted the Boston position effective June 1. On April 18, in a formal letter to the Secretary of Agriculture, Smith confirmed his resignation "to take effect after May 15, 1895."

> For reasons which I have stated in writing to Dr. Salmon, Chief of the Bureau, I ask to be relieved from my duties at the laboratory after May 1.
>
> I take the liberty of recommending the appointment of Dr. V.A. Moore, first assistant, to the position vacated by me.
>
> Permit me also to express my thanks to you for the courtesies shown me and my regrets at my separation from the Department under your administration.[144]

Sterling Morton officially accepted the resignation and approved the two weeks' leave of absence.[145]

Early in April, Smith completed his tenth annual spring course in bacteriology at the Columbian Medical School. "Last laboratory hour in bacteriology. 2 evenings per week since 1st of year. About 10 to 12 students in each section."[146] (Increased enrollment had entailed dividing the class into two laboratory sections). Then he visited Albany to address the Alumni Association of the Medical College on the antitoxic and bactericidal properties of the blood following immunization.[147] He emphasized the virtues of diphtheria antiserum, which represented "nature's remedy manufactured under artificial compulsion by the horse, and transferred by the ingenuity of man to the body of the feeble child," adding there were "other buds and blossoms on this tree of serum therapy which may ripen into good fruit." Dr. Van Derveer moved a rising vote of thanks.

Theobald's parting from Salmon and colleagues was amicable: "Presented today by Dr. Salmon in the name of co-workers in Bureau with a gold-headed cane and a silk umbrella."[148] On Saturday, May 4, accompanied by Lilian and the children, he bade farewell to the Experiment Station. His matter-of-fact notation for the next day was typical: "Last Sunday at home—weather beautifully clear and cool." And on May 6: "Left home for Boston to take new position and stopped over at Baltimore, but missed seeing Prof. Welch." On May 7, in New York City, he visited the Veterinary College on 57th Street near Third Avenue,

the center for diphtheria antitoxin production; the Carnegie Laboratory (operated by Hermann Biggs); Eimer and Armand (a laboratory supplies firm); and
his brother-in-law Melville. On the morning of the 8th, he arrived alone at
Boston, with one week of his terminal leave of absence from the B.A.I. still un-
expired.[149]

8

BEGINNINGS IN BOSTON AND
FIRST EUROPEAN TOUR

The treatment of diphtheria with specific antitoxin was based on discoveries by pupils of Koch and Pasteur, beginning in 1884, when Löffler reported the isolation of the causal bacillus. They came to a climax in 1894 when Roux reported to the Eighth International Congress of Hygiene and Demography at Budapest that the mortality of diphtheria could be halved through serum treatment.[1] Within four months of that meeting, 50,000 doses of diphtheria antitoxin had been produced at the Pasteur Institute.

In the United States, the Department of Health of New York City assumed the lead in diphtheria control. Hermann M. Biggs, Chief Inspector of the Division of Pathology, Bacteriology and Disinfection, arranged in 1893 for William H. Park, a pupil of Prudden, to be appointed "Bacteriological Diagnostician of Diphtheria." Biggs visited Koch's Institute in June 1894, and by mid-December thirty-five to forty horses were being immunized at the New York College of Veterinary Surgeons, 154 East 57th Street. Before the year-end, the cities of Newark and Boston followed suit, and delegates from other cities and representatives of commercial firms went to these sites to be initiated. Harold Ernst supervised the production of diphtheria antitoxin for the city of Boston from October 1894.[2] In the same month, Walcott appointed J.L. Goodale, a graduate of Harvard Medical School, who later studied bacteriology and pathology at Vienna and Berlin, to produce diphtheria antitoxin on behalf of the Massachusetts Board of Health. A small serum-processing laboratory was set up at the

State House in downtown Boston, and five horses were stabled in makeshift quarters near the Bussey Institution.

Benjamin Bussey (1757–1842) had left in trust to Harvard University a tract of nearly 400 acres in the Jamaica Plain section of West Roxbury for the development of a school of agriculture and horticulture. He built himself a mansion in southern plantation style on a part of the property known as Woodland Hill. When he died, his married daughter, Mrs. Thomas Motley, occupied the Bussey Mansion. As trustee of the legacy, she released seven acres, on which a three-storied, stone-faced rectangular structure was completed and partially furnished in the academic year 1871–72. This building, known as the Bussey Institution, was situated about five miles from Boston, near the Forest Hills Station on the New York, New Haven and Hartford Railroad. The faculty of five included the trustee's husband, Thomas Motley, Instructor of Farming; Francis Parkman (the famous historian), Professor of Horticulture; and Francis H. Storer, Professor of Agricultural Chemistry and Dean of the Bussey Institution. Parkman resigned soon because of ill health and was succeeded by Benjamin H. Watson. In 1874, Mrs. Motley, unable to pay the taxes assessed by the City of Boston, relinquished to Harvard her residual interest in the Bussey estate. She and her husband were granted free use of the buildings and lands in return for careful management.[3]

In 1872, a legacy by James Arnold (1781–1868), a whaling magnate of New England, for "the promotion of Agricultural and Horticultural improvements," was transferred to the President and Fellows of Harvard College and used to establish an Arboretum on a substantial portion of the Bussey land. The city of Boston undertook to maintain and police the Arboretum as a city park, leasing back the acreage to Harvard tax-free for 1,000 years for one dollar a year. Charles Sprague Sargent, a dynamic protege of the famed botanist Asa Gray, was Director of the Arnold Arboretum from 1874 until his death in 1927. The Arboretum flourished and became world-renowned, but at the Bussey the undergraduate teaching program languished. Although staff members conducted worthy researches, students were more attracted to the Harvard Veterinary School in Boston, the State Agricultural College at Amherst, or other land-grant colleges.

Dean Storer reacted to Goodale's antitoxin horses by insisting that "the Bussey Institution should be subjected to the least possible injury and annoyance," and that the Bussey Farm never be mentioned in connection with the work, lest fear of infection should divert business to "rival horse-boarding establishments."[4] The State Board of Health was prepared to rent from Harvard whatever space in the Bussey was needed for antitoxin production. Apparatus and equipment could be ordered through the State House office. This suited President Eliot who wanted the Bussey used more effectively. Charles William Eliot (1834–1926), president of Harvard since 1869, while professor of analytical chemistry at the Massachusetts Institute of Technology, had co-authored with Storer two textbooks on this subject. Storer and his small faculty were expected to make room hospitably for Theobald Smith, but his presence and function were unwelcome to the other inhabitants of the Bussey.

Initially, Theobald Smith lodged at Mrs. Fernald's boarding house in Jamaica Plain, at the corner of Pond and Centre Street. There was no lack of social engagements. He dined with Dr. William T. Councilman, Professor of Pathological Anatomy, who in March had written a very friendly note to Smith expressing pleasure at his appointment and putting his laboratory at Smith's disposal. Councilman is said to have resigned from Johns Hopkins University when that institution accepted half a million dollars from the Mary Garrett endowment on condition that women students be admitted to the medical school, for he definitely believed that woman's place was in the home. However, when one of his daughters later underwent nurse's training during World War I, he followed her career with close interest and respect.[5]

Smith frequently visited the Ernsts. Recently, Ernst had been promoted full Professor of Bacteriology. He and his wife, as Theobald wrote to Lilian, had "built themselves a little colonial home. The interior is well stocked with fine things. He practices here some & has done much outside work to swell his income. Evidently the absence of children puts a wholly different direction to life with the professional man."[6] The day after Smith's arrival, Ernst drove him out to the Bussey Farm and took him to tea. On May 17 (Smith's seventh wedding anniversary), President Eliot and Dr. Walcott came to inspect the Bussey. After this visit, Theobald informed Lilian, "The expenditures for apparatus alone will probably amount to $800 or more, excluding the fitting up of the Bussey rooms, of which I shall have two on the second floor, the only available ones just now. Tomorrow I expect to make plans for fitting them up. This will consume several weeks at least."[7]

In April 1895, President Eliot arranged that Smith be elected by the Fellows to the vacant Chair of Applied Zoology, an appointment which the Board of Overseers confirmed a few weeks later. Smith offered lectures on Rural Hygiene to Bussey students and prepared a course of lectures to begin the following February at the Harvard Veterinary School. But his aloof relationship with other Bussey inhabitants persisted. He was reticent and difficult to know. Despite a disarming, somewhat messianic air, he could be sarcastic and was scornful of carelessness, stupidity, and apathy. He wrote to his wife:

> I took luncheon with good Mr. Watson and met the botanist of the Bussey—a Mr. Kidder [Nathaniel T. Kidder]. He ah's the a's more than anyone I have heard here-

abouts. His duties are light. He comes to the Bussey once a week to teach botany. When he left, I found a fancy rig and a dressed-up footman waiting for him. I am trying still to find the man hereabouts who is working for a living—Ah no. He has a private yacht—he does not need to do it, and so on. If he does need to do it, he marries a million and continues to do it as his leisure.[8]

Theobald had recently run across the Coolidges (the wealthy in-laws of Councilman) "in their carriage," waiting for a lecture by "Mr. Jack of the Arboretum to close. Mr. Collidge invited me to call on them very warmly as a friend of William's [Councilman's]." Jack gave a popular series of lectures and outdoor exercises on trees "mostly to old ladies in silks and satins . . . Thus has the Bussey fallen."[9] John C. Jack, who was appointed jointly to the Bussey and the Arboretum in 1896, had offered this course annually since 1890.

There had been a timely partial replenishment of the Institution's shrunken funds: "Now the last heir died . . . & left enough to carry on the Institution, if I don't use it up in repairs."[10] (The last heir, Thomas Motley, eldest brother of John L. Motley, the historian, was still on the Bussey staff at the time of his death on March 9, 1895.) The necessary alterations were exasperatingly slow. "Unless the work is done on time there will be no antitoxin next winter," Theobald informed Lilian. "One of the antitoxin horses died the other day, after being ready to furnish serum. Dr. Goodale is still doing the work as my hands are tied until the lab. is ready."[11] The next Saturday Theobald bought four horses at an auction; and on June 17, just before the new horses received their first injection, his stable assistant Dowse went on a spree and caused him trouble. Laboratory work started at the Bussey on July 3, although inside renovations took another two months, and the stalls in the stables were not ready by mid-October.

Early in July, Smith was joined by J. Reverdy Stewart, his laboratory assistant at the Bureau of Animal Industry since 1889. Stewart, who was on friendly terms with the Smiths and had slept at their house on O Street to safeguard the family during Theobald's absence, was persuaded by Veranus Moore and Lilian Smith to accept the position despite a lower salary. Appointed Assistant in the Department of Comparative Pathology in 1898, Stewart stayed with Smith until 1900, when he began training in dentistry. He proved especially helpful in making culture media. Before the end of August, the first batch of sixty-five doses of antitoxin had been bottled. "During the winter we shall probably need 100 bottles a week for the State—excl. Boston which has its own plant."[12] By November, Theobald noted that "Bussey work on antitoxin continues absorbing and predominating."[13]

A bottle-washer and animal caretaker were required urgently. "Can you give me the name of any student," Smith inquired of Storer, "who would be willing to work for me on demand (possibly 10 or more hours a week at $.15 an hour) in cleaning glassware. I should like a careful man . . . I should like to have someone assist morning and afternoon in cleaning the horse stalls . . . I have thus far assumed voluntarily the work of caring for the horses although it belongs properly to the Institution charging the regular price for boarding horses."[14]

His parents-in-law turned up at the O Street house the day after Theobald left Washington for Boston. Mrs. Egleston, sixty-nine years old, had been ill for some months. Lilian expressed her loving concern for her mother: "She is so content and thankful to be here . . . I feel grateful every day that you gave me the chance to do her this last service."[15] For their wedding anniversary she had planned to send photographs of the two children, but the weather kept her from going downtown, so she dispatched a book instead. Although the day was noted in his diary, he failed to mention it to her, excusing himself lamely after she remonstrated, "I intended to send a telegram . . . but . . . you might have anticipated some accident."[16] He expressed "doubt about bringing you here before next spring."[17] He afterwards told her, "As it now appears, the burden of starting the Bussey work and that of setting up housekeeping will come together. How I shall manage the two I do not see just now . . . If you were in any condition to stand the strain now it would be easier."[18] Lilian was pregnant again, but spurned the suggestion that she should stay in Washington for another year. "The moving and the settling again is a good deal of an undertaking . . . but I have been getting along very well and feel in good shape . . . I should be where you are—the children and I need you . . . We cannot make a home without you!"[19]

Theobald first considered a house on the Bussey grounds, but then decided on Jamaica Plain, which had several houses for rent within convenient distance of the Bussey Institution. He sent Lilian detailed descriptions of the available properties, with floor plans and maps. The final choice was 41 Orchard Street, about half a mile from his boarding house. The property comprised some 10,000 square feet, about 1,000 square feet larger than their O Street lot.[20] Neighbors were at least fifty feet away, and there was an attractive outlook to a wooded hill. It had only three bedrooms, but Theobald assured his wife they would have enough room. There was "an asphalt horse shed attached to rear of house for children to play in." The walking times to important destinations were: stores, eight to ten minutes; electric tram, five to six; steam train depot, fifteen; Bussey (via Arboretum), fifteen. The annual rent was $500.

Theobald made a side trip home before attending a bacteriological convention at the New York Academy of Medicine on Friday, June 21, and returned to Washington late that evening. He and Lilian spent the Saturday arranging transportation and finished packing in a few days. They passed the weekend at the Buckingham Hotel on 15th Street where the Egleston parents had taken refuge.[21] The Smiths set out for Boston on Monday, July 9. Arriving at Jamaica Plain the next day, they stayed at Mrs. Fernald's boarding house until 41 Orchard Street was inhabitable. Very soon he began sleeping in the new home, "working morning and evening to get goods distributed."[22] On the 23rd, they all moved in.

Early in August, the Egleston parents descended on them and stayed for ten days. On the day they departed, Father and Mother Smith arrived from Albany for a week.[23] Their visit was more enjoyable, for the weather was kind,[24] they contentedly took daily drives in the parks around Jamaica Plain, and, unlike Mrs. Egleston, they were not ailing. Moreover, they insisted on leaving $40 for their household and personal board.

Early in September, Theobald received a despairing letter from his father-in-law in Williamstown saying that his wife's physician there had consulted with Dr. Van Derveer of Albany, and they concluded that she had an inoperable malignant tumor of the hip-bone. "My own condition I cannot describe . . . I can now only wait, and pray for light to come . . . Mother . . . does not know the real state of her case."[25] On September 23, she was taken to Massachusetts General Hospital where the diagnosis of tumor of the ilium was confirmed. After a few days, she was moved to Mrs. Fernald's boarding house where she died on September 30. The body was transferred to 41 Orchard Street for a brief private service and on the fourth day the coffin was taken to Williamstown for burial. In the middle of it all, Theobald found time for "removing all pears from tree, some ripe, others ready to ripen in house. Probably half bushel in the hall."[26]

Early in October, just as Father Egleston left for Elizabeth, his daughter-in-law Celia arrived to help out during Lilian's coming confinement. Six weeks later, the third Smith child was born. "Today Lilian gave birth to a boy of 8 3/4 lbs. at noon . . . Ether used for nearly 2 hours, then forceps used to extract the head."[27] Afterward, Lilian felt very low and suffered various post-partum complications. A nurse was hired for the customary month of convalescence while Celia stayed for three months. The boy was named "Philip" after his paternal grandfather, who sent a $25 draft to welcome the newcomer.

For nearly a year after beginning work at the Bussey, Smith still yearned for an appointment on the Cornell campus and was keenly interested in a possible chair at that College. After the New York State Legislature passed an appropriation of $100,000 to complete the construction of a new Veterinary College authorized in 1884,[28] Gage wrote Theobald that President Schurman had expressed to Wilder a continuing interest in him and Law had said that "one of the great features of the school was to be the bacteriology and that they had you in mind to make it great. I guess that if you wish, after . . . a taste of Harvard, you will have an opportunity to come here."[29] However, Lilian now dampened Theobald's enthusiasm for a return to Cornell. She had talked with a couple who recently found the campus very "provincial."[30] She expressed distaste for a possible early move from Jamaica Plain: "I mean to like our new home and take root in it."[31]

In August 1895, Gage described for Smith in considerable detail the third floor laboratories in the unfinished new building. As Professor of Microscopy, Histology and Embryology, he would share this area with the Professor of Pathology and Bacteriology, separated only by a cross-wall. The layout appeared very attractive; but Smith was in a quandary, for Dr. Walcott, who had proved a very good superior, anticipated early constitutional changes at the Harvard Veterinary School. If he were offered comparable positions at Harvard and Cornell, the decision would be difficult to make.[32] He had written to Gage that soon "the people" would return, "only those with above 5,000 annual income being considered, and moreover with a family tree resting back in the colonial era, or even farther back towards Old England." However, "these same people—the medical men I know—have been very cordial and have at once elected me an honorary alumnus of Harv. Med. School, and shown me other courtesies such as inviting me to respond to a toast at the alumni dinner."[33]

Toward the close of 1895, Eliot offered Smith the deanship of the Veterinary School. Smith agreed to think about it but suggested "that such a position would turn me into a correspondence clerk and I was adapted to other things. I had especially at heart a little research work to keep up my courage and supply the necessary motive power."[34] In January 1896, Eliot had come up with another proposition—an Institute of Comparative Pathology, for which funds were available, if he could get the proper Head. To such an institute the University might grant post-graduate status, and the State would use it for appropriate work.

Smith had until the end of February to think things over. By then he hoped Cornell might make him a definite offer. Gage sent him an outline plan of three "beautiful" rooms for Bacteriology and Pathology on the third floor of a building now under construction. The salaries were to be $3000 for the Head, and $1000 for his assistant. The professor would teach two lecture and laboratory courses—two hours weekly throughout the year in Bacteriology, and approximately twice as many hours in Pathology—a teaching load which Gage considered excessive for the research-minded. "There is no use hiding the fact," Theobald responded, "a position here means most of the energy devoted to teaching, scraps to investigation."[35] But in some institutions the pattern was worse. When Smith outlined an offer received from Philadelphia, Gage protested that this would reduce him to grinding out medical students. "You are a born investigator and do not want to be wasted in more teaching." If the Cornell possibilities fell through, he should pursue President Eliot's proposals. "Harvard is a good foster mother."[36]

To Smith's annoyance, rumors had started in Washington that he was going to Cornell, the result probably of President Schurman speaking with Trustee Salmon. To imagine Schurman failing to seek Salmon's advice about Smith is as difficult as to assume that Salmon would be enthusiastic about such an appointment. Smith authorized Gage to tell Schurman about the Harvard situation. In the Cornell position, he feared low entrance standards more than the labor and strain of teaching, and "a flood of future docs, vets etc. whose very manners would freeze the current of one's sympathy as well as intellect." Further, if newly appointed staff gave their time solely to the Veterinary College, "the grip of politicians would be upon them and there would be a State howl if the teaching is not ultra-practical."[37] Nathaniel Egleston wrote to Theobald that the Department of Agriculture was seething with rumors of an allegation by a Mr. Lisle that Smith, Salmon, de Schweinitz and Moore had disposed of departmental property to outsiders. The Secretary of Agriculture appointed a commission under General Irish which "entirely exculpated" Smith and Moore. The findings about Salmon and de Schweinitz were not mentioned.

President Schurman had resolved that new appointments could be made only after the State Legislature had voted funds specifically for them. At last, in April, he expected the whole Veterinary College Bill to become law within ten days, and he requested Gage to relay this news to Smith. If they were to open next fall, it would be necessary to proceed as soon as the bill was passed.[38] Gage conveyed an urgent official invitation to Smith to visit the campus the following week, after delivering his presidential address at Albany to the Medical College Alumni Association.

Smith replied that the invitation was too late. On April 6, President Eliot had disclosed that negotiations about founding a professorship of comparative pathology were practically completed. The salary was to be $3,500 with possible increase to $4,000 after five years. He had informed Eliot several months before about the Cornell possibilities, but after these vexatious delays he felt bound to Harvard and too obligated to Dr. Walcott to back out. Besides, advancement was more likely in Boston, and the work would be for a time less arduous there. It seemed cruel to want something for so long only to have duty call elsewhere. "To have been begging for a place in one's alma mater for years, and then to have it offered you without any solicitation by another University," was a little trying. "Please write to cheer us up."[39]

Smith and Gage continued to correspond without rancor. Veranus Moore was appointed as Professor of Pathology, Bacteriology and Meat Inspection at Cornell and began his duties at Ithaca in September 1896. Some months later, Smith alluded enviously to Moore's situation. "He has a fine laboratory while mine is still on paper—1 ft. ? 0.2 inch—as I drew it last summer. Harvard is poor, absolutely starving . . . If Dr. Schurman had said that February day—'we will take you when the position is created,'—instead of quizzing me about men from Koch's laboratory . . . perhaps it is better so."[40]

On March 21, Eliot had acknowledged Smith's "sketch of a proposed Institute of Comparative Pathology" whose main practical obligations would be to investigate the etiology and prevention of infectious animal diseases and their relation to human health, and to supply the State with selected biologic products of controlled quality. Soon thereafter, Eliot secured from Mr. George Francis Fabyan, a wealthy cotton broker of Boston—who preserved a temporary measure of anonymity as a "Merchant of Boston"—an initial payment of $25,000, another $75,000 being payable by July 1. Eliot conveyed these essentials in a private note to Theobald Smith, stating that Mr. Fabyan had contracted to provide a fund of $100,000 for a professorship of Comparative Pathology, to be named after his father, George Fabyan, M.D. "The next thing is to proceed to the appointment of the professor, but this is a mere formality. I congratulate you and the University on this important acquisition."[41]

When Prof. Edward S. Wood of the Department of Chemistry at the Harvard Medical School had first drawn George F. Fabyan's attention to the possibility of endowing a chair, the Professor of Medicine, Dr. F. C. Shattuck, and Dr. H.P. Walcott were consulted. The latter suggested a Chair of Comparative Pathology, knowing that Fabyan, like Eliot, was a lover of horses. In this enterprise, Fabyan received much help from his old friend, Major Henry L. Higginson, a wealthy lawyer-banker and member of the Harvard Corporation.

Early in April, Eliot wrote to the benefactor to confirm verbal assurances that "the right person, by common consent of those who know him and his work, is already in the service of the University." He was soon able to inform Fabyan that Smith had agreed in writing to accept the proposed chair[42] and that Walcott fully concurred. On April 10, Eliot accompanied Fabyan to meet Smith in the laboratory at the Bussey Institution. At a meeting of May 27, the President and Fellows of Harvard College, and the Board of Overseers duly elected and confirmed Theobald Smith as Professor of Comparative Pathology.

A cordial relationship with the Fabyan family was begun during the summer when George F. Fabyan invited Theobald for a weekend on his yacht. Lilian was unable to go. With Mrs. Fabyan and a son and daughter on board, they steamed northeast and supped at Marblehead Neck. Next day, a drive through Marblehead and along the coast brought them to Gloucester Harbor for dinner. Returning to Marblehead, they put up in the harbor overnight, and thence entrained for Boston.[43]

Eliot's official confirmatory letter again mentioned the Veterinary Department. "I hope you will . . . take the direction of our Veterinary Department," he related.[44] Theobald was promised substantial assistance provided that a scientific man, not a practitioner, headed it. Smith need not teach much, but rather should lay out the program and oversee its execution. Was it not desirable to get rid of the word "Veterinary" altogether? "Comparative Medicine" was a better term. Eliot stressed the desirability of "the closest affiliation between the Medical School and the School of Comparative Medicine."[45] The proposition did not appeal to Smith, but since the next letter urged him not to feel pressured, he made no vigorous protest. Having "lived for nearly twelve years in a place as turbulent and unsettled as a Spanish-American Republic,"[46] he had an obsession against politically motivated veterinarians. "I got so sick of it in W. that the dread of political vets may have had some influence on me."[47]

During his first trip to Europe, which was to follow, Smith visited veterinary schools and eventually joined the Harvard Veterinary Faculty. But he managed to escape the deanship. President Eliot's 1897–98 Report visualized an Advanced School of Comparative Medicine, comprising professorships for Comparative Anatomy and Physiology besides that of Comparative Pathology. This School, together with medical, dental and veterinary schools for training practitioners, should be under the direction of the Faculty of Medicine.[48] The concept was endorsed by the Medical Faculty in 1899. "In devising these improvements an active part was taken by Professors Bowditch, Whitney, Minot, Ernst and Theobald Smith of the Medical Faculty, all of whom were members of the Veterinary Faculty."[49]

At Eliot's request, Smith prepared a brief about the reorganization of the Veterinary School, which was published.[50] He asserted that comparative medicine differed from human medicine in shifting the emphasis to prevention. Since the principles of preventive medicine were scientifically derived from biological studies, the training in comparative medicine should be especially thorough, as the German schools recognized, in "the preliminaries"—physics, chemistry, anatomy, physiology, botany and zoology. These subjects should be accommodated in a separate, new building. Also, the admission requirements should include successful completion of four years' high school or its academic equivalent. The plans proved unacceptable because of prohibitive costs. By 1899 the Veterinary School and Hospital incurred an operating deficit of $4,200, which doubled in the next year. In 1901 the Harvarad Veterinary School was closed. The President bewailed that "the University has never before been compelled to abandon a department of instruction once adopted by it."[51]

In the spring, while discussing Smith's future at Harvard, President Eliot asked him to consider taking over in September the tenancy of the Bussey mansion at Woodland Hill, which on Thomas Motley's death had reverted to Harvard College. The rental was to be fifty dollars monthly, deductible from salary at source. Theobald accepted. In April 1896, Thomas's two unmarried sisters— the "Miss Motleys"—were given three months' notice to vacate by President Eliot. This caused some resentment. On June 18, 1896, the Harvard Corporation, eager to appease the four surviving Motley sisters, (there were two married ones, Mrs. Low and Mrs. Winthrop), granted them "full liberty to take any of the plants or shrubs about the Mansion House at Woodland Hill which you may wish to keep in memory of the old home."[52] The Corporation sent a man to remove any wanted flora, which proved to be not excessive.

The new Department of Comparative Pathology required more space. President Eliot's notification of this necessary expansion provoked a belligerent letter from Dean Storer, who claimed that "The vocation (and avocations) of Dr. T. Smith are wholly incongruous with those of the Bussey School."[53]

The policy now determined upon by the Corporation is a staggering blow to that school [which Mr. Bussey directed his Trustees to maintain] and to myself.

It is a curious commentary on human endeavor that when "means" came to the Bussey School, after years of abject poverty, those means should be perverted for the aggrandizement of other interests. I well know that there are those among you who hold that "the end justifies the means." Here speaks the Jesuit, from whom in the last analysis all evil flows.

Thus far, Dr. Smith has been devoting his energies to the preparation of a *drug* (a chemical product) which for months past, and during the whole period of his incumbency, has been prepared (of equally good quality) by several manufacturing druggists in this country. It is precisely as if I were to employ the resources of the Bussey Laboratory in preparing quinine, chloral, phenacetine—for the benefit of the poor and suffering *and* the glory of the distributor.

Dr. Smith's lectures on Rural Hygiene had no meaning for the Bussey School! In my opinion they should be dispensed with in the future. I cannot see any reason, rhyme or utility in forcing a continuation of Prof. Smith's connection with the Bussey, as a teacher in *its* School. Moreover, it is most desirable that Prof. Smith should employ and board his own men and provide for the whole care of his collections of animals, without having anything to do with any employee of the Bussey Farms . . . for boarding horses is no compensation for the friction and bother & the sense of uncertainty which the presence of these horses entails.

If Dr. Smith is to live in the Motley house, why shouldn't he keep his horses in the Motley stable—and have his own men look after them there? . . . I hold that Dr. Smith should procure from local dealers the hay and grain he needs and so relieve the Bussey Farm from any unpleasant entanglement, and that every effort should be made to keep his affairs distinct from ours.

More diatribes, increasingly aggressive and spiteful, were to come. Storer re-iterated that Smith should remove the Board of Health horses to the Motley sta-ble. He proposed a monetary allowance from the professorship of Comparative Pathology and the Board of Health, which "should be used for strengthening the teaching powers of the Bussey School." In winter, he refused to remove snow or to clear the avenue to the Motley house. "That work should be done under the personal direction of the occupant."

Despite Storer's resistance, Smith's accommodation in the Bussey was in-creased to "Three rooms of medium size . . . together with a small animal house—a transformed unused greenhouse attached to the building of the insti-tution."[54] In April 1897, a second story-room was officially assigned to Smith for conversion into a Laboratory of Comparative Pathology. Before the end of 1895, and again in 1898, the horse stables were expanded and improved. An unused barn on the grounds was taken over and adapted for studying animal infections and for related purposes.

Walcott and Eliot undertook to cover Smith's expenses for a six or seven weeks' journey to Europe, which he planned to take in midsummer or the fall of 1896. He tried to persuade Gage to go with him: "It will not cost very much. We can take a cattle steamer from here and live reasonably over there. Your compan-ion, who has always been a kind of stingy fellow, will show this quality to your satisfaction."[55] Gage regretfully was unable to accept.

On August 20, Theobald parted from Lilian and their three small children. "I hope that the journey will tear me away from too much absorption in work and give me a new start as husband and father," he wrote to her on the following day.[56] He stopped overnight in Albany with his parents and then continued on to New York. From the train, he assured Lilian he would count the days until his re-turn. He admitted he had been neglectful and self-centered, lavishing loyalty, time and leisure upon his work, yet seldom voicing appreciation of his wife's en-terprise and sacrifice. He was glad that her father would return to the Orchard Street address, and even if the old man proved more nuisance than help in Sep-tember when they moved into the Woodland Hill mansion, at least she would have his company.

On August 22, he sailed from New York on the S.S. *Manitoba* of the Atlantic Transport Line. He shared his cabin with a Baltimore doctor and found the ac-commodations comfortable. Besides forty-four passengers, cattle were stalled, fore, aft, and below. Off Sandy Hook they dropped the pilot and were soon in open water. Meeting adverse winds, the boat tossed in the rough swell, but Theobald was little bothered by sea-sickness. He played shuffleboard; ac-companied a Swedish vocalist at a charity concert; valiantly played "Lead, Kindly Light" at the Episcopal service on the second Sunday; and rendered first aid when the ship's carpenter had his arm accidentally crushed as he oiled the steering gear.

The boat took twelve days to reach London. The cattle were "honorably discharged" at Deptford. After several hours of maneuvering at different water levels past great merchantmen loading or unloading from all parts of the world and manned largely by red-turbaned Indians, they reached a vacant space for landing at the Royal Albert Docks. Theobald took a train to central London and went to The Great Eastern Railway terminus. He found the waiting rooms very inadequate. "And the Englishmen! About one half resemble Col. Hopkins and rest are an indescribable mixture. The women seem to dress very dowdily."[57]

Making no attempt to explore any part of that historic city, he caught the evening train to Harwich, crossed the North Sea the same night to the Hook of Holland, and then entrained for Cologne. He had worked out a *Rundreise,* with a sequence of stops that provided maximum exposure to important objectives in minimum time. He travelled second-class on fast trains, third-class on branch lines, stayed in modest hotels, ate and drank frugally, and accomplished the whole trip for less than $600, return passage included.

After lunching in Cologne's magnificent depot and admiring the nearby cathedral, Smith caught a one-horse car to the abattoirs, where he observed "the whole operation of taking vaccine from a calf." Next morning he toured the large slaughter-house to watch its customary activities. He objected to paying $1.12 for a six-course dinner and supped lightly in a cheaper place. Fat Germans sat over their glass of beer, glaring at the crowd. Dogs were harnessed to handcarts. He was intrigued by the quaint old houses, fine central buildings, and the wonderful Dom, with myriads of delicate pinnacles striving ever upward, until the mighty towers looked like immense inverted stalactites.[58]

On September 5, he left Cologne, heading southeast for several hours, through Bonn and the Rhine Valley, amidst sloping vineyards and fascinating castle ruins, to the historic city of Frankfurt-am-Main. The scientific part of his five-day stopover was completed in one morning visit to the adjacent town of Höchst, with its "immense chemical factory to which is attached the plant for the preparation of diphtheria antitoxin according to Behring. This is the largest plant in the world." The laboratory of light yellow brick, three stables containing fifty or sixty horses, and a covered paddock for exercise, were all of generous size; but nothing was really novel. "The new ideas are underground, i.e. only communicable by the men interested, and they are dead silent. Perhaps at Berlin, from whence the thing is managed, I may get a stray idea."[59] This secrecy was typical of Behring. After quarreling with Koch, he had moved as professor of hygiene to Marburg where he soon established the Behring Institute and made a fortune from the sale of biological products.

Smith's main interest now lay twenty to thirty miles to the northwest, beyond the Taunus mountains, in and around Limburg-an-der-Lahn, the old cathedral city in which his parents had worked and met, and "where all their memories live." A cousin, Franz Kexel, came by train from Oberursel, nine miles away, to greet him. Franz, a pharmacist, had set his comfortable house in a half-acre garden. His seventeen-year-old son, Heinrich, was training to be a teacher, and there was a daughter aged seven. Theobald stayed overnight. Next day, Franz's wife, a peasant girl, insisted on mending his woollen stockings and brought a large pear—one of four on a dwarf tree—and a bottle of wine.

From Limburg, Heinrich conducted him to two small villages, reached by local train and a long tramp from the railroad stop through wild, hilly country. On the first excursion they met two of his father's sisters, aged sixty-seven and seventy-seven. Most of the villagers, men and women, were out in the meadows raking the second crop of hay. Next morning, Theobald and Heinrich set out for his mother's birthplace. Her older sister, Franz's mother, now seventy-seven, was somewhat taken aback by Theobald. "The voyage is too stupendous for them to guess who I am. This aunt looks very much like mother and has her ways. She is a dear little old woman, living all by herself in a room of a small house . . . Yesterday she walked $1-1/2$ hours to a shrine or church and back again (10 miles)." The photos received from America were hung up where they sat. Everyone cried when he left. They still had "that deep-seated warm feeling, that emotional, religious nature which seems to go slowly with a higher mental growth." In Limburg, his mother had gone into service after being left an orphan at thirteen. Theobald asked Lilian to imagine their small daughters in a similar situation.

On September 10, Smith left Frankfurt for Stuttgart where his one-day stay was spent mostly at the large Veterinary School and the Vaccine Laboratory. The following morning he departed for Munich. He arrived on a Saturday evening, perforce spending the next day in sightseeing, first viewing the paintings in the Old and the New Pinakothek. While the churches and city-portals were venerable, nothing here equalled Limburg in quaintness. The restaurants and large gardens were packed with people drinking. He had drunk wine at times, but did "not intend to have it forced down my throat by these guzzlers, or to pay 50 to 76 cents for a glass, as I could only take a little."

The institutional visits of the next two days proved simple and rather perfunctory, as most people were on vacation. On September 14, he visited the Veterinary School at the other end of the city, and also the Pathological and Pharmacological Laboratories. In the afternoon he inspected the vaccine establishment. On the 15th he went through the Hygienic Institute, named after its founder,

Max von Pettenkofer, who now was seventy-eight years old and retired. Finally, he climbed up the round staircase inside the huge bronze statue of "Bavaria" and looked out through the little hole in her forehead.

From Munich, the route turned northward to Weimar, over 200 miles away. To break the journey and ensure sleep, Smith stopped overnight at a small hotel at Nurnberg, resuming his journey before noon on September 16. He reached Weimar in the evening, engaged a room for three nights at the Hotel Chemnitius, and treated himself to supper, his first meal of the day. In the morning, Theobald Smith called at the charming stone house of the Geheime Medizinal- und Hofrath Dr. Ludwig P. Pfeiffer, private physician to the Grand Duchess of Saxe-Weimar-Eisenach. Pfeiffer had published on many subjects, from cholera in Thuringia to the numismatic history of plague and the technique of vaccination. He was an ardent microscopist and amateur microbiologist and had built a small laboratory in his garden. Until he had finished visiting patients, his son showed Smith "microscopic slides of the vaccine microbe . . . described this spring" in a report that had provoked Smith to write to Pfeiffer. As Guarnieri had claimed in 1892, the rabbit's cornea inoculated with vaccinia exudate showed proliferation of a non-bacterial, intracellular parasite, whose final taxonomy remained unsettled, though Pfeiffer drew analogies between this and other such parasites as the protozoa of malaria and Texas fever.[60]

Finally the father came, a pleasant, hearty man, who greeted Theobald warmly and suggested that he return in the afternoon to show his Texas fever slides. Theobald stayed to supper with the family—the wife, son, two daughters, and a physician son-in-law. The next afternoon, Pfeiffer and Theobald tramped to a distant brook. "Here he fished with a net for Gammarus [a small crab-like crustacean], which in some cases contains interesting organisms like Texas fever protozoa." In the Belvedere, the Duchess's beautiful summer residence, they took coffee in a little garden restaurant with the son and his fiancee and then walked back to Weimar in the dusk through the orangeries and down a long avenue of horse chestnut trees. Smith visited the Goethe and Schiller houses, as well as the Library, which contained many busts of eminent people, paintings and works of art, arranged by Goethe himself. The simplicity of their death chambers moved him inexpressively. He wrote to Lilian, "The bedroom of Goethe and the armchair in which he died made a pathetic picture, still more so the small bedroom of Schiller."[61]

At Dresden, Theobald found the second-class hotel recommended by Pfeiffer expensive. The cheapest room was 87–1/2 cents per day. He wrote with the aid of a small electric drop light, now customary in most large city hotels. On the next day, a Sunday, he explored the chief buildings, among them the Gallery containing Raphael's impressive Sistine Madonna. He went to the Zoo and enjoyed a military band. When commencing a new letter to Lilian, Theobald told her that "Three weeks from date, dearest, I hope to be on the water again, face homewards."[62]

On Monday, after visiting the vaccine plant and the large abattoir, he made his way to the Royal Veterinary School (Königliche Tierarztliche Hochschule), where he met the Professor of Pathological Anatomy, H. Albert Johne. In the year preceding Smith's visit, Johne had published a paper about chronic bovine pseudo-tuberculous enteritis ("Johne's disease").[63] His co-author, Langdon Frothingham, a young veterinarian from Boston who later joined the Department of Bacteriology under Prof. Ernst at Harvard Medical School, was associated for a while with Theobald Smith, and maintained a lifelong interest in tuberculosis.[64] Johne invited Smith for the next afternoon to his summer home. This substantial house (about a half-hour by train from Dresden up the Elbe valley, followed by a steep climb), had a fine garden and a sweeping vista of the Bohemian mountains in the south. On the veranda, Johne and his youngest daughter, a schoolgirl, plied him with coffee, wine, tea and sandwiches. In the evening he saw a musical play at the Hoftheater.

Smith left Dresden on Wednesday, September 23, for the three-hour trip to Berlin, where it was wet and muddy. Out of compassion for the landlady, a professor's widow, he took a dark, miserably small room in a recommended pension. He disliked Berlin, which was large but unattractively cosmopolitan. People sat in open-air restaurants, drinking beer and smoking. He had been trying beer with meals and could now swallow about half a large glass. "I do it partly as an experiment, partly because from one end of Germany to the other people evidently regard one as a lunatic if you do not drink either beer or wine." At the Court Opera House, he enjoyed a poetic rendering of Dickens's *The Cricket on the Hearth,* with music by Goldmark.

Smith made his first call at Koch's Institute on Saturday morning, September 26. Just as the chief of the scientific division was about to hand him over to an assistant, he learnt that the visitor was the Texas fever expert. Then he talked freely and showed specimens. Smith did not expect them to tell him what they were working on directly, because he himself would hesitate to do so in a similar situation. He did not see Geheimrath Koch but made an appointment to call on him at 10 o'clock on the following Monday.

On Sunday, stores were open, teachers at work, and letters were delivered, at least in the morning. He had arranged to see Professor Dr. W. Schütz, Rector of the splendidly equipped Veterinary School. "He is also pathologist and his pathol. Institute is nearly twice as large as the Bussey . . . We were working 10 years ago on the same swine disease which is still interesting from here." In the afternoon, he visited the Hygienic Museum, and then the Zoo. As university vacations extended August to November, many professors were away.

On Monday, he returned to the Koch Institute for his appointment with Koch, who was very pleasant and courteous. "He reminds me very much of Prof. Welch in manner, even in a little faint lisp. I could not have pictured a more fascinating man to be with." Koch demonstrated some lepra bacilli. Smith spoke to him about Texas fever. The Texas fever monograph was regarded in Europe as his *chef d'oevre*. "In regard to tuberculosis, I spoke to him about the differences between the bovine and human types." Smith spent most of the morning in the Institute. Everybody was very cordial and anxious to show interesting things. On his last full day in Berlin, Theobald posted accumulated jottings to his wife, shopped a little, and went into the suburbs to see a calf inoculated with vaccine lymph. In the afternoon he paid 25 cents for "a real German dinner with sour crout, ham and mashed peas . . . served in four courses, and plenty of it."[65]

He left Berlin before noon on October 2 for the four-hour trip to Hamburg, whose "remarkably American physiognomy" impressed him favorably. "A little dirt in the streets, parks not very neat, no militia moving about, American gongs in place of bells in the trolley cars, people in a hurry and perhaps a little more slovenly, street vendors, etc." Hamburg had steam tramways and an abundance of asphalt pavements. The western sun shone full through his hotel window—quite different from the cave-like situation in Berlin—but in the chill of the evening he put on an overcoat and cap, and perched "like a priest reading mass . . . a candle on either side . . . I prefer to keep windows open & wear more clothing than to be shut up."[66]

Next day he visited Dr. William P. Dunbar, an American-born pupil of Gaffky, who was in charge of the Hygienic Institute of the State of Hamburg. Besides being expert in the bacteriology of water, Dunbar had published authoritative reports on hay fever, to which he was himself very susceptible. He had fourteen assistants, some of whom were detailed to show the visitor such features as the water filtration and disinfecting plants. In the evening Smith and about six others took dinner at Dunbar's house. He had evidently married a very wealthy girl, but had worked his own way in Germany since his fifteenth year. There was plenty to discuss, especially about the bacteriology of water; for only four years earlier, a great epidemic of water-borne cholera had centered in Hamburg, causing over 8,000 deaths. In consultation with Robert Koch, Dunbar efficiently supervised the intensive testing of water supplies.[67]

Smith's journey from Hamburg to Antwerp took thirteen hours, ending late on Sunday night, October 4, which left four clear days before the S.S. *Westernland* departed. As the rain would not let up, he visited the impressive cathedral, the fine Art Gallery with many Rubens paintings, and shopped. The cathedral had a sixty-bell set of chimes that rang almost continually. The peal, short when the hour began, increased until at the end of the hour it lasted several minutes, like "an outburst of a flock of bobolinks."

On the 6th he went to Brussels to inspect the vaccine institute, where he was compelled to speak French. Then he looked over the city and saw the Royal Palace, the Park, and the statues of Egmont and Hoorn before returning to Antwerp. On October 7, Lilian's birthday, he told her of a little "remembrancer" in his trunk, and of his regret not to be at home. "This is the port from which father and mother started out in life 42 years ago. Think of those poor young, shrinking people leaving for a new world—then battling with the waves in a sailing vessel for nine long weeks." On the same day, he sent a brief letter in German to his parents.

He made good use of the remaining time, which was sunny and warm, and also free day at the show-places. He looked over the Steen (Inquisitorial) Building of the later Middle Ages; inspected the treasures of the fine old Plantin-Moretus Building, the home and workshop of the family with the exclusive right to print Bibles; and revisited the Art Gallery to view its modern paintings. Finally he rode by horse car to the city boundary to see the remarkable fortifications.

As there were only thirty-six first-class passengers on the *Westernland,* Smith had a cabin to himself. On the second night the wind howled and the sea rose, and he became seasick. On the third night, the ship rolled and pitched until everything in the cabin fell to the floor. At about 5:30 A.M., unable to endure the turmoil, Theobald went to the saloon deck. Mountains of water rose and fell on all sides and it seemed as if the vessel must topple over. "I . . . thought our hours numbered." At last the sky cleared and the wind subsided; yet the water continued tumultuous all day—a grand sight, to be remembered forever.

When the storm subsided, Theobald assembled his notes on institutions, techniques, and interviews. During the voyage, he accompanied the hymns at Sunday episcopal service. On the day before landfall, he played dominoes for several hours with two young priests and a lawyer, which ended in a hot discussion on proofs for the existence of a soul. At 10:30 A.M. on October 14, Sandy Hook hove in sight.[68] Theobald hastened back to an affectionate family welcome in the new setting of Woodland Hill.

The family had settled in the "mansion" during Theobald's absence. He wrote to Gage from Antwerp:

However much I disliked to leave this burden on Mrs. Smith's shoulders, I could not well back out. I had expected to move in before leaving, but extensive repairs were found necessary at the last moment . . . the work is not yet completed. She is now lodged in it, however, and writes that every window is a joy. It is situated on a high knoll, and within the embrace of the Arboretum . . . I am looking forward to a healthful, quiet home.[69]

After Theobald left for Europe, Lilian was kept very busy sewing clothes for the children and visiting Woodland Hill almost daily to inform fifteen workmen what she wanted done. She also went to Boston several times to choose wallpapers and carpets. They moved on September 14 and 15, while the carpenters and painters were still around, and the parlor not yet papered. In mid-September, she wrote to her mother-in-law:

So many want to ask questions or be directed that I have to be here and there from morning till night and then I am too tired to sleep. But the little ones are so well and happy! Philip has four teeth and shouts and plays like an older child . . . He has his father's brown eyes and I think them very handsome. If he only grows up a good boy![70]

To Theobald she wrote that Stewart had proved resourceful, and her father had "been most useful in many little ways and I have enjoyed his stay greatly." Her husband in turn hoped that she had eased the situation by using both "Stewart and money" and urged her to do no more than was necessary for comfort until he returned.[71]

Having enjoyed the hospitality of Johne, Pfeiffer and Dunbar, he looked forward to receiving distinguished visitors himself in an appropriate setting. Besides, though the excessive scale of the grounds and the unaccustomed opulence of the mansion caused him some embarrassment, his appetite for domestic amenities had been piqued by the trappings of prosperity exhibited by some Harvard colleagues. The new tenants called their house Woodland Hill (its official post office address), while others knew it as the Bussey Mansion, the Motley House, or the Mansion House. In the Harvard University Calendar for 1896–7, Theobald Smith listed his address modestly as South St., Jamaica Plain.[72]

Theobald liked the landscaping with specimen trees and flowering shrubs, "hundreds of snowdrops near the house,"[73] "thousands" of crocuses "shivering in the mist and rain."[74] But he worried about the high maintenance costs. The lawn would need regular mowing and the road-bed of the avenue seasonal repairs; and that huge house must be heated for seven or eight months every year. Yet these commodious living quarters were near his main work-place; and while redolent of country life, they adjoined one of North America's most vibrant centers of education. The Forest Hills Station, eight minutes walk from the house, was reached from Boston either by electric or the less crowded steam train.

Gage sought to entice Smith for a visit to Ithaca and a bicycling trip through the Catskills. However, for nearly four years Theobald Smith had neither possessed nor ridden a bicycle. "I get my exercise on our ground, gardening, etc."[75] He persuaded Gage to try out Woodland Hill for a few days. There would be no bicycling and little walking. "There are electrics riddling the country here . . . besides the railroads and the boats . . . I am giving all my spare time to garden work of all kinds, from sawing down dead limbs and young trees to raking the drive."[76] Gage stayed at Woodland Hill during the next years on several occasions, beginning in July 1897. He showed thanks after the first visit by sending a box of maple sugar bricks. These proved so popular that the Smiths regularly ordered consignments from Gage's brother-in-law, at six to ten cents per pound.[77]

All three children first attended the private school of Miss Seeger—a distant relative of the American poet, Alan Seeger. Later, Dolly and Lilian went to a public school in Boston with high academic standards, the Girls' Latin School. Philip attended the Roxbury Latin School, the oldest school in continuous existence in the United States, founded in 1645, and endowed by John Eliot, the "Apostle to the Indians." Tuition was then free to residents of Jamaica Plain. James Bryant Conant, a pupil at the school, was Class Assistant in Physics and Chemistry in Philip's day. In later life, Smith professed agnosticism, but in Jamaica Plain he rented a family pew and attended the First Congregational Church. "Going to church won't do you any harm," he once assured his son.[78] The minister, the Rev. Charles F. Dole (related to the pineapple family), became friendly with the Smiths. His congregation included many who considered themselves Unitarians, among them Theobald Smith.

Theobald and Lilian enjoyed attending concerts by the Boston Symphony Orchestra in Cambridge at Sanders Theatre, as well as occasional theatrical performances. Nearly every evening after supper he played on the piano. They had a Steinway upright, which later was replaced by a Mason and Hamlin grand. He was intrigued by the mathematics and structure of music. In addition to classical Romantic music, he played the works of Edward MacDowell, then considered a "modern." MacDowell lived in Boston until 1896, when he moved to New York after composing the *Indian Suite*. As a pianist, Theobald's technique was rather heavy-handed, sometimes provoking his wife to mock dismay. This habit perhaps reflected his earlier organ-playing, or strumming at Delta Epsilon dance nights. His performances were later curbed by arthritis.[79]

They had many social invitations from a widening circle of acquaintances in the medical school and outside. The psychiatrist William Noyes and his family became firm friends, and they often had overseas visitors. In November 1896,

President Eliot notified Theobald of his election to membership in the Thursday Evening Club, which met fortnightly in Boston to hear a series of short papers, followed by "an excellent supper at ten. The cost of belonging to the Club is two or three dollars a year. It is a good place to meet men of influence in various walks of life . . . The rich members do the entertaining; the literary and scientific members furnish the papers; but no obligation rests on any member of the Club either to entertain or to speak."[80] Eliot also arranged that Theobald Smith be presented with an honorary A.M. degree at the 1901 Commencement exercises in Sanders Theatre.[81] Four years later, he was elected to life membership in the Harvard Union.

Theobald still kept details of all expenditures and income, and taught his children to do likewise. Their allowances ranged form $1 to $5 per month. Each child had an account book, and the balanced accounts were presented to the father on Sunday evenings. He tolerated but did not approve entries such as "unaccounted for." His own income was supplemented with dividends and interest from his investments. The accounts for July 1899, when he was forty years old, show total assets of roughly $13,150, including nearly $7,000 in savings banks and over $6,000 in sound securities.[82] Lilian had two maids, at monthly wages of $16 and $20 each. A wizened Irishman, named Roach, whose official duties by day involved care of the Arboretum's grassy pathways, was chief handyman, at 50 cents hourly. Philip eventually took over the lawn mowing at the going wage for young boys of one dime per hour.

The hot-air furnace was very extravagant and inefficient and required good management to hold the coal consumption to 15 tons. In February 1903, it was supplemented by an independent "steam heating plant." Unused rooms were closed off and left unheated, storm windows installed on the two lower floors, and folding wooden shutters closed during subzero temperatures. A stone building about thirty yards from the house contained an accumulation of nut coal and dust in two large bins. Theobald offered his son 10 cents for every scuttleful of coal sifted from the dust and brought to the kitchen bin. Both parties benefitted from this deal. Theobald gained at least a ton of good coal, and Philip made a sure profit until the mine gave out. A page in the contemporary account book, headed "Coal notes," announced that "kitchen scuttle holds 18 lbs. nut coal," and that Lilian had used three scuttles in one baking day in the kitchen. Theobald eventually took over the running of the furnace in the mornings and evenings, while Philip became responsible for tending it after school and, if need be, restarting it with logs before father came home.[83]

Family life pivoted around Theobald and his work. His wife made herself subservient to his interests. When Theobald came home from the laboratory, he would call upstairs, "Lilian?", and she would reply, "Yes, Theo!" from her sewing room. He would continue to his ground-floor study, seemingly relieved in his mind. At meals, to which they were summoned by a gong, Theobald encouraged conversation, whether topical, socio-political, or philosophical. He contributed maxims, such as, "If you fill your mind with trivia, there won't be room for the worthwhile." Sometimes he became lost in thought and missed part of a discussion. When the consequent misinterpretation provoked him to a protest or a caustic rebuttal, he would recover his equanimity—without apologies—if put to right.

One of Theobald Smith's convictions, from which perhaps stemmed in part his sparing use of experimental laboratory animals, was that life should not be wantonly wasted. Not only was he horrified by war between nations, he knew how to calm the frightened rabbit and the scurrying guinea-pig. Once he tamed a flock of white turkeys kept in a wired enclosure at Woodland Hill. He would enter their enclosure and talk to them, while they perched on his lap and shoulders. At home, the Smiths always kept a dog, first an ugly Boston bull, then a stray but very smart mongrel, and then Shawn, a beautiful Airedale. The whole family doted on Shawn, and mourned his tragic disappearance many years later. When a rat fastened on Shawn's nose, Lilian showed her devotion and courage by pulling the rat away.[84]

Skating was permitted when the ice was safe in winter, and they played lawn croquet in summer. In April 1902, a tennis court was installed,[85] so that Theobald and the children played foursomes. He took them to the Mechanics' Fair, the circus, or the "Muddy Pond" region, and walked them through the Arboretum to school or to church, botanizing on the way. Dolly collected butterflies, and they all observed tadpoles changing into little frogs or toads and learnt to identify bird songs. "A few days ago we heard the (presumably) Wilson's thrush singing his rippling melody in the hemlock woods," he informed Gage. "It took me back to my delightful summers at Ithaca with you when I heard this song in the Cascadilla woods."[86]

Seaside vacations provided the biggest thrills. While the children swam and searched for shells, the parents waded at low tide, took short walks, and picked blueberries. Theobald examined the local fauna and flora, caught mosquitoes, and corresponded daily about laboratory work.[87] On Christmas Day, a tree was set up in their father's study on the ground floor. Family and guests were assembled at one end of the long high-ceilinged room. Then the sliding doors separating the study and parlor opened—to reveal the candle-lit tree, "father standing nervously by, armed with a pail of water and a sponge-mounted stick."[88]

Early in 1899, Theobald visited his parents, who had "the grip—I found both quite sick and feeble though not in bed." He bought "food, wine and medicine," a commode, and a stove for the bedroom, to make them more comfortable.[89] Recalled to Albany after three weeks, he found his father "in bed; very weak . . . very much emaciated. Evidently no power of recuperation."[90] On February 2, a telegram brought news of his father's death. He returned to Albany for the funeral. His lawyer friend Montignani effected the necessary changes in his mother's will.[91] He subsequently wrote Gage, "To think of a father or a mother gone forever is a shock which no amount of anticipation can relieve."[92]

Philipp Schmitt died in his seventieth year. He left his widow an estate totalling about $15,000, some $6,350 savings in two banks, mortgages of $3,700, and two properties on Alexander and Lark Streets valued at $4,500. Theobald arranged for perpetual care of his father's grave in the Rural Cemetery and persuaded his mother to live at Woodland Hill, with some of her own furniture. She arrived at Jamaica Plain in May. "Mother comes from Albany to live with us. My study turned into chamber for her."[93] Her son-in-law Arthur Murphy and his three children stayed on in the Lark Street house, and she planned to spend the summer months with them. The daughter, Theresa, and one of the boys, Edward Theobald, visited Woodland Hill in 1898 and 1901, but gradually the Smiths lost touch with the Murphys.

The second-story bed-sitting room of Theobald's mother adjoined Philip's bedroom, which she tidied up for him. Unobtrusive, she was always punctual at meals, never initiated conversations, and left the table early. She not only mended and darned for anyone, but also knitted stockings, mittens and scarves. For her keep, she faithfully paid Theobald $20 monthly in advance. His birthdays were commemorated with presents of $25, sometimes $50, and in 1906 she made him an unsolicited gift of $2,050.[94]

Lilian's father, who had been unhappy in a Washington boarding house, came to Woodland Hill in 1898, and remained until he died in 1912. Installed on the second floor in the sunniest room, he was never on time for meals and regularly had to be fetched by Philip, but was always about when visitors came.[95] Neither of his sons wanted him to join their own domestic establishment. Melville's sporadic contributions towards his father's keep averaged less than $100 a year. Howard paid nothing although he still owed Theobald money. In calculating income and expenditures for April 1898, Theobald entered this reference: "N.H. Egleston Jr's worthless a/c of 1891, deduct $310.00 (leaving balance of $9957.02)."[96]

9

IN THE SERVICE OF MASSACHUSETTS
AND HARVARD (1896–1903)

Public Health Laboratory Activities

Theobald Smith believed his prime obligation was to produce sufficient diphtheria antitoxin to meet the growing demands of the State Board of Health. Initially he did everything from buying, inoculating and bleeding the horses, to testing, bottling and labelling the final product. He ordered the laboratory supplies (mostly from Messrs. Eimer and Amend of New York, but occasionally from Germany) and personally complained to the shipper about broken and missing items, or to the College Treasurer if a case of apparatus did not clear Customs. The stable hand continued his drunken sprees and was discharged in December 1895. Bypassing the State Board of Health procedures, Smith engaged N.W. Mitchell for the seven-day a week job, at $36 a month, deducting $17 for meals taken at the Bussey.[1]

Despite the unstinted enthusiasm of President Eliot and Dr. Walcott for Theobald Smith's work, and his own efforts to spare animals needless suffering, he was hampered by local zealots who would eliminate animal experimentation entirely. Smith knew that "comparative pathology . . . draws its breath of life in an atmosphere of experimentation," and contributed with Eliot, Walcott and twenty-seven other citizens of Massachusetts to a booklet stressing the importance of such experimentation to biological and medical sciences. The publication included remonstrations against the antivivisectionists by doctors of divinity, as well as doctors of medicine and philosophy. In his article, Smith likened civilization to "a great dike which protects us from an external sea of disease," where leaks must be stopped. "This dike has been thrown up by the medical profession. I think it unsafe to meddle with their work . . . Man's power is finite enough; let us not use his weakness and failures as an argument to limit it still more."[2]

The continued hostility of Storer was particularly worrisome. Smith complained to President Eliot in June 1898 that the horses needed more space, and that Storer disputed the Bussey's obligation to share the costs of currying the horses and cleaning the stables. Eliot reviewed the situation on the spot, and then wrote to Storer:

> Dear Frank, Professor Smith would like to have an enlarged paddock made at the Home Barn for the occupation of his horses . . . It seems to me that 10 horses really require more room, & that they should also be given some shade during the hot weather. Will you please look at Professor Smith's plan, and give your assent to the necessary changes, unless indeed you can suggest improvements in the plan.
>
> He asks that the Bussey provide a competent man for two hours each morning, and he believes that this amount of labour may reasonably be considered paid for in the three dollars per week which the Bussey charges for each horse. So far as I know the customs and the charges of boarding places for horses in the country, I agree with him.[3]

Eliot also relayed a request for "a wooden dust-proof closet in the cellar of the stone building for storing antitoxin and other materials in a cool place where the bottles and flasks will not get dirty."

The President interested himself personally in various details, such as the Woodland Hill gate-house, which was to be occupied by Mr. Stearns, the Bussey greenhouse assistant, "without plumbing at his own risk and charges." This concern for details about situations demanding presidential approval, and also Harvard's penury at this period, are illustrated by the fact that when young Stearns married, he moved to an old farmhouse on Motley Avenue, after Harvard had repaired "an old fashion privy in the woodshed" and laid a water pipe on to the kitchen sink, following a suggestion made by Storer to Eliot.[4]

The City of Boston gave up manufacturing antitoxin in 1899, although the *Annual Reports* of the Massachusetts State Board of Health indicated a mounting demand for diphtheria antitoxin. A ten-year review of the production and distribution of the serum, compiled by Smith in 1906, showed the average monthly requirement increasing from fewer than 300 doses in the first six months of

1897, to more than 6,000 doses in the corresponding period of 1905. From eight to fourteen horses had to be stabled at a time to meet demands.[5]

By 1900, when A.L Reagh joined the Bussey group (as the first Austin Fellow), the staff consisted of Smith and his assistant J.R. Stewart; the Board's bacteriologist, E.L. Walker; Miss Adams, who with one assistant did routine laboratory tests and kept the office records; Mitchell, the stable attendant, and his assistant; and a "*Diener*" who tended the guinea pigs and served as janitor.[6] When Stewart left to study dentistry, the horse-bleeding task reverted to his chief. Occasionally, a graduate student did his researches at the Bussey Institute.

Theobald Smith was not content merely to produce antitoxin. He improved the quality by selecting consistently toxigenic strains for immunization. Samples of potent diphtheria toxin were solicited from other workers in this field, such as B.M. Bolton and J.J. Kinyoun. In 1897, using dextrose-free medium, Smith and Walker found that none of forty-two cultures of diphtheria bacilli obtained from throat swabs in Massachusetts surpassed in toxin production the "Park-Williams No. 8" strain of diphtheria bacillus.[7] This culture had been isolated in 1894 by Anna Williams in W.H. Park's laboratory in New York. Early in 1896, Smith wrote to Park: "I am still using the culture received from you. It has given me a toxin of which .01-.02 cc. represents the minimum fatal dose, but only in certain kinds of bouillon."[8] Further investigations of the relationships between toxin production and the pH of the medium and its dextrose and peptone contents showed that a certain amount of free dextrose was essential, but that the medium must be low in natural muscle-sugar.[9]

By Smith's devoted and sustained efforts, the average potency of the diphtheria antitoxic serum distributed in Massachusetts was increased from 100 units per ml. in 1896 to 425 units in 1900.[10] And by 1902 he could boast, "the diphtheria antitoxin supplied . . . by the State Board of Health . . . is the best made in the country."[11] Although his name was not attached to the thirty-fourth *Annual Report* of the State Board of Health, which reviewed production for the seven years ending March 31, 1902, Theobald doubtless accounted for its impressive statistical data. The number of packages of antitoxin distributed annually increased from 1,724 in 1895–96 to 40,211 in 1901–02. Total distribution for this period was estimated at 200 million units of antitoxin. For the two latest years reviewed, the costs of production did not exceed $14,000 or about one-tenth the minimum retail price of an equivalent commercial product. It was estimated that in seven years some 10,700 lives were saved in 158 cities and towns of the State.

Smith gained much satisfaction from anonymously saving lives through the manufacture of the specific antitoxin for free distribution. He had encountered this prevalent and often tragic disease since his high school days, when his friend

William Shaver recovered from diphtheria. Lilian had been moved by the fate of the Grand Duchess Alice of Hesse, Queen Victoria's second daughter, who in 1890 lost "her life after a struggle single-handed with the diphtheria that attacked her husband and four children at once."[12]

Every lot of serum released from a reputable laboratory was labelled in terms of antitoxic units, indicating its specific toxin-neutralizing capacity. At first, one (1) antitoxic unit was designated arbitrarily as the amount just capable of neutralizing 100 minimal lethal doses (M.L.D.) of toxin, using 250-gram guinea pigs. That unit proved unsatisfactory, since crude toxins were unstable. In 1896, the Prussian Ministry of Education and Medical Affairs appointed Paul Ehrlich director of the Institut für Serumforschung und Serumprüfung, a ramshackle one-story building in the Berlin suburb of Steglitz. In 1897, Ehrlich reported a new method of standardizing diphtheria antitoxin.[13] Antitoxins proved more stable than crude toxins, especially when sealed as dried powder in glass tubes *in vacuo,* stored at low temperatures away from light, and when finally taken into solution with glycerinated saline. Ehrlich therefore concluded that an unknown serum should be assayed by comparing its neutralizing capacity for a fixed dose of crude toxin with that of a standard serum. The fixed dose of toxin ("test dose") should not be based on the labile M.L.D., but upon the minimum amount that, *when added to one standard unit of antitoxin,* killed within four days a 250-gram guinea-pig injected with the mixture.

Ehrlich's designation, L^t (Limes-Tod), for this "test dose" gained wide and lasting approval; and his vials of standardized serum from the Steglitz establishment, and after 1898 from his Institute for Experimental Therapy at Frankfurt, were accepted internationally. In 1898, Ehrlich introduced the confusing concept that every batch of crude toxin had its own "spectrum" of arithmetically proportioned components.[14] In devising, naming, and renaming the components of these spectra, his imaginative fertility eventually outstripped the supporting scientific data. In letters to his cousin Carl Weigert, he expressed growing disenchantment with the problem. "I shall be glad when I am finished with this business; one can't get much fame out of it either . . . I distinguish now pro-, syn,- meso-, epi-, transtoxoids quite a lot, but I cannot do it any cheaper . . . This is a damned tricky field."[15]

Smith was probably the first American bacteriologist to adopt Ehrlich's standards and general methods. In a paper on "The Antitoxin Unit in Diphtheria," published in October 1900, Smith stated that he had been supplied regularly with standardized antitoxin by Ehrlich for more than three years. Ehrlich's serum and principles of titration had given remarkably satisfactory results, but he deplored the "exceedingly tedious and expensive" method. He felt that the neutralization phenomena have shown "so great a complexity . . . that my hypothesis fails to explain them." Nonetheless, he concluded that "The action of antitoxin upon toxin appears more and more in the light of a true chemical reaction."[16] Although he stressed that the antitoxin-manufacturing plant was still too experimental to be imitated,[17] Smith's preeminence in this field in the United States, and the cooperative arrangements between the State Board of Health and Harvard University, drew many visitors. Early in 1903, he was elected chairman of an "antitoxin committee" formed at Philadelphia.[18]

Ten or more horses stabled near a public park are bound to arouse curiosity in a State riddled with antivivisectionist sentiment. At the legislative committee hearings on animal experimentation early in 1896, President Eliot consented to the university laboratories being viewed in action by someone with appropriate credentials. Accordingly, a representative of the *Boston Sunday Journal* visited the Bussey Institute, where several times he was "freely admitted to the laboratories and operating rooms." The resulting article[19] was an accurate and sympathetic account of antitoxin production, describing in layman's language all steps from the preparation of toxin and its injection into horses, to the testing of the harvested serum on guinea-pigs. With photographic illustrations the article occupied practically a whole page of the newspaper. "The experimenters" made a small concession to the antivivisectionists by expressing the hope that eventually the antitoxin could be determined and tested chemically, "and the trouble of using animals done away with."

The booklet illustrating the important advances in biological and medical sciences made possible by animal experimentation included testimony given before the 1900–1901 legislative committees that held hearings on antitvivisection bills.[20] The controversy waxed and waned. Smith vigorously defended his activities at the 1902 annual meeting of the Massachusetts Boards of Health, where there was a "Discussion as to value of Antitoxin work of Board and its intended abolition by the Legisl."[21] But although the tenacity of the campaign gradually subsided, Smith judged that a local eruption of the issue in 1905 demanded his involvement: "Speak at anti-vivisection hearing at State House," he noted in his diary that year.[22] The successful production of diphtheria antitoxin naturally led Smith to consider the feasibility of preparing the pioneer and (when properly manufactured and stored) most effective of immunological agents yet known—namely, the vaccine virus.

In Massachusetts in 1901 there were 717 cases of smallpox. total cases rose to 2,305 in 1903, with 274 deaths. In February 1902, a bill had been introduced in the Legislature which would authorize the State Board of Health to produce vaccine lymph as well as diphtheria antitoxin.[23] Smith, Walcott, Eliot, Ernst, and leading members of the Harvard Medical Faculty strongly favored this measure. An editorial in *The Boston Medical and Surgical Journal,* probably written by Ernst, claimed that sharp rivalry, or the sudden demand of a smallpox epidemic, "occasionally leads producers to unscrupulous methods, not only of production, but also of advertising their wares."[24] When a physician questioned the journal's preference for "political bureaus" over "reliable pharmaceutical houses" to prepare prophylactic agents, another editorial cited the Massachusetts State Board of Health's life-saving work on diphtheria antitoxin, and the inferior quality of some privately manufactured antitoxins offered for sale within the State.[25]

Private manufacturers mounted a strenuous defense, which began with an attack upon Smith's manufacture of diphtheria antitoxin. On March 11, 1903, W.W. Bartlett, the "legal representative" of the Massachusetts Pharmaceutical Association, read a report to the Legislature's Committee on Public Health. Based on a brief visit to the State's Antitoxin Laboratory, it began: "This Biologic Laboratory consisted of two very dirty stables . . . Dirt and filth seemed to be the order of the day." It concluded: "Massachusetts in this respect is crude, primitive, and far, far behind the times in the methods of manufacture of these products and should stick to inspecting and not attempt to manufacture them."[26]

Letters to Boston newspapers publicized the matter. The *Boston Evening Transcript* printed the full text of the report, also embodied by Bartlett in an information circular to physicians. Theobald Smith dispatched an indignant letter of refutation to *The Boston Medical and Surgical Journal* (in which his name was given as Theodore Smith), stating that "Everything was done in the simplest manner compatible with the safety and efficiency of the product." A week, rather than the fifteen to thirty minutes spent by Bartlett on his visit, "would have barely acquainted him (even if he were trained) with those processes which form the true safeguards of a biological product." Private manufacturers had "thus far not contributed anything of value to the problem of serum therapy and vaccines. If they have, it is kept as a trade secret, and neither scientist nor physician could be in a position to gauge its value."[27] And he also noted, "The public plant finds in the promotion of science its chief incentive, the private plant finds the same necessarily in making money."

The manufacturer of diphtheria antitoxin entailed bacteriological tests incidental to diphtheria control. Physicians within twenty-five miles of Boston received a sterile swab and a slant of Loeffler's serum medium, with instructions for taking a throat specimen for bacterial diagnosis of diphtheria and for returning it to the State House by hand or express. In six years from April 1896 to March 1902, no fewer than 17,814 cultures were received from 118 towns and cities in Massachusetts. Of these, 8,301 were concerned with diagnosis, the others with release of convalescents from quarantine. Analysis of the positive cases illustrated the benefits of antitoxin therapy at various stages, and on the duration of infectivity.[28]

In 1896, Smith and Walker compared the clinical severity of the diphtheria cases with the bacillary morphology and toxin production of forty-six cultures isolated therefrom. Four were non-toxigenic cultures of "pseudo-diphtheria bacilli." Using Löffler's alkaline mehthylene blue stain, the authors noted three morphologically distinguishable types of bacilli, all virulent for guinea pigs, in the remaining forty-two cultures. The data reported are insufficient to warrant the assumption, but does not exclude the possibility, that these three types corresponded to the *gravis, intermedius,* and *mitis* types described in 1931 by McLeod and his colleagues in a classification now widely accepted.[29]

In June 1902, Smith presented a paper on the preparation of animal vaccine to the Massachusetts Medical Society, contending that a State that strongly advocated vaccination should also manufacture the vaccine and safeguard its quality.[30] Nevertheless, private firms soon began to displace public plants as sources of "biological products." The Massachusetts State Board of Health did not follow this general trend, largely because of Theobald Smith's efforts. He did his best to shepherd bills through the Legislature which would authorize "a permanent plant for the State production of antitoxin and vaccine under the Board of Health." He assumed this heavy responsibility, he wrote to Simon Flexner, "because it has done much good for the State and has helped medicine."[31] The letter was occasioned by a rumor that the newly established Rockefeller Institute for Medical Research had assigned a research fund of $100,000 for the manufacture and testing of anti-dysentery serum by a private firm. Flexner at once took steps to dispel the allegation.[32] Near the end of the 1903 session of the Legislature, the Board of Health was authorized to diversify its output of biological products.

Theobald Smith's duties included various diagnostic public health laboratory procedures, many of which he introduced. He began classifying hog cholera and related bacilli by their agglutination reactions in 1898, at first with J.R. Stewart's occasional assistance, and since 1901 in association with A.L Reagh. He published two fundamental discoveries with Reagh. Their first paper showed the importance of the agglutination reaction in bacterial classification—incidentally confirming that Sanarelli's *B. icteroides* was *B. cholerae suis.* The second paper reported that different agglutinins acted upon the flagella and the body of *B. cholerae suis,* thus revealing an antigenic complexity which provided the basis for the Kauffmann-White Schema for differentiating and identifying species of the so-called *Salmonella* genus.[33] And, in 1900, "the . . . 'Widal, Agglutinative or Serum Test' was . . . begun by Dr. Arthur L. Reagh in Dr. Smith's laboratory."[34]

Until 1901, Smith withheld the Widal "agglutinative" test from practicing physicians, lest they "place too much reliance upon a test so frequently negative in the first week of typhoid fever." During the first three months of that year, eighteen out of sixty-two such tests were positive in serum dilutions of 1:20 or higher.[35] The Widal test outfit comprised a small, weighed square of white paper, and a wire loop for placing several individual drops of blood near the paper's edge. When dry, the paper was folded and returned to the laboratory with the loop and a completed questionnaire. The latter had instructed the physician how to interpret the results and prevent the spread of typhoid fever, and reminded him that in doubtful cases early blood cultures might yield diagnostic results.

Beginning in 1896, physicians in malarious regions could request and return by mail small tin boxes containing two glass slides for blood films, which Smith himself searched for malaria parasites. Later that year, glass vials were made available to physicians for sputum samples from cases of suspected pulmonary tuberculosis. Until 1897, specimens collected at the State House were transported daily to the Bussey. Thereafter, Walker, Reagh, or Smith himself went into the city to examine the daily accumulation at the State House laboratory. Any unusual specimen, e.g. from a suspected source of anthrax, glanders or trichinosis, was examined by Smith personally. Such miscellaneous examinations might provide both incentive and momentum for new research projects, as in two parasitological investigations of the period.[36]

Teaching and Research in Comparative Pathology

Early in 1896, Theobald Smith outlined at President Eliot's request a Proposed Plan of Work for a Department of Comparative Pathology. An undated draft of a five-page brief (with a four-page addendum dated 1898), all in smith's handwriting, emphasized both the utilitarian and educational aims, and their inseparability,[37] and a polished revised version was dated April 1898.[38] If practical services were offered first, the department would become a public necessity and its educational facilities assured. "The more work such a department can accomplish for the State, the more material it will control for educational purposes." The department could supply the State with tuberculin, mallein and reliable vaccines of controlled quality; and the State Board of Agriculture would be provided with expert consultative advice in disease emergencies. A liberal endowment or regular appropriations from the State would be required. Further, instruction and research required suitable laboratories, accommodation for infected animals, breeding quarters for small animals, an autopsy room, and museum space. In his outline, Theobald expressed his belief that "Each kind of work destined for a practical end involves, when properly done, the highest kind of scientific thought."

At a dinner address to the Harvard Medical Alumni Association soon after arriving in Boston, Smith suggested that comparative pathology might launch researches in three fields: 1. Problems ancillary to human medicine, but not solvable by it alone. 2. Agricultural economies, particularly livestock conservation. 3. Problems in general biology and pathology. He did not reject "the demand for so-called practical studies which is penetrating into the halls of the colleges . . . My own conviction is that there is as much pure gold of science to be gathered in the working out of problems applicable to the every-day life of the individual and of the State as in other kinds of inquiry aimed much higher."[39] Here he echoed Pasteur's repudiation of the opinion that "Science could be divided into 'theoretical' and 'applied'." Nothing could be more erroneous. *Il y a la science et les applications de la science,* linked together like the fruit to the tree that has borne it."[40]

Smith's failure to mention veterinary medicine did not indicate the preclusion of research into infectious diseases of animals. A report by himself and Stewart on the isolation of a rare pathogenic bacillus from a guinea-pig began, "No excuse need be offered for the study of infectious disease of the smaller mammals. The history of bacteriology is a sufficient witness of their importance in furnishing information upon etiology."[41] But he was anxious to be personally dissociated from veterinary medicine. To a request for data about himself as a Cornellian who had contributed substantially to this field, he responded: "My affiliations and interests are with human medicine and not with comparative (veterinary) medicine, although my chief work is to approach general pathology from the comparative side. I have achieved nothing in comparative or veterinary medicine as my work has been in pathology simply. I am interested in medicine as a science rather than an art."[42]

Although Smith decided soon enough that in basic sciences the Harvard Medical School facilities were "too good to be in any way duplicated,"[43] at the end of 1896 he applied to the Faculty of Medicine Committee on Fourth-Year electives to give a course entitled "The Etiology of Infectious Diseases." The Committee approved it as a second-term Comparative Pathology elective. E.E. Tyzzer, who in time succeeded Smith in the chair, praised the course. Students found that "disjointed subjects . . . fell into place, and for the first time a conception of disease as a whole dawned upon the mind."[44] And Smith, for his part, exclaimed, "What a job it is to teach medicine any way, even to well-prepared students."[45] But the course had few registrants and the lecturer found that troublesome. In Smith's view, if the student lacked basic knowledge of the subject, "You might as well talk into a fog . . . I have acquired the habit of reading all accessible material on a subject, or trying to do so before lecturing. It is this mania (which I hope will pass away), which makes any course so burdensome to me."[46]

Beginning in January 1900, he gave an obligatory course in "Medical Protozoology" or "Parasitology." Six one-hour lectures, each followed by an hour in the laboratory, were given twice-weekly as part of the Second-Year course in Pathology. The following year, the total number of sessions was raised to ten, presented daily, so that a more concentrated series was over in two weeks instead of three. He still found that "teaching, conscientiously done, is laborious work . . . Nowadays a professor should create his lectures by his own researches . . . Research, therefore, should form the background of every teacher's life; and I trust that in comparative pathology that background will not be obscured by too many students' heads in the foreground."[47]

He considered the lecture a necessary shortcut to the acquisition of information. But in some subjects, *methods* were more vitalizing, and the facts could repose in handbooks; while in others, *facts* were the all-important stimulators of thought. All reservations notwithstanding, preparations for the new course began at least two months beforehand. Yet, despite excellent content, the lectures were dull and uninspiring, so that "Parasitology" was rated the most unpopular course in the Medical School curriculum. "He did not try to establish contact with the ordinary student, and even failed to ask whether there were any questions after his lectures," one long-time Harvard faculty member remembered.[48]

Theobald Smith thought highly enough of his course to send an outline of it to Washington in 1899, entitled "Animal Parasites and their Relation to Pathological Processes. Syllabus,"[49] to be copyrighted at the Library of Congress.[50] In the same year he rejected a request from Appleton, the New York publisher, to compile a Bacteriology text. His chronic lack of assistance largely governed this decision. For his first ten years as a Harvard professor, he had no full-time departmental Instructor or Class Assistant. An Austin teaching Fellow assigned in 1900 had only half-time teaching duties and the appointment was short-term.

In December 1898, three members of the American Society of Naturalists, A.C. Abbott, University of Pennsylvania, E.O. Jordan, and H.W. Conn (father of H.J. Conn) of Wesleyan University, agreed that the developing science of bacteriology should have its own organization.[51] They circularized potential members and arranged a meeting, which would include a scientific program at New Haven on December 27–29, 1899. Of fifty-nine would-be members, about thirty were present, and seventeen papers read, including one by Theobald Smith on bacterial variation.[52] He was appointed to a Committee on the Constitution of the Society, along with Abbott, Conn, Jordan, and Wyatt Johnston. W.T. Sedgwick was elected President for the ensuing year, and Theobald Smith to the council, together with Ernst, Jordan, and E.A. de Schweinitz. C.-E.A. Winslow recalled forty years later that rarely had "a new organization enjoyed the leadership of so distinguished a band of sponsors." Among them, he singled out Theobald Smith for special tribute: "Incomparable scientist, sparse and dry and black-bearded, so imaginative that he anticipated in the nineties many of the 'discoveries' made by others for a quarter of a century, so uncannily clear-headed a thinker and so meticulous an investigator that he left no errors for his successors to correct."[53]

Welch was elected President for 1901, H.W. Conn for 1902, and Theobald Smith for 1903. None of them published an official address, but Smith preserved the corrected manuscript of his "Introduction" to the scientific presentations, composed during the Christmas holidays and given at Philadelphia on December 29, 1903. Discovered among his papers, it was published in full nearly eighty years later.[54] The address (short by standards then prevailing) developed two favorite themes—the host-parasite relationship and the importance of comparative pathology. The true cause of disease lay neither in microbe nor in host, but in a delicate, specific equilibrium, changeable by factors influencing either host or microbe and different for every host species. Generalizations entailed comparative study of these differences, and "As long as the stupid distinction between human and animal pathology is maintained . . . progress will be slow." In the second paragraph of his address, Smith defined "science" in simple but memorable terms: "Science does not cling tenaciously to one aspect of a subject, take sides, and exhort and entreat its votaries to share its views, but its true essence consists in presenting as many aspects, as many conflicting theories which have any standing, as possible. Science can never sermonize, but it can and must raise doubts and lead to further searching enquiries."

Theobald Smith had no personal drive to establish new professional organizations; but he willingly joined the more promising enterprises started by others. In April 1900, he attended the founding and became a member of the American Association of Pathologists and Bacteriologists, now known as the American Association of Pathologists, Inc. He presided over the 1924 meeting at Buffalo and was awarded the Association's Gold-Headed Cane in 1930.[55] In 1913, he was one of twenty-five charter members of the American Society for Experimental Pathology, whose purpose was "to bring the productive investigators in pathology, working essentially by experimental methods, in closer affiliation with the workers in other fields of experimental medicine." The Society met in Boston at the end of 1914, when Smith became its second President. His successor was Simon Flexner. This Society merged with the American Association of Pathologists and Bacteriologists in 1976.[56]

Those Societies, in which Theobald Smith soon rose to prominence, were formed largely because of the microbiological discoveries of the nineteenth century's last quarter. Cohen has suggested that birth of the Society of American Bacteriologists was also "facilitated by the participation, two months previously, of thirty-two of its thirty-nine founders in the organization of the Section on Bacteriology and Chemistry . . . of the American Public Health Association."[57] Theobald recalled in 1931 that "I was a member of the Association for ten or fifteen years, and was at one time Chairman of the Laboratory Section."[58]

The formation of a Laboratory Section of this Association was instigated mainly by Wyatt Johnston of Montreal. He urged that a Report on "Procedures Recommended for the Study of Bacteria," prepared by a group comprising George Adami as Chairman, with William Welch, W.T. Sedgwick, and Theobald Smith among the seven other bacteriologist-authors, should be presented at the Association's annual meeting at Philadelphia in September 1897. This was done and the Report published in 1898.[59] Smith's fermentation tube, and his methods of preparing nutrient media, featured in the text. At its next annual meeting (Ottawa, 1898), the Association appointed a Committee, under Wyatt Johnston's chairmanship, to report on "Laboratory Work and Methods" at the Minneapolis meeting in 1899. There the proposal to form a Laboratory Section won enthusiastic approval. Theobald Smith, in absentia, was elected sectional chairman for the following year. (The Laboratory Section was designated Section on Bacteriology and Chemistry for the first two years of its existence.)

One morning in late October 1900, in Indianapolis, after having supped the night before with the State Governor and his wife at the suburban Hospital for the Insane,[60] Smith introduced the new Section's scientific program with a keynote address on "Public Health Laboratories." He stressed that the worker in such a laboratory should be "very cautious concerning the conclusion he may publish and maintain." In reporting results, "Conservatism is of the utmost importance . . . we should always clearly state the limitations governing our work." Mingled with these exhortations to caution was a warning that "crystallized methods" might be "both a safeguard and a danger. They guide us and make our results homogeneous. They may also petrify our modes of thought if we too slavishly adhere to them." Characteristically, he interspersed these admonitions with a philosophic deduction from the history of science:

> The most commanding geniuses have always created new methods rather than use those of their contemporaries or predecessors . . . Every discovery of a new fact demands a new method, or at least a profound modification of existing methods. From this point of view, methods and procedures are of very high significance in science.[61]

Theobald regularly attended the Association's meetings for several years, but eventually quietly resigned because, as he explained to the unwitting head-office secretary who had invited him to apply for membership, it had become "the organ of public health officials."[62]

In 1901, he was elected to Fellowship in the American Academy of Arts and Sciences and soon represented its Section of Medicine and Surgery as Councillor. In 1902, to secure membership in the Massachusetts Medical Society, he went to the trouble of taking the written and oral examinations. Now in his early forties, Theobald Smith was recognized by most professional and academic colleagues as an eloquent apostle of science as well as an eminent bacteriologist. To the initiated, he was *primus inter pares*. But despite these semblances of success, and in marked contrast to the balanced authority of his address to the Laboratory Section of the American Public Health Association, Smith had to battle for his conception of the needed area and facilities for research at Harvard. Every yard of floor space, every item of equipment, appeared to be disputed. Institutional poverty was interpreted as loss of confidence, and he felt very discouraged.

In April 1897, the President and Fellows of Harvard College had assigned the "finished North room" in the second story of the Bussey to Theobald Smith. Storer protested to Eliot in vain: "I should regard the act of alienating this North room as of the nature of an utter misconception on the part of the Corporation of the plan and purpose of the Bussey Institution."[63] The total cost of alterations and installations ($435) roughly equalled the difference between the interest on the endowment of $100,000 and the Fabyan professor's salary, and was charged to the George Fabyan fund. This fund had provided Smith already with $200 for a microscope and pathological materials, and with $25 monthly "to employ an additional servant." Another $250 was voted in June 1897 for apparatus and expenses in the new laboratory.[64] These sums were still inadequate for Smith's envisaged research and teaching program. Further correspondence ensued with Dr. Arthur Tracy Cabot, a distinguished surgeon and Fellow of the Harvard Corporation,[65] in which smith detailed his needs, stating that he "could profitably spend $200 a year on salaries and maintenance, in place of the $300 hitherto used;" but Cabot's support notwithstanding—"The desire of the Corporation is that your laboratory shall be so fitted out that you can devote yourself to any scientific work towards which you are drawn"[66]—the protest proved fruitless.

Then the situation became more promising. Hearts were touched and consciences troubled, and earmarked funds and equipment for Theobald Smith's department began to flow. Smith continued to deposit small sums himself, usually $25, received from the sale of tuberculin or mallein, with the Corporation for the Department's credit. In August 1900, George F. Fabyan and Prof. F.C. Shattuck each sent $250 "to aid in the equipment of the laboratory of Comparative Pathology." Within two years, additional donations included $100 from the newly created Rockefeller Institute; a Zeiss microscope and several pieces of optical equipment, through Dr. Austin Peters on behalf of the Massachusetts Society for Promoting Agriculture; an anonymous gift of $500, through Dr. F.C. Shattuck; and, in 1902, an additional $25,000 for the endowment of the Chair from its founder.[67]

Before cessation of the flow of gifts had been followed by more disgruntlement, Walcott and Eliot planned to benefit the State Board of Health, and also to recapture Smith's enthusiasm for his job, by erecting on the Bussey estate a new and separate laboratory building, to be designed by Smith, for the production of diphtheria antitoxin and the manufacture of vaccine virus. Further, the Department of Comparative Pathology would retain the expanded quarters assigned to it, under vigorous protest, by the Bussey Institution.

Smith wrote retrospectively: "To obtain a suitable site for the State Laboratory . . . would have been impossible without acquiring a large and expensive tract."[68] To overcome this difficulty, he later remembered, "the Corporation of Harvard University came to the aid of the State, and agreed to use a portion of the land of the Bussey Institution adjoining the Arnold Arboretum . . . and build a laboratory in which the preparation of diphtheria antitoxin and animal vaccine could be carried on together."[69]

Walcott and Eliot had agreed, moreover, that Theobald Smith should be granted leave of absence on full salary during the summer of 1903 to visit vaccine manufacturing plants in Europe. He would be accompanied by Marshal Fabyan, a third-year medical student at Harvard, and second son of George F. Fabyan, who had offered to finance the whole trip. The anxiety to retain Smith's loyalty reflected more than the conviction that he had exceptional gifts to dedicate and services to offer. As he had recently rejected an invitation to become director of the laboratory of the newly-formed Rockefeller Institute for Medical Research, the account of Theobald Smith's second visit to Europe should postdate an outline of the founding of that Institute. Chronology also dictates that other developments should be given primary consideration.

Smith's momentous discovery that bovine and human types of tubercle bacilli could be differentiated made it necessary to reappraise the public health significance of cattle tuberculosis. Since this work began while he was still employed at the B.A.I. in Washington, renewed attention will first be focused on bovine tuberculosis and the ramifications these studies underwent in his first decade at Jamaica Plain. Theobald Smith's impatient researches on endemic malaria in the Boston area soon after he arrived there are less well-known and were sooner completed, but they certainly help to correct any impression that his frequent appeals for more space and equipment, and for trained laboratory assistants, were issued by a querulous empire-builder. Smith at this time should rather be viewed as a frustrated, over-committed scientist, eager to investigate problems of obvious public health consequence, far beyond those relating to diphtheria antitoxin production and assay, and to simple diagnostic laboratory procedures.

10

BOVINE TUBERCULOSIS

S almon's instruction to de Schweinitz to begin the manufacture of tuberculin, and that chemist's decision (without consulting Theobald Smith) to send out a questionnaire with this product, hastened Smith's decision to leave the Bureau of Animal Industry. An intolerable invasion of his own field of research was threatened, and either he or de Schweinitz must go. Recently he had observed and reported (1886) distinct differences between a "human" and a "bovine" type of tubercle bacillus. (The adjectival designations "human" and "bovine" have survived many reforms of bacterial nomenclature.) Among the attractions of a move to Boston were the ambitious plans of the State of Massachusetts for combatting both human and bovine tuberculosis.

The State Board of Health was especially concerned about the high incidence of "consumption." More than a decade before Koch's discovery of the causal bacillus, the Board's secretary, Dr. George Derby, had discussed this "terrible scourge" and its chief deterrents. "Fresh air by day and by night . . . Let in the sunlight, and never mind the carpets; better they should fade than the health of the family."[1] In 1895, soon after Smith's arrival, a circular from the State Board of Health informed the public about the nature of consumption and its mode of spread. Three years later, following a bill passed by the Legislature, the Massachusetts State Sanatorium opened at Rutland for tubercular patients "not too far advanced for reasonable hope of radical improvement." This was the nation's first State sanatorium. Late in 1896, sputum vials were offered for distribution by local Boards of Health.[2] Initially, roughly one-half of specimens reaching the laboratory were positive, but this proportion was reduced when detection of occult pulmonary tuberculosis became the main objectives, so that multiple specimens arrived from suspected or convalescent cases.

Smith was unenthusiastic about personal involvement in antituberculosis campaigns sponsored by public health organizations. Later, contact with famous clinicians especially involved in the control of this disease such as E.L. Trudeau, William Osler, and E.G. Janeway warmed him to the human applications of his laboratory researches. Thereafter, he faithfully attended advisory council meetings of the Henry Phipps Institute, became secretary of the United States Society for the Study and Prevention of Tuberculosis, and eventually was elected president of that Society's replacement, the National Tuberculosis Association.

Koch's initial declarations that tubercle bacilli from all mammalian sources were indistinguishable gave rise to the mistaken belief that tuberculous cows and phthisical human beings were reciprocal reservoirs of infection, and exaggerated fears of the bovine disease developed. Full control of tuberculosis would be impossible without cooperation between the human and veterinary professions. When Harold Ernst, M.D., and Austin Peters, D.V.M., reported to the Massachusetts Legislature that tubercle bacilli were detectable in milk from cows without palpable mammitis, the State Board of Cattle Commissioners, led by Dr. F.H. Osgood and Dean C.P. Lyman of the Harvard School of Veterinary Medicine, recommended drastic action. The Legislature passed a bill aimed at total eradication of bovine tuberculosis from the state through rigid scrutiny and tuberculin-testing of herds at frequent intervals, followed by destruction of infected animals and meat inspection in abattoirs. Herds rendered tuberculosis-free would be subjected to strict inter-herd quarantine, until the whole State was "accredited."[3]

By 1896, a state-wide tuberculin-testing program was in full swing. "During these few years of active warfare, beginning in 1893," Smith reported later, "I was able to make autopsies on about 350 head of cattle which had reacted to tuberculin." The finding that many of the world's best dairy cattle were reactors evoked "astonishment and consternation . . . [and] some ill-considered laws were passed to destroy all reacting cows and their flesh, for the purpose of eradicating the disease."[4]

The policy provoked opposition because of the high costs entailed in the bill's recommendations and also because "the importance of the strictly human source of tuberculosis, the sputum, was being pushed to the background and our State was appropriating not less than a quarter of a million dollars a year for the eradication of bovine tuberculosis."[5] Five experts, including Theobald Smith, were appointed to evaluate the tuberculin test. Each of them examined the carcasses of 130 reactors slaughtered at the Brighton abattoirs in April 1897 and submitted his own report. Theobald smith, Harold Ernst, and a veterinarian, George

Kinnell, reported the test to be very dependable.[6] A minority report by two veterinarians, Charles Wood and the vituperative Frank S. Billings, disparaged the whole legislation.[7]

The bill was abandoned in June 1897 because a committee representing the Senate and House advocated a more conservative program, which restricted the compulsory tuberculin test to cattle entering the Commonwealth. In 1898, an editorial by Theobald Smith in a local journal on "The Waste and Destruction of Wholesome Meat" pointed out that "50 to 80 percent of all cattle which react to tuberculin have only one or several thoracic lymph glands affected. Traces of disease cannot be found elsewhere."[8] ("By now," he told Gage, "I am deep in tuberculosis. The trunk I attacked 4 years ago has now divided into half-a-dozen stout branches. I am climbing up several of these at a time.")[9] The Cattle Commission, now under the chairmanship of Austin Peters, was empowered, through a proper inspection system, to end this waste of wholesome meat.

In Massachusetts, the Cattle Commissioners (three to five men appointed by the Legislature) had assumed the consulting function elsewhere performed by the State Veterinarian. Despite various kindnesses received from the Commission, Smith implied in a brief to President Eliot in 1899 that the Department of Comparative Pathology should take over this role. The Board should only "execute the laws of the State. Its mandates should come from a scientific institution not directly interested in the practical execution of the work, and not from its own agitation."[10] In 1902, the Board of Cattle Commissioners was succeeded by a one-man State Cattle Bureau, with Austin Peters as its Chief.[11] Twenty years later, the Tuberculosis Eradication Division was established federally at the Bureau of Animal Industry to deal with the problem of bovine tuberculosis.[12]

In May 1897, Smith resumed researches on cultures of tubercle bacilli of human or bovine origin. "Some of the work was done in the newly established laboratory of comparative pathology of the Harvard Medical School," i.e. in the Bussey Institution. Further, President Eliot reported that "the stable belonging to the Mansion House of the Bussey Institution was assigned in March 1897 to Professor Theobald Smith for the accommodation of cattle under observation while suffering with bovine tuberculosis."[13] The Board of Cattle Commissioners offered to furnish cattle and provide fodder for their maintenance.

A preliminary account, which included the Washington experiments involving two bacillary cultures and two heifers, was appended to the Cattle Commissioners' Annual Report for 1897. The new studies related to ten freshly isolated cultures, tested on ten healthy tuberculin-negative head of cattle. Each animal received intrathoracically 2 cc. of a bouillon suspension of a single strain of tubercle bacillus, whose turbidity matched "a bouillon culture of typhoid or hog-cholera bacilli about 24–26 hours old." Survivors were killed after two months and carefully examined post-mortem.

The six head that received human (sputum) bacilli gained weight and stayed afebrile. At autopsy, one showed no disease, two had slight local lesions, and three had more marked local lesions, but without dissemination. Five animals received bovine bacilli, and one a culture (probably of bovine origin) isolated from swine. These either lost weight or remained stationary, and were febrile for about three weeks. Two died of generalized tuberculosis, three showed extensive lesions, and one had severe but less extensive involvement. Smith concluded that "bovine tubercle bacilli and human bacilli as found in sputum are not identical," and that human sputum was neither especially dangerous to cattle nor a factor in the introduction of tuberculosis into a healthy herd.[14]

In September 1898, the *Journal of Experimental Medicine* (edited by William Welch) published an expanded, sixty-page account of this work, which included the cultural methods, the results on rabbits and guinea-pigs, and the pathological changes in all inoculated animal species. Smith had delivered the gist of his findings early in May, before the Association of American Physicians, in whose *Transactions* it was also published. In the same month, he summarized the investigations before the Boston Society of Medical Sciences, and his presentation appeared in its *Journal* as well. Finally, in 1937, the complete report was reprinted in the first volume of *Medical Classics*.[15]

The work involved seven cultures from human sputum, one from a *Nasua* pet (presumably human in origin), six isolated from cattle, and one each from pig, horse, and cat—the last two received from Dr. Langdon Frothingham. The pig and cat cultures acted like bovine strains, the horse culture gave equivocal results. Cultures were grown on coagulated dog serum. The opening paragraph described the quandary posed by the dissimilar pathogenicities:

> The adaptation of a highly parasitic organism to one of these species for centuries may possibly deprive it of much of its power to multiply in the other. Or the reverse may be true. The adaptation of the bovine bacillus to a longer, more vigorous organization may thereby render it more dangerous to man. Assumptions of this sort stimulate inquiry but do not furnish us with positive information.

Theobald repeatedly examined hundreds of slides, and concluded that most strains of human tubercle bacilli grew more vigorously and attained greater length than bovine bacilli. Softer medium, coagulated at 71°C instead of 75°C, yielded feebly-staining organisms. On firmer serum, round, subterminal, deeply-stained bodies developed. Theobald conjectured that Koch, when upholding in his remarkable monograph "the unity of the tubercle bacille which he obtained from human beings as well as from a variety of mammalia," had mistaken these for spores, but they were not dismissed by Smith as probably a degenerative or involution form of unsolved significance.

"The most important means of demonstrating identity or divergence of characters of pathogenic bacteria is the test upon animals," Theobald contended. To secure maximum differentiation between human and bovine cultures in pathogenicity tests, guinea-pigs should be inoculated subcutaneously and rabbits intravenously. Both animal species showed greater susceptibility to bovine than to human sputum cultures, but the difference was more pronounced in rabbits. In guinea-pigs receiving large doses of bovine or human cultures intra-abdominally, the disease progressed so rapidly that these types appeared equally virulent. However, under suitable conditions, animals given bovine cultures died sooner and their more extensive lesions contained greater numbers of bacilli. Koch had failed "to recognize any differences worth mentioning" in the virulence of tubercle bacilli from different mammalian species, as he was then "endeavoring to prove to the world that the tubercle bacillus is the cause of tuberculosis. Minor details received no attention because of the great and difficult task before him." That generous explanation stands in marked contrast to Koch's refusal for many years to mention Smith's clear-cut observations and conclusions conveyed in 1896, both as published report and in personal conversation.

In Theobald Smith's experience, tubercle bacilli from human sputum and from bovine sources were clearly distinguishable. The recurring hypothesis that the bovine type could convert into the sputum type in the human body was unsupported by bacteriological evidence. The crucial issue, the possible infection of the human subject by bovine bacilli, could not be settled by direct experiment, but the time had come "to study with care the tubercle bacilli from cases of supposed animal origin, so that some experimental, trustworthy basis may be formed on which to found statistics." He himself set about that tedious and intricate task. A whole decade later, Theobald Smith presented his views on type conversion at the Sixth International Congress on tuberculosis, held at Washington in 1908. He was even then reluctant to gainsay the hypothesis completely—"The time has not yet come for us to state that one type can or cannot be transformed into the other."[16] However, his own and corroborative data had convinced him that bovine and human types of tubercle bacilli were not interconvertible within reasonable experimental time limits. He was also certain that the bovine type was potentially pathogenic for man.

While skeptical about *transformation* in this species, Smith recognized that *variation* might occur. Indeed, at the inaugural meeting of the Society of American Bacteriologists at New Haven in 1899, he included mammalian tubercle bacilli among many examples of pathogenic bacteria in which he had observed variation[17]—a pioneering step. He cited the recent report of K. Vagadez, a former assistant to Koch, who noted a wide range of virulence for rabbits shown by twenty-eight cultures of human tubercle bacilli and two *Perlsucht* strains.[18] Previously, in September 1898, as guest speaker at the annual meeting of the American Climatological Association (an anti-tuberculosis society dedicated to open-air sanatorium treatment), Smith had compared the virulence of tubercle bacilli to the varied toxigenic capacities of diphtheria cultures. Variations of the tubercle bacillus had been little studied, he contended, "mainly because it seems to have been taken for granted that varieties do not exist." He had isolated a strain of low pathogenicity for rabbits and guinea-pigs from a cervical abscess in a man. Although in "diseases of slow progress,"[19] attention must be given to the factor of host resistance, in this instance the strain itself was of intrinsically low virulence. Smith had previously detailed that particular situation and grasped the opportunity to caution against assigning such a patient to a hospital ward for consumptives.[20]

Always mindful of the practical consequences of his theoretical conclusions, and impressed by the hazard of ingesting raw milk from tuberculous herds, Theobald Smith reemphasized the importance of pasteurizing cow's milk as a public health measure. He resumed his studies on the heat susceptibility of tubercle bacilli.[21] Smith selected six cultures of bovine and one of porcine origin, and two from human sputum, all isolated by himself, and tested the infectivity of the samples by intraperitoneal injection into guinea-pigs, confirmed by autopsy. Emulsified in various fluids, including milk, most of the bacilli, regardless of type, were destroyed in five to ten minutes at 60°C. There were no survivors after fifteen to twenty minutes at this temperature. However, the pellicle which formed during exposure of the milk suspensions to 60°C. might contain living tubercle bacilli, even after sixty minutes.[22]

The potential pathogenicity of bovine tubercle bacilli for man did not weaken Smith's opinion that in the campaign against tuberculosis of cattle, dairy farmers in general were not pulling their weight. On balance, in his view, bovine tuberculosis should be regarded as mainly a problem of agricultural economics, for which the livestock owner rather than the taxpayer ought to assume the chief fiscal responsibility. "Bovine tuberculosis is at best an agricultural calamity and its widespread diffusion and frightful ravages should arouse even the most conservative to bring about by individual effort rather than with the help of the public purse the rehabilitation of the dairy-cow."[23]

At the British Congress on Tuberculosis, held in London on July 22–26, 1901, the keynote address, entitled "The Fight Against Tuberculosis," was delivered by

Robert Koch. His message in that setting guaranteed a sensational response. Koch denied the unicity of tubercle bacilli, and asserted that the bovine bacillus was harmless to man. Queen Victoria had died six months before. Her cousin, the venerable Duke of Cambridge, a retired field marshal, represented King Edward VII and presided over the opening ceremonies, including a series of short addresses by distinguished delegates. William Osler, spokesman for the United States, assured his audience that the 2,500 registrants were determined to reduce "the captain of the men of death .. to the ranks."[24] The Duke invited Osler to sit and chat. He liked Americans: they were "so joky."[25]

Several international experts among the delegates had become skeptical of Koch's original claim that tubercle bacilli from different animal hosts were indistinguishable; nevertheless, they had sponsored public health regulations aimed at protecting the customer against bovine tuberculosis. The incidence of apparently milk-borne tuberculosis remained particularly high in the United Kingdom. Koch's clever but grievously flawed address now negated all these efforts.[26]

He sought to cloak the reversal of his well-known stand on the unicity of tubercle bacilli by stating that in his earlier work, verifications of the distinctiveness or otherwise of the two forms were unavailable, so he had left this question undecided. Inoculated guinea-pigs and rabbits also yielded inconclusive results, but indications of differences between the two forms of tuberculosis "probably were not wanting." Recent access to experimental cattle enable him and Prof. Schütz, Director of Pathology at the Berlin Veterinary College, to show that bovine and human cultures were strikingly different. Acknowledging neither the information imparted by Theobald Smith in 1896, nor the more detailed findings published by him in 1898, three years before this address, Koch condescendingly stated: "Comparative investigations regarding human and bovine tuberculosis have been made very recently in North America by Smith, Dinwiddie, Frothingham and Repp, and their result agrees with ours." Owing to the great importance of the question, the German Government had appointed a Commission to make further inquiries.

To the acceptable contention that his experimental cattle resisted inocula of human sputum bacilli, Koch added the astonishing claim that bovine cultures were of negligible infectivity for man: "I should estimate the extent of the infection by the milk and flesh of tuberculous cattle, and the butter made of their milk, as hardly greater than that of hereditary transmission, and I therefore do not deem it advisable to take any measures against it."[27] Lord Lister, who chaired the meeting (at the age of seventy-four), in thanking Koch, disputed "the startling thesis that bovine tubercle could not develop in the human body . . . The Congress would probably require a more searching inquiry into the subject before accepting this doctrine." Professors Nocard, Bang, and Sims Woodhead quickly announced that Prof. Koch's arguments left them unconvinced. Section III of the Congress ("Pathology and Bacteriology") unanimously passed a resolution submitted by Woodhead, its president: "This Section considers that, in the light of the work which has been presented at its sittings, Medical Officers of Health should continue to use all the powers at their disposal, and relax no effort to prevent the possible spread of tuberculosis by meat or milk." Woodhead also urged that the Minister of Agriculture be advised to appoint another Royal Commission to settle this issue, meanwhile continuing the current measures as recommended by the previous commission, dating from 1895.

A new five-man Royal Commission on Tuberculosis was appointed soon after the British Congress disbanded. Throughout its prolonged existence, Professor G. Sims Woodhead (later Sir German Sims Woodhead), played a leading role. The other members were Sir Michael Foster (Chairman), Profs. Sidney Martin, J. (later Sir John) MacFadyean, and R. (later Sir Rubert) Boyce. Before the Commission's Final Report was published in 1911, Chairman Foster and Commissioner Boyce were dead; and so was Koch.

Two contributors to the program of Section III properly acknowledged Smith's prior work. The bacteriologist M.P. Ravenel, at the Laboratory of the State Live Stock Sanitary Board, Philadelphia, had followed the methods and confirmed the recent findings and conclusions of Theobald Smith. Peculiarities of growth and morphology, and marked differences in pathogenicity for various animal species, permitted human and bovine types to be differentiated. Ravenel considered the evidence also warranted the assumption that "the bovine bacillus has a high degree of pathogenic power for man . . . especially manifest in the early years of life."[28] D.B. Bang of Copenhagen recorded observations on the thermal death-point of tubercle bacilli in milk.[29] Using rabbits, his results were similar to those reported by Smith two years before, with guinea-pigs as indicators of bacillary survival.

As W.H. Welch did not attend the Congress, William Osler was probably the only person there who had heard Theobald Smith address the Association of American Physicians in 1896 on the differences between bovine and human cultures. Osler's sense of fairness may have impelled him to draw the attention of journalists to Smith's priority. Hence, perhaps, the lengthy article with its arresting headline, "KOCH SIMPLY FOLLOWS, BOSTON DOCTOR LEADS," which appeared in the *Boston Post* about a week after Koch's address.[30] Using statistics on death rates from tuberculosis in some of the world's largest cities, borrowed from another periodical, the journalist accused Koch of outright plagiarism, although "scientists to whom the *Post* has submitted the question emphatically deny that this is the case, none more so than Dr. Theobald Smith, who is most concerned." The issue might have "slumbered unnoticed, had not Professor Koch attracted the attention of the world to it."

Other newspapers took up the story and Smith found himself in the limelight. In a major headline, the *Boston Journal* of August 4 asked: "DID DR. KOCH USE A BOSTONIAN'S THEORIES?" The answer was given in a subsidiary heading: "Dr. Theobald Smith of Harvard the Real Pioneer in the Investigation of Bovine and Human Tuberculous Bacilli—His Theories Published in 1898." To a reporter seeking further enlightenment at Smith's "beautiful estate in the midst of the Arnold Arboretum," who inquired whether bovine tubercle bacilli were harmless to human beings, Theobald responded that removing the restrictions on infected cattle would appear "unwise and perhaps dangerous."[31]

The *Brooklyn Eagle* of August 11, 1901, under the headline "American Forestalled Dr. Koch in Tuberculosis Discovery," mentioned Theobald Smith's priority in differentiating human and bovine cultures, "publicly recalled within the last few days by Professor Welch . . . and a number of other well known bacteriologists." Smith had concurred that the primary aim of efforts to control tuberculosis should be to diminish infection through human sputum, and had advocated isolation of patients either in hospitals or sanatoria.[32] But while he agreed with Koch, even in the public press, that the sputum of careless consumptives was the main vehicle of human tuberculosis, he could not consider sputum the *only* source. He took pains to stress this point in his addresses to professional colleagues.

Dr. E.G. Janeway, a former Commissioner of Health of New York, attended the Congress in London, and four months later he described the highlights to the New York Academy of Medicine. He had invited Theobald Smith to address the Academy on the relationship between bovine and human tuberculosis: "You have been working so earnestly in this matter that I am sure a resume of your work would greatly interest the members."[33] In clarifying complex issues, Smith displayed remarkable personal detachment and magnanimity: it required the authority of a Koch, reversing his own long-standing conclusion, to awaken the lethargy of investigators, start new commissions, and arouse the opposition of public-health and other officials. Smith nevertheless maintained his own conclusions, rejecting "the sweeping, and what appear to me hasty, inferences drawn by Koch from his experiments that the bovine bacillus cannot invade the human body."[34]

Koch reiterated his London theme at the International Conference on Tuberculosis held in Berlin toward the end of 1902. Dismissing as of no significance all ostensible bovine-type infections in man, he announced that

The battle against tuberculosis must aim at shutting off the chief, indeed we may say almost the only, source of infection. This is those consumptives who in consequence of the unfavourable conditions under which they live, or because they obstinately set aside the simples rules for the prevention of infection, are a danger to their companions.[35]

This prompted Theobald to point out diplomatically that "his [Koch's] views exercised a salutary influence in forceably drawing the attention . . . from a minor to a major source of disease."[36]

At the time of the British Congress on Tuberculosis, belief in the potential pathogenicity for men of the bovine tubercle bacillus rested chiefly upon recognizing the soundness of Smith's work on type differentiation, and upon the fact established by Smith and several others that the bovine bacillus could be secreted and sold in the milk of tuberculous cows. This type, according to Smith, should be sought in primary intestinal tuberculosis of infants and young children. He cautioned that "The cultivation of tubercle bacilli requires, even under the best circumstances, constant personal attention and those not prepared to give it had better not attempt it seriously."[37] Further, verification of identity must be bacteriological, i.e. "based on the isolation of tubercle bacilli having the characteristics of the bovine variety."[38] Smith was surprised by the low incidence of bovine isolates in the selected human infections. Near the outset, he confided to Gage, "Precious little has been demonstrably traced to cattle. It reminds me of the Chinese gong ringing for dinner and the slim repast we sit down to afterwards."[39]

Eighteen months later, still baffled by his failure to isolate bovine bacilli from selected human cases, Theobald Smith again grumbled to Gage: "I have been busy at my Bussey workshop—spreading out thin on a number of subjects—I do not feel sure of any perceptible progress."[40] However, he was encouraged by the discovery of the paper by Vagadez[41] in a journal edited by Koch. Smith surmised that the Vagadez strain "W.XX," which had been isolated from a fifteen-year-old girl with pulmonary tuberculosis, was of bovine type. However, the first generally accepted bovine-type culture from a human case was the "BB" strain of Ravenel, from the mesenteric glands of a child aged seventeen months, who died of tuberculous meningitis. This strain proved very virulent for experimental cattle. Since 1897, Ravenel had zealously urged the dangers to human health of bovine tuberculosis.[42]

During the period 1903–07, Theobald Smith published three papers detailing his cultural studies of tubercle bacilli. The first and longest of the series was read to the Sixth Congress of American Physicians and Surgeons at Washington in May 1903.[43] This centered upon the isolation of two tubercle cultures (by passage through guinea-pigs) from the mediastinal glands of two children aged three years, both of whom died in the same Boston hospital with generalized tuberculosis. One culture was of human, the other of bovine type. Additional strains from two patients proved of human type, while two cat strains were of bovine type. A canine strain, provisionally of human type, was lost before tests were completed.

In order to test the revived notion that bovine strains were modifiable in the human host to human-type bacilli, Theobald Smith had attempted unsuccessfully to transform cultures by passage through rabbits. He also described here for the first time his "reaction-curve" for differentiating human from bovine bacilli *in vitro*. Grown for up to three months in acidified beef bouillon containing 3–5 percent of glycerol, human strains tended to make the medium more acidic, bovine strains to render it alkaline, using phenophthalein as indicator. The curves that resulted from plotting the medium's reaction at suitable intervals had type-identifying characteristics. Smith and his disciples advocated and refined the method for several years,[44] but it proved too complex for routine use. Sometimes he got so "deep in tuberculosis" that would-be followers found themselves out of their depth.

In 1904, Theobald Smith described three cultures isolated from fatal cases of generalized tuberculosis, considered to be food-borne. The human subjects were respectively an eight-month-old infant, a Chinese male, aged twenty-six years, and a thirty-nine-year-old Negro cook. The isolated cultures were all of human type. He presented his detailed findings in February to the Boston Society of Medical Sciences, and in May to the Association of American Physicians in Washington.[45]

In May 1905, Smith addressed the first Annual Meeting of the National Association for the Study and Prevention of Tuberculosis. Among the explored branches of the tuberculosis tree, whose trunk Theobald Smith had climbed in the mid-1890's, was the significance and constancy of capsule formation by the various types of tubercle bacilli. In Smith's hand, parallel cultures from human and bovine sources showed more abundant capsular substance in human-type bacilli, especially after longer growth periods. In this bacterial species, pathogenic power and capsule formation seemed unrelated. Provided their conditions of growth were controlled carefully, he concluded, "The characters of the several races of tubercle bacilli . . . still a burning question in some quarters . . . are remarkable constant."[46]

In 1907, with his assistant H.R. Brown as coauthor, Theobald Smith again reported bovine-type tubercle bacilli as human pathogens. They studied eight cultures from selected cases of human tuberculosis, using a freshly isolated cattle strain for comparison. Of four bovine-type cultures isolated from children aged two to five years, three were from tonsils removed by Dr. J.L. Goodale—first producer of diphtheria antitoxin at Jamaica Plain—while the fourth was from a case of tuberculous meningitis with caseous lymph nodes.[47] Four human-type cultures were isolated from adults, one from the urine of a case of genito-urinary tuberculosis, the other three from patients who died with generalized tuberculosis.

By now, individual reports had strengthened the evidence which Smith and Brown undertook to submit to "a summary and critical analysis . . . in a subsequent paper."[48] They did not do so, presumably because of the unequivocal verdicts of the Royal Commission on Tuberculosis, which began issuing reports and supplementary documents contradicting Koch's pronouncements at the Sixth International Congress. Sir Michael Foster's successor as Chairman of the Royal Commission was W.M. (later Sir William) Power, medical officer of the Local Government Board. The Commission's specific assignments were to determine:

1. Whether tuberculosis in animals and man is one and the same disease.
2. Whether animals and man can be reciprocally infected with tuberculosis.
3. The conditions, if any, under which tuberculosis is transmitted from animals to man, and what circumstances favor or discourage such transmission.

The first Royal Commission on Tuberculosis (1890–95) had been considered dilatory. The second Commission (appointed in 1901) took twice as long to produce its fifty-four-page *Final Report*. However, it issued three *Interim Reports* (in 1904, 1907, and 1909) as well as several volumes of Appendices, for a net expenditure of about £75,000. Eventually all concerned found patience rewarded, and the taxpayer got his money's worth. The public purse was spared and science rendered a great service through the generosity of Sir James Blyth, whose farms at Stanstead, Kent, were placed at the Commission's disposal for laboratory work and cattle experiments.

The new Royal Commission's methodology was thorough, its scope broad, and its recommendations forthright. Koch's contention that bovine-type tubercle bacilli played no significant role in human tuberculosis was vigorously opposed—"The Royal Commission to inquire into the relations of human and animal tuberculosis . . . has obtained striking experimental results which contravert Professor Koch's hypothesis."[49] Other national groups (including those at the Gesundheitsamt, Koch's own headquarters) had similar findings. There was complete agreement that bovine and human strains of tubercle bacilli, although related, were nevertheless different in growth properties and in pathogenicity for laboratory animals; that in suitable dosages, bovine-type bacilli proved virulent for cattle and rabbits, whereas human-type cultures were practically harmless for these animals; and that bovine cultures might be pathogenic and even lethal for humans, young children being especially liable to tuberculous cervical and mesenteric lymphadenitis due to ingestion of raw cow's milk. That all these findings had been reported or foretold by Theobald Smith in the preceding decade was forgotten or overlooked at the Sixth International Congress on Tuberculosis, held at Washington from September 21 to October 12, 1908, when the situation came to a head.

Koch and his wife were in Japan, basking in his fame, prior to resuming their world tour, when he received instructions from Berlin to lead the German delegation to the Congress. In his main address, entitled "The Relations of Human and Bovine Tuberculosis," Koch at last acknowledged that Theobald Smith (present in the audience) had first drawn his attention to differences in the two types of bacilli. But neither in the address, nor in the *in camera* discussion that took place later (at Koch's request), did he modify his contentions as to the negligible pathogenicity of bovine bacilli for man.[50] Theobald Smith and Sims Woodhead were conciliatory in approach; Hermann Biggs tried flattery; many of those present became impatient; and some were outspokenly hostile.

Leonard Pearson, the State veterinarian of Pennsylvania, and Ravenal's nominal chief, upbraided Koch for interfering "most seriously with the control of bovine tuberculosis, and hence with the danger to man due to its prevalence." If the firmness and unity of the opposition surprised Koch, he stood his ground undaunted and alone, with strident obstinacy and militaristic arrogance defending the wrong. A leading British textbook of bacteriology has extended the chidings of Leonard Pearson into a timeless denunciation of that false doctrine which exonerated "cows from all blame in the causation of tuberculosis in man;" so that "the public health expert has to fight a continuous battle against the ignorance and prejudice resulting from an authoritative statement made on inadequate evidence"[51] over a century ago.

Although his scientific position was unassailable, Theobald Smith preferred to avoid contention and to be self-effacing. His own paper, entitled "The Relation Between Human and Animal Tuberculosis, with Special Reference to the Question of the Transformation of Human and Other Types of the Tubercle Bacillus,"[52] could be read without defiantly introducing new instances of bovine-type isolates from human cases. Smith's former assistant, Paul Lewis (now working under Simon Flexner at the Rockefeller Institute), felt no such constraint. He reported on a series of fifteen consecutive cases of tuberculous cervical adenitis seen at the Harvard Medical School. Bovine-type cultures had been isolated from the surgically-removed tissue of nine children, while the other six cases had yielded human-type cultures.[53] Shortly after the Congress, Marshal Fabyan reported from Smith's department three clinically diverse cases of tuberculosis due to bovine-type bacilli.[54]

Smith's own paper stated that investigators were practically unanimous in acknowledging "a sharp, easily recognized difference" involving morphological, cultural and pathogenic features between the types of specific bacilli isolated from human consumptive sputum and from tuberculous cattle. While the possibility of interconvertibility of the human, bovine and avian types of tubercle bacilli was undeniable, the phenomenon had not been demonstrated and was unlikely to be of any practical significance. The bovine type had been detected in man, but almost exclusively in infections pointing to the digestive tract as a portal of entry. However, contrary to Behring's claim that all human tuberculosis was acquired by alimentary route, Smith advanced evidence that human tuberculosis existed in regions having little or no chance of conveyance by cattle. Such situations obtained in Japan, according to Kitasato; in northern Sweden; and on the Labrador Coast, as reported by his former Cornell contemporary Dr. Alfreda Withington, who had spent a recent season with the Grenfell Mission.[55] Under H.M. Biggs' chairmanship, an informal *in camera* conference of leading international experts convened at Koch's request after the Congress, but failed to reach common ground, mainly because of Koch's intransigence.

Koch's attitude at the Congress was the reverse of Smith's. Annoyed at the interruption of his triumphant world tour, Koch seemed more than usually overconfident and blind to his own vulnerability. He cancelled his tour and returned to Germany where he resumed researches and promulgated his doctrines, despite signs of cardiac weakness. In April 1910, a few nights after lecturing on the epidemiology of tuberculosis to the Berlin Academy of Sciences, he suffered a severe anginal attack. Six weeks later, on May 27, he died suddenly and quietly while dozing in his chair at a sanitorium.

Koch had stayed in New York for several days after the Congress. On October 15, Flexner sought Smith's advice about the Rockefeller Institute's possible participation in an investigation of pulmonary tuberculosis which Koch would carry out on returning to Germany. Koch's main purpose was to ascertain whether bovine bacilli were ever involved, and if so, had been repeatedly isolated in cases of pulmonary tuberculosis. If Theobald Smith thought the Institute should participate, "the chief work would fall on Lewis." The response, if any, is not on record. The project was never activated because of Koch's increasing ill-health.

Two further group reports on bovine and human types of tubercle bacilli were published after Koch's death. In October 1910, Park and Krumwiede[56] reviewed recent work and reported their observations on unselected specimens from New York hospitals. They implicated bovine-type infections in twelve of eighteen cases of cervical adenitis and in eight of twenty cases of abdominal or generalized tuberculosis, all in children aged under five years. In the five to sixteen years age group, cases of cervical adenitis yielded eight bovine-type strains among a total of twenty-seven cultures. By contrast, only one bovine-type strain was identified in four cultures isolated from adults and adolescents with genito-urinary tuberculosis, while none was present in 291 cultures from cases of pul-monary tuberculosis.

In July 1911, the Royal Commission issued its *Final Report.* A.S. Griffith's two-volume Appendix soon followed, detailing the bacillary types involved in vari-ous forms of the human disease.[57] Griffith extended his work in this field for many years after the last technical appendix appeared in 1913. The Commis-sion's elaborate inquiries reached certain main conclusions, which merit a brief summary.

1. *General Technical Principles:* Type conversion, though theoretically possible, seldom if ever occurred under ordinary circumstances and hence did not affect the identification of human and bovine types of tubercle bacilli. Avian bacilli were very rarely pathogenic for human subjects. Other consensual findings were the growth stimulating (*eugonic*) effect of glycerol-containing medium upon hu-man cultures, and the absence of such effect (*dysgonic*) upon bovine cultures. Many experimental animal species, particularly rabbits and cattle, were more susceptible to bovine than to human cultures. In some hands, rabbits proved more reliable for type differentiation by virulence tests.

2. *Distribution and Incidence of Bovine Cultures in Human Subjects:* The first official refutation of the claim that *Perlsucht* bacilli were practically non-infective for man came from the Kossel team at the Gesundheitsamt in Berlin.[58] Among sixteen cultures isolated from young children with cervical lymphadenitis or abdominal tuberculosis, ten were of bovine type. In the Royal Commission's *Second Report* (1907), three of nine cultures isolated from cases of cervical lymphadenitis, and ten out of nineteen from abdominal tuberculosis, again affecting young children, were of bovine type. Thus bovine bacilli were responsible for about one-half of cases in sample groups of these two clinical forms of the disease.

Theobald Smith forecast in 1898 that the bovine bacillus might infect human beings through inhalation as well as by ingestion, and that persons closely associ-ated with cattle should be susceptible to this mode of infection. "If bovine bacilli may invade the human body without let or hindrance, we have not only food in-fection through milk and milk products to guard against, but also the inhalation disease to which men are exposed in stables containing tuberculous cattle."[59] Many years elapsed before this prophecy was fulfilled, but in 1932 Lange re-ported some regional figures from Germany, showing an incidence of 0.7 per-cent bovine type in 281 cultures isolated from the sputum of adults with pulmo-nary tuberculosis, whereas the corresponding figure in forty occupationally-exposed adults was 20 percent.[60] At the same meeting, Griffith reported that of 548 cultures isolated from patients with pulmonary phthisis in Scotland, 3 percent were identified as bovine-type.[61] More data on this question are furnished by Myers and Steele.[62] Koch would have been astounded by such figures.

3. *Preventive Measures:* The Royal Commission urged that better security should be provided against alimentary infection conveyed by foodstuffs from tuberculous animals. In particular, public health regulations should ban "the milk of the recognizably tuberculous cow, irrespective of the site of the disease, whether in the udder or internal organs."[63] In Britain, preventive measures initially failed, not due to their inherent complexity, but because apathy, ignorance and prejudice interfered with their implementation. As late as 1944, bovine-type cultures were responsible for 30–35 percent of cases of non-pulmonary tuberculosis in persons under fifteen years old. Since then, tuberculosis has been virtually eliminated from cattle in Britain; almost all supplies of liquid milk have become subject to heat treatment, and the bovine type of infection in man has disappeared.

In Germany, where the incidence of bovine tuberculosis in man was never as high, the disease came sooner under control. In the United States, the incidence has varied according to the knowledge and zeal of state and municipal health authorities. A campaign against tuberculosis was conducted with special vigor and success in New York City under the leadership of Hermann L. Biggs, General Medical Officer to its Board of Health from 1902 to 1913. In 1904, at the newly established Henry Phipps Institute, Biggs gave an outstanding address on the administrative control of tuberculosis.[64] This campaign, and the further improvements in New York City's anti-tuberculosis measures reported by Biggs at the Sixth International Congress at Washington in 1908, were strongly commended by Koch. The states of Massachusetts, Pennsylvania, and New York showed special initiative in their anti-tuberculosis campaigns. The State of New York addressed the particular problem of bovine tuberculosis control. In November 1914, the Legislature appointed a twenty-person committee of experts to investigate the causes, incidence and prevention of bovine tuberculosis. Biggs and V. Moore were members, and Theobald Smith was nominated chairman of the Commission. After five or six meetings, the Commission published a report in March 1915.[65] Its main recommendations were the pasteurization of all market milk and cream from herds not proven tuberculin-negative; and the pasteurization of all skimmed milk and whey to be fed to calves and swine. However, a bill embodying these measures was rejected by the Legislature (For further details, see Chapter 21).

Among the fruits garnered by Theobald Smith in climbing the tuberculosis tree were improvements in cultural techniques; the distinction of bovine from human types of tubercle bacilli; the recognition of a range of virulence within these types, especially among human strains; the isolation of bovine-type strains from human patients; the demonstration of type stability; and the effectiveness of pasteurization (properly conducted) on tuberculous milk. Few younger microbiologists would be aware of Smith's role in any of these accomplishments, justifying his own pronouncement that "We must not be discouraged if the products of our labor are not read or even known to exist."[66]

It has been asserted that the eclipse of Smith's fame "testifies partly to his self-effacing character."[67] Certainly he lacked the flamboyance of Ronald Ross and the aggressiveness of Robert Koch.[68] Toward much of his own work on tuberculosis, he appeared at times even self-abnegatory. Yet he knew the value of his contributions and resented attempts to belittle them. For instance, in 1931, Simon Flexner forwarded to Smith for comment an excerpt from a paper on "bacteriological typing" by F. Neufeld of Berlin, which claimed, "Through Theobald Smith and Robert Koch, the causative agents of mammalian tuberculosis were separated into human and bovine types."[69] Smith's response was tinged with smoldering resentment rather than lofty indifference. He outlined thus the historic sequence of events:

> 1st paper 1896. Talk with Koch in Berlin 1896 (he entirely quiet and noncommittal). 2nd paper 1898. Koch's address 1901. Koch acknowledges my giving him *the idea* (in 1896)—in Koch's address to 1908 Congress in Washington—a statement found in his collected papers. Neufeld's adding Koch's name is pure nationalism to which they are so inclined in the face of clear-cut data. It's all on record, even in Koch's own words.

Smith charitably added: "Possibly Neufeld never read Koch's address here in Washington."[70] The persistent adulation of Koch perhaps provoked after all some personal envy in Theobald Smith, who showed the very human trait of preserving scrapbook reminders of Koch's plagiarisms and about-faces.

Resentment might have changed to anger if Smith read Lange's claim, presented a few months later at the Centenary Meeting in London of the British Medical Association. "It has been possible since Koch's day to confirm thoroughly his opinion that bovine tubercle bacilli can be definitely distinguished from human bacilli by laboratory investigation, and that the types are constant."[71] Nor can such distortions be blamed always upon over-zealous nationalism. At the same commemorative meeting in 1932, Griffith discussed the bovine tubercle bacillus in relation to human tuberculosis. He made several allusions to Koch, but did not once mention Theobald Smith.[72]

At the outset of his bacteriological career, Smith picturesquely confided to Gage his obsession of always covering his candle light with a bushel basket. Fourteen years later, when launching sustained researches into tuberculosis, he expressed again this peculiar diffidence to his old friend: "There is something in the exuberant productiveness in our special field of work going on all over the world which at times make one feel paralyzed, especially when the time comes to take some definite stand on any practical problem."[73] If that "paralysis" assumed the form of withdrawal from a confrontation with Koch, a sensitive observer would understand and even applaud the reaction. But fellow-members of committees were less patient when Theobald Smith's compulsive pondering of all sides of an issue rendered him altogether mute, or at least reduced his ability to help colleagues make up their minds.

To his chosen disciples, Theobald Smith was unequalled in his capacity to inspire, and to be inspired, by the atmosphere of pure science. A close and personal assistant felt always grateful for having shared the experience with him. Smith constantly reminded himself and other workers at the bench of "the importance of steadying the flights of our imagination by chaining it to patient research within and without the laboratory, and accepting only those premises which have successfully passed a severe scientific scrutiny."[74] Hypotheses were anathema, unless supported by adequate experimental evidence. If his researches produced conflicting results, a conclusive report might be long delayed.

Soon after his pioneer studies on the bovine type of tubercle bacillus had been established, Smith had to interrupt his researches on tuberculosis. Before long, he resumed climbing the tree, hoping to discover a way to induce specific immunity against the bacillus. His fruitless exploration of this branch will be outlined in a later chapter. Though he turned to less disappointing fields of experimentation, Theobald Smith maintained a constructive and life-long interest in tuberculosis. In his seventy-fifth year, still at work, he penned some sagacious and relevant advice to younger generations of microbiologists:

> No research will answer all questions that the future may raise . . . It is not profitable to enter into controversies, especially with those working in another geographic area or continent . . . even the prizes do not always go to the discoveries to which we would assign them . . . The individual worker finds the problem too large, not too difficult. He must learn to work with others.[75]

11

MALARIA AND SANITATION

Malaria

Throughout the nineteenth century, malaria retarded the white man's advances in almost every direction on the North American continent. From the St. Lawrence Valley to the Mississippi and beyond, from the southernmost states of the Union to Alaska, this disease was often a bane to the immigrant and a brake on development. During the 1850's, a few years before Theobald Smith was born, malaria repeatedly interrupted the completion by the Royal Engineers of the Rideau Canal linking Kingston and Ottawa, the future capital of Canada. In the first decade of the present century, construction of the much better-known and far more important Panama Canal hinged upon mastery of regional malaria and yellow fever. Theobald Smith's trail-blazing work on Texas fever prepared the way for the discoveries of Ronald Ross and Walter Reed, and the consequent vigorous anti-mosquito measures at the Isthmus by William Gorgas.

At Constantine, Algeria, late in 1880, Alphonse Laveran declared the causal agent of malaria to be a hematozoon, which destroyed the host's red blood cells during its asexual multiplication. Several subsequent papers by Laveran confirmed and expanded his observations, culminating in 1891 in a treatise entitled *Du Paludisme et de son Hematozoaire*[1] which was translated into English by J. W. Martin and republished in 1893 as *Paludism*.[2] Laveran described four distinctive components of a parasitic life-cycle in blood films from malaria patients, but made no attempt to connect them sequentially. The commonest elements, capable of amoeboid movement, were hyaline, spherical, expansile bodies, free-floating or attached to red blood cells. Mobile fragments ("flagella") might protrude from the periphery of these bodies and break away in a fashion that convinced Laveran of their living nature. The more severe cases showed crescent-shaped, cylindrical bodies, often with central collections of granular pigment. Occasional red cells were occupied by a spherical segmented "rosette" body, again with pigment in the center.

Laveran's "haematozoon of paludism" became a fiercely controversial topic in Europe and North America for several years. Indian Medical Service pundits who seldom or never looked down the barrel of a microscope, dismissed belief in the parasitic theory of malaria as "Laveranity." In 1882, the Frenchman took his specimens to Rome, where malaria was common and oil-immersion objectives were plentiful. Among those who saw his blood films were the pathologists E. Marchiafava and A. Bignami, the clinician G. Bastianelli, the hygienist A. Celli, the parasitologist G.B. Grassi, and C. Golgi, a visiting neurologist from the University of Pavia. Laveran contended that Marchiafava and Celli, after initial skepticism, plagiarized his discovery. A deplorable scramble for credit ensued. Eventually, Laveran was awarded the 1907 Nobel Prize in Medicine "for his works on the importance of protozoa in the origin of diseases."

At the inaugural meeting of the Association of American Physicians in June 1886 W.T. Councilman, then assistant to William Welch in the Pathology Laboratory at Johns Hopkins University, gave a paper on the blood in malaria patients,[3] partly confirming Marchiafava and Celli's observations on an intracorpuscular amoeboid body which they had named *Plasmodium malariae*. William Osler, a skilled microscopist, although initially skeptical about the specific nature of the hyaline, amoeboid bodies noted by Councilman, became an enthusiastic convert to the protozoal origin of malaria after intensive study of blood smears from seventy patients with the disease at the Blockley Hospital in Philadelphia. He observed a convincing number of crescentic, flagellate and rosette forms, and attempted to differentiate the parasites associated with the three clinical types of the disease—quotidian, tertian and quartan. Osler's findings were communicated to the Pathological Society of Philadelphia at the end of October 1886, and were published widely within a few months;[4] by 1890, he was prompted to exclaim, "It takes away one's breath to see . . . long flagella develop under the eye."[5]

Golgi finally characterized the tertian and quartan parasites (1885–88) and in 1889 foretold that the aestivo-autumnal fever would prove to be associated with crescentic and unpigmented amoeboid forms of the parasite. Marchiafava and Celli confirmed this prophecy later that year. Welch proposed the term *Haematozoon falciparum* for the crescent-producing species, and the specific term "*falciparum*" is still used. By the end of the 1880–90 decade, whether one viewed *Plasmodium malariae* pluralistically or not, the protozoal origin of malarial infection was generally accepted. The mode of conveyance remained unsolved. In

1922, J.W.W. Stephens observed a fourth species of malarial parasite, *Plasmodium ovale,* in a human blood smear from West Africa.

Patrick Manson arrived in 1871 as a young doctor at Amoy, in southern China, to be medical officer to the Chinese Imperial Maritime Customs Service, in whose Medical Reports (1877) he recorded his remarkable findings "On the Development of *Filaria sanguinis hominis.*" After twelve years he moved to Hong Kong, becoming Dean of the College of Medicine in 1887. He saw Laveran's parasite only after he had settled in London, where it was demonstrated to him in 1892 by the protozoologist H.G. Plimmer. Surgeon-Major Ronald Ross of the Indian Medical Service went to London on leave in 1892. He was befriended by Manson, who revealed the haematozoon to him, along with the concept that mosquitoes carried the malaria parasite, much as they carried filaria. Manson considered that the ex-flagellation process represented the malarial parasite's struggle to escape from the blood stream of the human host in order to establish itself in another environment—probably water. Manson guided Ross to triumph, largely through correspondence, within four years.

The hypothesis linking mosquitoes with malaria did not originate with Manson. Early in 1882, A.F.A. King startled the Philosophical Society of Washington by producing arguments (not all of them valid) "in support of the mosquital origin of malarial disease," through "the bites or punctures of these insects—The punctures of proboscidian insects . . . by which bacteria and other germs may be inoculated into human bodies."[6] King cited the recent work of Manson in China and of Finlay in Cuba, linking mosquitoes with filariasis and yellow fever, respectively. He made the suggestion, presumably in the unrecorded discussion that followed, to protect the city against malaria by surrounding it with a fine-mesh screen as high as the Washington Monument. At that time, Theobald Smith was working as an assistant in Newell Martin's Biological Laboratory at Johns Hopkins University, and the malarial fevers of Baltimore[7] were at least as rampant as those of Washington. But King's proposal for a circumferential mosquito-proof screen was not viewed seriously by the denizens of either city. By August 1884, when Smith knew his way around the capital, the only precaution he seems to have taken was to secure lodgings "on the fourth floor, breezy and far above malaria."[8]

Shortly after Theobald Smith moved to Boston, he found that malaria was endemic in certain parts of Massachusetts. In the affected regions, the disease was associated often with stagnant waters and excavations; but he rejected the local hypothesis that the germs of malaria were latent in the soil and became airborne when the ground was disturbed. This concept was too reminiscent of the discredited theory advanced from Rome in 1879 E. Klebs and C. Tommasi-

Crudeli, that a sporulating bacillus, present in the air, water and soil of malarial regions, gave rise to the disease when inhaled or ingested by susceptible individuals. In his address to the Association of American Physicians in 1893, Smith had referred to Texas fever as "this interesting malarial disease of cattle," and concluded that "The agency of parasites in transferring the microbes of protozoan diseases should henceforth receive more attention." Although he suspected that Texas fever and malaria were conveyed comparably, the conviction that human malaria was mosquito-borne probably did not dawn on him until the middle of 1896—he afterward reported that "The relation of mosquitos to malaria as carriers became a definite working hypothesis with me in 1896."[9]

Meanwhile, the State Board of Health turned to physicians, with their unequalled opportunities of becoming "cognizant of cases of this ephemeral and sporadic disease," expressing the hope that afflicted communities might free themselves from odium by cooperating in studies of causation. The Board would do its part by instituting laboratory facilities for the microscopic detection of malaria.[10] In May 1896, the State House in Boston distributed to physicians an instructional circular on making blood films for this purpose, together with ten-point requisition forms for patients. Besides the usual information regarding the specimen's source, the physician was asked the date of the last previous attack, the interval between any chill and the preparation of the blood film, and whether quinine or other drug had been administered beforehand. Theobald Smith played a key part in the implementation of these official plans, which were presumably instigated then because he had started the diagnostic facility unofficially in 1895.

Late in the summer of 1895, Smith noted: "Went to Uxbridge, Mass, to investigate malaria for S. Board of Health. Returned in the evening."[11] Clinical tertian malaria was known to be endemic in Uxbridge. Smith urged Dr. L.D. White, the Health Officer of Uxbridge, that multiple blood films should be sent from all suspects. "I shall keep you supplied with glasses and may soon make another visit to see how the work is progressing."[12] On October 21, 1895, his diary noted, "Saw tertian malarial organisms today for first time."

Before the 1896 malaria season began, Smith badgered White to keep an account of early cases, particularly their date of onset.[13] He sent a supply of "schedules" (one to be filled out for each malarial patient), coverglasses with pill-box containers, and return envelopes. If the completed schedule and pillbox were returned in the sealed envelope, "the postage for one case will be 2 cents."[14] White had sent a newspaper clipping about sanitary violations in the area. Smith reciprocated by confiding his working hypothesis that "the malaria germ is carried by mosquitoes; not all mosquitoes to be sure, but only those in infected localities." This hypothesis should not be published or discussed at present, as it lacked supporting evidence. "I simply make the suggestions for your own use as Health Officer."

> Anything that favors the breeding of these pests like stagnant ponds, pools, sewers etc would favor the disease . . . In your work of supporession [sic], I would suggest that you keep your mind on these insects. Advise protection by window screens, indoor life after sundown, abandonment of barrels, tubs, etc about the house that contain water in which they breed abundantly.
>
> How far this hypothesis will be found true I do not at present know. The State Board is not prepared to make any public statements, so I wish you to keep the letter a confidential matter. I regret that my work here does not permit me to spend more time at Uxbridge. But if you keep me informed, I can make suggestions from here.

Smith asked White to send him preparations whenever opportunity offered. He hoped that his boy would catch "some of the Uxbridge mosquitoes and send them to me alive in a box with pinholes . . . I wish to compare them with those in this non-infected neighborhood."[15] But White was becoming uncooperative. He merely sent blood films from three patients, of which one was positive. Then he ceased sending preparations altogether, despite the reiterated request for material. Smith resolved to gather further evidence about the mosquito hypothesis during the 1897 malaria season. White then offered to cooperate—at a price. Smith asked what he would consider "reasonable compensation for doing the work you suggest in your last letter." Smith wished the Uxbridge program to continue along the following lines:

> 1. Sending coverslip films whenever possible. 2. Filling out blanks like those sent you last year. 3. Plotting the cases on a map which I had prepared for you last year. 4. Sending me at certain times mosquitoes for study. (These are easily caught in a pillbox by clapping the box and cover over each one by itself.) The Board has but a comparatively small appropriation but Dr. Walcott will, I think, be ready to pay something for such work.[16]

No reply, if any, has been found. White sent blood preparations sporadically, but no mosquitoes. For the remainder of 1897, Smith sent out a supplementary questionnaire with the blood film outfits. In December, a printed supply replaced the handwritten seventeen-point, double-page form. Two of the new queries concerned the water supply and sewerage, and another three related directly to the possibility that malaria was mosquito-borne. "Is patient out much after dark? Are mosquitoes about house? Are windows screened?"[17] The final outcome of the investigation is unrecorded. However, in the year ending April

1897, among fifty-seven patients, twenty-eight yielded positive films, of which twenty-four were from forty-one individuals who lived at Uxbridge.

On August 20, 1897, after many false trails on another continent, an excited, exhausted Ross found the evidence he sought in the stomach wall of a previously unused species of dappled-winged mosquitoes (probably *Anopheles stephensi*).[18] These insects had fed on a malaria patient a few days earlier. Within their gastric cells parasites were growing, which contained clusters of black pigment granules. Ross thus identified the alternative host for the malaria plasmodium: it could thrive in the stomach-wall of certain mosquito species, confirming Manson's earlier prediction that "The malaria germ does not go into the mosquito for nothing, for fun or for the confusion of the pathologist."[19]

Unaccountably, Ross was now posted for military duty to a small station in Rajputana. In February 1898, largely owing to Manson's efforts, he was assigned to a Calcutta laboratory to complete his researches. Because of a local scarcity of suitable cases of human malaria, he finally followed Manson's earlier advice to continue his task on avian malaria. Manson urged him to "do the best you can with the poor opportunities at your command."

> Much can be learned from analogy and comparative pathology, and I am not sure that you could not do a great deal, especially in the experimental line, by working on the lower animals. Don't forget that mosquitoes bite birds and that the plasmodia of birds are just as likely to be conveyed through mosquitoes as are the plasmodia of man.[20]

Further justification for turning to avian malaria had come from Welch's laboratory at Johns Hopkins Medical School, where W.G. MacCallum followed in crows the life-cycle of *Halteridium* (A. Labbe), a hematozoon infesting birds. While studying the ex-flagellation process, he noted the pointed end of a flagellum penetrate one of the non-flagellating spherules. He surmised that the free-swimming flagella were in fact "sperms" seeking to complete a sexual cycle outside the avian host, in the stomach of an engorged *Culex* mosquito.[21] Manson urged Ross to check MacCallum's observations.

Beginning in March 1898, Ross studied another malaria-like parasite, *Proteosoma,* infecting larks and sparrows. He noted that the fertilized female parasite, or zygote, penetrated the mosquito's gastric epithelium, expanded and ultimately ruptured, releasing a multitude of rods or threads which were conveyed by the mosquito's blood to its salivary gland. He now expressed confidence that "Malaria is conveyed from a diseased person or bird to a healthy one by the proper species of mosquito, and is inoculated by its bite." But, before he could confirm the findings for human malaria, Ross was sent to Assam to investigate kala-azar. An Italian team, Bastianelli, Bignami and Grassi, extended his avian observations to human malaria.

After leaving the Indian Medical Service, Ross became Lecturer at the Liverpool School of Tropical Medicine and devoted the rest of his life to improving the standards of sanitation in tropical regions. In 1926, the Ross Institute was founded to promote studies and interest in tropical medicine. It was chronically short of funds. Theobald Smith was among those who subscribed to the Institute's maintenance.

Ross had not read Theobald Smith's Texas Fever Bulletin before he did his work, but in due time paid this handsome tribute to its author:

> The discovery of the parasite opened a new chapter in the study of parasitic Protozoa . . . the first instance in which a protozoan parasite was shown to be communicable by the agency of intermediary hosts . . . Men will gradually perceive the importance of this work and . . . feel due sentiments of gratitude to the distinguished man who performed it.[22]

In 1931, Ross sent Smith a copy of the new (third) edition of *In Exile,* "the poem which I was writing in India when I discovered the malaria parasite living in mosquitoes in 1897."[23] The following year, Smith conveyed seventy-fifth birthday greetings to the very sick Ross, who died poor.[24] His abrasive personality and vanity annoyed many of the powers that be, but Ross received the Nobel Prize in 1902, and was knighted in 1911.

Meanwhile, at Jamaica Plain, Theobald Smith "became imbued with the idea that malaria is introduced to human beings, and that the mosquito only becomes infected through its food obtained as blood from infected individuals." Infected laborers, "huddled together in open camps at night near sluggishly-running or stagnant water," provided conditions favoring an epidemic among them and the local population.[25] In an autobiographical sketch requested by the Liverpool School of Tropical Medicine in connection with his Mary Kingsley Medal award, he reiterated that two hypotheses dominated his field inquiries into malaria. 1. The dissemination of the disease by mosquitoes. 2. The introduction of the infection by migratory workmen.[26] Smith did not attempt laboratory confirmation of the mosquito-borne hypothesis. The 1903 Shattuck Lecture emphasized "the hopelessness of making any progress in this subject in a latitude usually free from malaria and only sporadically invaded by it"[27]—"the opportunities for investigation in this climate . . . were very unsatisfactory."[28]

Smith therefore turned to other aspects of the local problem. He was convinced, he informed the New York Academy of Medicine in 1899, "that the time has come for public health authorities to take some stand on . . . the spreading of tertian malaria in our own climate."

Much of the evil which manifests itself in the increasing prevalence of the mosquito is due to the carelessness and indifference of private persons, corporations, and even public authorities who create and perpetuate the conditions which favor the silting up and the partial drying up of our streams and smaller water courses and the stagnation of surface water.[29]

The essence of the problem was to prevent access of the potential vector to an infected individual, by minimizing the human sources of infection, by markedly reducing contacts between mosquito and man, and by applying kerosene or copper sulphate as larvicide to known breeding places, especially of the *Anopheles* species. From late in 1895 until at least 1904, Smith promoted every element of this campaign. By formulating and driving home the principles and techniques which were to rid Massachusetts of the disease, Theobald Smith won recognition as a leading American authority on malaria control in temperate climes.

He lost no opportunity of demonstrating that the local situation met the larger claims respecting the vector role of *Anopheles* mosquitoes in human malaria. In the identification of mosquito species, Theobald Smith himself caught most of the specimens, although colleagues, neighbors and family cooperated. If the insects settled on the childrens' skin, they were walloped without being killed, and kept for their father to examine. Lilian wrote from Woodland Hill in midsummer 1903: "oh such a plague of mosquitoes! We cannot sit outdoors at all . . . I sew and slap—slap and sew."[30] In the Boston area, about 90% of those caught were *Culex,* but representatives of two *Anopheles* species were discovered in or near the Bussey Institution, while *A. quadrimaculatus* was captured indoors at Woodland Hill and in Smith's own laboratory.

During August 1902, Theobald travelled to Millbury, Watertown, Freeway, Clinton and South Lancaster in quest of *Anopheles* breeding-places. The following are selected entries from his September diary:

Sept 2, 1902	Visit Concord to study distrib. of Anopheles & Malaria.
15	To Springfield . . . Spend 16th in trolley rides to find breedingplaces of mosquitoes.
17	Spend the day at Pittsfield. Visit New Lenox dam . . . where I found many Anoph. larvae.
19–30	Return to Boston . . . Spend considerable time in inspecting the territory of Chas. River for mosquitoes.

On some trips, the local doctor drove Smith around, and perhaps offered a bed at home. His total expenses, amounting to $39.29 for August and $28.79 for

September, were paid by the State Board of Health. He stimulated the anti-malaria campaign by talks and demonstrations to various lay and professional groups. The climactic effort was on June 9, 1903, when he delivered the Shattuck Lecture to the Massachusetts Medical Society. Theobald Smith was nominated for this lectureship two years beforehand and it took four months of active preparation.

In March 1902, Smith was appointed consultant to the Charles River Dam Committee. Nearly ten years before, a commission representing the State Board of Health and the Metropolitan Park Commission "reported favorably upon the plan for beautifying the Charles River by building locks to control the water level."[32] The Committee's revived mandate included an assessment of the probable effect of the dam upon mosquitoes and malaria. For Theobald Smith, the assignment involved reading, travel in the prospective Charles River basin inspecting for mosquitoes, and considerable laboratory work. For example, as one diary entry in June told, "Spent most of day with Charles River Dam Committee, on a launch on Charles River."[33] He trained his teaching fellow, C.H. Boxmeyer, to assist in testing water samples and identifying mosquitoes. Shortly after completion of the survey, Boxmeyer went to Saranac Lake for treatment of pulmonary tuberculosis.

Smith finished his report in November 1902. About a year later it appeared in print as an eighteen-page appendix to the main report of the Charles River Dam Committee. He had thoroughly investigated the present sources of pollution of the Charles River and the probable future effects of impounding its water, concluding that "The substitution of a fresh-water basin for the present tidal reservoir would not tend to intensify malarial influences, provided the present breeding-places of mosquitoes are properly dealt with. There would be material improvement over present conditions, both as regards mosquitoes and malaria."[34]

For several years, wealthy Bostonians consulted him regarding mosquito abatement on their suburban estates. "We have had almost no mosquitoes here" wrote a prominent lawyer who had sought his advise in 1904, "I find the blue vitriol works very well . . . Since the last week of Aug. when I put it in pools on my Island, I have found no larvae."[35] Theobald ignored requests to be billed for his services. But he willingly accepted honoraria of $200 for the Shattuck lectureship, and of $500 for his consultant services to the Charles River Dam Committee.

Theobald Smith and Ronald Ross were in character very unlike. In the same setting, Smith's remarkable patience, tenacity, and methodical approach might have solved sooner and with less turmoil the mysterious mechanism of malaria transmission. He was far better grounded than Ross in histological and general laboratory techniques, and his bent for solitary research was deeply rooted. Ross was handicapped by the impoverished library resources of the Indian Medical Service, which was especially deficient in literature on malaria and mosquitoes; whereas Smith had ready access to the authoritative knowledge of the mosquito possessed by the entomologist Leland O. Howard,[36] his former Delta Epsilon confrere at Cornell. Trumpeted Ross from Bangalore, "Great is Sanitation—the greatest work, except discovery, I think, that a man can do."[37]

If Ross's true vocation were "discovery," he should have gone to greater length to pursue it, both before and after the champion venture. Instead, he proclaimed sanitary improvement as the paramount objective of his working life. "I did not undertake this work on malaria in the interests of zoology," he noted in his Memoirs, "but . . . of practical sanitation."[38] By contrast, in his last testamentary letter to microbiologists-at-large, Theobald Smith declared: "The joy of research must be found in doing, since every other harvest is uncertain, and even the prizes do not always go to the discoveries to which we would assign them . . . My interest in a problem usually lagged when certain results could be clearly formulated or practically applied."[39]

Sanitation

The sanitary reform movement of the nineteenth century's second and third quarters was led by persons convinced that the high mortality, poor physique, and excessive proliferation of the working population were due to such squalid concomitants of the industrial revolution as polluted water, dirty milk, messy drainage, rudimentary sewage disposal, and all-pervading filth. The sanitary reformers were followed by "germ theory" pioneers, including such well-known North American physicians as G.M. Sternberg, W.H. Welch, W. Osler, M.T. Prudden, H.M. Biggs, and L.E. Holt—and, of course, Theobald Smith himself. Disease "germs" became grist to the mill of the new generation of sanitarians, while the bacteriologists willingly advocated sanitation as a means of controlling pathogenic microorganisms. This interdependence grew during Smith's years at the B.A.I., during which many enlarging cities, including Washington, used untreated river water for drinking purposes, despite clear evidence that typhoid fever and cholera were often conveyed by water supplies.

Starting from his 1886 note on the bacterial counts of Potomac River samples from the laboratory tap, about a dozen of Theobald Smith's publications over the next several years dealt with the bacteriology of water and the hazards of waterborne disease; and it was fitting that thirty years later, when he received the Kober Medal, appreciation was voiced for his pioneer work on the improvement of public water supplies. Smith's work in this field while he was attached to the

Bureau of Animal Industry has already been reviewed in Chapter VII. One of Theobald Smith's obituary tributes appropriately reminded readers that his interests in sanitation extended beyond the purification of water supplies.[40] He himself recorded that in preparing his annual lectures and demonstrations as professor of bacteriology in the medical department of the Columbian University, "The great possibilities in the applications of medical bacteriology to preventative medicine and hygiene were early impressed upon me. And these I attempted to bring out."[41]

If circumstances seemed to require that his views on some matter of public health concern were to be more widely communicated than by a scientific report in a professional journal, Theobald Smith would step into the breach—particularly in his earlier years—sometimes clearly and effectively, as newspaper clippings in his scrapbooks indicate. But misunderstanding or misinterpretations often resulted; mistakes were apt to be made by reporters; and undertakings not kept; but for Smith the fun of such forays did not outweigh the inaccuracies and other complications. He tried to explain the situation to Gage, that the pleasure of being busy could be marred by the distraction of having people around, even when the work directly involved them—"When the work directly affects people and the public health . . . the added worry rather spoils it and crowds the mere pleasure of being busy out of sight."[42]

Within two years of arriving in Boston, Theobald Smith prepared five papers bearing on water as a vehicle for infection. Two of these recorded laboratory work done before he left Washington; a third was an illustrated nineteen-page pamphlet on farm and rural hygiene, issued by the U.S. Department of Agriculture in its series of *Farmer's Bulletins,*[43] and a fourth, similar to the third, was based on a lecture entitled "Sanitation on the Farm," given to a local Farmer's Club.[44] The other publication was an address presented in January 1896 as guest speaker at a meeting of the New England Water Works Association, in which he made skeptical comments on water as a direct vehicle for malaria—one of Manson's hypotheses:

> I doubt very much whether such a germ can have two ways of entering the body . . . If it can be shown, as I think it has been shown abundantly, that malaria is contracted when drinking water is not implicated, I believe that fact is almost of itself sufficient . . . to counterbalance the argument that malaria is carried in water.

He also stressed the indispensability of laboratory tests in the control of water supplies, by emphasizing the significance of convalescent and healthy carriers of cholera vibrios and typhoid bacilli, the reduced susceptibility of the partially-immune but pathogen-excreting individual, and the importance of bacterial counts (total and coliform).[45]

Afterwards, he was complimented for an admirable presentation by W.T. Sedgwick, whom he had first met in the spring of 1882. Smith was then a temporary assistant in Henry Newell Martin's biology laboratory and Sedgwick had just completed his Ph.D. course in biology and physiology. In 1883, Sedgwick became assistant professor of biology at the Massachusetts Institute of Technology. The Massachusetts State Board of Health under Walcott in 1887 established the Lawrence Experiment Station for the study of water purification methods, and Sedgwick developed the laboratories as a supplementary training ground for students in sanitary biology and chemistry. He became consulting biologist to the Board in 1888, and began directing the evolution of systematic chemical and bacteriological tests for water and sewage control.

The State of Massachusetts was obviously fortunate in the quality of expert advice and effective mechanisms for supervising its public water supplies and its sewage disposal arrangements. Theobald Smith took care to avoid flaunting his own qualifications in this field of sanitation, and soon turned to other areas. In 1930, he was the second recipient of the Sedgwick Memorial Medal, awarded annually through the American Public Health Association for "distinguished service in public health." Two cordial letters from Sedgwick, dated 1895 and 1903, are among Smith's papers. The first told of his election (on Sedgwick's nomination) to the Boston Society of Medical Sciences. The other, sent to Smith as retiring president of the Society of American Bacteriologists, suggested that E.O. Jordan, "even if he was one of my 'boys'," would make a suitable successor. F.G. Novy was elected president as Theobald's immediate successor for 1904, but Jordan's turn came in 1905.

Theobald Smith could be eloquent, forthright, and exhortative, although in later life these qualities faded or were repressed. In April 1896, as president of the Albany Medical College Alumni Association, he addressed the graduating class and admitted them to the Association. Here, amidst reminders of his boyhood and of his early professional life, from boating on the Hudson to sampling it for bacteriological tests, his endeavor to convey the significance of the *prevention* of disease naturally focused on the sanitation of water.

A lengthy passage from John Ruskin illustrated "the thoughtlessness and indifference of the bulk of the people to pure water." He also quoted C.W. Eliot, H.P. Walcott, W.T. Sedgwick, Virchow and others. He warned that perhaps some great war would reveal "the quiet and almost frictionless work of sanitary organization holding the reins of a number of restive disease germs whose power over society is by no means extinct." The budding physicians were urged to cultivate "a liberal, receptive mind, free from the bigotry of the old as well as the conceit of the new." Alexander Pope's shallow advice, "Be not the first by whom the new are tried / Nor yet the last to lay the old aside," was denounced as more suitable for fashion than for medicine. "If your judgment tells you that the newest is best, you should not hesitate to use it. In your prognosis you will show your mastery or your ignorance and neither will be forgotten."[46]

Although Theobald Smith's address at Albany was the last of his series on water-borne diseases, references to such outbreaks intruded when he strayed into the field of general sanitation. For instance, early in 1904, he spoke before the Massachusetts Association of Boards of Health on various modes of spreading infection. The press had reported multiple accounts of water-borne outbreaks of typhoid fever, particularly the 1903 outbreak at Ithaca, where fifty-one died among 681 cases, including twenty-nine fatalities in 291 Cornell students affected. No cases occurred among those who used only the university's treated supply.[47] Such episodes, according to Smith, resulted from half-way sanitation. "The public has acknowledged the necessity for pure water but it has not yet torn itself away from the filthy habit of polluting its rivers whence the water is taken." Besides, he declared on another occasion, it was "a biological necessity for disease germs to be transmitted . . . the entire mechanism of infection is directed towards this necessity of being eliminated or set free to invade another host."[48] Organized public health thus gained a clearly-defined, prophylactic purpose—to *prevent* the passage of pathogens from a known or suspected source to a new susceptible host. The clinician's province was to cope with disease germs that had entered the individual.

Theobald Smith's reports on milk sanitation were likewise broadly-based, although perhaps less fundamental than his studies on the sanitation of public water supplies. His interests in milk as a vehicle of human infection ranged from causation to prevention. Cow's milk was shown to be a good nutrient medium for various pathogenic bacteria, whose source might be either exogenous, from the milker (Group A hemolytic streptococcus, typhoid bacillus) or endogenous, from the cow (bovine turbercle bacillus, Bacillus abortus). He also demonstrated and firmly proclaimed that infected milk was rendered safe by exposure to adequate heat, as in proper pasteurization, for which he determined standards. His forecast that raw milk would cease to be a beverage within a decade was wildly optimistic. Many factors probably account for the comparative lack of recognition stemming from Theobald Smith's contributions to current knowledge of milk hygiene. Among them must be reckoned those competitive and often conflicting reports from numerous experts hired because of the very commercialized and politicized character of the dairying industry; the reversal of attitude toward such polices as the slaughter of all tuberculin-positive cattle; and Koch's controversial contention that the bovine type of tubercle bacillus was without public health significance.

Finally, Smith's concern for better sanitation ended a few years later with a brief swat at the housefly as a potential transmitter of infective agents. To insect vectors of disease which provided essential biological links in the life cycles of certain specific parasites, he now added such passive transmitters as the ubiquitous house-fly, *Musca domestica,* "the one insect next to the mosquito . . . to which we should direct our attention."[49] In 1908, Smith addressed the same group on the housefly as disseminator of infectious diseases, and urged attacks upon its breeding places.[50] The campaign aroused the enthusiasm of health officials of Massachusetts, Rhode Island and New York and was described in an article in the *Boston Post* (duly pasted into the scrapbook) entitled "Death to the House Fly! . . . Bay State Heads War on Germ-Carrying Insect."[51] Truly Smith lived up to the motto "Non curare sed praevenire"—Not to cure but to prevent—of the New Jersey Health and Sanitary Association which was inscribed on the bronze plaque presented to him in November 1934.

12

ESTABLISHMENT OF THE ROCKEFELLER INSTITUTE FOR MEDICAL RESEARCH, AND EUROPE REVISITED

The Rockefeller Institute (1901–1906)

The Rockefeller Institute's successful start was conditioned by the coexistence of three crucial factors. The first was an enormous fortune in the hands of one individual, who believed that the ability to make money was as God-given as the obligation to use it for the benefit of his fellow man. This belief underlay John D. Rockefeller's skill and ruthlessness in amassing incalculable wealth, and his carefulness in dispensing it. The second factor was Frederick L. Gates, an ambitious, able and eloquent minister of Rockefeller's own sectarian faith, who in 1888 exchanged a struggling pastorate in Minneapolis for the executive secretaryship of the American Baptist Education Society. In 1889, he persuaded Rockefeller to donate $600,000 to the University of Chicago to make it a center of leadership for the denominational colleges of the Midwest. By 1910, the university had received 45 million dollars.

In the early 1890's, Gates moved to New York as Rockefeller's investment counsellor and confidential almoner. Here he renewed his long-standing interest in medicine. In response to Gates's inquiry into the current quality of medicine and how it might be improved, a former member of his congregation, now qualifying as a physician, recommended Osler's *Principles and Practice of Medicine* as preeminent in style and content. Gates purchased a copy of the second edition (1896) and during the summer of 1897 read every line of its 1,000 pages, with the aid of a small medical dictionary. He gathered two indelible impressions— the lack of specific remedies for most diseases, and North America's relative neglect of the scientific aspects of medicine. Gates prepared a memorandum urging the establishment and endowment of an institute for medical research, particularly into infectious disease, comparable to those erected for Koch in Berlin and Pasteur in Paris. He left this document in Rockefeller's desk and never saw it again.

When John D. Rockefeller, Jr., who had just graduated from Brown University, began to devote himself to thorough appraisal of the philanthropic projects submitted to his father (now approaching sixty), Gates selected a lawyer neighbor, Starr J. Murphy, to assist him in collecting ideas and information for the institute. Murphy pursued his assignment with quiet efficiency and eventually became Rockefeller's personal attorney. In 1915, Gates complied with Starr's request for his recollections of the founding of the Institute. This account has been reproduced in full as an appendix in Corner's *History of the Rockefeller Institute, 1901–1953*.[1] The Rockefellers pondered the accumulating data for nearly three years and then acknowledged the need for continuing advice from professional experts.

The third prerequisite to a successful launching of the project were congenial and competent advisers. Dr. L. Emmett Holt, a fellow parishioner of Rockefeller, Jr. at the Fifth Avenue Baptist church, was a prominent pediatrician whose efforts to practice scientific medicine were often foiled by critical gaps in bacteriological or biochemical knowledge. His friend Christian A. Herter, a summertime neighbor of Rockefeller, Sr. on Mount Desert Island, Maine, was a professor at Bellevue Hospital Medical School and at the College of Physicians and Surgeons of Columbia University. He was a sensitive, philosophical, and cultivated man whose private wealth permitted him and assistants to operate his Madison Avenue residence as a laboratory for research in basic medical sciences, especially in pathological chemistry, pharmacology and bacteriology.[2]

On a train journey from Cleveland to New York, Holt explained to Rockefeller, Jr. that diphtheria antitoxin resulted from the deliberate application of scientific principles in planned experiments. Shortly afterward, the small son of Rockefeller, Jr.'s sister, Edith McCormick, died of scarlet fever. Following this untimely death of his first grandson from a disease of unknown causation, with no specific remedy, Rockefeller, Sr. overrode his personal homeopathic leanings and activated the proposal for an institute. In March 1901, Herter and Holt recommended William Welch, their old teacher at Johns Hopkins, as their first choice for fellow-adviser, and amongst other names included Hermann M. Biggs and T. Mitchell Prudden, both from New York, and Theobald Smith at Boston.

On March 15, 1901, Herter wrote to Welch soliciting his support for the project which would start in a small way, unconnected with any hospital or university. He named nine additional possibilities as advisers and invited his views on the size and constitution of the advisory board. Until its own quarters were built, space might be found in the prospective laboratories of the New York City Health Department at the foot of East 16th Street, where they would be free from interference. Welch expressed satisfaction with the proposals and suggested a meeting in New York of the six advisers already selected, including himself, to consider the Board's ultimate size. He would gladly join the Board, but not as chairman, as he lacked the time. A New York man, such as Prudden or Biggs, would be preferable for the chairmanship. To find a highly-trained, competent director was essential for success of the undertaking.[3]

This correspondence was forwarded to Rockefeller, Jr., who notified Holt on April 27, 1901 that his father was willing to give up to $20,000 a year for ten years for medical research to be distributed by a committee "empowered to formulate the policy and direct the organization of the work." Holt, Herter, Prudden, Biggs and Welch met in Washington during the annual meeting of the Association of American Physicians on April 30-May 2, 1901. Theobald Smith did not attend the meeting. By common consent, William Welch assumed the chairmanship, despite his earlier demurral, and filled this difficult role with distinction throughout his life. The group decided that the new institute should be in New York City, and Smith was invited to become its first laboratory director.

Welch promptly communicated with Smith about "a matter which promises to be of considerable importance."[4]

> It is the establishment by Mr. Rockefeller of provision for research in this country, especially along the lines of infectious diseases and preventive medicine . . . I was asked last summer by President Low [of Columbia University] to answer in writing a series of questions [put by Rockefeller, Jr.] considering the foundation of a laboratory which seemed to contemplate something with the scope and resources of the Pasteur Institute in Paris . . . It seems that Mr. Rockefeller is not prepared to provide at present for a laboratory on such a scale as I inferred from President Low's letter last summer . . . but Dr. Holt, who has conversed with him, thinks that the possibilities for the future are immense . . . We were unanimous in the opinion that you were the best man—indeed it seemed to us the only man in this country possibly available—to take charge as director of the new laboratory.

While Welch knew "the possibilities for scientific work and doing good" would be the determining factor, Smith's name had been so enthusiastically received that Holt thought the projected director's salary of $5,000 could be doubled— "in fact that any pecuniary arrangements which you might suggest as to salary would be met." Although the matter was confidential at the moment, "Dr. Walcott knows about it, and if you like, you can confer with him."

Next day, Herter followed up Welch's letter, inviting Theobald Smith "as a member of our Committee" to meet Mr. Rockefeller at dinner at the University Club on May 10, 1901 to discuss with him "the establishment of a research laboratory in New York City." Smith's diary for that day simple recorded: "Leave for N.Y. Stop at Murray Hill [Hotel]. Dinner at Univ. Club given by Mr. Rockefeller Jr., followed by organization of Rockefeller Institute with Welch, Prudden, Holt, Herter, Biggs and myself." There is no documentary evidence, but despite the fact that Smith afterwards told Simon Gage that "I anticipate much good from this new Institute and eventually it will be richly endowed, I believe,"[5] he presumably informed Welch verbally that he would decline the laboratory directorship. The appointment was left in abeyance while other matters went ahead. Mr. Rockefeller consented to have the Institute named after him, simple bylaws were adopted, the consultants began to designate themselves "Directors," and the Board of Directors was expanded to seven.

Simon Flexner, Welch's former assistant, now professor of pathology at the University of Pennsylvania, needed little persuasion to accept his election to the Board. Herter and Dr. E.K. Dunham called on Smith at home in June 1901, perhaps hoping to change his mind. A friendship developed, and during visits to New York City in the Board's earlier years, Smith often stayed overnight at the Herter residence, 819 Madison Avenue. Throughout the next three years, Smith seldom missed a meeting. In due course these were held quarterly, but organizational problems at the outset required more frequent conferences. The directors received a rounded figure for travel expenses—$25.00 per trip in Smith's case—without honoraria.

In reply to Gage's written comment that the newspapers reported very favorably on Rockefeller's benefaction, Theobald Smith informed his old friend that "the first plan was to start a laboratory at once in New York and for a week I was seriously considering a very urgent letter from Professor Welch to become the director."

But the conditions were uncertain and I did not feel sufficient confidence in my own management of people . . . So the temporary plan goes through for this year and I do not believe my candidacy will be seriously considered again, either by myself or the Board. Probably the possibilities will induce our Corporation to make more efforts to develop the work here. It was in fact a member of our Corporation [presumably Walcott] who brought me the first news of my candidacy. The funds are in the hands of 7 directors, Welch, Prudden, Biggs, Herter, Holt, Flexner and myself. I shall have this year $650 to use for salary & expenses in research . . . So much for the personal element . . . But after all you and I know that research cannot be forced very much—there is always danger of too much foliage & too little fruit.[6]

The Board of Directors decided to distribute about one-half of the annual allocation in grants-in-aid, tenable in existing laboratories. The grants ranged from $250 to $1,500 each. The response from applicants was both "pathetic in its eagerness and inspiring in its revelation of the devotion with which many young men . . . were struggling on with inadequate facilities and support."[7] In each of the first two years of the arrangement, about two dozen grants-in-aid were apportioned to universities such as Harvard, Pennsylvania, Yale, Chicago, Western Reserve, Michigan and Stanford, where suitable research projects could be launched under sound leadership. Holt was the Board's official secretary, and Herter was treasurer. Welch dealt in long hand with every application. Grantees were encouraged to publish their findings, and the Board purchased reprints for binding in *Studies from the Rockefeller Institute*. Theobald Smith was favorably impressed by these arrangements and passed his approval to Simon Flexner following the June, 1904 meeting of the Board of Directors:

> The results of last year's grants were evidently very satisfactory, and I think the future promises well. To be sure, no great discoveries need be looked for from small grants, for the former are generally unpremeditated and cannot be laid out beforehand. The new laboratory must be looked upon as the true storm centre of work and discovery.[8]

The $650 mentioned in Smith's letter to Gage was allocated to A.L. Reagh, who collaborated with his chief in two papers on the agglutination reactions of the "hog-cholera bacillus" (*B. cholerae suis,* or *Salmonella cholerae suis* as it is termed today). In the first, Reagh was designated "Research Scholar, Rockefeller Institute, 1901–02;" while the second paper, on flagellar and body antigens of Salmonella, was annotated as "aided by the Rockefeller Institute for Medical Research." Reagh stayed on to reach senior rank in the State Board of Health laboratory service. The careers of other pupil-collaborators of Smith were launched with grants from the Rockefeller Institute for Medical Research: for example, Paul A. Lewis, subsequently an Austin Teaching Fellow in Smith's department, joined the full-time staff of the Institute in 1908, and Herbert R.

Brown assisted in the Department of Comparative Pathology for several years before going to the University of Rochester. The grants diminished in number when the Institute's own laboratories began to function, and were discontinued entirely after 1917.

Gates was impatient at this cautious beginning with small individual research grants. A larger-scale project was initiated by Hermann Biggs, who proposed that the Rockefeller Institute assign unexpended funds for an investigation of the quality of milk sold in metropolitan New York. A bacteriologist, a biochemist, supporting staff, and laboratory animals were provided for a study under the combined direction of the bacteriologist W.H. Park and the pediatrician L.E. Holt. Park had previously reported some shocking findings in a survey of New York City's market milk supplies. He was confident that this gross bacterial contamination could be markedly lessened by the action of health authorities. Farmers and shippers did not realize the extent of the risks of contamination, or the rapidity with which harmful bacteria could multiply in milk, especially in summer heat.[9]

Park and Holt now showed that the high infant mortality in New York City from diarrheal diseases ("cholera infantum") was due largely to the milk supply. Their studies, published at the end of 1903,[10] greatly improved the sanitary control of milk in the metropolis. The resulting publicity demonstrated that medical science, when put to use, could yield great benefits. This idea appealed to the practical-minded Rockefeller and Gates.

The Board met again on January 11, 1902. Welch had been assured, at a dinner beforehand with Rockefeller, Jr., that a laboratory would be permanently endowed. The Directors decided to go ahead, believing that "The most important matter is to secure a man of first-rate scientific and administrative ability to direct the work of the laboratory."[11] At the meeting, Theobald Smith was invited to consider heading the bacteriological department—the Institute's core—and to formulate his ideas about the whole undertaking. Two days later, Welch wrote to Herter, describing his meetings with Rockefeller, Jr., as "most satisfactory." Welch thought "if we can get together a good working staff for a laboratory, this seems to be our next move."[12] At the same time he wrote to Rockefeller, Jr., himself, urging continuation of the research grants program, along with a modest start upon the laboratory. Experience would indicate its future organization and development.

Nearly three weeks had passed without word from Smith, so Welch reminded him that the Directors could not proceed until they knew his decision. Judging from this delay and from Smith's reaction to the initial offer, Welch expected his final response to be negative, so he wrote to Herter on January 30: "I think we should next learn whether Flexner would consider a proposal." Smith mean-while brooded over the renewed offer until he prepared a provisional reply on February 10. Next day the final document was sent off, typed on a recently ac-quired machine. His diary, summarizing February's activities with unusual lo-quacity, indicates the careful thoughtfulness behind the decision: "Gave much time to a consideration of the offer of the Rockefeller Inst. for me to take charge of the Rockefeller laboratory. After due consideration the offer declined in a let-ter preserved." Colleagues on the Board were given three chief reasons for his decision not to accept "this tempting and highly honorable offer."

> First, I feel a strong sense of gratitude to the President and Fellows of Harvard University and to Mr. George F. Fabyan for the sacrifices they have made in found-ing and maintaining a chair of comparative pathology which is only now beginning to show signs of fruitage. Second, I should lose the accumulated labors of at least several years here and several years would be spent in finding the right place for a new laboratory in any large community . . . Third, my interest for years in animal pathology and my firm belief in its great usefulness in the study of problems in hu-man pathology might give an impress to the work of the laboratory which might eventually arouse adverse criticism.[13]

Smith felt that the organization of the new laboratory should crystallize around the study of the infectious diseases. Initially the director should have charge of three integrated laboratories, devoted respectively to morphological studies, especially protozoology and parasitology; pathological physiology, in-cluding bacteriology and immunology; and physiological and pathological chem-istry. Growth in other directions would occur inevitably. "By beginning with a small program and a few problems the laboratory is in the best position to make organic growth as contrasted with mere accretion which leads to sterility and extravagance." A budget of at least $40,000 - $50,000 should be available.

Because Welch had stated earlier that the Rockefeller's favored a New York City location for their institute, Theobald did not believe that it was worthwhile to discuss any other place. However, in expressing his views about the project, Smith challenged this position.

> The prime need in carrying out such a laboratory is the proper provision for ani-mals both large and small which are under observation and experiment. That this may be accomplished within a large city is open to doubt. I therefore strongly urge the establishment of the laboratory where gradual extension is possible with special reference to the shelter of large animals and the breeding of small ones needed in the investigations. The suburbs of a large city are in my experience very satisfactory.[14]

This problem does not appear to have been discussed by the other Directors.

Welch forwarded Smith's letter to his former pupil, Simon Flexner, requesting him to let him know by the next Board meeting whether he would "consider favorably such as offer as was made to Smith." He also asked Smith to attend the next Board meeting. To hear his letter read need occasion no personal embarrassment, he believed. Board members would consider his decision final. Should Flexner decline, they would have to take up other names, or discuss a program for the coming year, "and for this we especially need your advice and help . . . There is no chance of our wanting under any circumstances to lose you from the Board."[15] Theobald Smith's letter was inscribed upon the minutes of the Board meeting on March 8, 1902, followed by the comment: "It was voted to ask Dr. Simon Flexner to consider under what circumstances he could be induced to take charge of a laboratory."

Flexner was not altogether happy at Philadelphia, despite good friendships and a new laboratory of his own design. The University of Pennsylvania in those days had a strong antisemitic faction. Flexner was advised by his close friend L.F. Baker to accept the Rockefeller offer if certain conditions could be met. "The only three men who could be considered for the position are Theobald Smith, Herter, and yourself, and in my opinion you have more of the desirable qualities than either of the other two."[16] Whereas Smith had envisaged mainly an expansion of his own areas of research, Flexner drafted a plan encompassing "the whole field of medical research in respect both to men and animals." Flexner, Prudden and Holt drew up a budget for submission to the Rockefellers totalling $137,640. This covered the operating expenses, maintenance, and salaries of three laboratory departments and a hospital, including $10,000 for the director of the laboratories. The costs of land, buildings and equipment would be additional.

The Board met on May 10, 1902, at which time the Directors expressed their conviction that "there is yet a field of far higher promise in the permanent establishment of an institute of wider scope"[17] and approved Flexner's general plan for the organization and activities of the laboratory, as well as this budgetary estimate, for submission to Rockefeller, Jr. Theobald Smith had no wish to contest alone the Institute's location in New York City. Although the ambitious scope of this budget and the accompanying text epitomized Flexner's views, the memorandum incorporated several of Smith's recommendations. The following paragraph was lifted almost verbatim from his March 4 letter to Welch:

> The dominant note of medical research today is the study of infectious diseases from all points of view. They are the great threatening dangers of our present social system. Hence in the Institute, the organization might at first wisely crystal-

lize about this general subject. In a broad sense the direction and methods for the study of disease may be classified as morphological, physiological and clinical; and the Institute should include departments providing for these divisions of the subject.

This excerpt and the section immediately following largely reproduced Theobald Smith's ideas.

In June 1902, Rockefeller, Sr. pledged one million dollars for the Institute; and at the October meeting of the Board of Directors, Flexner was nominated director of the laboratories. In the fall of 1903, Flexner went to Europe for a year to review the operation of research laboratories and to study biochemistry in Berlin. He returned to New York in the fall of 1904, recruited from various sources a staff of four senior scientists and several juniors, and moved with them into two converted brownstone houses at the corner of Lexington Avenue and Fiftieth Street. These quarters had been rented and equipped for temporary laboratory use, after being approved for the purpose by Mitchell Prudden and Theobald Smith. The four pioneers were Eugene L. Opie, a pathologist from Welch's department at Johns Hopkins; Samuel E. Meltzer, trained as a physiologist in Germany; P.A.T. Levene, a trainee of Emil Fischer in biochemistry; and Hideyo Noguchi, a Japanese microbiologist who had become Flexner's protege at Philadelphia. In 1907, when the Board officially ranked the scientific staff, three of the above-named were designated Members of the Rockefeller Institute for Medical Research, while Noguchi was made an Associate Member. The term "Professor" was thus avoided. The lower ranks were Assistants, Fellows, or Scholars. Surprisingly soon, publishable material of high quality came from this band of enthusiasts.

Meanwhile, a tract of about thirteen acres of farm land, between east 64th and 68th Streets, had been bought for the Institute. A Boston firm of architects, Shepley, Rutan, and Coolidge, recommended by Rockefeller, Jr. had been hired to erect buildings on this site, as nucleus for an Institute destined to expand. The structures, of simple functional design, comprised the main laboratory, a building for experimental animals, and the powerhouse. The five-storied laboratory was based on a floor plan drawn by Prudden, with outside dimensions of 136 by 50 feet. The ground floor was reserved for the library and administrative offices, with some unassigned space; the second, third and fourth floors were for chemical research, experimental pathology, and bacteriology and parasitology, respectively; and on the fifth floor, just under the roof, were the surgical operating rooms, and accommodation for test animals. The total cost was about $300,000.

Prompt completion of this core of Rockefeller Institute buildings was spurred perhaps by a competitive element. At that time, large fortunes could still be amassed by individuals. In 1903, Henry Phipps began his philanthropic involvement in the control of tuberculosis, at Philadelphia, culminating in 1910 in the erection and endowment of the Phipps Institute, on whose Council Theobald Smith served faithfully for many years. Again, in January 1902, another tycoon, Andrew Carnegie, had incorporated the Carnegie Institution of Washington, with a capital endowment of ten million dollars, to further the "investigation, research and discovery and the application of knowledge to the improvement of mankind." The Directors of the Rockefeller Institute for Medical Research were human enough to foresee overlapping objectives here, and hence possible rivalry in accomplishment and prestige. Corner states[17] that Rockefeller, Jr. sought and received an assurance from Carnegie that his Institution would not enter the realm of medical research.

Flexner and his group left their temporary quarters after only eighteen months and in April 1906 moved into the new main building by the East River. The formal dedication ceremonies, which took place on May 11, 1906, featured addresses by Emmett Holt and William Welch, representing the Board of Directors, and by Presidents Nicholas M. Butler of Columbia University and Charles W. Eliot of Harvard. An evening banquet capped the day. A sense of propriety obviously prevailed in both the issuance and the acceptance of invitations to the banquet. Theobald Smith's diary entry for the day reads: "Leave for N.Y. to attend dedication of Rockefeller Institute Laboratory. Banquet in evening attended by J.D. Rockef. Jr., Carnegie, Phipps & many disting. doctors." A few weeks later, Flexner became engaged to Helen Thomas, a woman of remarkable intelligence and quality. The story of their courtship and marriage has been told by their younger son.[18]

A hospital was envisaged in Flexner's original prospectus—"There should be attached to the Institute a hospital for the study of special groups of cases of diseases"[19]—and in January 1902, Flexner told Christian Herter that the whole board favored him as chief physician.[20] But Herter was inconsolably depressed by the death of his two-year old son, Forel, named after Herter's teacher, the Swiss neurologist Auguste Forel, who had died in 1890, when less than three years old. Herter described this summer to Smith as the hardest of his life. He planned to go to California for three months. "I hope a change in surroundings will give me courage to go on."[21] Smith's answer was prompt:

Have you tried the comforts of reading good literature, especially that which puts one far away from one's own field and leads to an attitude of mind which tends to accept the things of life as our forefathers did? I think the painful character of the life today is due to our belief that we can or could alter our lives, whereas in fact the unknown and unknowable elements are, to me, just as preponderating.[22]

Flexner, Welch and Theobald Smith tried to provoke resumption of Herter's normal enthusiasm and energy, and he himself in sundry ways valiantly attempted to recapture a zest for life. For instance, he wrote a short biography of Pasteur, emphasizing his mode of thought and discovery, which Smith agreed to criticize. Smith corrected a few errors, improved words and phrases, and harped with gentle irony on Pasteur's rivalry with Koch. Pasteur's technique would have been less irritating "if it had not kept the old pace long after better methods had been introduced for staining & cultivating bacteria. They, however, originated across the Rhine." Pasteur's ideas on microbic variability and adaptability "proved true although he may have gone a little too far at times . . . Koch and his school were very rigid and conservative until within a few years. Now they have fully but tacitly accepted the doctrine." As for Pasteur's simplicity and transparency, "How could the genuine man of science have been otherwise and yet successful? For we cannot juggle with Nature and if there are such tendencies in us to make the worse appear the better reason they must be eliminated, and will be through the pure contact with science."[23] Herter used this sketch on Pasteur in delivering the 1903 commencement Address at Johns Hopkins University Medical School.[24]

On his way to a holiday in California, Herter wrote several letters to Theobald Smith. He helped to persuade Jacques Loeb, the mechanistic philosopher, professor of physiology at the University of Chicago, to join the Rockefeller Institute, though this decision was not effective until 1910. Smith questioned how Loeb's investigations of sea urchin eggs and other low forms of living matter were connected with medical research.

Herter's letters to Smith from California reported Santa Barbara to be extremely beautiful. Stanford University had many admirable features, but represented a very strange mixture of medieval and modern tendencies. Although faculty and students were progressive, the university government was despotic. No doubt conditions would improve ultimately. Meanwhile "Research is almost unknown here . . . Immense sums are expanded on a cathedral while the library goes begging."[25] Then Herter arranged to spend several months of the 1903–1904 winter at the Frankfurt Institute, where "Ehrlich has kept me pretty busy, without himself being conscious of the fact, but I . . . shall always feel that I did the right thing to go to him."[26] Ehrlich is reputed to have commented, "I have had many brilliant Americans come to work with me; but Christian I loved."[27]

Despite such changes of scene, Herter's health did not improve. He and his wife donated $25,000 to the Johns Hopkins University to establish an annual lectureship in memory of their youngest child. The three-person selection committee (chaired by Welch for many years) chose Paul Ehrlich as the first Herter Foundation Lecturer. At Baltimore, in April 1904, Ehrlich delivered three lectures on various forms and aspects of immunity. Twelve years later, in May 1916, Theobald Smith was the first American to give the Herter lectures. He delivered three (unpublished) lectures at Baltimore in May 1916 on certain aspects of parasitism, including "Immunity and Parasitism."

During the next two or three years, Herter's bouts of depression and physical weakness recurred and worsened. With Flexner's encouragement, he rallied and made estimates of the operating costs for the hospital. They would be "not far from $5.00 a day for each patient," he wrote to Flexner. "This looks pretty stiff, but I do not see how we are to get what we need for less expense."[28] By May 1908, Rockefeller had pledged sufficient funds to warrant proceeding with the Hospital, but Herter was obviously too ill to direct it; Rufus Cole, aged thirty-six, a graduate of Johns Hopkins Medical School, was named Director of the Rockefeller Institute Hospital, while Herter was appointed Physician to the Hospital and Member of the Institute. Herter's apathy merged into increasing physical weakness, which was recognized as organic only when wasting paralysis developed, variously diagnosed as myasthenia gravis or amyotrophic lateral sclerosis (then termed Charcot's, later Lou Gehrig's disease). In retrospect, the latter seems the more likely diagnosis. Herter died, aged forty-five, on December 5, 1910, only a few weeks after the official inauguration of the Hospital. By then, a handsome addition to the endowment brought the total capital invested by Rockefeller in the Institute to more than six million dollars.[29]

Among innumerable messages of condolence to Susan Herter was one from Welch. "Especially shall we miss Christian in our circle of scientific directors of the Rockefeller Institute, now for the first time broken."[30] Jacques Loeb's tribute to the gallant Herter was truly eloquent: "One of the most lovable human beings, a piece of poetry in a too prosaic world, and the most sympathetic of all my friends . . . I have no consolation to offer to you—except that we all cherish and keep alive his memory."[31]

In March 1903, having informed President Eliot and Dr. Walcott of his decisions about the Rockefeller Institute directorship, Smith sent a copy of the letter of declination to G.F. Fabyan, asking that the document be preserved, as he wanted to keep the only other copy among his posthumous effects.[32] All the arrangements for his leave of absence had been officially approved, enabling him and Marshal Fabyan to make a tour of Europe in quest of scientific information. On June 9, he delivered the Shattuck lecture on "Malaria in Massachusetts." Then he added to his wardrobe. Every purchase was itemized and priced, from a new suit, bathrobe and shoes, to four pairs of socks ($1.00) and a tie (25 cents). The June accounts also listed a passport ($1.28), "$24.70 in gold in Europe," and total assets of $20,817.89. On June 30, Smith and his young companion left Boston as saloon passengers for Liverpool, on R.M.S. *Saxonia*.

Europe Revisited, 1902

Among Smith's papers was a leather-bound booklet labeled "MARSHAL FABYAN—his book—June 30, 1902." In this book, Theobald Smith, as controller of the treasury, entered expenditures and meticulously recorded every transaction, especially those relating to his letters of credit in Liverpool, London and Copenhagen—until complications arose, whereafter "Highlights Only" were noted. On their return, Fabyan senior was so astonished by the modest overall outlay ($854.56, excluding transatlantic fares) that he would not inspect the accounts submitted. Smith later redressed a minor imbalance by sending $25 to the Harvard Treasurer's office for the George Fabyan Fund.

The *Saxonia* reached Liverpool on the morning of July 9. Smith and Marshall made for the North-West Railway Hotel. That afternoon they met "Ross, Boyce, Grünbaum & others" while visiting the Thomson-Yates Laboratory and the School of Tropical Medicine. Ross had recently received the Nobel Prize. Three months before Smith's visit, the directors of the Liverpool School of Tropical Medicine decided to strike a medallion commemorating the West African explorer, Mary H. Kingsley, who died in 1900. The medallion was awarded intermittently "to distinguished scientists who had specialized in the field of tropical medicine and kindred subjects." In 1907 Theobald Smith, Professors Danielevsky and Golgi, Dr. Charles Finlay, Dr. W.M. Haffkine and Colonel Gorgas were all listed as recipients. In 1906, 1908 and 1909, there were no awards.

Next morning, Smith and Fabyan caught a southbound train, and began what proved to be largely a kaleidoscopic sightseeing trip. Leaving the train at Leamington, they drove to Kenilworth Castle, and stayed overnight in Warwick. A side-trip to Stratford-on-Avon on the 11th permitted them to scan all the Shakespeariana, including the grave. Returning to Warwick, they visited the Castle and then entrained for Paddington. At High Holborn, the First Avenue Hotel accommodated them both for a whole week for £8–12–7. As July 12 was a Sunday, they attended matins at St. Paul's Cathedral and evensong at Westminster Abbey.

Next day the Tower was visited in the morning and the Jenner Institute of Preventive Medicine in the afternoon. The Institute, founded in 1891 as the British Institute of Preventive Medicine, had been renamed in 1897 to commemorate the centenary of the first vaccination against smallpox. To avoid a lawsuit from another manufacturer of the Jennerian product, the name was changed again in 1903 to the Lister Institute. The headquarters in southwest London is still known by this name. With Baedeker as guide, July 14 was a day of pilgrimages: to Hampton Court by rail, on foot through Busy Park to Teddington, by electric underground to Richmond, and aboard a bus to Kew Gardens, returning to the hotel by another underground route.

On July 5, Smith discussed tuberculosis with E. J. Steegmann, Secretary of the Royal Commission appointed in 1901; lunched at the Jenner Institute with Drs. A. MacFadyean and H. G. Plimmer; and met Dr. F.R. Blaxall, director of the Local Government Board's vaccine lymph laboratory, who invited him to that establishment. On the 16th, after jointly exploring the City near the Bank of England, Smith went to the Royal Commission's farms at Bishop's Stratford, while Fabyan patronized the Hippodrome. Next morning, Smith looked over the Local Government Board's vaccine plant and in the afternoon visited the London Hospital. Finally, on July 18 they toured the Jenner Institute's antitoxin farm at Elstree before leaving that night for Copenhagen via Harwich and the Hook of Holland.

After crossing Holland and passing through Hamburg and Bremen, they stopped overnight at Kiel. Next morning they inspected the Canal and continued on to Copenhagen by train and ferry. On the 21st, with Prof. S. Arrhenius of the Staatenseruminstitut, they viewed the new friezes in the Glyptothek sculpture gallery and walked through the woods near the Baltic shoreline before dining outdoors. The following day, the itinerary included the Kommune and the Infectious Diseases Hospitals, the Thorvaldsen and Moltke Museums, Hansen's Carlsberg Laboratorium and the Tivoli "amusement garden." Copenhagen's architecture was fascinating and Theobald purchased statuary models for the children. The morning of the 23rd was spent in Madsen's laboratory, and the afternoon at the vaccine establishment. At the evening "dinner & supper with Dr. Madsen," the other guests included Salomonsen and Arrhenius.

On Friday, July 24th, they left for Berlin where they stayed at the Hotel Bristol. The weekend was spent sightseeing in the Old and New Museums, the National Gallery, the Royal Palace and stables, the Arsenal, the Thiergarten, and the Zoo. They dined at Kroll's restaurant and listened to the Thiergarten band. On Monday, they visited an abattoir and Dr. Schultz's vaccine plant. Later they made a courtesy call at the Institut für Infektionskrankheiten, whose Director, Robert Koch, was in Bulawayo, investigating "redwater" in cattle and "horsesickness." On the 28th, they went to Koch's former laboratory in the Imperial Health Office and conferred at the Institute with Dr. W. Dönitz. The following morning, having toured the Reichstag, they inspected the Veterinary School before entraining for Frankfurt, where the 30th was spent at Ehrlich's institute. Ehrlich's American pupil, the Rockefeller Institute Scholar, Dr. Preston Kyes, drove them to the Palmengarten and around the city before they dined with Ehrlich and his family. On July 31, Smith's forty-fourth birthday, they took a steamer down the Rhine to Coblenz and returned by rail. After his death, on December 14, 1934, Marshal Fabyan wrote to Lilian Smith:

> Dr. Smith did not find it so easy to be hitched to an active young man on his first trip to Europe, but the effort he made to keep the pace did him real good; as he told me the next Spring, he had never got through the winter's work so easily, or felt less tired at the end . . . I remember a birthday we spent on the Rhine (we attempted to see it all in one day), and at the close he said feelingly he hoped he would never have another birthday like that one.

On August 1, after bidding Ehrlich goodbye, they left for Switzerland. They stayed three nights in Lucerne, took a cable ride to the Sonnenberg, a lake steamer to Vitznau, the cogwheel railway up the Rigi, and roamed about. They continued on to Interlaken, toured the Schynige Platte and circled the Kleine Rugen. During an interlude at Grindelwald ("tramp to upper glacier, enter ice grotto, return 4–5 P.M."), Theobald was photographed by Marshal, resolutely treading an alpine trail toward distant peaks, impeccably attired in a three-piece suit and bowler hats, and clutching his furled umbrella. On August 8, Berne was reached by steamer via Lake Thun and the River Aar. They attended Sunday service at the Protestant Munster on the 9th, visited the "bearpit" and climbed a nearby hill. Next morning, after going over a vaccine and serum laboratory, they caught the train for Lausanne and Geneva. Arriving in Paris on the 12th, they stayed at the Grand Hotel, Boulevard des Capucins, near the Opera.

During the first two days in Paris, their itinerary covered visits to the Eiffel Tower and the Louvre, the museum of the old Luxembourg palace, the musée de Cluny (French antiquities), the Pantheon, the church of St. Etienne du Mont (completed under Louis XIII), the Sorbonne, and the Latin Quarter. On the 15th, they called at the Pasteur Institute, and talked to Roux, Metchnikoff, Levaditi and Marmorek. On Sunday the 16th, they went to Versailles, afterwards viewing in Paris the Greek and Russian Churches, the Bois de Boulogne, the Jardin d'Acclimatisation and the Zoo, and surmounting the Arc de Triomphe de l'Etoile. Next day they saw Les Halles Centrales and Notre Dame, where the church's deep bell, *le bourdon,* was tolling at the funeral ceremonies for victims of a recent subway disaster. On the last day they revisited the Louvre, looked over a vaccine institute, and dined at Pousset's.

They left Paris on the 19th for another three nights in London. Smith noted on August 20: "Rainy. Visit vaccine establishment to see children vacc. Visit royal

Soc. & lunch with Sir Michael Foster at some club. visit Tate Gallery 4–5 P.M."
Foster was vice-president of the Royal Society and chairman of the Royal Commission on Tuberculosis; the club was probably The Athenaeum. Smith returned
to the Local Government Board's plant on the 21st to see calves vaccinated. He
and Marshall bought clothing, leather goods, miscellaneous presents—and a
"vaccine bulb 1/6." The boat train left London on the 22nd for Liverpool where
they boarded the Cunard Line's *Lucania,* which was bigger and faster than the
Saxonia. Theobald Smith, the only "Prof" on board, was confined to his cabin by
sore throat and seasickness. Among the passengers was Signor G. Marconi, already famous and wealthy. Both steamers were fitted with his "system of wireless
telegraphy."[33] Smith's account book for July 2 shows a "marconigram" sent to the
U.S.A. for 10 shillings. This message, transmitted to a westbound sister-ship,
R.M.S. *Ivernia,* was relayed to Lilian five days later when the *Ivernia* docked in
New York.

Theobald had sent her five or six letters, one card, and a picture of Kenilworth
Castle for Dolly, while Lilian wrote him two or three letters a week. Her comments personified the affectionate, intelligent wife who stayed at home to care
for children and household. "How strange it was to watch you go! the in-
evitableness of it is like death—no turning back when the time comes!" She had
paid the bill for his *American Medicine* subscription, looked over the Bussey[34] and
checked and returned the Shattuck lecture proof.[35]

The girls had been invited for ten days to "Miradero," the Herters's establishment near Bar Harbor, Maine, on Mt. Desert Island where they formed a happy
quartet with the Herter daughters. Lilian packed "Plenty of good suitable clothing . . . Sixteen little gowns, some made-overs, but I *made* eleven gowns." The
"Miradero" had fourteen servants, including a governess, a coachman, and at
least two "sailors" for a boat, the *Suzetta.* There were three riding-horses, two
ponies and a cart, a goat with a cart, and a small laboratory. Simon Flexner and
his fiancée, Helen Thomas, soon to be married, were also guests. Their host,
though obviously unwell, was very hospitable, and did his best to enjoy the company and the setting.

Lilian had declined an invitation from the Fabyans to their summer home in
Cohasset, about twenty-five miles south of Boston. Marshal's sister mentioned
long and enthusiastic letters from him. The family "pitied you for having such an
indefatigable sightseer with you—they feared you would not come back
rested."[36] The *Laconia* reached New York on August 30. Marshal's brother
George greeted the two travelers at the dock and conducted them to a train for
Boston.

13

THE NEW ANTITOXIN AND
VACCINE LABORATORY
EHRLICH AND DIPHTHERIA RESEARCHES
THE "THEOBALD SMITH PHENOMENON"

Within a month of returning from overseas at the end of August 1903, Theobald Smith was "planning the new vaccine and antitoxin building on Bussey grounds; searching thro' numerous catalogues and ordering apparatus from 6 or more foreign firms."[1] By October, in addition to outlining a lecture course on bacteria as parasites, he recorded "hunting up calves and horses, besides carrying on routine work and overseeing Beyer, Reagh and Brown in lab."[2] (Beyer, a medical officer in the U.S. Navy, had leave to work under Smith at the Bussey Institute.) The imported apparatus began arriving in January 1904. Smith insisted on unpacking it himself. Now in his forty-fifth year, he had started to wear bifocal spectacles. He looked and felt his age.

The building plans were entirely his, except for details of stalls for vaccinated calves. The structure was defined by President Eliot as "a laboratory of Comparative Pathology [built] under the skilful direction of Professor Theobald Smith." Financed from Bussey Institution funds, the laboratory cost about $20,000 and was rented by the Commonwealth of Massachusetts for $1,000 a year. "In the barns and paddocks adjoining are kept the horses and cows which furnish material for these two life-saving products of medical research"[3]—diphtheria antitoxin and vaccine virus for prevention of smallpox. They were cheap for the

State Board of Health, but this diversionary investment of the already inadequate Bussey endowment provoked some further caustic criticism from Dean Storer.

A less cautious and conscientious person than Theobald Smith might have envisaged a larger structure, arguing that demands for public health services had always outstripped the experts' anticipations, particularly in a community as progressive as the State of Massachusetts. A more opportunistic individual, realizing that his presence in the Bussey building was unwelcome, would have seized the chance to move out into roomier quarters. But Smith did not abuse his express assignment. The new laboratory was designed solely for the routine production, testing and storage of diphtheria antitoxin and vaccine lymph, with some provision for work on minor problems concerned with maintaining or improving standards. The unpretentious brick structure, which Theobald believed would be more healthful than a building of damp stone,[4] was to be 42–1/2 feet square with two floors and basement. An additional wing for calf-stables, extending backward, involved the first floor and basement only. The specifications included cement floors, covered with asphalt, except in the basement; walls and ceilings finished with hard plaster, enamel-painted for easy washing and disinfection; doors tin-covered and iron-framed.

The inclement 1903–04 winter caused suspension of construction, much to Smith's annoyance, until late March. Calves began arriving around the middle of July and by the end of the month some of the staff moved in. The first packages of antitoxin were issued from the new laboratory in September 1904, and in October a small batch of vaccine was forthcoming. The exasperating delays—a mild foretaste of wartime frustrations more than a decade later—persuaded him to urge patience upon Simon Flexner, who was also fretting to move into expanded laboratory quarters.[5]

Smith requested authorization from President Eliot to spend up to $500 from Fabyan funds on apparatus for his laboratory in the Bussey Institute.

> The transfer of the antitoxin work to our new building has completely stripped my laboratory of all apparatus but that used in histological work. The apparatus belonged to the State.
>
> The work this summer has been very arduous. In the first place I had to give much time, fully a month, to directing personally the workmen. Then came the moving, with the maintenance of the antitoxin output, the establishment of the vaccine work and the training of the needed servants. We have now vaccine ready for a preliminary test on children.

On the whole, he was very gratified with the new quarters. Early in 1904, he described the new laboratory's lay-out and objectives,[6] and in 1906 gave details of the production and State-wide distribution of diphtheria antitoxin during the preceding decade.[7]

An inquirer about a possible diphtheria antitoxin plant for the State of Wisconsin was assured that in Massachusetts the free supply of this agent had led to the use of larger doses. Theobald Smith estimated that the people of Massachusetts were saved about $50,000 a year. Costs could be minimized through University affiliation, by utilizing available laboratories, stables, paddocks, and trained personnel attached to faculties. The laboratory director was responsible for the product's safety, and therefore must exercise complete operating control, and should have sole rights to appoint and dismiss: "Political appointees would be very unsafe persons in such an establishment."[8] In his 1902 address on the preparation of vaccine, Smith had emphasized that "Efficiency is not the only consideration. Purity and safety are of still greater importance."[9]

Preparation of the vaccine was not free from start-up troubles. Material from the New York Vaccine Laboratory took well at first, but proved heavily contaminated with skin micro-organisms. Seed vaccine sent by the Government Lymph laboratories in London lost its potency through building delays and summer heat, so that it failed to take when tried in the fall of 1904. The best take, and excellent subsequent results, were shown by a small sample of "Pfeiffer retro-vaccine," presumably from a German establishment.[10] (Retro-vaccines were products harvested from a calf inoculated with lymph from human vaccine pustules, either directly, or indirectly through a series of calves.)

Smith's interest in vaccine did not cease with its manufacture and release—as witness his comments about plans for setting up a "vaccine station" in a new hospital:

> There is at present no satisfactory vaccine station in Boston. Whatever can be done to safeguard the operation and make it more attractive to the mass of people will be in the interest of public health. There should be several stations in a city as large as this so that it would not be necessary for people to bring small children long distances . . . in times of threatening epidemics the present facilities are wholly inadequate to safeguard vaccinations when so many have to be made rapidly.[11]

As a distributor and manufacturer of diphtheria antitoxin in Massachusetts, Theobald Smith was already familiar with the work of Paul Ehrlich, whose earlier claim to fame derived from his theoretical and practical concern with the standardization of this product. As it happened, despite some extreme differences in temperament, they became friendly and candid correspondents. Most of this chapter will be devoted to their revealing associations with the interactions between diphtheria toxin and antitoxin.

Correspondence between Smith and Ehrlich started in the spring of 1897, when Smith sent Ehrlich a report on the potency of some commercial antitoxins. This was acknowledged on May 20 by Ehrlich's colleague, W. Dönitz, who enclosed a list of changes approved by the Ministry of Health in the method of testing. Later in 1897, Smith sent reprints of his own reports on diphtheria[12] to Ehrlich, who reciprocated by inviting Smith's opinion of the proposals for providing a more satisfactory system of standardizing antitoxic sera, as outlined in his difficult paper, "The assay of the activity of diphtheria-curative serum and its theoretical basis."[13]

This was the paper "about the theory of the tests for diphtheria," which Ehrlich hoped had clarified the "so dark" field. (It had "required an unbelievable amount of work and experimental animals," Ehrlich told Smith, adding "I hope at least to have brought some clarity into that so dark field.")[14] One of the paper's main proposals was that toxin attenuation occurred through step-like degradations, whose products bore simple arithmetic relationships (e.g., one-half, two-thirds) to the postulated total of 200 units. Ehrlich contended that one standard unit of antitoxin would neutralize this "absolute total" unitage of crude toxin—including toxoids or toxones that had lost all lethality for guinea-pigs, but retained their antitoxin-binding capacities. Specific antibody formation was explained in terms of Weigert's side-chain hypothesis.

Dönitz had sent Smith a vial of freshly prepared standard serum of 1700-unit strength in order to facilitate comparisons between the old method of estimating the potency of antitoxic sera and Ehrlich's innovations—use of a standardized antitoxin and the "$L_?$ dose" of toxin. The figures given by the two methods of titration showed wide discrepancies, which were to Ehrlich inexplicably "colossal" when contrasted with the results obtained by him and Dönitz at Steglitz, and by Madsen at Copenhagen. "In any case, such differences between various investigations suggest that the old method with its subjective determination had to be abandoned and replaced by a purely objective one, such as the present method."[15] Ehrlich wondered if this gross disparity was due to the lower potencies of European toxins. Smith responded that stronger toxins did seem to deteriorate more rapidly, citing one test toxin that in about seven weeks lost one-third of its potency. As the State Department of Health had authorized him to accept Ehrlich's offer to maintain a supply of standardized serum, he requested a quarterly shipment of "a vial of the 17-fold serum."[16]

A few months later, Theobald outlined Ehrlich's "very ingenious theory" in an address on diphtheria toxin and antitoxin at the annual meeting of the Massachusetts Medical Society. Smith correlated the symptomatology of the human disease with the paralytic and other effects of diphtheria toxin upon 188 guinea-pigs which had survived injections of toxin or toxin-antitoxin mixtures, and expressed "the conviction that toxins and antitoxins are realities, entities, whose obscure nature and action need not stand in the way of our belief that we have reached the right path in studying them."[17]

In another report,[18] Ehrlich postulated several break-down products of toxin, each with its own pattern of toxicity and antitoxin-binding power. The Lo and L+ doses of a toxin permitted its constitution ("spectrum") to be determined numerically and represented graphically. Smith requested Ehrlich to suggest the spectra of two toxins whose stated Lo and L+ doses had been determined in the Bussey laboratory. Ehrlich painstakingly responded.[19] His first published references to toxophore and haptophore groups, which embellished the side-chain theory (to be more fully expounded in the Croonian Lecture in 1900),[20] were followed by this assertion to Smith: "I do believe that only the assumption of toxophore and haptophore groups can give us an insight into the nature and genesis of immunity."[21] Smith still applauded the side-chain concept in 1934. "Though derided in recent years, the side-chain hypothesis has been highly stimulating and suggestive . . . As long as life is not reduced to a formula, those who study living things are compelled to assume something more in their behalf than what is offered at present by physico-chemical research."[22]

In 1899, Theobald Smith reported that "Animals from some sources seem to be much more susceptible to diphtheria toxin than those from others."[23] Guinea-pigs from a dealer had proved more vulnerable than home-bred pigs. The latter exhibited "a remarkably uniform susceptibility." Smith cited Behring as stating that "Ehrlich obtained from a breeder a race of diphtheria-immune guinea-pigs"—a fact which Ehrlich never published but affirmed in a letter to Smith over five years later. In 1900, Smith recorded his detection of four such immune guinea-pigs out of 600 to 700, "all from the same mother in two litters."[24] This was his initial reference to the phenomenon of transmitted passive immunity, which he later investigated thoroughly.[25] The same paper contained the first published observation that guinea-pigs were more susceptible to the toxin in winter than in summer. Ehrlich confided that he had also observed this fact: "According to my own experience, the summer animals are most constant. Therefore I have best performed my main experiments on the spectrum during the summer months."[26]

Smith informed Ehrlich in 1902 that a recently received vial of standard dry serum showed deterioration in neutralizing capacity. Ehrlich acknowledged in an agitated letter that they had noted a similar decline: "Our standard dry serum, in contrast to the experience of long years, had changed its titre." A new standard, now being put up, would be sent at once, and the situation was being investigated. While they hoped to hear the results of any tests, "I beg you to consider this information in friendliest fashion as *confidential.*"

Our purpose has been only to clarify the situation for you, and to prove to you that we ourselves act with the most absolute care in the preparation of the standard, and that only a completely unforeseeable mishap caused the disturbance. It will interest you that *you* are the only one who discovered this occurrence by newly testing the standard.[27]

In his letter, Ehrlich also told Theobald that "I am as convinced of the absolute trustworthiness of your reports as if I myself had made the experiments." Smith replied reassuringly. Ehrlich expressed heartfelt thanks and relief: "I am glad you have retained full faith in our trustworthiness," he responded.[28] He thanked Theobald later for a "report on the question of the test serum" and solicited a culture of outstanding toxigenicity. "We believe here that generally you in America are in this respect superior to us all."[29]

In 1900, Smith had stated that studies of toxin-antitoxin mixtures "indicate such complex relationships that a theoretical unit cannot be looked for in the near future."[30] However, in 1903, a few weeks before Smith's European tour, Ehrlich wrote to Smith, telling him

That the normal unit can be reconstructed according to the principles evolved by me, and also approved by you, was pointed out in my letter only to verify that it is not altogether an arbitrary standard unit that is in question, but one which is basically reconstructable. The case here is similar to that of determining the meter, which in the beginning was a definite fraction of the earth's diameter . . . My efforts were intended only to fashion, through exact determinations, a unit that is scientifically more closely definable.

Such an undertaking would become necessary only if a unit were lost completely—a most unlikely event.[31]

Ehrlich was perplexed by the contrast between the wide acceptance of his practical contributions to the problem of antitoxin assay and the antagonism aroused in some quarters by the theoretical considerations which in his view underlay and justified this system. The more readily understood parts of his toxophore and haptophore group concepts, and of the side-chain theory, were also generally welcomed innovations. But the increasing number and variety of hypothetical break-down products eluded the average grasp. Despite growing confusion, he plunged deeper and deeper into the forest. He did not stop at postulating proto-, syn-, and epi-toxoids, with their lost lethality and increased, unchanged, and diminished antitoxin-binding powers. He substituted the term toxones, which supposedly caused retarded paralyses of guinea-pigs. His letters and publications were sprinkled with spectra carrying such designations as hemi-, deutero-, and trito-toxins. Yet his goal of a general formula covering all toxin-antitoxin neutralization phenomena remained elusive.

Almost seven years before, soon after launching his quest, Ehrlich had written prophetically to Weigert: "Everything wobbles here and it is as if one wanted to build a palace in a bog . . . I shall be glad when I am finished with the business; one can't get much fame out of it either."[32] Now, Prof. Max Gruber of Munich (and Clemens von Pirquet of Vienna) had brought a defamatory verbal campaign to a head with a published letter, parodying Ehrlich's theories, signed "Dr. Peter Phantasus, M.D. Chemist by the Grace of God," and claiming that sulfuric acid, and even water, had toxic spectra.[33] Ehrlich had taken up the cudgels, pointing out that Gruber's "ten-minute experiments" were "absolutely worthless."[34] The exchange of insults ended late in 1903.[35]

At the Steglitz Institute, Ehrlich had put Thorvald Madsen to work on the interactions of tetanolysin and antitetanolysin, a system which had the advantage of being assessable *in vitro*. Madsen found, to Ehrlich's satisfaction, that the specific neutralization of tetanolysin was represented by a continuous hyperbolic curve. After returning from an American tour, during which he met Theobald Smith, Madsen continued his researches at the Danish State Serum Institute in cooperation with Svante Arrhenius, a leading physical chemist. In a classic paper replete with columns of figures, abstruse formulae and graphs, they showed that the neutralization curve for tetanolysin resembled those depicting dissociating solutes and their respective products, according to the mass-effect law of Guldberg and Waage.[36]

Ehrlich maintained that this law was not applicable to the diphtheria toxin-antitoxin relationship, where the affinity was strong. He was confident that neutralization of pure diphtheria toxin by antitoxin would proceed in a straight-line form. Any deviations expressed the fact that crude toxin comprised various toxoid-like substances, preformed and of different affinities. "The natural aim of physical chemistry" [in which he acknowledged Arrhenius's leadership] must always be to introduce as few factors as possible for purposes of calculation, whereas biological analysis always seeks to pay due regard to the wonderful multiplicity of organic matter."[37] He believed that "If the mathematicians set aside all precautions . . . [and] . . . neglect the facts of plurality, as determined biologically, then we will fall under a tyranny of figures."[38] However, in July 1903, Madsen, who remained scrupulously respectful to Ehrlich, showed by guinea-pig experiment that the process of diphtheria toxin-antitoxin combination also followed the Guldberg-Waage law.[39]

Ehrlich wrote to Smith in November 1903, seeking Smith's consent to his citing "the factual part" of a letter sent "some time ago about the absolute determination of the value of the immunity unit (1 International Unit - 200 Lethal Doses)." He was then "perfectly aware that my toxin investigations made possible a new evaluation of the I.U. . . . . The last publication of Arrhenius and

Madsen . . . could easily make it appear to outsiders that Madsen had discovered the principle of newly determining the immunity unit." Ehrlich added a few points to show Smith "on whose side is the right in this battle over curve or spectrum." If the mathematicians prevailed, they "eventually must devastate our entire field."[40] Ehrlich soon wrote again, requesting another reprint of Smith's work on "the constitution of diphtheria toxin." Arrhenius had reported to him that Madsen had made a miscalculation in their recent paper.

> I am most astonished about this. Here a toxin is estimated, which ought to have been so accurately investigated as never before, and the calculated figures supposedly prove a curve-like saturation analogous to the ammonia-boric acid poison. Now it turns out that the whole calculation is absolutely false, and that actually there was no ground for attacking my views on the basis of this poison.[41]

Further experiments by Arrhenius and Madsen confirmed their earlier work and showed that, contrary to Ehrlich's views, aging toxin was homogeneous. In a footnote, Arrhenius denied that their data had been miscalculated.

Paul Ehrlich was invited by Herter to give the first series of Christian A. Herter Lectures at Baltimore on April 12, 13 and 14, 1904. On April 2, after inspecting the quarters proposed as the Rockefeller Institute's temporary laboratories, Theobald Smith attended a dinner given in Ehrlich's honor at the home of Samuel J. Meltzer. Meltzer, three years older than Ehrlich, had studied medicine in Germany, and emigrated to America in 1884, because, as a Jew, like Ehrlich and his cousin Weigert, he could not hope for a university chair. After practicing medicine in New York City for twenty years, Meltzer was invited by Simon Flexner to become a Research Member of the Rockefeller Institute. He grew to fame as the Institute's leading physiologist.

Ehrlich's wife, who accompanied him, was fluent in English, but he himself knew none and delivered the lecture in German. In his second lecture, he referred to Theobald Smith, who had investigated a toxin "with the utmost precision." Ehrlich ended the lecture by expressing the conviction that what he had "established through long years of work concerning the nature of the diphtheria poison will withstand the Northern storm and with the course of time prove itself to be real and vital."[42] He was guest at the annual meeting of the American Association of Pathologists and Bacteriologists, also attended by Smith and Meltzer, both charter members.[43] Smith wrote to Flexner on March 31: "Ehrlich will be there and I have no doubt he will be an inspiration to the men to stick to their work until something permanent is born." A few days later, Ehrlich was made an Honorary Member of the New York Academy of Medicine. Several years after his death, when Ehrlich's wife took up residence in the United States, the Academy accepted custody of some of her husband's memorabilia, including his Privy Councillor uniform.

On April 19, Walcott inspected the State Board of Health laboratory in preparation for the distinguished visitor. A dinner was given that night in Ehrlich's honor at the Somerset Hotel. Next day, accompanied by his wife and a *Diener,* presumably Kadereit, his general factotum at the Frankfurt Institute,[44] he called on Smith at the Bussey Institution and stayed for lunch at Woodland Hill. Despite a snowstorm, the crocuses were out. The scope and methodology of Theobald Smith's researches left an indelible impression. During his subsequent tour, Ehrlich received an honorary doctorate from the University of Chicago. He appeared more immediately impressed by shredded wheat biscuits served at breakfast, and above all by a box of super-strength cigars presented to him at Ann Arbor.[45]

Soon after returning to Frankfurt, Ehrlich thanked Smith for the friendly reception by his family, and praised his thorough methodology.

> I was extremely delighted with what I saw in your laboratory and my conviction that in no Institute in the world—unfortunately, not even in my own—is better and more reliable work done than in yours, was fully and completely confirmed. You weave the net of your experiments so fine that nothing essential can escape you, while the rest of us have always to rely on a certain amount of luck.

Ehrlich had battled recently with Arrhenius at a meeting of physical chemists in Bonn, where he had found "quite wonderful support from Nernst, who produced proof that the formulae of Arrhenius are based on inaccurate and in part quite false premises; it appears that Arrhenius *completely ignored* the main point, that with these substances their colloidal nature plays a major role."[46] Two weeks later, Ehrlich informed Smith that Nernst's article[47] had appeared in print. "You will perceive from it how untenable are all the formulae of Arrhenius . . . It is a veritable cuckoo's egg that the authors have laid for us in the nest of immunity."[48]

In a postscript to the preceding letter, Ehrlich Added: "Friend Herter will bring you a small medallion of me, which my pupils dedicated to me on my 50th birthday." Herter forwarded the medallion by mail from Seal Harbor, Maine on July 2, 1904. This was a small replica of a bronze plaque showing Ehrlich's head in profile, presented to him by assistants and collaborators on March 14, 1904. The plaque hangs on the wall of Smith's elder daughter's apartment in New York in the group photograph of Mrs. Stefanie Schwerin and her two sons, taken in December, 1964.[49] Herter did not find the medallion to his liking. In his covering note to Smith he wrote: "The refined alert look of Ehrlich is not in this profile; at least I cannot see it. Still I hope it will be a welcome to you for his sake." A few days later, Herter wrote again to Smith: "Ehrlich's nature contains so much of the spirituelle, and [he] is so capable of concentration on the topic that happens to fill his mind that he becomes extraordinarily oblivious to what [occurs] about him; and I think this explains his forgetfulness and impractibility. I enjoyed my contact with him greatly and never learned so much in so short a time."[50]

Two weeks later, Ehrlich drew Smith's attention to an article by Madsen and Walbum on the reactions between ricin and antiricin, which behaved like the tetanolysin-complex.[51] Ehrlich found the article "extremely weak . . . ricin has an extraordinarily complex composition . . . permeated with a colossal quantity of toxoids . . . I absolutely do not understand how one can draw any biding conclusions from such an unsuitable toxin!" Ehrlich expressed pleasure that Smith "had begun the great task of assembling all your diphtheria paralyses." He had found, like Smith, that paralyses were rare after subcutaneous injection of toxin. "It was precisely this circumstance which first led to the assumption of the existence of special toxins [toxones]."[52]

Ehrlich continued to try to engage Smith in the controversy with Arrhenius. "Your material, which has been examined with such wonderful exactitude, is probably more suitable than anything else for clarifying the inadmissibility of this calculation." He asked permission, which was given, to refer to Smith's work.[53] Smith, in German, wrote that "my experiments with guinea pigs do not entice me to exact mathematical calculation. Unfortunately, I do not have large-scale experiments . . . My principle has always been few animals, but well observed."[54]

Smith's paper on the irregular susceptibility of guinea-pigs to diphtheria toxin appeared in February 1905.[55] He testified to the uniformity of Ehrlich's antitoxin standard, but the uniformity was gauged by the death of guinea-pigs, which "do not respond with mathematical accuracy to the minimum fatal dose . . . irregularities were the rule rather than the exception." He ascertained, from careful records, that they represented an inheritable tendency, transmissible by the same mother to several litters. Unless the guinea-pigs were "better controlled and made more constant, neutralization experiments cannot very well lead to mathematically accurate formulae. In the practice of testing antitoxins both inaccuracy and cost are increased by variations in the susceptibility of guinea-pigs."[56]

In 1907, Smith demonstrated that the increased resistance shown by some young guinea-pigs resulted from the mother developing a relatively high level of circulating antitoxin in response to the subcutaneous injection of diphtheria toxin-antitoxin mixture, and transferring this passively to the offspring through the placenta, and also possibly through the milk. He referred to work by

Wernicke, published in 1895 in an unusual commemorative volume, that female guinea-pigs, injected alternately with diphtheria toxin and antitoxin, transmitted immunity to successive litters.[57] (Ehrlich himself had reported earlier, in 1892, that the progeny of a ricin- or abrin-immunized mouse inherited a specific transient immunity;[58] but he failed to perceive the analogy with the guinea-pigs resistant to diphtheria toxin.)

Theobald Smith further determined the important principle that "there is apparently no immediate relation between the severity of reaction . . . and the degree of immunity produced." Indeed, harmless toxin-antitoxin mixtures conferred far better immunity than an injection of damaging toxin. He raised the possibility of using "similar neutral mixtures for producing an active immunity in the human subject . . . It would be of great value to substitute for a passive immunity in exposed children an active immunity extending over a considerable period, provided such an immunity is attainable as easily and without any more difficulties than in the guinea-pig."[59]

Smith later verified that high levels of lasting immunity to diphtheria toxin could be induced in guinea-pigs by the injection of apparently innocuous toxin-antitoxin mixtures.[60] The acquired immunity was demonstrated indirectly by the enhanced resistance to toxin of litters produced several months after the mother was immunized with a single subcutaneous injection. Smith thus established that suckling guinea-pigs gained no immunity through maternal milk; that a sublethal injection of toxin alone provoked no detectable immunity; that mixtures containing an excess of toxin produced more immunity than neutral or "balanced" mixtures, while excessive antitoxin reduced the antigenic efficiency; and that the neutral mixtures were effective, having been held at room temperature, over a time range of fifteen minutes to five days after their preparation.

He concluded that "a practical, easily-controlled method" could be worked out for active immunization of the human subject. Smith also noted the theoretical difficulty of reconciling his findings with "current theories of the relation between toxins and antitoxins in mixtures." Apparently four to five days after preparation, a mixture whose toxin content was initially well below the Lo or neutral level, still contained enough free antigen for the production of immunity in the guinea pig. "These toxins may be free, either because uncombined *in vitro,* or else because the mixture is partially dissociated *in vivo,* or there may be a third possibility . . . namely that toxin and antitoxin took time to unite into a firm union that did not dissociate."[61]

Smith's last paper on this question was presented with H.R. Brown as co-author at a meeting of the Association of American Physicians in 1910. The authors formulated the hypothesis that a good antibody response depends upon the widespread reaction of various tissues to antigen released there in small quantities from mixtures incompletely saturated with antitoxin, and therefore loosely bound. "The antitoxin, as it were, smuggles the toxin into the body by disguising it. This procedure, which gives us an easier way to immunity, is likewise a source of danger, since it may bring the toxin to the nervous system and lead to paralysis."[62]

The report by Smith and Brown did not mention the practical use of toxin-antitoxin mixtures in producing active immunity in human beings. Theobald Smith's natural prudence no doubt helped to restrain him from direct personal involvement in experimentation on humans. Perhaps the restraint was reinforced here by his own perception of this procedure as potentially dangerous. Another possible factor was Smith's liability to lose personal interest in a discovery, if and when its practical applicability became plain. No such inhibitions affected Behring, who reported in 1913, at the Congress of Internal Medicine at Wiesbaden, that he had directed the immunization of forty-one children with a diphtheria toxin-antitoxin mixture of unspecified composition.[63] Terming this a "new diphtheria-defense remedy," he omitted any reference to Theobald Smith's extensive work on guinea-pigs as an obvious preliminary to trial of such mixtures in children. By characteristic failure to carry his laboratory findings into clinical practice, Theobald Smith perhaps lost opportunities of wider renown. But he shunned publicity (although sometimes seeming to court it), and in any event could not muster the bravado needed to cajole a clinician into cooperative ventures in which the laboratory investigator would hold the reins.

Ehrlich also sensed the gulf between the results of animal experiments and human therapy; but unlike Smith, sought to bridge it himself. Although Ehrlich leaned closer to the clinician—toward the direct cure of existing disease—he appreciated Smith's more philosophical outlook, which favored preventive medicine and the public health. Both were talented selectors of suitable research projects, and abandoners of problems that proved too unyielding or tiresome. Ehrlich "was always particularly proud of 'the art of marching off'," he wrote to Meltzer on March 9, 1910.

> Everything which did not really suit me, I always tried as far as possible to keep away from me, and I have always done only those things that pleased me and were therefore easy for me . . . I only got into real difficulties in a very few instances (as, for example, over the constitution of diphtheria toxin).[64]

The "real difficulties" over the constitution of diphtheria toxin contrast with his 1897 boast of pleasure, love and understanding. "In the end, I am still the only one who has pleasure, love and understanding for this very difficult field."[65] To announce a change from infatuation to bewilderment in such a scientific context took courage and candor.

During Ehrlich's visit to Boston, Smith mentioned the sudden death of guinea-pigs following a second injection of horse-serum, given after an interval of several days or weeks. He did not want to pursue a problem that would cause many deaths in his guinea-pig colony. The visitor had not encountered the phenomenon, but thought it should be investigated, so Smith invited Ehrlich to assign the problem to an assistant at the Frankfurt Institute. Just over a year later, Ehrlich wrote:

> Surgeon-Major Otto has carried out these experiments on quite a large scale, and perhaps will take the opportunity some time to publish his investigations . . . About one-half of the test animals die after a later injection of horse serum, while the other half becomes severely ill. The injurious action is induced, however, only by horse serum, not by other sera, e.g. goat serum, and is thus always specific . . . Your phenomenon . . . we have of course found to be exactly as you have described it."[66]

Otto's publication appeared early in 1906 in the memorial volume to Surgeon-General R. von Leuthold.[67] He showed that the serum in the toxin-antitoxin test mixture made the guinea-pig hypersensitive to serum of the same animal species, administered after an interval of at least ten days. The phenomenon is now considered a key example of "anaphylaxis," a term coined by Charles Richet in 1902.[68]

Shortly after Otto's report, M.J. Rosenau and J.F. Anderson of the United States Hygienic Laboratory published a detailed study of the very occasional instances of sudden death following an injection of horse serum in man.[69] In August 1906, the same authors published a second, shorter bulletin on two subjects: 1. the maternal transmission in guinea-pigs of immunity to diphtheria toxin; 2. the hypersensitivity to horse serum developed by guinea-pigs after an injection of diphtheria toxin-antitoxin mixture. The first part of this report dealt, on a larger scale, with the passive transfer of immunity in guinea-pigs noted by Smith in 1905, whose pioneer work in the field was duly acknowledged. The second part concerned the "Theobald Smith phenomenon," already defined by Otto earlier that year, unknown to Rosenau and Anderson.[70]

In June 1906, Rosenau and Anderson gave an address to the Section on Pathology and Physiology of the American Medical Association on "hypersusceptibility," which considered the relationship between guinea-pig anaphylaxis and human sensitivity to horse serum. A detailed abstract appeared in September,[71] containing two errors that had eluded proof-reading. Both the toxic and the sensitizing principle in horse serum were placed in Ehrlich's "hat-pin group" of substances (instead of *haptin* or *haptene*), and Theobald Smith allegedly stipulated an interval of two or three "minutes" (instead of *weeks*) between the first and second injections of horse serum. Smith was quoted as saying that "the subject had interested him since 1902." Subsequently, Sir Henry Dale suggested that Smith's statement established him as the first observer of "anaphylactic shock," a term originally applied to a harmful reaction to the reinjection, after a suitable interval, of a normally innocuous protein. "Portier and Richet, at the time of their publication in 1902, and for some time afterwards, still thought that what they had observed in the dog was an accentuated reaction, due to an abnormal, acquired sensitiveness to a natural poisonous foreign protein."[72]

Simon Flexner's isolated and undeveloped observation that guinea-pigs might succumb to a second dose of dog serum injected after an interval of several days or weeks[73] was resuscitated after fourteen years by Paul Lewis, an Austin Teaching Fellow to whom Smith had assigned the task (after Rosenau and Anderson's presentation) of further elucidating the induced susceptibility of the guinea-pig to horse serum. Lewis's paper[74] brought him to Flexner's favorable attention and he joined the staff of the Rockefeller Institute for Medical Research in 1908. In his report, Lewis alluded "to tests and experiments commenced in April 1903," when it was customary to inject guinea-pigs with samples of serum before its release for human use, as a safeguard against contamination.

Early in 1910 Smith wrote to congratulate Ehrlich on the progress being made in the drive for a cure for syphilis. Ehrlich was pleased. "You know yourself how extraordinarily high I place your judgment in scientific matters," he replied.[75] He was particularly grateful for the generous aid received from the Rockefeller Institute. "I only beg your pardon for not having yet thanked you especially for it."[76]

After working at Frankfurt for nearly a year, S. Hata demonstrated the outstanding spirocheticidal properties of the compound "606" in fowl spirillosis and rabbit syphilis. Supplies of the drug were distributed for human trials. Ehrlich had hoped that "in spirillosis the new substance which has been tried out by Hata will confirm itself in practice."[77] "But now the question will arise whether in a large number of cases hyper-sensitivities make the use of the remedy impossible. The hypersensitivity is just the stumbling-block which obstructs direct connection between animal experiments and human therapy!"

Smith thanked Ehrlich for the first volume of the *Encyclopädie der Mikroskopischen Technik,* separately sent. He thought the therapeutic experiments could be transferred more easily from man to animals if "monkeys were not so expensive. Man is phylogenetically too far from our laboratory and domestic animals to give us confidence in our own experiments." Civilized man had less resistance than animals. Ehrlich's discovery of drug-resistant strains perhaps helped to explain the many variants amongst bacteria, which probably belonged to a genus that had accommodated itself to many hosts. "Only he who does comparative pathology will be able to understand the importance of this theory of adaptation."[78] Ehrlich answered: "Your remarks about the monkey experiments are extraordinarily pertinent . . . In Germany we have the greatest difficulties both in the procuring of monkeys as well as with their maintenance, and Neisser in Breslau can sing a song about this. He finally got so far that he keeps the animals in his private house and his wife keeps the animals in her personal car."[79]

Ehrlich was extremely happy that the discovery of recidivist strains seemed so important to Smith. He also believed analogous conditions existed for bacteria and that chronic infections (tuberculosis), or such recurring sicknesses as Malta fever, would be best for these studies.

> But I believe the technical difficulties are extraordinarily great here and require a bacteriologist of your type! As you certainly know from our discussions, my own relevant acquirements are insufficient for the solution of this question. Therefore I have steered away from this course and have confined myself to the protozoa and parasites which are much easier to work with in this respect.

Ehrlich's letter closed on a sad personal note: "my grandson Herbert Landau, the son of my daughter Marianne a wonderfully talented boy of 4 years, succumbed to a septic laryngitis."

> The child fell ill one morning with a slight sore throat, which the specialists in the field considered unimportant; at 2 P.M. there was already laryngeal stenosis, and at 5 oclock tracheotomy had to be done, which helped little. I went at once to Göttingen at the first news, but could not help at all and found the child already in the worst condition; after another 24 hours death occurred from heart failure. Diphtheria bacilli could not be found despite a most intensive and careful investigation; so it must have been a very acute septic bronchitis.

He supposed they were dealing with a very specific hypersensitivity against a bacterial type which perhaps was usually quite harmless.[80] Three weeks later, along with Hata and various clinicians, Ehrlich addressed the Congress of Internal Medicine at Wiesbaden on the successes and pitfalls of the chemotherapy of syphilis. His grief at the diphtheria-like death of the small grandson was drowned in the turmoil, tragedy and triumph of the last five years of his own life.[81]

Theobald Smith and Paul Ehrlich were in many respects antithetical. In particular, the childlike ebullience, verbal extravagances, and egocentric impulsiveness of Ehrlich's letters were alien to the faint, dry sallies occasionally ventured by Smith; for example, in his note to Simon Flexner of March 31, 1904, just before

Ehrlich's arrival in the New World, Smith wrote: "I hope that you are not growing impatient to get into your own laboratories, for a little holding back is thoroughly good for the indefatigable worker."[82] Again, Smith's reluctance to follow up clinically the antigenic properties of his diphtheria toxin-antitoxin mixtures did not reflect disdain for the practical aspect of his researches—most of which at least began as mission-oriented projects. He genuinely preferred to work at the laboratory bench, either alone or with an initiated assistant. "Laboratory work will give not only a steadiness of the judgment, but also an abiding sense of the circumscription of knowledge," he believed.[83] Those days were gone, when researches led "straight to Public Health regulations . . . we must be content with the vision of future usefulness;"[84] but his personal preference for the laboratory was undiminished.

This preference carried the hazard that some unguarded remark to a newspaper reporter could be distorted by him into a fanciful solution of one of the world's big problems. For instance, in 1904 Theobald Smith published a paper on the osmotic fragility of the red blood cells of horses, which he embellished in 1906 with the assistance of H.R. Brown, a Rockefeller Institute Research Fellow. The osmotic fragility of red cells was shown to be remarkably constant for the individual horse, and although the fragility increased in horses bled repeatedly for diphtheria antitoxin, these change were less than the inherent difference between horses.[85] This work found exaggerated mention in the *New York Tribune* and other newspapers. A paragraph in the *Tribune,* headlined "FINDS HEREDITY'S LAW," asserted that Theobald Smith "says he has made an important discovery which seems likely to solve the secret of heredity . . . while experimenting with the blood of horses in making serum."[86] And eighteen months later, the *Chicago Inter-Ocean* of March 27, 1907 suggested that "the personal equation in blood corpuscles" would make it feasible to identify an individual by microscopic examination of his blood corpuscles. However the blame for such a fiasco should be apportioned; Theobald Smith's contemporary ventures into more speculative, philosophic aspects of his field marked a successful departure from his customary sparse style.

In the previous month, September 1904, Smith gave a lecture, entitled "Some Problems in the Life History of Pathogenic Microorganisms" to the Section on Bacteriology of the International Congress of Arts and Science at the Universal Exposition held at St. Louis. This Universal Exposition celebrated the centenary of the purchase of Louisiana in 1804 from France, and was commonly referred to as the Louisiana Purchase Exposition. Theobald Smith had been invited by a vice-president of the Congress, Hugo Münsterberg, Professor of Philosophy at Harvard from 1892 to 1916, to become a member of the Congress and to participate in the proceedings. Celli (Rome) and Ross (Liverpool) were invited to address the Section of Preventive Medicine. Smith spent much time on his speech. His day-cards indicate that for at least three weeks he devoted from one to two hours almost daily to preparation of the address. He received an honorarium of $150, and a year later the President of the Exposition sent him a Commemorative Diploma and a Medal.

In his lecture, Smith bolstered, with bacteriological, immunological, and epidemiological data, the following two hypotheses. First, that bacterial parasitisms tended to evolve slowly through the ages toward states in which the hosts ultimately ceased to manifest infection. Invading microorganisms would act defensively, seeking chances to multiply and escape to other hosts. The less adapted parasites provoked the more acute diseases. In grave epidemics, involving very susceptible hosts and virulent bacteria, both host and parasite might perish through mutual destruction. Secondly, that the process of mutual adaptation between microorganism and host could be jeopardized, interrupted, and even reversed by interferences with "natural law" attributable to civilization.

> The social and industrial development of the human race is continually leading to disturbances of equilibrium in nature, one of whose direct or indirect manifestations is augmentation of disease . . . It is the true function of medical science to discover and put into effect those compensatory movements which will counterbalance the temporary ill-effects of what, for want of a more illuminating term, we call human progress.

The paper appeared in *Science* by invitation, as well as in another American journal, and in excerpted form in a German periodical.[87]

November 1904 may be cited as a very busy month, socially and scientifically, in Theobald's life. Gage came from Ithaca to carry out some research on leucocytes, which commanded Smith's attention at the Bussey for several weeks. The Pneumonia Committee met in New York City and Smith dined with Welch and Osler afterwards at the University Club. He and Lilian were invited by President Eliot to a luncheon honoring Charles Darwin's son William. Near the end of November, he gave a paper on "Medical Research: Its Place in the University Medical School" to the Harvard Medical Alumni Association of New York. "The aims of research are not culture, not miscellaneous information, not a mood of leisure meditation upon the origin of things, but mainly utility and service to mankind . . . We describe carefully and minutely, not for the sake of the picture and its details, but chiefly to be able to recognize the change." But, quoting Claude Bernard: "He who does not know what he is looking for will not lay hold of what he has found when he gets it." Personnel should be selected with great care, especially since the costs of medical research were mounting.

There is danger just now that some of the flotsam and jetsam caught in an eddy or else afraid of the current of practical life may seek the quiet of the laboratory because of some imagined taste or capacity which fails to materialize later on. It is far better not to have any research worker than poor ones.

The medical school's duties were "to train practical men, physicians and health officers, and to encourage the few who incline to research." He pleaded for the development of preventive medicine and sanitary science. Efforts should be encouraged "to evade or mitigate the penalty incidental to advancing civilization" through more preventive medicine, which "attempts to arrest disease before its momentum has carried it beyond the means of help. It is the truly modern as contrasted with the medieval point of view."[88]

In May, 1905, Smith spoke on "Research into the Causes and Antecedents of Disease. Its Importance to Society," to the American Social Science Association. The more links in the chain of causality identified for any given disease, the greater the likelihood of discovering a removable or breakable link, thus making possible the prevention or abortion of that disease. The minute analysis of disease-promoting factors demanded careful observation and animal experimentation. Many antivivisectionists were well-intentioned but were either uninformed or badly misinformed. "Over-development of physique, which is often taken for health, is at present among certain classes something of a fetish which dominates and to a certain extent causes atrophy of more important faculties." Again, the noise, dirt and smoke that vitiated city air were products of social evolution, and could be mitigated, but not eradicated. If we insisted upon urban conveniences and luxuries, we must be content with less pure air than our forefathers enjoyed. The overriding truism was that "for society to control causes of disease is infinitely less burdensome than to palliate effects."[89]

Theobald Smith was the sole or senior author of more than 300 publications. Most of them recorded the unchallenged findings of his scrupulously planned experiments. This body of work established his reputation as the leading North American microbiologist of that era. On suitable occasions he could be eloquently philosophical, yet strictly rational, about problems as diverse as the evolution of parasitism, and the selection and training of medical research workers. Three such thought-provoking addresses within a year (he subsequently gave several isolated lectures of this type) naturally brought his qualifications to the attention of the Harvard Medical School authorities, who were wrestling with the question of how best to introduce public health and preventive medicine into the curriculum. Smith thus became a favored candidate for the supervision of that field. But he, preferring the prophetic to the messianic role, withdrew his candidacy in advance.

14

HARVARD MEDICAL CENTER
THEOBALD SMITH'S HARVARD
CONNECTION

The transformation of the Harvard Medical School from a proprietary agency, whose connection with the University was only nominal, into an institution under the university's administrative control, and providing scientific medical education of superior quality, was due mainly to the efforts of Charles W. Eliot, the long-term president (1869–1909) of Harvard college.[1] President Eliot's greatness derived from a liberal outlook on the world at large, coupled with his ability to discern whose individual talents and aspirations could best fit Harvard's immediate or long-term needs. When he reached his seventieth birthday on March 20, 1904, the Faculty of Medicine gave him a silver tankard to mark the occasion. On the initiative of President Theodore Roosevelt, H.P. Walcott, and four other prominent members of the Harvard corporation, all faculties presented a formal address. Theobald Smith was among the Harvard alumni who signed it.[2]

In a surprisingly short period, the Faculty of Medicine accepted Eliot's educational doctrines, adopted the elective system previously introduced at Harvard College, and came under the University's administrative control. At Eliot's insistence, would-be medical students lacking a college degree were required after 1877 to pass an entrance examination, and by 1900 a bachelor's degree became mandatory. Instruction in chemistry, physiology and pathology was expanded and first-hand experimentation introduced. Clinical section teaching was replaced by the clerkship, in which a student was involved in every aspect of his patient's care.

A new medical school building had been erected on Boylston Street in 1883 with $200,000 raised almost entirely from professional and business sources in Boston, in a campaign led by two young faculty members, the surgeon J.C. Warren, whose great-grandfather had been among Harvard's first medical professors, and the physiologist H.P. Bowditch.[3] By the mid-1890's, the inadequacies of this building were vividly apparent. Existing departments could not expand, and there was no room for a new department such as Smith's. As adjacent land was not available for additional construction, planning for a larger medical school began in 1899. There was general agreement that this medical center should comprise several substantial buildings, and that the site chosen ought to accommodate a fully equipped general hospital, as well as other hospitals or acceptable paramedical institutions that might want an adjacent location.

An official building committee, of which Theobald Smith was a member from the outset, met frequently to evaluate and promulgate the changing image of Harvard's Medical School. This would be an institution for disseminating and extending professional knowledge; for training investigators as well as practitioners; for multiplying and reaping the benefits of medical research. "We want to have a school," wrote President Eliot, "which is going not only to train men learned and skilful in what is known and applied, but expectant of progress and desirous to contribute to new discovery."

The medical faculty, again led by the redoubtable Warren and Bowditch, launched their second fund-raising drive in March 1901, this time for three million dollars.[4] The previous drive's total had been reached through modest contributions from many Bostonians. The second drive raised during its first year nearly $600,000 from the Boston community, including $100,000 from James Stillman of the First National Bank, as well as $50,000 from Henry Higginson, a Fellow of the Harvard Corporation, who from the outset showed a lively interest in Theobald Smith's welfare and accomplishments.

But the huge sum now envisaged required large donations from a few carefully selected philanthropists. These people were approached individually. In June, J. Pierpont Morgan, fresh from his triumphant organization of the United States Steel Corporation, donated $1,135,000 for construction of three of the proposed medical school buildings, in memory of his father, a one-time resident of Boston.[5] John D. Rockefeller responded only after his attorney, Starr J. Murphy, had made an exhaustive appraisal of the project and Welch had reassured him that expansion of the Harvard Medical School would help rather than interfere with the usefulness of the Rockefeller Institute for Medical Research.[6] In February 1902, the senior Rockefeller offered Harvard University $1,000,000 with the proviso that by the following Commencement an additional $765,000 for the new Medical School should be raised from other contributors.[7] The momentum that had been achieved was epitomized by J.C. Warren, who, in a letter to George F. Fabyan, wrote, "I believe now is the time to strike with horse, foot and artillery and make this great school a reality."[8]

The stipulation was met. Donations included $250,000 from Mrs. Arabella Huntington, widow of Collis P. Huntington, the Central Pacific railroad baron. The following excerpt from J.C. Warren's letter to George Fabyan illustrates the unabashed approach made to the wealthy:

> I suppose you have seen in the papers that Mr. Rockefeller has matched Mr. Morgan's gift to the Medical School. We are expected to raise in the neighbourhood of half a million more to be able to avail ourselves of this money. I have already $167,000 subscribed. Fred Shattuck gave $50,000 this morning for certain professorships as endowment . . . I shall be glad to call on you at any time with Dr. Bowditch if you still contemplate to do what you alluded to last summer.

Fabyan did not react immediately, but early in March 1903, he added $25,000 to the George Fabyan Fund. In June 1906, he gave a further $75,000.

Henry Higginson formed a syndicate of some twenty friends of Harvard. They bought a twenty-six-acre estate near Longwood Avenue for the future Harvard Medical Center. About ten acres were set aside for a School comprising five separate but connected buildings, for which the Boston architectural firm of Shepley, Rutan and Coolidge prepared plans. These plans were reviewed by Drs. Warren and Bowditch and then by the department heads. Finally the working drawings were scrutinized by President Eliot, and by Drs. H.P. Walcott and A.T. Cabot representing the Harvard Corporation.

The Longwood Avenue Medical Center, completed in 1906, comprised an imposing high-terraced Administration Building, designated on the architect's plans as "A," flanked symmetrically by four matching-fronted laboratory buildings, "B" to "E," two on each side, linked by a lower-level terrace and enclosed corridors. All five structures were constructed of Vermont marble, in simple classic Greek style. This impressive grouping of white marble structures thus enclosed a spacious quadrangle 215 by 415 feet, with the Administration Building on slightly higher ground in the center of the south end of the quadrangle. The connecting corridor passed through the basement of Building A, but was on the ground floor level elsewhere. A Power House, whose tall chimney dominated the landscape about 800 feet away, supplied heat, electric light and power, ventilation, refrigeration, steam, vacuum and compressed air to the whole complex.

Building A housed the administrative staff. It also provided faculty and student common rooms and a large amphitheater. Above the second floor were arranged the well-lit exhibits of the Warren Museum, some of them historically famous and dating back to the Medical School's early days. The basement contained three X-ray machines, rooms for instruction in bandaging, storage space, and a dark-room. Each laboratory building housed two or more related departments, distributed wherever possible in separate wings extending to the rear. The wings were connected by a central portion fronting on the courtyard, comprising the lecture theater, departmental libraries, and other shared services. To allow for libraries and lecture theaters, these central portions were generally two floors' height above the ground level. The wings often included mezzanines, which permitted more rooms to be set aside for individual research.

The dimensions of teaching laboratories for twenty-four students were set at 23 × 30 feet, representing three "window units" based on a 10-foot module. Most professors had two window-unit laboratories, while other research workers rated the one window-unit size. Building B accommodated the departments of Anatomy and Histology, with space allocated to Operative Surgery and the undeveloped department of Comparative Anatomy. Building C was for Physiology and Physiological Chemistry. Building D was assigned to Bacteriology and Pathology, with quarters for Surgical Pathology and Photography. Animals for these two departments were kept in a wood and plaster shed, also classic in style, to the rear of Building D.

Theobald Smith's department was in Building E, known as the Hygiene and Pharmacology Building. Its southerly wing accommodated the Department of Pharmacology and Therapeutics, with space assigned to Surgical Research on the top floor. The northerly wing was divided vertically between the Departments of Hygiene and of Comparative Pathology. Theobald Smith's department was distributed on all four floors of the rear portion of this wing. Plans to house the department in an entire wing had been rejected. By inserting a mezzanine between his two top floors, Smith provided quarters for small laboratory animals and also an operating room. The allocation of space to his department presented difficulties which the final arrangement did not complete resolve. Building E had to house a very heterogeneous group of departments.

The main architectural features of the new Medical School buildings on Longwood Avenue were summarized, and the entire group of five structures well illustrated, in a commemorative volume, *The Harvard Medical School 1782–1906*, compiled and distributed by the Faculty of the Harvard Medical School.[9] Further details are given in an article (subsequently reprinted) in a contemporary issue of the *Harvard Graduates' Magazine*.[10]

Before the erection of this imposing cluster of buildings began, a leading professional journal had pointed out that the tasks of fostering investigators, developing teachers and training technicians "in the completest way" would prove far more difficult than the construction and equipment of "any number of buildings and laboratories."[11] About seven years had elapsed since Theobald Smith had joined the Harvard staff; and two since the Medical Faculty had approved of H.P. Bowditch's resolution that the Corporation should secure sufficient land to accommodate "all Departments of the Medical School, the Veterinary School, the Dental School, the Graduate School of Comparative Medicine, and also for a Hospital to be connected with the Medical School." Already it was evident that this resolution could not be fulfilled. The Veterinary School had been abolished, and the Graduate School of Comparative Medicine (a dream project of President Eliot) had vanished, largely because Theobald Smith did not wish to be involved in improvement of the former or in development of the latter. Soon after Bowditch's resolution was passed, the Dental School had merged with the Medical School to form the Faculty of Medicine. The lack of a hospital that would entrust the nomination of its chief physicians and surgeons to the University Corporation continued to handicap the Harvard Medical School for several years after the preclinical buildings were completed in 1906. However, a Dental Hospital was erected on Longwood Avenue in 1909; and three years later, at long last, the Peter Bent Brigham Hospital was completed as an affiliated organization on Harvard Medical Center land.

The professorial staff had access to their freshly finished quarters in May 1906. Near the end of that month, Theobald Smith visited his "new lab." On June 7, an Open House was staged for physicians and their families and he joined the "multitude" for afternoon tea on the "esplanade."[12] Between then and the end of September, when the new buildings were officially dedicated, was a period of domestic and workaday unsettlement. On June 6, eleven-year-old Philip had an emergency appendectomy, and for several days was visited in hospital each morning by his father, who nevertheless managed to produce a "Demonstration of blood hemolysis in salt sol & diluted serum before section of A.M.A.,"[13] and also to attend the regular meeting of the Rockefeller Institute directors in New York on the 9th. On June 12, he accepted a dinner invitation from Dr. F.C. Shattuck in honor of Victor C. Vaughan, Dean of Medicine at the University of Michigan, who then delivered the Shattuck Lecture. Smith had met Vaughan two years previously, when returning from Chicago from testifying in support of Prof. E.O. Jordan in a court battle over the Chicago Drainage Canal. It was a noteworthy occasion, duly recorded in Theobald's diary: "Meet Dr. & Mrs. Vaughan on train and I remain their guest during day. Visit Medical School. Dinner at Vaughan's in evening to which faculty invited."[14]

On the 22nd, Theobald went to his daughters' school for Class Day Exercises. Despite the succession of guests at home, including Prof. Gage and his sister (Dr. Isobel Day) and Prof. E.O. Jordan from Chicago,[15] he still found time to investigate protozoan turkey disease and to continue his experiments on hemolysis.

The harassed life continued into July. "Working on disease of turkeys, blood-corp-resistance tests, guinea-pig resistance to diphtheria toxin, tubercle cults., ordering apparatus, arr. my pamphlets to go into new med. buildings, planning changes in new lab. Substituting for assistants on vacation."[16] He also began "to teach Dorothea chemistry," and examined a candidate for the post of City Physician. In August, the daughters were invited for two weeks to Seal Harbor by the Herters. Theobald spent part of August and September in Montana, as expert witness for the Anaconda Copper Mining Company. He returned on September 19, in time to attend the official opening of the Harvard Medical Center.

Dedicatory Exercises were held on September 25, 1906, on site at Longwood Avenue. Theobald recorded the event with the terse notation, "Dedication of new buildings, wear gown & sit on terrace among faculty."[17] Outstanding among the speeches of the day was the address by Dr. Frederick C. Shattuck, Professor of Clinical Medicine. "These ample, beautiful buildings" would be mere shells unless endowed financially for their maintenance, and "for the support of workers therein whose discoveries . . . by an unwritten but immutable law may not be patented." They represented only a subordinate portion of the "necessary means for furthering progressive medicine . . . Where are the hospitals? what relation do they bear to the Medical School?" Shattuck deplored the separateness of hospital and medical school development, which often remained a bar to progress. "The patients under the charge of a teacher of medicine, surrounded by sharp-eyed and critical young men, are sure to receive more careful study than patients not so guarded."

> In the laboratories about us healthy animals are the subjects of experiments made . . . for the purpose of ascertaining what disease is, in order the better to prevent and cure it. A wise benefactor has provided a foundation for Comparative Pathology . . . Whatever the source of a hopeful suggestion for relief or cure, the final test and proof lie in the hands of the clinician, who deals with human beings, allied to but not identical with other animals . . . [He] should be as animated by the scientific spirit as his brother of the laboratory . . . The two are interdependent.[18]

(As previously mentioned, Shattuck's plea was answered favorably in 1912.)

The Dedicatory Exercises continued next day in the Sanders Theater in Cambridge. President Eliot spoke on "The Future of Medicine." Medicine must become more preventive. Curricular changes would include improvements in "popular exposition concerning water supplies, foods, drinks, drugs, the parasitic causes or consequences of disease in men, plants, and animals," and modes of disease communication. Knowledge of man's relationships to the animal and plant kingdoms could be broadened at Harvard, with its separate chairs in comparative Anatomy, Physiology and Pathology. Exposure to psychology and religion was liberalizing and enlightening. A useful naturalistic outlook might result. The future physician should have "mastered the elements of biology, chemistry and physics before he enters a medical school." Future medical discoveries might depend largely on cooperative approaches to a problem by specialists in different sciences, medical and non-medical or by individuals with a working knowledge of several sciences.[19]

William H. Welch's felicitous address showed him at his best—scholarly, timely, and prophetic. He mentioned Harvard Medical School's fine record, including "medicine's supreme gift to suffering humanity of surgical anaesthesia." The union with Harvard University assured stability and growth. "The remarkable growth of laboratories for the cultivation of the various medical sciences" initiated by Liebig and Virchow were cause and result of the recent rapid progress of medicine. "Especially urgent is full recognition of the unity and cooperation of the clinic and the laboratory." The exploration of fields opened by Pasteur and Koch had provided "the power to restrain and in some instances to exterminate such diseases as cholera, plague, yellow fever, malaria, typhoid fever, tuberculosis and other infections." These "noble" buildings were obviously adaptable to research as well as to educational uses. He applauded "this dual function of imparting and of advancing knowledge." The capital invested in buildings, equipment, and operating expenses would yield rich returns. Yet creative men with a talent for research counted "more than stately edifices and all the pride and pomp of outward life . . . Search for them far and wide . . . and when found cherish them as a possession beyond all price . . . Rare indeed are the thinkers, born with the genius for discovery, and with the gift of the scientific imagination to interpret . . . the phenomena of nature."[20]

Theobald Smith attended all official functions on the two ceremonial days. Woodland Hill meanwhile was astir with visitors. On the 23rd (Sunday), the Noyes family brought with them H.H. Donaldson, recently appointed Professor of Neurology at the Wistar Institute in Philadelphia. Smith and Donaldson first met in 1882, almost a quarter-century before, in Newell Martin's biology laboratory at Johns Hopkins University. Simon Flexner arrived as an overnight guest on the 26th, after the exercises in Sanders Theater. The following Sunday, the "Herters came out (5 strong) & stayed for lunch. All have a good time."[21]

Since the headquarters of the Department of Comparative Pathology were to be in Building E at the Medical Center, Theobald Smith resolved to commute each day between the Forest Hills Station at Jamaica Plain and Longwood Avenue. This took about two hours daily from door to door. By the end of September, the transfer of essential equipment from the Bussey Laboratory to the Center was completed. He also deposited there "about 3000 pamphlets and over 50 large reprints."

Smith's relations with the Faculty of Medicine now grew closer. He attended faculty meetings and served faithfully on the Advanced Education and Boylson Prize committees; championed animal research in opposition to the still rampant antivivisectionists; and vigorously advocated teaching preventive medicine and sanitary science in medical schools. He viewed preliminary exposure to the physical sciences as essential to the medical student. "I have the impression that we are not getting the best students," he wrote to Gage, "and with the silly requirement of the bachelor's degree without any restrictions as to what the degree stands for, we are not satisfied."[22] But he retained his personal preference for a broad non-professional education, such as Cornell had provided. In 1908, the Secretary of Harvard's Faculty of Arts and Sciences notified Smith that he had been appointed Chairman of the Division of Medical Sciences.[23] The Division represented a group of Medical School courses open under certain conditions to members of the Graduate School of Arts and Sciences.

At the start of the twentieth century, faculty members of the Harvard Medical School had an opportunity to meet many distinguished medical scientists from abroad. The characteristic pilgrimage of earlier decades from North America to Europe was beginning to reverse. Pioneers who had been observed initially in their home setting might now cross the ocean westward to expound concepts and display techniques. The Herter Lectures facilitated this trend. Ehrlich's visit in 1904 to New York, Baltimore and Boston had cemented the mutual admiration between himself and Theobald Smith and provided them both with much scientific satisfaction. The second series of Herter Lectures at Baltimore had been given in 1905 by the experimental pharmacologist Hans Meyer, with whom Herter had studied briefly in 1903. Welch invited Sir Almroth Wright to give the 1906 lectures, which were entitled "The Therapeutic Inoculation of Bacterial Vaccines and Its Application in Connection with the Treatment of Bacterial Disease."

Almroth Wright (1861–1947) had just been knighted for his work on antityphoid vaccination in the British Army. Son of an Irish clergyman and a Swedish mother, Wright was an iconoclast who lived unpeacefully the dictum of Emerson—"God offers to every mind its choice between Truth and Repose." As some military authorities disputed the efficacy of his heat-killed vaccine, in 1902 Wright resigned his Professorship at the Army Medical School, Netley, to become Pathologist and Bacteriologist at St. Mary's Hospital, Paddington. Stimulated by his friends Ehrlich and Metchnikoff, helped by W.B. Leishman and S.R. Douglas, and provoked by George Bernard Shaw, a fellow-Irishman, Almroth Wright expanded, propounded and defended the doctrine of vaccine therapy with eloquence, ingenuity and tenacity. "The physician of the future," he proclaimed, "will be an immunisator."

Wright and his followers contended that the phagocytic power of the polymorphonuclear leucocytes of the blood depended upon a specific heat-labile entity in the serum, which Wright named "opsonin" (from the Greek "opsono," *I prepare food for, I make tasty*). The opsonic content of the patient's blood, and his phagocytic capacity for a particular bacterium, could be increased by injections of heat-killed vaccine of that species. The *opsonic index* was the ratio between the number of specific microorganisms ingested by 100 washed polymorphs mixed with the patient's serum and the number ingested in the presence of normal serum.[24]

Before going to Baltimore, Wright proposed to "spend a week or two first in the Canadian woods with one of the best of my pupils, Ross, a son of the late Prime Minister of Ontario."[25] While there, Wright delivered a well-received lecture on "The Opsonic Theory"[26] to the medical students of the University of Toronto. More skeptical audiences in Baltimore, New York and Boston, including the percipient Welch, responded with mixed feelings: "The impression he made here was that of a strong character with traits of real genius, but with eccentricities and streaks of unsoundness rather baffling to some of the young men who are accustomed to more uniform excellence in a great leader."[27] Theobald Smith first met Wright in New York on October 13. After an all-day meeting of the Rockefeller Institute directors, followed by dinner at Holt's residence, he attended a reception held by the Flexners for Wright and his assistant, G. W. Ross. Flexner engaged Ross to give a five-week course of lectures and demonstrations on opsonins and vaccine therapy at the Rockefeller Institute, which was not received enthusiastically by registrants.

Almroth Wright came to Boston on October 17 and 18. Smith surrendered the 17th to the visitor. They lunched at the St. Botolph's Club with Faculty of Medicine representatives. In the evening Wright lectured on opsonins, and next day demonstrated his methods at the Harvard Medical School. Although Smith had heeded opsonin crusaders—in January 1906, for example, he recorded "Dr. N.B. Potter of New York visits laboratory in heavy snow storm conferring about opsonins in tuberculosis"[28]—he did not accept the importance of opsonin in host defense against tuberculosis. Six months before Wright's New York lecture, Smith addressed the Harvey Society on "The Parasitism of the Tubercle Bacillus and its Bearing on Infection and Immunity." After alluding respectfully to "the theory of opsonins which Wright had developed with so much skill and industry since 1902," he denied that blood leucocytes played any special part in the body's defenses against tuberculosis. The tissue reaction to the tubercle bacillus did not favor this role.[29]

During his American tour Almroth Wright made no reference to Theobald Smith's pioneer work of twenty years before on the specific immunization of pigeons by a heat-killed vaccine of hog cholera bacilli. Smith had looked forward to meeting this celebrated contemporary, two years his junior. But apart from their common desire to "attract to the work of research a proportion of the best ability in every country,"[30] and their mutual friendship with Paul Ehrlich, the two men differed widely in personality, approach, and technical methods. Wright's comments on scientific matters were usually provocative, whereas Smith became more cautious in speech and print as he grew older. He deplored Wright's failure to champion *prevention* over *cure*. Wright abhorred statistical considerations and interpreted clinical responses subjectively, while Smith enjoyed mathematical conundrums and viewed his own findings skeptically, repeating experiments if results were equivocal. The forceful personality and dialectical combativeness that ensured Wright both devoted disciples and fanatical detractors contrasted with the general modesty and self-effacing, almost reclusive habits of Smith.

For nearly four years, Smith ruminated over Wright's doctrines before appraising them in an address to the Massachusetts Medical Society, entitled "What is the Experimental Basis for Vaccine Therapy?"[31] Suppression of the great plagues of animal life by vaccination "furnished the experimental basis for human preventive inoculation," Theobald told his physician audience, observing that "Experimental medicine has very little to offer . . . in deciding upon the efficacy or harmfulness of vaccination during disease."

> Unfortunately the most effective methods devised to protect animals cannot be safely used on the human subject, because they . . . might, occasionally jeopardize life. Our methods must be so toned down as to fit the weakest and most susceptible. In animal life this is not necessary, for it is desirable that the weakest be eliminated and that it shall not propagate its kind.

Smith readily distinguished between the usefulness of vaccines in averting infection, at least temporarily, about which "there is no longer any reasonable doubt," and their applicability in an already existing infection. "The presence of virulent living bacteria makes it seem absurd to add dead ones. Why are not the former stimulus enough?"[32] His conclusions remained substantially unaltered three years later when he attempted to interpret "Present-Day Uses of Vaccine" for the Philadelphia Pathological Society;[33] and likewise in 1921, when he gave the Second Pasteur Lecture at Chicago, on "Theories of Susceptibility and Resistance in Relation to Methods of Artificial Immunization."[34] Eventually Wright himself closed that chapter in 1941, at eighty years of age, by an address to the Royal Society of Medicine "On the Need for Abandoning Much in Immunology that has been Regarded as Assured."[35] The content, like the title, showed the peculiar blend of forthrightness and circumlocution that characterized most of Almroth Wright's utterances and published works.

Theobald Smith did not seek, and often spurned, any opportunity for enlarging his academic responsibilities. He effected no important change without having consulted President Eliot, who held him in highest regard and seldom disagreed with him on important issues. With the tacit consent of Eliot, Walcott and Fabyan, he limited his main activities to the duties of State pathologist, and to laboratory research on microbiological problems which he chose himself. The lecture courses and demonstrations which he gave to medical students were too brief in duration, or too disdainfully delivered, to be allowed (with a few exceptions) an important "Harvard Connection." The scope and thoroughness of his researches, and the bond between the president and the Fabyan professor, comprised the main "connection."

Eliot enjoyed offering detailed budgetary advice. He suggested to Theobald Smith that he consider spending most of an accumulated surplus of around $3,000 in the Fabyan Fund partly on glassware and partly on the training of two laboratory helpers who would be needed in the new quarters. Early in November 1904, Smith reported the purchase of $200-$300 worth of apparatus and glassware, and the hiring of a woman laboratory servant "who can keep accounts, make card catalogues and who is learning to make culture medica, cut and stain histologic sections. She receives $25 per month, with a promise of $30 after 3 or more months." A young person who could manage rougher work was still needed. The costs of operating the Bussey laboratory had risen despite the removal of antitoxin production, because now Theobald could use only occasionally the services of any of the seven persons employed by the State Board of Health.[36]

Both Eliot and Cabot had dropped broad hints that Smith should delegate more of the daily operation of the State laboratories. President Eliot had to accept at face value Smith's reasons for spending so much of the working day at Jamaica Plain. After all, it was he who had planted Smith in the Bussey Institution and offered him the Woodland Hill residence. Part-time appointees usually find it difficult to divide fairly their loyalty and effort. Theobald Smith found this especially hard to do because Harvard University (through presidential initiative based on Eliot's friendship with Walcott) so often smoothed the path of the Massachusetts State Board of Health. On the whole, Smith benefited from this policy; but he never exploited it, and in some ways may have been its victim.

The imbalance began when Harvard supplied at nominal rent, through the Bussey Institution, the basic laboratory and stabling facilities for diphtheria antitoxin production. The fractious Dean of that Institution, F.H. Storer, resented the intrusion and was very uncooperative with the president and his protege, although he had been Eliot's former colleague in chemistry. Within a year or two of Smith's arrival, Eliot arranged his appointment to a new chair of comparative pathology, endowed by George F. Fabyan. Eliot also offered Smith and his family the tenancy, at low rental, of the spacious living quarters and grounds of the Bussey Mansion (Woodland Hill). In vain President Eliot then urged Theobald Smith to assume the deanship of the languishing Veterinary School. As that school was overstraining the University's resources, it was abolished in 1901, much to the personal disappointment of the horse-loving president.

Eliot profoundly admired Smith, and shared similar outlooks on sanitation, public health and preventive medicine. The former made repeated efforts to improve the working space within the Bussey Institution. When disaffection remained, he requested A.T. Cabot—one of Harvard's most distinguished Fellows—to look into Theobald Smith's laboratory necessities. In particular, Cabot was asked to assess the possibility of establishing, within the Bussey Institution, a satisfactory Laboratory of Comparative Pathology. Cabot seemed to find Smith's difficulties somewhat diffuse, involving deficiencies of assistance as well as of space and equipment. His chief recommendation, with Eliot's concurrence, was that Smith should delegate a substantial portion of the routine public health laboratory work, and thus secure more time for personal researches.

Meanwhile, Eliot and Walcott planned to provide Smith with a new laboratory for diphtheria antitoxin and vaccine virus production and research, to be constructed on Bussey land, according to Smith's design and under his supervision. He would first review the latest European developments in this field, the expenses of the trip to be covered by Fabyan, whose youngest son, Marshal, a medical undergraduate at Harvard, would go along. Before Theobald Smith had become accustomed to his new building, the handsome Harvard Medical School complex was dedicated, and he found himself and his department spread on all four floors of Building E. Since his department was henceforth to be headquartered in this building, Smith transferred there some workers and material, and a vast collection of pamphlets and reprints. It was understood that the department should maintain the Laboratory of Comparative Pathology in the Bussey Institution—a decision that of course provoked a further vigorous protest from Storer.

Theobald Smith was now expected to spend much of his time downtown in Building E, although he was apt to be still anchored at the Bussey. Besides, each journey between laboratories, or between Woodland Hill and Longwood Avenue, took nearly one hour. To Smith, these trips were relaxing and refreshing; they encouraged free play of the mind. Some of his colleagues, who likewise pre-

ferred suburban amenities and rural charms to city noise and pollution, understood and sympathized. Others, more envious, may have suspected that he took
advantage of a cushy job.

Eliot's admiration and encouragement of Smith's outstanding research abilities were shared by George Fabyan. In June 1906, shortly after the new laboratory quarters at Longwood Avenue were opened to the Medical Faculty, Fabyan
wrote as follows to the President and Fellows of Harvard College:

> In testimony of my interest in and satisfaction with the work thus far done by Pro-
> fessor Theobald Smith in the Department of Comparative Pathology, and with the
> desire that he and his successors may be enabled to work even more fruitfully in
> the future without overtaxing the resources of the University or of the Medical
> School, I have the pleasure of offering you the further sum of $75,000 to be added
> to the sums which I have already given.[37]

Any income (from the total principal of $200,000) in excess of $8,000 per annum was to be added yearly to the principal until it reached the sum of
$250,000. Fabyan hoped that this endowment, besides paying the salary of the
incumbent professor, would "furnish him with such material, apparatus and assistance . . . as may be required in prosecution of the work." The future designation of the fund should be the *George Fabyan Foundation for Comparative Pathology*.
At their next meeting two weeks later, the President and Fellows gratefully accepted the offer.

Shortly afterwards, when Theobald Smith received a copy of Fabyan's letter,
he promptly wrote Eliot a lengthy, meticulously detailed prospectus of "plans for
developing the new laboratory."[38] In addition to the woman and the boy who had
been trained in his laboratory, he proposed to employ a third laboratory helper,
"A mature man who will take charge of the experimental animals both at the
laboratory and at the Bussey Barn, repair apparatus, assist at autopsies, operations, etc. and learn to cut microscopic sections." There was such a man at the
antitoxin laboratory, receiving $55 monthly from the State Board of Health. "To
cover carfares," Smith proposed to offer him $60. Expensive apparatus, includ-
ing a Zeiss microscope, microtome, centrifuge, animal cages, and thermostats
(incubators) would be needed to put the laboratory into working condition. The
operating costs could not be estimated from the Bussey experience, for there his
researches had been on problems connected with public health and sanitation,
largely funded by the State. "In the new laboratory there will be more advanced
teaching of small classes, the cost of keeping animals will be greater, and there
will be more research." He was anxious to verify that the total amount available
from the Fabyan Foundation in 1906 for equipment and running expenses would
be about $3,500, besides an unused surplus of some $3,000.

He also sought permission to spend about $100 in making repairs and installing more windows in the upper barn at Woodland Hill. This barn would then be suitable for rabbit breeding pens. He wished to study the transmission of acquired immunity to disease in rabbits, for which project he had a $500 Rockefeller Institute grant. In the preceding two years, his guinea-pig experiments had shown that the progeny of female guinea-pigs treated once with diphtheria toxin in their youth possessed a life-long increased resistance to this toxin, which was not present in the next generation, unless their mothers were inoculated in turn.

He emphatically stated that he could carry no more teaching load without an assistant. The students' greatest need were courses intermediate between elementary and "the more or less unguided work of the beginning investigator." Such courses were "very trying, because the work of preparation falls wholly upon the teacher." He wanted to set up a small library for the use of advanced workers, to which he would contribute several volumes of two German journals. "Probably $100 annually will pay for the necessary journals and books to aid the workers in tracing the literature before consulting large libraries. To put the library into shape, bind the volumes on hand, supply the table and chairs, another $100 will be needed this year."

Finally, "Mr. Fabyan has repeatedly told me that he wished me to furnish properly the little study I have reserved. It is a room 10 feet wide. I shall try to please him without being extravagant. I have hinted several times that I should prefer apparatus and supplies to furniture, but his mind was made up on that point." Eliot consented to every proposal. "All the arrangements you propose in your letter of July 8 seem to me judicious and frugal and I hereby authorize you to carry them out as soon as you conveniently can." He suggested slightly higher wage scales for the three permanent helpers. Intermediate courses were not in question for the coming year.[39]

In November 1906, Smith sought an opportunity within the next two or three months to discuss his future work with the president: "We have come to the parting of the ways in some respects. It will be necessary to decide whether my work shall be chiefly advanced teaching or research. I shall endeavor to think the subject out as clearly as possible before consulting you."[40] Eliot quickly reassured Smith, telling him, "I shall be glad to talk over with you . . . the future of your work."[41] He visualized that Smith should supervise some advanced teaching, but assign the greater part of his time to research, "the teaching to be given chiefly to assistants in your researches." Smith wanted to retain the Laboratory of Comparative Pathology in the Bussey Building because there "work of an objectionable or perhaps dangerous character can be done not far from the living animals." He also proposed to retain the old greenhouse attached to the main building, now used for small animals.[42] Eliot agreed and undertook to notify Dean Storer.

The Bussey Institute was in the meantime undergoing major changes. In March 1907, the governing authorities decided to transform it "from an undergraduate school of agriculture into an institution for advanced instruction and research in the scientific problems that relate and contribute to practical agriculture and horticulture." It thus became one of the component parts of the Graduate School of Applied Science, whose Dean was W.C. Sabine, a physicist. In the reorganization, Dr. Carroll Dunham tried to play a part. His credentials, and the extent to which his recommendations were incorporated in the final plan, are unclear. Soon after Dunham began looking into Bussey affairs, Storer got wind of his involvement and expressed disdain in a letter to President Eliot: "You do not mention . . . that C. Dunham first graduated from a Homeopathic Medical College. I believe his ideas about helping the Bussey are wild."[43]

Dunham and Smith were in contact. In October 1905, following a directors' meeting of the Rockefeller Institute in New York, Theobald Smith went northward along the Hudson "to Irvington, where I visit Dr. Carroll Dunham for sev. hours to discuss the Bussey Institution." A few days later he recorded, "writing a short paper on a proposed change in the Bussey Institute to Dr. Dunham."[44] On June 15 1906, Smith's diary noted, "Dr. Carroll Dunham & wife call on us." Later, a day card announced that two evening hours had been devoted to "Dr. Dunham's Bussey reorg. plan."[45]

The Board of Overseers (who share with the Corporation the governance of Harvard University) had appointed a committee to investigate Bussey affairs. Storer assumed that this committee would be influenced by Dunham's proposals. He wrote to Eliot "about an unpleasant bit of intrigue bearing on the C. Dunham proposition—whatever that may be . . . I feel that someone on that Committee should know what kind of underhand wire-pulling is 'in action' to influence the Committee."[46] On February 15, 1907, Eliot notified Storer that the Committee on Visitations had reported adversely on his administration of the Bussey Institution, so that his resignation as Dean would be acceptable. Storer thought he had been dismissed and intemperately rejected his pension rights, adding "You will naturally inform me in due course to whom I shall turn over . . . all matters relating to students who are now with us."[47] On learning that he was not dismissed from his professorial appointment, he asserted:

> I *know* that . . . up to the present time, I have been doing good service in the work of admitting and encouraging students . . . and in putting the school on a firm basis. I am confident that—because of experience—I am better fitted to perform these duties now than I ever was before. I presume the Committee men knew nothing of my services in these particulars.[48]

Storer offered to assist a new Dean as "a mere professor" until he had familiarized himself with his duties. He expected to stay perhaps until the end of November, unless "something unforeseen should prompt an earlier departure." During the first six weeks of term, "a spare hand who knows the ropes can hardly fail to be helpful. Of course I should expect no remuneration for this service other than the satisfaction of knowing that the School had been left in good condition."[49]

The Institution began a more productive and harmonious phase of activity in 1908. The staff expanded and student enrollment increased. Theobald Smith retained his foothold there for a while, and his name, attached to the Department of *Comparative Pathology,* featured in the Bussey Institution's printed letterhead, along with the names of the transferred representatives of *Entomology* and of *Genetics (Animal* and *Plant).* Before 1914, he left the Bussey and confined his State Board of Health work to the Antitoxin Building. He kept aloof, except for occasional lunches in the graduate students' mess, maintained by the Bussey Institution during World War I.[50] In 1915, the Institution became designated officially the Graduate School of Applied Biology, with Professor W.M. Wheeler as its first Dean.[51]

The Institution was closed in 1938 until World War II, during and after which it was occupied by the Army Medical Corps. In 1949, the Massachusetts Department of Public Health Laboratory moved back into the Bussey Building. The State purchased the Bussey grounds and laboratory buildings from Harvard University, and in December 1963 conducted ground-breaking ceremonies on adjacent land for the new State Laboratory Institute. By the time the new building was ready for occupancy in 1974, the wrecker's ball had destroyed the old Bussey Institution.[52]

In 1906, Smith's patron, George Fabyan, began to fail in health. His blood count fell, and at least twice Theobald Smith cultured specimens. He paid many visits to the Fabyan household, alone or with Lilian. A ten-year history of the chair of comparative pathology, initiated early in 1906, was brought up to date for Fabyan to peruse before his death on January 18, 1907. Theobald Smith served as honorary pall-bearer at the Trinity church funeral. He and his wife kept in touch with the Fabyan family. The daughter married in June 1908, and the widow died in April 1909. The elder son, George, who prospered in Chicago with the stockyards, belatedly made some misguided protests at what he interpreted as Harvard's shabby treatment of Theobald Smith. The younger son, Marshal, became a physician, and served for many years as Smith's unsalaried second-in-command in the Department of Comparative Pathology.

15

THE ANACONDA SUIT
TRIPS TO ANACONDA AND BUTTE,
MONTANA (1906–1907)

In February 1905, some 100 farmers owning over 90% of the agricultural lands in the Deer Lodge Valley formed an Association to sue the Anaconda Copper Mining Company near Butte, Montana, and its amalgamated Washoe Copper Company for alleged damages to livestock, vegetable crops and forage plants caused by poisonous smelter emissions containing arsenic and sulfur dioxide. If damages estimated at about $1,175,000[1] were not settled within three months, the Association warned, it would seek a permanent injunction against operation of the Washoe smelter. As the amalgamated companies failed to comply, suit was filed on May 4, 1905.

The plaintiff was Fred J. Bliss, selected as the only non-resident property owner in the valley entitled to sue in the Federal District Court at Helena, Montana, where political pressures would be less formidable. In December 1905, the presiding judge, W.H. Hunt, delegated Master-in-Chancery O.T. Crane to hold hearings in the Federal Building in Butte. The "Bliss Suit" or the "Smoke Case," as the legal action came to be called in local newspapers, was of hitherto unparallel duration and litigious complexity. In all, over 25,000 pages of typed evidence (more than 6 million words) were recorded, involving the testimony of nearly 250 individual witnesses, including from twenty-five to thirty experts, and 737 exhibits were displayed.[2]

The defendants had several advantages. Their chief lawyer, Cornelius F. Kelley, was also the Company's Secretary. He was exceptionally alert, shrewd and urbane. In 1911, only a few years after these events, he was named Vice-President of the Company, by which time its annual production was 20 million pounds of copper, or 15 percent of the world's total supply. He became its President in 1918. Whereas the Company hired an impressive array of leading scientists, the Association could raise only $40,000 to support its present case. Besides, the Company had paid $330,000 in compensation for alleged smoke damage to the farmers' livestock in 1903 (some claims being false and exaggerated) and had rebuilt the Washoe smelter stack to a height of 1,100 feet above the valley floor, remodelled the flues, and constructed dust chambers to render the emissions harmless, at a cost of $750,000. Nevertheless, contended the plaintiff, the situation had not improved; cattle, horses and sheep were unthrifty, with high mortality rates; the yields of hay and other forage crops were poor; vegetables were puny; and the value of farm lands throughout the valley had depreciated. In rebuttal, the company claimed that the valley's "rich and fertile" soil was actually thin and in certain regions naturally too alkaline. The limited areas of rich natural soil, if properly tilled, remained fertile.

The economic factors were stressed powerfully. Anaconda, a city of some 10,000 to 12,000 people, depended entirely on the continued operation of the smelter. The 60,000 inhabitants of Butte, one-fifth the total population of the State of Montana, likewise prospered with its mines. If the smelter were closed, some 8,000 men would lose their livelihood, involving more than $7 million in annual wages. Indeed, such a shutdown would entail a world-wide copper shortage, with higher prices for many commodities. Replacement of the smelter would cost at least $10 million, and there was no suitable alternative site for it. The smelter's manager, E.P. Mathewson, contended that his company's precautions were "greater than those taken at any other smelting plant in the world."[3] These arguments and threats were uttered openly, and company agents warned the farmers that the court fight would continue until they lacked enough money to buy breakfast.[4] Finally, the defendant's chief counsel claimed "we have a perfect right to carry on a legitimate business, and if incidentally we should pollute the atmosphere nobody has the right to complain until specific damage gives him a cause of action."[5]

In January 1906, the plaintiff's experts introduced technical evidence bearing on chemical pollution.[6] A grayish powder with a high arsenic content could be shaken from hay and vegetation in the "smoke zone" to windward of the stack. Although subjacent soil samples showed a low retentivity for arsenic, and plant life apparently did not selectively absorb this element, the chemists contended that arsenical dust deposited on plants could be toxic and even lethal for animals ingesting it. Sheep fed daily doses of arsenic trioxide eventually died, and scrapings from the ulcerated nose of a horse showed a high concentration of arsenic.

In February 1906, Theobald Smith received a letter from Dr. D. McEachran, a retired professor of veterinary science at McGill University, on behalf of the Anaconda Copper Mining Company. "I write," McEachran explained, "to ask if you could undertake an investigation of some conditions occurring in horses, in connection with a lawsuit in which the Company are defendants."[7] The company had retained McEachran and others to make investigations "including chemical analyses of soil, water, plants, and stomachs and intestinal contents, tissues and fluids of animals, as well as pathological and clinical evidences of disease." Smith should state what he would consider a satisfactory retaining fee and per diem allowance in addition to expenses; a bacteriological laboratory and animal house were available, supervised by Dr. W.R. Wherry, who in 1902 had worked in Smith's laboratory.

A subsequent letter from Wherry assured Smith that the Company would pay liberally and "is perfectly fair in its attitude towards its scientific workers— simply asking for facts." Smith would have an enjoyable vacation with bracing climate and excellent accommodation. They were particularly concerned about "a peculiar sort of nasal ulceration, with fungoid out-growths, in the horse."[8] McEachran also wrote about the necrosis and perforation of the cartilaginous septum of the nose of horses, which the plaintiffs attributed to arsenic dust, though they had failed to reproduce it experimentally. He asserted that the climate, at 5,000 feet above sea level, was "most beneficial to an eastern man's health."[9] Smith tentatively accepted the invitation, subject of course to President Eliot's approval, but he was not "hardened to western winters or to much outdoor work in cold weather and I will have to exercise some care during my stay, at least at first."[10] President Eliot's approval for leave was secured early in March. Mathewson, the Company's manager, and Smith agreed on a fee of $50 per diem, in addition to all travelling and hotel expenses. He was invited to bring a competent technician, whose expenses and reasonable fees would be covered.[11] Smith hired one of Gage's assistants, a second-year medical student named Earle V. Sweet, who was able to cut tissue sections, for $100 monthly.

Theobald Smith visualized a single leave of at most three or four weeks duration; but actually, between March 1906 and March 1907, he took five trips to Montana for a total absence of four months. The dates of the trips were: 1. March 21 to April 21, 1906; 2. August 21 to September 19, 1906; 3. November 14 to December 3, 1906; 4. December 14 to January 2, 1907; 5. February 28 to March 19, 1907. He had not expected such a prolonged court case so closely involving him and other expert witnesses and subjecting him to summonses for repeated hearings. To the Harvard administration, he expressed his increasing reluctance to return to Montana and eventually rejected the Company's requests to do so.

Theobald Smith proved to be the defendent company's star witness. His experimental approach and dry testimony were no doubt important factors in determining the final judgement. Five long absences in the Far West, totalling some four months in duration, emphasized the dispensability of his lectures to the Second- and Third-year students at Harvard Medical School; but it is arguable that, in this century at least, Harvard University's fame has derived as much from its ability to furnish experts of Theobald Smith's caliber as on the success of its basic professional training programs.

The first two excursions to Anaconda were routed through Albany, so that he could visit his mother and the Murphy family. All trips went through Chicago, where he often spent a few hours with George Fabyan, elder son of George F. Fabyan. From there westward he took the Chicago, Minneapolis and St. Paul line as far as it went. From St. Paul the "North Coast Limited" of the Northern Pacific brought him to Butte. The city of Anaconda, entirely a company town, was about twenty-five miles further west, dominated by a 585-foot smelter. Visitors traveled to and fro by a Marcus Daly enterprise, the Butte, Anaconda and Pacific Railway. Marcus Daly's syndicate had owned the Anaconda mine from 1881 to 1899. His miners, sinking a shaft in 1882, hoping to replenish the gold and silver reserves, hit instead a rich vein of copper ore, a veritable copper mountain, which by 1891 made Anaconda the world's largest single source of copper.

Smith left Boston in the early morning of March 21, 1906 and arrived at Butte on Saturday evening the 24th, where he conferred at the Hotel Thornton with C.F. Kelley, director of the legal defense. Next morning he proceeded to the Hotel Montana at Anaconda. This Hotel, completed by Marcus Daly along grandiose lines in 1889, soon became known as the largest hotel between Minneapolis and the Pacific Coast.

At Anaconda, Theobald Smith soon learned to his surprise that D.E. Salmon, former chief of the Bureau of Animal Industry, was retained by the plaintiff to conduct investigations. Early in September 1905, Salmon had submitted his resignation from the B.A.I. He was said to have been pressured into resigning by President Theodore Roosevelt, who held that the B.A.I.'s inefficient inspections were largely responsible for recurrent scandals involving the Chicago stockyards. Hoping to recuperate his health and equanimity, Salmon had gone to high-altitude Montana with a recently-acquired second wife prior to beginning duties as Head of the Department of Veterinary Science at the University of Montevideo, Uruguay, in the summer of 1906.

Smith planned to autopsy all livestock dying or slaughtered on or near the Company ranch. By carefully studying the gross anatomy and histological structure of their viscera and tissues, he could renew familiarity with the naked-eye and microscopic appearances of normal organs of horses, cattle and sheep, and correlate any abnormality with previous symptoms of acute or chronic intoxication. For almost three weeks his daily activities were governed by those arrangements. The autopsies began early in the morning at the ranch, to which he was driven, generally staying for lunch.[12] In the afternoons, he went to the laboratory, to examine microscopically the tissue sections prepared by Earle Sweet. Twice he inoculated the nasal mucosa of two horses with scrapings from an ulcer in the nares of an autopsied horse. He autopsied "2 horses and 2 cows which had been fed arsenic in large doses," trying to resolve inconsistencies in textbook accounts of tissue changes in arsenic poisoning. The evenings were spent in his hotel room, correcting autopsy notes, writing letters, and "reading on topics connected with the work."

Occasionally he relaxed a little. On Palm Sunday (April 8), he and Dr. Wherry were driven ten miles up the valley to the Warm Springs Station of the Montana Insane Hospital. On Easter Sunday he worked in the laboratory until 4 P.M. with Sweet, arranging tissues for him to section. Then they "tramped to Daly's race course" to watch clay-pigeon shooting. Theobald Smith left Montana on the evening of Easter Monday, April 16, after a full day's work. At the University of Minnesota in Minneapolis, he reciprocated an earlier visit to Boston from the bacteriologist H.W. Hill. In Chicago, on the 19th he met George Fabyan, and called at the University of Chicago and the Rush Medical College. He arrived in New York on the 21st in time for the meeting of the Rockefeller Institute Directors, took lunch with the Herters, and reached home at midnight.[13]

He promptly reported to President Eliot. He had autopsied "about 35 horses and 8 cows to determine any abnormal conditions. Every facility was afforded . . . During this stay I worked in the open air nearly half of the time. The autopsies were made on a ranch about 6 miles from Anaconda . . . The country is semi-arid, 5200 feet above sea level . . . The other half of the time was spent in a well-equipped laboratory of the company, where I made a preliminary examination of tissues from the animals autopsied."[14]

On his second trip, Smith inspected fifteen steers and a large dairy herd on the Bliss ranch. He examined the stained sections prepared by Earle Sweet during his absence, paying particular attention to tissues from horses and cows treated with arsenic for some months, and autopsied by Dr. H.C. Gardiner, a competent local veterinarian hired by the Company. Most of September 1, a beautiful Saturday, was spent at the Butte Fair and Racing Association's Annual Meeting.

Smith enjoyed the "Eight Big Races" on this Eleventh or Miner's Day.[15] Sunday morning was devoted to the microscope.

In the afternoon he was driven twenty miles along the west side of Deer Lodge Valley, returning on the east side. Livestock seemed flourishing everywhere he went. Toxic plants grew abundantly on many untended ranches and might account for the occasional carcass, which showed no evidence of arsenical poisoning. Next morning (Labor Day) the Warm Springs Valley was explored similarly.[16] During the remainder of his second visit, Smith autopsied three horses and two sheep at different ranches, studying the microscopy of their tissues in the laboratory. He also renewed acquaintanceship with his former colleague and successor at the B.A.I., Veranus A. Moore, Professor of Comparative Pathology at Cornell University, who had been invited by Mathewson to join the Company's team of experts. (Local newsmen insisted on naming him *Uranus Moore.*) He made full use of Sweet's services.

With Lilian's encouragement, Theobald Smith returned via Yellowstone Park, accompanied by Moore. They entrained for Livingston, Montana, from where they headed south by road for Gardiner, at the north entrance of the Park. Thence they shared with other visitors a four-horse sightseeing coach, for a five-day circuit of more than 100 miles. The main spectacles that impressed them included the terraces, hot springs and pools, a buffalo herd, innumerable geysers, the Continental Divide and the Grand Canyon. Then, back at Livingston, they boarded a Northern Pacific sleeper. After four uncomfortably hot days in transit, Theobald Smith arrived in Boston in the evening of the 19th.

The slides he brought back from Anaconda were supplemented by two mailed boxes of kidney sections from horses, cattle and sheep. Over the next six weeks, whenever he could spare an hour or two, he worked on these slides. He forecast to President Eliot that he would have to return to Montana to testify. The University might feel compensated for his absence if it were presented afterwards with about 500 microscopic slides and some gross specimens, valuable "for special investigations and as types of normal tissues of horses, cattle and sheep."[17]

On November 14, a telegram summoned Theobald Smith to Butte to testify as expert witness for the defense. In Chicago, during the afternoon of November 15, George Fabyan entertained him between trains. At St. Paul, Smith met another distinguished comparative pathologist, Leonard Pearson, State Veterinarian of Pennsylvania, and Dean of the Veterinary Faculty of the University of Pennsylvania, whose consultant services the Company had likewise hired. They travelled together to Butte on the North Coast Limited. Extreme cold delayed their arrival until the 19th. Smith appeared briefly in court on the 20th and testified continuously from November 21 to 27, except for Sunday the 25th and the afternoon of the 26th, when he was incapacitated with a bad cold.

The scientific evidence overwhelmingly favored the defendants. Since October 1906, J.W. Blankenship, professor of botany at Bozeman Agricultural College, had produced 1,000 plant samples, arranged in thirteen books, to support his contention that no injury to Deer Lodge vegetation (with the possible exception of some trees near the smelter) was attributable to toxic smoke. C.A. Daremus, a toxicologist at the Bellevue Medical College and the American Veterinary College of New York, found only negligible traces of arsenic in twenty-nine analyses of tissues and fluids from dead animals in the valley. He had observed no evidence of arsenical poisoning, acute or chronic, among livestock there. The regional veterinary surgeon, H.C. Gardiner, had fattened cattle and sheep on hay grown in areas exposed to smelter emanations. In one experiment cows and horses actually gained weight while fed relatively small doses of arsenic over a period of several months. When a ranch owner complained that his sheep flocks were destroyed, and other stock badly injured by smelter smoke, no trace of dead or damaged animals could be found on repeated inspection. However, the sheep once showed signs of locoweed intoxication. Other poisonous plants, such as lupine and death camass, grew in uncultivated ranch areas. On the basis of numerous autopsies of horses and cattle, principally from the Deer Lodge Valley, and intimate personal knowledge of the local livestock, Gardiner disbelieved that the Washoe smelter emanations had been injurious to farm animals.

The two veterinary experts, V.A. Moore and D.A. McEachran, testified just before Theobald Smith's arrival. Moore displayed a large collection of normal-histology slides of specimens from health farm animals, contrasting them with the fatty degeneration in specimens from animals deliberately poisoned by arsenic. McEachran had visited several ranches in the Valley to detect abnormal mortality rates during the preceding two years. Some cattle had died from tuberculosis, others from established conditions. Initially he had suspected that smelter smoke was injurious, but his investigations since June 1905 had convinced him otherwise. He and Moore considered the nasal ulcers due to bacteria and denied any contributory role for arsenic.

W.H. Wherry, who had spent three months in 1902 studying pathology and bacteriology under Theobald Smith before taking up a laboratory appointment in Manilla, had cultured a mixture of pyogenic micrococci from the ulcerating nostrils of affected horses. When inoculated into the healthy nasal mucosa of horses, or of other experimental animals, these mixed cultures caused similar ulcers. No such effects could be produced by either arsenic or smelter deposits.[18]

Pearson, who testified after Theobald Smith, had studied the morbidity and mortality rates of animals in the Deer Lodge and other valleys of Montana. He had inspected 3,351 horses and cattle, which were generally in good, and sometimes in excellent condition, the few poor specimens being undernourished or badly fed. The only animals he examined which showed arsenical poisoning were seven experimental horses. Pearson, an authority on bovine tuberculosis, denied that the disease was caused by smelter smoke. Asked by Kelley for an opinion of Theobald Smith, he termed him "a very eminent authority on comparative pathology . . . at the head of his profession in the United States."[19]

On November 21 Smith began his evidence, which reportedly resembled a lecture, but "was listened to by the court and scientists present with the closest attention."[20] He had participated in at least half of the postmortems of Deer Lodge Valley farm animals killed for study purposes; and examined microscopically about 1,000 tissue sections of animals that he had personally autopsied, namely twenty-nine horses, eight cows and three sheep. Of the horses, twenty-one had received no poison and their tissues were normal; the remainder, fed either arsenic or flue dust from the smelter, showed fatty degeneration, especially in liver and kidneys, of a type ascribed to arsenical poisoning.

Altogether the four hired experts—Moore, McEachran, Pearson and Theobald Smith—had autopsied over eighty horses and cows, of which at least one-quarter had been fed arsenic or flue dust experimentally. Smith had suggested these experiments "to secure facts concerning effects of arsenic, in view of the contradictory statements in veterinary literature." He found no evidence from fresh post-mortem specimens, microscopic slides of tissues, or livestock inspection that Deer Lodge Valley Ranch animals suffered injuries from arsenical or other smelter emanations. The nasal sores of horses did not result from corrosive action, but from infection following abrasion. Minor traumata due to some sharp agent, such as foxtail awns, could incite invasion by pyogenic bacteria of species already isolated from these lesions.

During cross-examination by Attorney Clinton, Theobald Smith was asked if he considered himself an authority on arsenic poisoning. Smith replied (with a flash of the eyes) in the negative; indeed he knew of no established authorities in the field. "I don't think anybody has done enough work on the subject to be an authority." Attorney Kelley promptly inquired if he thought Salmon an authority on arsenical poisoning. The witness reportedly snapped in reply, "No sir!" Whereupon Kelley demanded, "Or an authority on anything?" Smith responded—while his eyes flashed again—"Not on any pathological subject."[21]

Smith informed Eliot from Montana that he would have to return yet another time to Butte.

A witness will be introduced on the complainant's side who though not qualified as a pathologist and bacteriologist will have considerable influence owing to the fact that he was for many years the Chief of the Bureau of Animal Industry, during my stay in Washington and subsequently. The defendants fear that he may ride roughshod through our testimony in the absence of anyone qualified to assist counsel in the cross-examination. I strongly urged them to call back a former Washington Assistant of mine (now Professor at Cornell) . . . But they insist on my presence . . . I could not divest myself of a certain sense of duty in protecting evidence laboriously built up by the best men the Company could find.[22]

Since Smith left Washington, Salmon had continued to belittle or try to discredit him. Smith had not resorted to any kind of retaliation, but he disliked being associated with someone he now despised. Only the year before, in 1905, Smith had rejected, pleading his basic interest in human medicine, a request to be grouped in the *Alumni News,* along with Salmon, Moore and another veterinarian, in a proposed tribute to distinguished Cornell graduates in comparative medicine. To V.A. Moore, as one of those involved, he imparted his real objective. "I have written to Dr. Hughes several letters that my interest & affiliation are now with human medicine and that I should rather be left out and come in, if ever, under preventive medicine. The fact is I am not desirous of joining with Dr. Salmon. I would rather be excused from this juxtaposition. I hope you will explain if explanation is needed."[23]

Smith reached Boston on the evening of December 3. After ten extremely busy days, on December 14 he set off again for Butte, with the latest German text on veterinary pathology for company, knowing that this journey would separate him from his family for the Christmas and New Year season. The two Lilians sent affectionate messages almost daily. "Dearest darling Father," young Lilian wrote on December 16, "I do hope you are not terribly mournfully dying of travelling." Her mother wrote on the 20th: "We miss you dreadfully . . . But we'll do our best and be thankful that nothing but temporary separation has to be borne—so many . . . cannot look forward as we can." And again, on Christmas Day: "We cannot *bear* to have you away!" Theobald had only one chance to write before Christmas, for next day he would be in Court:

> The window of my room faces Butte hill directly with its odd dressing of buildings, great mounds of earth and belching smokestacks, and huge derricks over the mineshafts.
>
> I hope that Christmas day and the vacation will be pleasant for you and the children and that you will give them whatever gifts you think advisable. Do go to some play or other attraction with them during the week and see about pianos to fill up the time.[24]

In January 1907, Theobald and Lilian splurged $700 of his fees from the lawsuit on a "Mason & Hamlin Grand Piano," plus their "Steinway upright allowed $200."[25] He billed the Anaconda Copper Mining Co. for a total of $5,650 for consultative services, plus travel expenses. It included time on trains, as well as $300 for the equivalent of six days' "work done at Boston, Mass. between Oct. 1 and Nov. 14, '06 . . . studying 800 to 1000 slides sent from Anaconda." Within the family, the piano became known as the "Anaconda."

On December 19 and 20, Salmon was allowed by Judge Crane to submit new evidence accumulated since his main testimony in the spring of the year, after which Theobald recorded "Working on Dr. Salmon's evidence & assisting Counsel in cross-ex. him."[26] Then, between December 21, 1906 and January 8, 1907, on twelve successive court days, he was cross-examined relentlessly to the point of complete exhaustion. Salmon testified that he had performed some sixty autopsies in Deer Lodge Valley between December 1905 and November 1906. Many sheep in the valley suffered from a malady resembling the sore noses of horses, which he attributed to arsenical flue dust lodging in their nostrils. The congested trachea of a sheep, and other preserved specimens, were introduced as evidence of irritation, reflecting the alleged presence of arsenic in the liver, kidneys and other tissues of animals from the Deer Lodge Valley, as demonstrated by a chemist. Salmon himself claimed to be a microscopist, and undertook to show histological injuries in various tissues from animals killed for post-mortem purposes.[27] Next day, he produced slides purporting to reveal abnormalities due to arsenic in the tissues of eight autopsied animals.

Under cross-examination by a substitute for Attorney Kelley, Salmon admitted that until this trial began he had not performed any recent autopsies. Further, for more than fifteen years he had made no tissue sections and had needed to consult scientific friends in their preparation. Asked why he had resigned from the B.A.I., Salmon gave as reasons that "The appropriation was not sufficient to carry on the work expected of the Department. Another was that I had been in the position too long. In carrying out the law I had opposed large interests, and that made enemies . . . The responsibilities of the place were too great and . . . I could not do justice to the work. It took up too much of my time in taking care of the attacks of my enemies."[28] He denied that his resignation was requested or that President Roosevelt had threatened to ask for it if necessary.

Kelley himself grilled Salmon for the last ten days. With a good-tempered mixture of cajolery, raillery and obduracy, he showed up Salmon's inexpertness. Asked if he agreed with Dr. Chaney, a veterinary witness for the plaintiff, that "black teeth are an evidence of arsenical poisoning," Salmon replied "I don't agree or disagree with him. I don't know." Confronted with the B.A.I.'s own approved list of questions for government meat inspectorships, Salmon could not say how many teeth a calf had at birth; he had paid no attention for years to such things as whether the teeth of a cow were "immovable;"[29] and he believed that a cow had fifteen ribs on each side. When Kelley responded, "Chauvaux says there are thirteen on each side," his victim agreed, "If Chauvaux says thirteen."[30] Asked to reconcile an authoritative textbook's statement that mucus in the stomach was normal with his own claim that its presence signified arsenical poisoning, Salmon explained "there was a difference in the color, one pink and the other transparent."[31]

He floundered in the new embarrassments created for him daily by the indefatigable Kelley. When some slides of tissues were produced for microscopic identification, Salmon's morale sagged to a new low. He complained that the light was very poor and that his nervous condition after the long cross-examination made it impossible to do himself justice. After prolonged study, he identified a slide of thyroid as "a piece of kidney." He refused to look at other slides, on the grounds that apart from the bad light, he had neither the animal's history nor information on how the specimen was prepared.[32] When Salmon denied that tuberculosis in cows led to "bronchitis with heavy catarrhal secretions," Kelley showed him a circular on the subject, issued while Salmon was head of the B.A.I., which said that tuberculosis frequently led to "bronchitis with heavy catarrhal secretions."

His testimony thoroughly discredited and his reputation tattered, Salmon then left to serve as head of the Department of Veterinary Science at the University of Montevideo. At the end of a five-year contract, having assisted in the establishment of a School of Veterinary Medicine in Uruguay, he returned to the United States and eventually found employment in a plant producing hog-cholera serum at Butte, Montana. There he died of pneumonia in August 1914, aged sixty-four. He was buried in the Rock Creek Cemetery, Washington, D.C.[33]

Smith left Butte on December 29, not staying to observe Salmon's discomfiture on the witness stand in the early days of January 1907. On the way home he visited Chicago's Art Museum, and on January 3 began a very full day's work at the Harvard Medical School. However, as explained in yet another letter to President Eliot, a final trip to Montana was required. The judge's authorization of new rebuttal evidence from Salmon had "reopened the case to the extent that the Master now allows retreatment of this testimony by the defendants . . . They are rather insistent as I was the only expert called last December to assist in the cross-examination of Dr. Salmon."

> While I feel less desirous of going than at any previous time . . . I realize that each trip has seen some gain in health and in knowledge of my field of work. The long journey affords considerable opportunity for study and thinking—a condition not attainable here in this formative state of the laboratory . . . Mrs. Smith hopes that you may have some good reason for keeping me at home.[34]

The President telephoned that the trip was "desirable," and Smith set out for the "surrebuttal" at Butte on February 28. At Chicago he was again "entertained" during the afternoon of March 1 by George Fabyan. Testifying from March 8 until noon of March 13, he left that night for Chicago, where he visited the notorious stockyards. The weekend was spent at George Fabyan's country home at Geneva, Illinois, where they discussed protective measures for the remnants of Fabyan's pet poultry flock, which was suffering unexplained losses.

Theodore Roosevelt's personal sympathies were against the smelter company. He wrote to Attorney General C.J. Bonaparte: "If my administration were to continue, I should direct that the suit against the companies be immediately prosecuted."[35] Hence Smith reported to President Eliot from Butte that his arrival in Boston would be somewhat delayed "because the federal Government, or perhaps more specifically President Roosevelt, has taken a hand in the litigation and sent five experts who testified against the defendant Company."

> This made it necessary to go over a larger amount of testimony than I had anticipated. The Government experts did not however do themselves much credit and perhaps injured the side which they were to support.
>
> I am packing up about 1300 slides and the paraffin blocks from which the sections were made . . . The slides represent about a year's work of the average trained laboratory man . . . I trust I shall not have occasion to ask for any leave of absence for some time to come, except perhaps to attend the Congress of Physicians and Surgeons which meets this year in Washington, D.C. during May.[36]

In May 1907, the case reopened before Judge Crane for "argument on the evidence" by the opposing counsel, which was limited to eighteen working days, to be divided equally between Bliss and the defendant companies. Judge Crane's draft of his findings was made public on October 5, 1907, and confirmed by Judge Hunt in May 1909. The amounts of arsenic then being discharged from the Washoe Smelter were deemed not harmful to either animals or plants; the sulphur emissions had caused no damage to the plaintiff; and he [Bliss] was entitled to damages of $350, a sum representing the actual loss suffered by him in depreciated rental value of his land.[37]

Early in June 1910, C.F. Kelley began to urge Theobald Smith to resume his expert assistance to the Smelter Company in a new suit brought by the United States Government under President Taft. Smith declined the invitation: "The fact that Dr. Moore will be on hand will go far towards making my presence unnecessary."[38] He offered to return the material sent him from the former case if it would be useful to anyone, and asked "whether the question of the effect of SO_2 on the body will be brought up this time and whether the effect of the smoke on the human beings has been injected into the case. These are new prob-

lems and any prospective witnesses should be familiar with the data."[39] The correspondence ended abruptly. Theobald Smith did not go again to Butte or Anaconda City. The governmental suit eventually failed.

The Anaconda interlude was a purposeful, down-to-earth venture illustrating
Theobald Smith's natural modesty, straightforwardness and common touch as
well as his scientific competence, integrity and enterprise. His reactions to this
unusual situation need no embellishment by moralistic reflections. Attention is
drawn, however, to the points not directly related to Smith. First, the remarkable change in general attitude toward atmospheric pollution. "Evidence of
specific damage" may still be a legal prerequisite to judgement favoring a plaintiff; but such evidence certainly need *not* precede "the right to complain," as the
Anaconda Copper Mining Company contended. Secondly, in opposing that
company, despite the lack of evidence of damage, Presidents Theodore Roosevelt and Howard Taft displayed notable prescience and political astuteness far
ahead of their time.

16

PUBLIC HEALTH, PREVENTIVE MEDICINE, AND LABORATORY RESEARCH— ATTEMPTED IMMUNIZATION OF CATTLE AGAINST TUBERCULOSIS

"To those who have the need to do research . . .
discovery should come as an adventure . . .
the job of research must be found in the doing."[1]

Lecturer, Investigator, Reluctant Administrator

Nearly forty-eight years old in spring 1907, Theobald Smith had completed twelve years of dual service—to a state department of health with narrow but exacting demands, and to a fast-expanding university, whose expectations were great and aspirations almost unlimited. But even though larger and more suitable laboratory space was now available, the financial restrictions which hobbled these employers still cramped his researches. He missed the counsel of Dr. S.W. Abbott, Secretary of the State Board of Health, his close associate for nearly a decade—"found dead in bed," October 22, 1904—and also of George F. Fabyan, his friendly and trusting benefactor, gone more recently.

With much of his research enthusiasm frustrated, and energy apt to be drained by conflicting obligations, he sometimes seemed unfulfilled, petulant and fault-finding. The Faculty of Medicine accepted one of his two courses as an elective. The other course was parasitology, which students generally disliked. He undertook other types of lectures as well. Smith's semi-technical lectures to specialized groups were well received and read impressively in print; but their preparation was very time-consuming, and to him they sounded hollow if they chiefly recorded the work of others. Although it was his great fortune to have a president with compatible convictions, he had to tread warily when emphasizing the significance of comparative pathology, lest he should seem to endorse the re-establishment of veterinary medicine in some form at Harvard; for President Eliot's interest in this field was almost obsessive. An editorial in the *Boston Medical and Surgical Journal* stated that the publications listed in the president's report for the year 1905–6 implied "that medicine and surgery for human beings are hereafter to be furthered largely by the study of the other animals with which man is in contact, the other animals ranging from bacilli and microscopic parasites to large animals. Mr. Eliot is evidently a friend of laboratories and of such departments as those of comparative anatomy, comparative physiology and comparative pathology."[2] The chair of comparative anatomy was endowed in 1902 with Charles S. Minot the first incumbent. A department of comparative physiology did not yet exist.

At President Eliot's instigation, the Harvard Medical Faculty offered a comprehensive course of twenty-four free public lectures on health education twice-weekly during the first four months of 1908. Theobald Smith participated, his topic being "The Relation of Animal Life to Human Diseases."[3] The series began with Walter B. Cannon's revelations on "Some Recent Discoveries in the Physiology of Digestion" and ended with William T. Councilman discussing "Tumors." There were separate exhibits on chronic rheumatic disorders and bacterial parasites. Notwithstanding E.P. Joslin's praise of "The Modern Crusade Against Typhoid Fever" on January 18, the war's spotty effectiveness was illustrated by this entry in Theobald Smith's diary of April 13: "Meeting in Eliot Hall of Med. Soc. to discuss Jamaica Plain typhoid epidemic, over 300 cases."

The attendance at these lectures averaged 190, so the experiment was repeated. Eliot reported exuberantly: "Many of the lectures were thronged, and it was sometimes necessary to exclude hundreds of persons who desired admission."[4] The Harvard Medical School continued to offer to the public a free series of medical lectures annually, up to and including 1914. Theobald Smith made another contribution in February 1911 on "The Duties of the Individual in the Maintenance and Improvement of the Public Health."[5] Moreover, he gave the 1909 series of public lectures in the Lowell Institute, Boston, on "Our Defenses

Against the Micro-Organisms of Disease." The following topics were covered sequentially in twice-weekly evening lectures from March 16 to April 9, 1909. 1. The Evolution of Disease. 2. How Micro-organisms Produce Disease. 3. How the Body Protects Itself. 4. Immunity and Vaccination. 5. How Infection is Disseminated. 6. Animals as Sources of Disease. Tropical Disease. 7. Lessons from the Plagues of the Past. 8. Public Education and Preventive Medicine. With three lectures still to go, he noted in his diary: "The work of month consists chiefly in preparing & delivering a portion of the Lowell lecture course. During the day of lecture, staid at home, wrote & rested. Used lantern slides in each lecture. Audience 1 / 3 to 1 / 2 full after first. The days between lectures spent at lab. all day. Working regularly at night."[6]

Smith's Lowell lectures were praised as "notable" for their non-sensational presentation of the relation of epidemic diseases to microorganisms, and the broader bearing of these problems upon civilization. He "has rendered the public a service of no mean value in thus presenting a subject, about which much popular ignorance still prevails, in so lucid a manner and in so philosophic a spirit."[7] Three days after completing the Lowell lecture, Theobald Smith fulfilled an invitation to take part in a series of twenty-four public lectures on "Sanitary Science and Public Health" offered by the medical department of Columbia University. His address, entitled "Animal Disease Transmissible to Man. The Relation of Insects to Disease,"[8] appeared in modified form as separate articles in two consecutive issues of the *Monthly Bulletin of the Massachusetts Board of Health.*[9]

The Harvard Medical School had not provided for the teaching of "tropical diseases." Smith's acknowledged authority on insect-borne diseases, and their obvious link to tropical infections, led to a vote of the Faculty of Medicine in December 1908 which resulted in his official appointment by the President and Fellows of Harvard College "to supervise instruction in tropical diseases." Smith was not flattered by this appointment despite its informal and temporary nature. It casually imposed a union between an expanding, exotic discipline of high importance and an individual whose only experience in that field was an early, self-taught foray into endemic malaria in Massachusetts.

Smith had been impressed by the remarkable success of Gorgas in controlling yellow fever in Havana, and later in the Panama Canal Zone, by systematic elimination of the mosquito *Stegomyia fasciatta.* Early in May 1909, he visited ex-Private John R. Kissinger of the U.S. Army at South Bend, Indiana. Kissinger was the first volunteer bitten by an infected mosquito at Camp Lazear in 1900. He recovered from severe yellow fever, declining any remuneration for a service performed "solely in the interest of humanity and in the cause of science." After leaving the Army, he married and settled in Indiana, but developed myelitis. Confined to a wheelchair, he and his wife had to live on a pension of $12 monthly, augmented by her earnings as laundress. Two weeks before his visit, Councilman, Smith and Ernst published a joint appeal for cash contributions to provide an annuity for Kissinger.[10]

As already recounted, Theobald Smith had to struggle, to the point of causing serious friction, in order to procure sufficient space for his research activities in the Bussey Institute. He was left largely to his own devices for solving the problems of devising suitable accommodations for large experimental animals, from cows involved in tuberculosis researches to the increasing numbers of horses needed to meet the demand for diphtheria antitoxin. Old barns were patched up, and paddocks and stables improvised in the vicinity of the antitoxin and smallpox vaccine laboratory. To the critical eye, the jumble of makeshift shanties must have seemed unkempt.

During reorganization of the Bussey Institute in 1908, complaints were voiced by a committee of the Board of Overseers about the appearance of Smith's buildings. C.S. Sargent, the masterful custodian of the Arnold Arboretum, had urged removal of "the old stable at the foot of your avenue." Believing that "It is time for us to consider what new buildings we shall need, and how much land we shall plan to occupy or use," Eliot suggested that the offending structures could be covered with vines, while the conspicuous large stones in the adjacent horse paddock might be replaced with some darker, cinder-like material. "Across South Street you made a temporary paddock, I believe. The Committee took some alarm from that lest all the ground between South Street and the Dedham branch of the R.R. should be put to unsightly uses."[11] Eliot also inquired whether Smith had any employee who could watch on the Bussey building while it was empty. "At your convenience," he smoothly ended his letter to Smith, "I should like to hear what further provision for keeping and studying animals at the Bussey you would think it desirable to make."

Smith had a man employed by the Antitoxin and Vaccine Laboratory, living in the cottage at the foot of the avenue, who could inspect the building periodically. He himself would give some personal attention to the buildings. As for the old barn on the Woodland Hill estate, this had been in use since 1896. "I carried on in it my experiments on bovine tuberculosis which antedated Koch by three years," he told President Eliot.

> I have made all my postmortems in its shadow. Last year I had sheep there. Now we are breeding rabbits on the second floor. Pens have been constructed rat-proof at a cost of more than $100 two years ago. We also store hay for the animals from the estate there. I am not anxious to keep it if there is the remotest chance of getting anything in its place. It can only be used in the summer because the water supply freezes up in winter. It needs repairs and is poorly fitted for any modern

experimentation on infectious diseases . . . If the environment is to match the Arboretum in appearance an abandoned farm not far away might solve the whole difficulty.[12]

Eliot reassured Smith. "The Corporation will not be willing to have removed any building of which you are making use."[13] He then proposed, "Let us arrange the old stable with a water-heater so that work can be carried on there comfortably in winter. The cost would be inconsiderable and I should think the gain would be great. To lose the sequence of experiments for four months out of the year looks to me like a very serious hindrance." Nonetheless, in May 1909, the old barn was finally torn down.

The Antitoxin and Vaccine Laboratory was itself a culprit in the clutter of brick and wooden structures that appeared in recent years near the three-storied Bussey. The building was a focus of esthetic disapproval for Sargent and his committee. Even more recently completed nearby was a two-storied horse stable, almost 100 feet in overall length. In his 1903–1904 plans for a new laboratory, in order to avoid excessive expense for Harvard, Theobald Smith had not incorporated a modern horse stable; however, he soon realized the need and visualized the remedy several months before he broached the subject with President Eliot in a letter stating that he had noted the great "contrast between the operating room in the old stable and our new quarters." He proposed writing to Dr. John S. Billings, whom he knew well "for some money for a modern stable in which both my future work and the antitoxin horses may be accommodated."[14]

Billings was chief adviser to Andrew Carnegie. By mid-October 1905, word arrived that Carnegie funds would be forthcoming for the new stable. The detailed plans were left entirely to Smith. More than two years later, he noted: "New stable practically done."[15] The sprawling stable was no architectural jewel: it was more than twice the length of the antitoxin and vaccine building. The central area (about 25-feet frontage and 47-feet depth), contained an operating room, office, and general services on the ground floor, and cages for small animals (guinea-pigs and mice) on the second floor. This area had access to symmetrically disposed wings—each about 36 feet in length and 24 feet in depth—which provided stalls for twenty-four horses on the ground floor. On the second floor the wings were used for storage of hay, with feeding chutes to the stalls below.

Still unmet was Smith's need for an adequate infectious disease laboratory, where some animal infection could be studied in isolation. The 1906–07 report to the Dean of Medicine from the Department of Comparative Pathology contained the following statement:

There is furthermore needed at the Bussey Institution a small building were some one spontaneous infectious disease of the domestic animals may be studied at a time. This should include a small laboratory for work which must be done near the animals under observation, an autopsy room for large animals, and shelter for a few animals affected with spontaneous or induced disease . . . Such a small plant would make accessible to study important problems of disease not now within reach of the human pathologist.

According to Smith, such an addition would help to differentiate the activities of the Department of Comparative Pathology from those of other departments; would provide course material for its own use, as well as for sanitary science and agricultures; and would "bring the student into context with actual disease as much needed inspiration for painstaking research." This clear definition of a desideratum drew no response—and there is no evidence that a reminder was sent.

Beginning about the year 1904 also, there were cumulative hints that University representatives, including President Eliot, felt that Theobald Smith should delegate to qualified assistants much of the routine Board of Health work—diphtheria antitoxin and smallpox vaccine production and public health laboratory tests—in order to secure more time for his own cherished researches, as well as for the teaching and training of future research workers. Theobald Smith himself had expressed disappointment that his hopes for an early reduction in the detailed supervision required by the antitoxin and vaccine service had not materialized. Eliot assured him: "In general, you will find the Corporation disposed to assist you in getting rid of minor duties in order that you may have time and strength for research work."[16] However, he was unwilling to relinquish full responsibility for the State laboratory.

In June 1905 Smith's routine work comprised directing the work of seven Board of Health employees; the ordering and purchasing of all supplies, including laboratory animals; testing toxin and antitoxin samples; vaccinating calves and removing the vaccine. The Harvard laboratory staff consisted of "2 lab. servants and Mr. Brown, who begins to work for State Bd. of Health on oysters, mosquitoes, etc."[17] When nearly four years passed with little improvement, Eliot proposed an obvious solution: "You seem to me to need an assistant director for the State laboratory, to assume full charge of the details of the work."[18] An assistant was never provided, however, and Smith eventually confined himself to early morning checks, but not before he had been thoroughly scolded by Eliot for a dearth of followers: "You ought to be bringing up some other disciples," the president admonished. "The investigator who does not accomplish that has only a very partial success, no matter what he himself discovers."[19]

The special bond between President Eliot and Theobald Smith derived from Eliot's long-held conviction that medical research yielded results of incomparably greater benefit to mankind than any other category of cumulative knowledge or scholarship. "The laboratory should form a far more important part of education of the student than the didactic lecture," he believed.[20] As early as 1898, Eliot had "observed with pleasure that the Harvard Medical School had been converted into a nest of laboratories," and regretfully noted there some residual lecture-rooms. In talks with the president, or in letters to him, Smith sometimes would unburden himself very candidly, underlining rather than deprecating his work, as though needing legitimization, or reassurance that his position was not unduly privileged. Eliot sought Smith's opinion on various questions—though seldom as sole consultant, and quite often without taking the advice given.

To choose a suitable Dean of the Medical Faculty, following the resignation of W.L. Richardson in 1907, was an onerous task. Eliot's letters to Smith implied that he already held firm views on the relevant facts. "The right kind of man is almost sure to be under 40 . . . Dr. John Warren would do very well for Secretary. He has declined election as Dean. Would Dr. Cannon make a good Dean, or Dr. Christian?" Several of the older Professors of the School advocated the appointment of Dr. G-, the Secretary who had been Acting Dean. "That . . . would be merely marking time instead of marching. Dr. G- is at least 55 years old and never was a research man."[21] (President Eliot at the time was over seventy-three.) Smith favored Cannon and advocated a five-year term as diminishing the danger of a man getting out of date and ossified.[22] Eliot agreed that Cannon would make a good Dean, but considered "Dr. Christian . . . to be very promising." As for the suggested five-year term of appointment, Eliot believed that only a rash man would consider "running the risk of being dropped at the end of a comparatively short term of service with a very injurious stain of failure on him."[23] Eventually, the job went to Christian.

Preventive medicine was also a subject very much on President Eliot's mind at that time. A few months before his retirement, Eliot addressed the annual meeting of the Aesculapian Club of Boston on the "Coming Change in the Medical Profession." He warned that medical practice would be seriously affected if preventive medicine became successful, and asked rhetorically: "Shall we not welcome the coming change? Is not the function of the medical profession regarded as preventive, higher, better, happier than the function of the medical and surgical profession regarded as curative?" Eliot's fellow-speaker was Simon Flexner, who discussed the "Relation of Independent Institutions for Medical Research to Medical Education." Flexner was content to suggest that the medical profession would benefit if more representatives took up laboratory careers, and if others could carry back into practice the principles and ideals of the laboratory.

Despite that sort of pressure, the medical student of those days showed little inclination for research electives. One editorial pointed out that the choice of electives by fourth-year students "continued to show a strong preference for the more practical and traditional subjects of instruction, and a wholesome disinclination to specialize at the early stage of the medical career."[24] Nor was preventive medicine rated any higher. At the Harvard Medical School, Charles Harrington was part-time Professor of Hygiene, and also successor to S.W. Abbott as Secretary to the State Board of Health under Walcott. Nonetheless, Walcott informed Eliot, "I have at times had visions of a large department of preventive medicine with Theobald Smith at the head, but they are very vague."[25]

Eliot called a conference for the afternoon of May 5, 1909, to consider instituting such a department and surveying candidates for the post. Theobald smith excused himself in order to attend an out-of-town meeting, but wrote a letter to the president designed to forestall any attempt to nominate him for the vacancy. "I do not believe it would be wise for me to make a change of such magnitude at my age," he told Eliot. "I should have to give up nearly all my present work," he protested. "It would be necessary for me to spend some time, six months or longer, in study and travel, and finally begin all over again to build another department." Instead, he could help the new Department in the study of animal foods and of animal diseases transmissible to man; and "by working on the causation of disease on a comparative basis," develop principles applicable to human life.[26] The Faculty of Medicine, to whom the whole matter was referred, resolved to establish a full-time professorship of Preventive Medicine and Hygiene. Milton J. Rosenau, Director of the Hygienic Laboratory in Washington, D.C., was offered this new chair in June 1909 by President A.L. Lowell, who had succeeded Eliot soon after the middle of May.

Aside from his personal reluctance, Theobald Smith's suitability for this undertaking could be questioned on too many grounds. First, he was not physically robust. Colds and sore throats, intestinal upsets, transitory fevers and dental visits recurred frequently. Although mumps in middle age, and the bouts of sacro-iliac disease which laid him really low, rated only matter-of-fact comments, he occasionally lapsed into a morbid analysis of his physical condition. He was very health-conscious, at times almost hypochondriacal. Secondly, Smith apparently could not or would not devote much time and attention to medical undergraduate teaching. Allegations that he was hard to please, remote and unfriendly, and somewhat of a martinet, were not disturbing to the administration, which opposed the fashionable crumbling of barriers between faculty members and students. More serious deficiencies would be real indifference, or inability to concentrate upon teaching or research because of preoccupation with petty administrative duties that should be delegated. Theobald Smith had been admonished by President Eliot for just such tendencies. The Harvard administration was also confused by Smith's reiterated need for additional departmental staff before he could undertake any new teaching load. His complaints about under-staffing had been followed sometimes by rejection of an offer to increase his laboratory help.

There was of course another side to the question. Although Smith's undergraduate teaching lacked sparkle, his diaries indicate how thoroughly each year he revised the lectures and prepared the laboratory work for both courses. The "laboratory servant" and the part-time Teaching Fellow helped in laboratory preparation, but the professor planned and rehearsed the exercises and experiments, and did all the marking. His Harvard staff was limited to two laboratory servants and one part-time Teaching Fellow, each receiving $500 per annum. What he needed was *not* the offered third diener, but an academically qualified full-time assistant, at a minimum salary of $1,500—which Harvard could not afford. With many successive part-time Fellows, such as Arthur Reagh, Herbert Brown and Paul Lewis, and assistants like the unpaid Marshal Fabyan, he took endless pains, taught them techniques, and conveyed attitudes to problem-solving that stayed with them for life and anchored their loyalty. He also gave bench space and strict short-term training to diverse graduates or postgraduates, who came with appropriate backgrounds and laudable aims, and left as ardent disciples.

From 1907–08 onwards, Theobald Smith no longer doubted that for him the betterment of human health demanded exacting, unrelenting research. The university administration accepted the situation because Smith's increasing fame, which redounded to Harvard's credit, derived from his microbiological researches. The honorary degrees and medals awarded, the numerous invitations to ceremonial occasions, the many distinguished visitors to his laboratories, and the vigorous flow of publications therefrom, symbolized and reinforced that fame. During August 1907, for example, Smith was "working on sketch of my life & list of papers for Liverpool School of Tropical Med. who are to confer on me Mary Kingsley Medal for my researches on Texas fever." In mid-December 1907, he entrained for Chicago via Albany: "3 P.M. attend convocation exercises with Mrs. Fabyan & sister. Degree of LL.D. conferred on me." He was the only recipient of that honor, and his wife made much of it: "We think you are now nearing Chicago and hope you have had a comfortable trip—you and your gown! Dear me, *how* I would like to see you on Tuesday!"[27] Lilian eventually got almost blasé about Theobald's honorary degrees but did not forget to tell the children about each new honor that came to him.

Attempted Immunization Against Tuberculosis

In 1890, shortly after Koch announced his discovery of tuberculin, Trudeau reported attempts to immunize small laboratory animals against tuberculosis. Rabbits and guinea-pigs acquired no protection against virulent tubercle bacilli from previous intravenous injections of a fortuitously attenuated human strain,[28] which he later identified as of avian type. The course of ocular tuberculosis in the rabbit following inoculation of virulent culture into the anterior chamber of the eye could be modified or aborted by "preventive inoculations of bird bacilli."[29] In 1894, de Schweinitz claimed that guinea-pigs, and also a cow and a calf, were protected against infection with bovine organisms by previous injections of an attenuated human culture procured from Trudeau. Trudeau's persistent efforts culminated in his 1897 report on the successful protection of guinea-pigs by "cultures of mammalian bacilli attenuated by prolonged growth on artificial media."[30] Behring struggled for leadership in the immunization of cattle. He repeatedly "improved" the antigens, and in 1902 reported the "Jennerization" of calves through inoculations of attenuated human bacilli, which firmly protected against virulent bovine strains.[31] Pearson and Gilliland[32] had equally good results in Pennsylvania, using similar techniques.

At this juncture, in an article entitled "Immunization from Tuberculosis," Simon Flexner paid tribute to "those patient and intrepid spirits who, like Trudeau, toil successfully and incessantly in remote places," and whose labors were liable to be forgotten or disregarded.[33] Flexner also lauded Theobald Smith's discovery that bovine and human tubercle bacilli had different properties. Four months later, in the same journal under the identical title, appeared a rebuttal by D.E. Salmon, complaining of the inclusion of Smith's own work and omission of the work by de Schweinitz. Salmon thought it "unfortunate that he [Flexner] should portion out the credit for a notable discovery in a manner which might be in the least suggestive of unfairness or bias."[34] To Flexner's assurance in a letter that he would gladly rectify any injustice done unintentionally to de Schweinitz, Salmon replied that the credit due to Trudeau and de Schweinitz had now been apportioned properly; but in his opinion the type differentiation done by Smith, which Flexner had termed an essential prerequisite, had little if any influence on the success achieved by Pearson and Gilliland.[35]

Smith began immunity experiments on guinea-pigs in 1898, hoping to improve upon Trudeau's results, believing that "The discovery of the tubercle bacillus . . . left the whole question of its complex relation to a given host untouched."[36] His findings, though inconclusive and incomplete, indicated the superior effectiveness of whole cultures killed at 60°C. Until the most effective antigen was identified "we must inject all of them." He recommended that the bacillary strain used should have been isolated recently, and grown on blood serum "to which pieces of sterile animal tissues may be added." Many years before, Smith had advocated a chopped-tissue medium for the cultivation of anaerobes without resort to inert gases, a method Noguchi later adapted to cultivating spirochetes.[37] Smith believed that the tubercle bacillus exuded a self-protective capsule,[38] and "the more recently isolated the culture and the more nearly the culture medium approximates the living body the more likely the active production of this envelope." The contention that attenuated strains gave the best immune response had not been pursued, as he lacked protective equipment against live bacilli. He had no opportunities for testing such products on tuberculous patients and they could not be "successfully tested on any animals, except perhaps monkeys and cattle," which presented major problems of expense and accommodation.[39] Despite all the anticipated obstacles, Theobald Smith resolved to tackle the problem.

Near the end of November 1904, Smith addressed the New York branch of the Harvard Medical Alumni Association on "Medical Research." He had "Dinner at Univ. Club beforehand with Drs. Wilcox, Nathl Bowditch, Potter (my guide)."[40] Nathaniel I. Bowditch represented a distinguished Boston family, which included Henry Ingersol Bowditch (1808–1892), co-founder (1869) and first chairman of the Massachusetts Department of Health,[41] and his newphew the physiologist Henry Pickering Bowditch, Harvard's Dean of Medicine from 1883 to 1893, who ran a substantial farm at Framingham, Massachusetts, about twenty miles west of Boston. Early in 1906, in his Harvey Society address, Theobald Smith called specific immunity to tuberculosis "the overshadowing problem before society today."[42] Later that year, he arranged with the Trustees of the Massachusetts Society for Promoting Agriculture, who were willing to cover the major costs, to begin immunization experiments of cattle against tuberculosis on the farm of Nathaniel Bowditch.

The first trials lasted from October 1906 to November 1907, and they were reported in June 1908 under the title "The Vaccination of Cattle against Tuberculosis. I."[43] The article tabulated the injection data and the results of challenging vaccinated and control calves with virulent bovine bacilli. Smith divided the animals into five experimental groups, of which group A, totalling twenty-one animals, was split into seven sub-groups of three calves—each sub-group being vaccinated with a different human-type culture. Group E comprised five unvaccinated controls, for testing the adequacy of the challenge dose. Groups B, C, and D (three calves each) were injected respectively with Behring's bovovaccine, virulent but dead bovine bacilli (heat-killed at 60°C), and an attenuated bovine culture. Every strain, except Behring's, had been isolated by Smith. All calves in groups A to D received two doses of vaccine intravenously, with an interval between doses of two to three months. Vaccinated calves not submitted to this severe challenge were distributed among infected herds for exposure to natural infection, and remained under observation.

The results of this complex experiment were far less explicit and dramatic than Pasteur's triumphant vaccination of sheep against anthrax nearly thirty years before at Pouilly-le-Fort. Smith was dealing with a host-parasite contest of much lower acuteness and tried to settle an issue involving many variables with too few animals. Hence his conclusions were hedged with reservations and incertitudes. On the whole, the results favored attenuated bovine strains over human-type bacilli. Vaccines could be easily prepared, but the immunity induced by vaccination was of uncertain degree and duration; and when insufficient, might prove dangerous through discharge of tubercle bacilli from small pulmonary foci.

Smith outlined several future research projects. Could breeds of cattle possessing high natural resistance to tuberculosis be selected by injecting them with attenuated bovine bacilli? Perhaps the order of responsiveness to the antigen among different breeds could be usefully determined. And since the survival of human or bovine bacilli in the lungs and udders of animals vaccinated intravenously would obviously be potentially hazardous to man, the frequency of this occurrence should be ascertained. Smith sent a copy of the report to President Eliot together with an article on the tetanus bacillus. The latter he had presented at a joint meeting of the Pathological and Medical Societies of Chicago,[44] on the day after he received his honorary doctorate from the University of Chicago in December 1907.

From Eliot's summer home (at Asticou, Maine) came a handwritten acknowledgement:

> I have just read your Vaccination of Cattle against tuberculosis I. There is promise in that I! I am eager to make sure that you have the means of conducting the five investigations indicated in your conclusions . . . as regards buildings, land, assistants, servants, and money . . . How much money did the Trustees of the Mass. Soc. for Promoting Agriculture spend on this Investigation I? Your tetanus paper is also important, but it gives warning rather than raises hope.[45]

Smith replied promptly: "The 'I' means that there are some 15 or more vaccinated animals exposed . . . to the natural infection." Such investigations were costly—the calves must be milk-fed, and might be under observation for long periods. Unfortunately the antigen prepared from human bacillary strains (which he could make for 10–15 cents per dose) did not confer a lasting immunity. The purchase price of Behring's bovo-vaccine was $2.50 per dose.

We are, of course, always in danger of being swamped by the U.S. Agricultural Department [B.A.I.], which takes up any such problem on a large scale when others are known to be at work on it. My plan therefore has always been to work at something quite new and not let it be known until I have reached certain definite results. After it has been taken up generally my interest in it is lost, except to defend my work when it is under fire.

To accomplish anything in the field of animal disease, notably the infectious diseases, an expenditure of from $1000 to $2000 per year would not be extravagant.[46]

Eliot wrote to the Treasurer of the Trustees of the Massachusetts Society for Promoting Agriculture, Mr. Saltonstall, who was well known to both Smith and Eliot as a fellow-member of the Thursday Evening Club, and favorable action followed. On April 16, 1909, the Treasurer of the Society offered the Corporation a grant of $1,200 per annum for three years, commencing July 1, 1909, "to enable Professor Theobald Smith to continue his experiments on bovine tuberculosis."

The Bussey Farm was much closer than Framingham to the laboratory and Smith persuaded Dean Sabine that calves might be kept there for the duration of his next vaccination experiment. The second and third reports on the vaccination of cattle against tuberculosis were published in September 1911 and July 1915. The promise which President Eliot had found in report No. I was not fulfilled in Nos. II and III. The second account, with the subtitle "The Pathogenic Effect of Certain Cultures of the Human Type on Calves," reported that of the nine calves given their first intravenous inoculations with one human strain, four died of tuberculous pneumonia within one or two months, and another became blind in both eyes and developed tuberculous lesions which would have proved fatal. Calves which survived the initial dose coped with larger second or third doses of the same strain. The third and final report, with M. Fabyan's collaboration, was subheaded "The Occasional Persistence of the Human Type of Bacillus in Cattle." This finding (persistence of living bacilli after vaccination) obviously circumscribed the practice of bovo-vaccination.[47]

In the spring of 1908, Robert Koch and his wife embarked on a long trip intended as a world tour, which would afford much-needed rest from his labors and enjoyment of the honors every country was eager to lavish upon him. In the United States, he proposed to visit his two brothers and other relatives in Chicago and in Iowa. In New York, he visited the City of New York Health Department, various hospitals, and the Staten Island Quarantine Station. As soon as Simon Flexner heard that the German Medical Society planned to fete Koch at a dinner in New York on Saturday, April 11, 1908, he arranged with John D. Rockefeller, Jr. to host a dinner on the preceding Friday, which all the Scientific Directors of the Rockefeller Institute for Medical Research would attend. Theobald Smith received an urgent telegram from Flexner: DINNER TO PROFESSOR KOCH BOARD OF INSTITUTE AND MR. ROCKEFELLER ARRANGED FOR FRIDAY EVENING PLEASE PLAN CERTAINLY TO BE PRESENT.[48]

Smith left for New York at noon the next day and attended both the dinner given by Mr. Rockefeller at the University Club that evening and the sumptuous banquet at the Waldorf-Astoria Hotel on the following night. He and Koch had plenty of opportunities to renew their acquaintanceship on this first quiet occasion. The second encounter was a formal affair, with about 500 guests and a Banquet Committee of ten officers and senior members of the German Medical Society of New York under the chairmanship of the Society's president, Dr. Carl Beck. The fifty-four member Honorary Committee included university Presidents C.W. Eliot and N.M. Butler, Andrew Carnegie, and Drs. W.H. Welch, Theobald Smith, Hermann M. Biggs and Simon Flexner and was headed by the German Imperial Ambassador to the United States, Baron von Sternburg. Regrets were read from E.L. Trudeau, who was too unwell to be present. A telegram was sent to him on motion of Koch, seconded by Carnegie.

Koch responded feelingly to florid speeches of tribute given by William Welch, Abraham Jacobi and Andrew Carnegie. He seemed more modest than usual, asking his hosts, "Am I really entitled to such homage?"

> I believe that I can accept with a clear conscience many of the laudatory things said about me. But I have done no more than you do daily. I have worked as hard as I could, and have fulfilled my duty. If the success was greater than usual, the reason is that in my wanderings through the medical field I came upon regions where gold still lay by the wayside. Good luck is necessary in distinguishing gold from the base metals, but there is no special merit in that.[49]

In the fight against tuberculosis, they could hardly hope for more success without new research. Such researches would be possible in the Robert Koch Institute for Tuberculosis in Berlin—"a foundation which Andrew Carnegie has so munificently endowed"—where international investigations would be made to the benefit of all mankind.[50] The proceedings closed with the chairman proposing the health of Koch's wife, who sat with many other ladies in the balconies.

Theobald Smith took no active part in the proceedings. His Day Cards for April 10th and 11th baldly stated: "10. lve for N.Y. at noon—dinner to Dr. Robert Koch at night. Rain. 11. Rockefeller Inst. meeting, banquet to Koch at Waldorf Astoria. colder." The entry for April 11 in his monthly account book was only slightly more informative: "Rockefeller Inst. Directors' meeting 10 to 5, banquet to Koch in evening at Waldorf Astoria. sit at invited guest table, and on honorary committee."

After visiting his brothers and other relatives in Chicago and the mid-West, Koch and his wife traveled via Honolulu to Japan, to which S. Kitasato, his favorite pupil, had returned fifteen years before. They were welcomed at Yokohama on board ship by Kitasato and Prof. M. Miyajima, a leading research scientist, who together escorted the Kochs on a triumphal tour of the country. Koch received the honors befitting a demigod, including presentation to the Mikado. After six weeks Koch prepared reluctantly to leave for China, when a telegram from Berlin early in August recalled him to lead his country's delegation to the Sixth International Congress on Tuberculosis at Washington, September 28 to October 12, 1908. There the heady but relaxing atmosphere of his sojourn in Japan was not to be found.

Although Koch received the respect and deference from the international delegates that was his due, the doctrines he promulgated at the British Tuberculosis Congress in 1901, to the effect that bovine tubercle bacilli were a negligible cause of human tuberculosis, had become unacceptable to an increasing number of authorities in several countries. His paper on "The Relations of Human and Bovine tuberculosis" provocatively confronted that same issue and stirred up very strong opposition to his unrelenting insistence that the bovine bacillus was not significantly pathogenic for man.[51] The English version was reproduced in German, with commentary by G. Pannwitz.[52] Koch now acknowledged that Theobald Smith had first called his attention to differences between human and bovine tubercle bacilli. "It was his work which induced me to take up the same study."

Smith maintained an active interest in tuberculosis for the rest of his life. During the quarter-century 1910 to 1934, Smith published thirteen papers about various laboratory or experimental aspects of tuberculosis, including the second Mellon Lecture (1916–17),[53] the two Thayer Lectures (1933),[54] and two presidential addresses[55] delivered in Washington in the fall of 1926. He also served for many years on committees, councils or boards of organizations concerned with tuberculosis control. He was a particularly honored member of the council of the University of Pennsylvania's Henry Phipps Institute at Philadelphia. Late in life he was nominated to the Trudeau Medal Committee, having been the first recipient of this award.

His discourse on "The Problem of Natural and Acquired Resistance of Tuberculosis"[56] revealed the quandary of the immunologist still facing the many problems created by a versatile parasite in a sensitized host. His "Remarks on the Co-operation of Science and Practice in Tuberculosis" reminisced charitably.

> It is 18 years ago that some of us here present met in this city during the International Congress on Tuberculosis . . . Among the important problems still agitating the members at that time was the relation between human and animal tuberculosis, and it was our good fortune to have as one of our distinguished guests Robert Koch, whom we could meet face to face and ply with questions *ad libitum* to bring out his point of view.[57]

Finally, Theobald Smith's review for the Historical Section of the Philadelphia College of Physicians on March 14, 1932, the fiftieth anniversary of the discovery of the tubercle bacillus, was described by one listener as "a classic . . . The audience would have been delighted to have you continue in the same vein for hours."[58]

17

CHANGE OF HARVARD PRESIDENTS
AND THE DARWIN CENTENARY

The tercentenary of the birth of John Harvard was celebrated by a dinner on November 26, 1907 under the aegis of the Harvard Memorial Society with appropriate college songs and the Harvard Hymn. The Cambridge Historical Society organized a dinner on April 27, 1909 for the centenary of the birth of Oliver Wendell Holmes. Despite a meager appetite and a spare stature, Theobald Smith liked to commit to his scrapbooks the menus interspersed with speeches and songs of those gargantuan feasts of food and drink. Such events were male-dominated; when ladies accompanied their men folk, they usually dined separately. These dinners may be classed as ceremonial, to which category belong also the banquet arranged at the Waldorf-Astoria in New York in honor of Robert Koch on his first visit to the United States.

There were other types of dinner affairs which at this period Theobald Smith seemed quite willing to attend—the annual dinners of fraternities and of alumni associations. On April 15, 1908, Smith was invited to the Phi Rho Sigma Fraternity dinner in a Boston hotel, at which each of nine official toasts was preceded by a speech. Walter B. Cannon toasted "Fraternity Ideals" and Henry A. Christian "Study Abroad;" Theobald Smith's assignment was "Science." All three were Honorary Members of the fraternity. Another notable get-together took place on May 19, 1908 at the Hotel Ten Eyck, Albany—the 35th Annual Dinner of the Alumni Association of the Albany Medical College. One of Theobald's scrapbooks contains an elaborate, printed program, autographed by Smith's old classmates, listing the Association's current officers and providing the words of several rather beery songs. On this instance, Smith decided to attend because it marked the twenty-fifth anniversary of his own graduation from Albany Medical College. On May 17, between the last two dinners, occurred his and Lilian's twentieth wedding anniversary. Lilian saw to it that Theobald should not forget. On the 16th, they left for Williamstown, where he spent two days and nights before entraining alone for Albany. For the 17th, a Sunday, his diary read: "20th wedding anniversary. Tramp about town & visit old friends. Attend chapel prayers at 5."

Honors from outside organizations began coming Theobald's way. In 1908, he was elected a Fellow of the London Society of Tropical Medicine and Hygiene, and also an Honorary member of La Société de Pathologie Exotique, Institut Pasteur, Paris.[1] He was particularly gratified by the news of his election to the National Academy of Sciences on April 23, 1908. Pasted into one of his five scrapbooks is a telegram from Welch, "Heartiest congratulations on your unanimous election," and also pleasant notes from two distinguished Harvard colleagues and fellow-academicians—W.M. Davis, the geologist, on his "unanimous first-in-the-list election," and B.O. Peirce, the physicist and mathematician, on being elected "without one blank or dissenting ballot." At this same meeting of the Academy, Simon Flexner was elected to membership.

His own university started to recognize the breadth of his knowledgeableness. In 1908, he was nominated to membership of the Brewer Croft Cancer Commission,[2] and a few months later was appointed Chairman of the Division of Medical Sciences, representing a group of the Graduate School of Arts and Sciences. In April 1909, at a meeting of the President and Fellows of Harvard College, in accordance with a vote of the Faculty of Medicine on December 1908, he was officially appointed "to supervise instruction in tropical disease."[3] This action reflected the increasing conviction that departments of tropical medicine be established in the larger North American medical schools.[4]

On October 26, 1908, Charles W. Eliot announced that his resignation would take effect on May 19, 1909, exactly forty years after his inauguration as President of Harvard. Despite the veneration felt for him by most of his faculty and administrative colleagues, a man of quite different views and outlook was elected as his successor. A. Lawrence Lowell was not only a generation younger;

as professor of history and government at Harvard, he had written most of the 1903 Report of the Faculty Committee on Improving Instruction which attacked the increasingly undemanding standards for the A.B. degree. Eliot in his last annual Report (1907–08) contended that a reduction in length of the A.B. program was essential to save the College, but Lowell posed an alternative in his Inaugural Address: "May we not feel that the most vital measure for saving the college is not to shorten its duration, but to ensure that it shall be worth saving?" Lowell also distanced himself from his predecessor by proclaiming his strong belief "in the physical and moral value of athletic sports, and of intercollegiate contests conducted in a spirit of generous rivalry."[5] Eliot had repeatedly denounced college baseball and football, the latter as "a brutal, cheating, demoralizing game."[6]

The last meeting of the Faculty of Medicine over which Eliot presided was scheduled for May 1, 1909. On this occasion, Dr. Shattuck assured President Eliot that the faculty fully appreciated what he had done for medical education and for medicine in the large sense. "You heard the fetal heart, watched over the pregnancy, assisted at the birth, promoted and rejoiced over the phenomenal growth of modern medicine. You have converted the position of the layman into a vantage point, and your horizon has sometimes been wider than that of us specialists." As a parting gift to the President, the Charles W. Eliot Fund was launched about six months before his retirement. The total exceeded $150,000. Donors of $5 or less numbered nearly 900, while thirty-one had donated $1000 or more. Theobald Smith gave $50. The Fund was to be invested and held "for the benefit of President Eliot, and after his death, of his widow."[7] Eventually the residue was expected to pass to the University. A Charles Eliot Club was formed by his friends for occasional dinners and the reading of papers on various topics. Theobald Smith was a charter member of its Executive Committee and soon was made Vice-President.

In response to an invitation to send an official representative to the ceremonies commemorating the Centenary of Charles Darwin's Birth and the Fiftieth Anniversary of the Publication of the Origin of Species, to be held at the University of Cambridge, England, June 22–24, 1909, the President and Fellows of Harvard College appointed "Mr. Alexander Agassiz and Professor Theobald Smith delegates from Harvard University to the Darwin Celebrations.[8] Agassiz was in his seventy-fourth year and unable to go. Smith added one month of vacation allowance to his month's leave of absence so that he could take his wife with him on a sightseeing expedition. In May, Dr. Charles S. Minot, Professor of Histology and Embryology, requested Smith to serve as his substitute from the Boston society of National History, of which Minot was president. The Provisional Programme,[9] which arrived well before their departure, ordained academic robes for all five ceremonial occasions and evening dress and orders for the Chancellor's Reception and the Banquet.

In February 1909, the New York Academy of Science had presented a bust of Darwin to the American Museum of Natural History. A bronze replica was offered now to Christ's College (of which Darwin had been an undergraduate member, 1828–1831) as a suitable gesture acknowledging his influence on American thought and science. The casting, transportation and installation of this memento at Cambridge was estimated to require about $1,000. Theobald Smith, who subscribed $25, was one of fourteen individual and twelve institutional contributors. The bust was donated and formally accepted at the Garden Party given by Christ's College on June 23.

The Smiths left Boston on June 1, 1909 by the Cunard Line's *Ivernia,* which reached Liverpool on the 10th. En route to London by train, they stayed overnight at centers of interest—Liverpool, Chester, Shrewsbury and Warwick. They drove from Warwick to Kenilworth and back on the morning of June 14, and took an afternoon excursion to Stratford, where Theobald's diary reveals that they saw the skylark and heard the cuckoo, but omits all mention of Shakespeare. Warwick Castle and St. Mary's Church at Leamington impressed them. Then came a week of shopping and sightseeing in London. They stayed at the Kingsley Hotel, Bloomsbury Square, while visiting the National Gallery, the Horse Guards, the Tower, Westminster Abbey, and the Wallace Art Collection. On Sunday the 20th they attended the morning service at Temple Church and went to St. Paul's Cathedral in the afternoon.

Arriving at Cambridge on June 22, they found among the twenty-eight delegates from the United States several whom Smith knew well, including H.M. Biggs, representing New York University; R.H. Chittenden (Yale University); L.O. Howard (National Academy of Sciences, Washington); H. Fairfield Osborn (American Philosophical Society); Jacques Loeb (University of California); and J.G. Schurman (Cornell University). In all, 431 delegates and other guests invited by the University were accommodated in colleges or private houses in Cambridge. Charles Darwin had married Emma Wedgwood, daughter of Josiah, founder of the pottery firm, and among the final List of Delegates and Other Guests[10] were twenty-one Darwins and eight Wedgwoods. Theobald Smith's name appeared as sole representative of both Harvard University and the Boston Society of Natural History. The Smiths were assigned lodging at the home of the Woodheads, where Dr. W.A. Jamieson, President of the Royal College of Physicians of Edinburgh, and Mrs. Jamieson, were fellow guests. They all attended the University Chancellor's Reception at the Fitzwilliam Museum that evening.

G. Sims Woodhead, Professor of Pathology at Cambridge since 1899 (and a prominent member of the British Tuberculosis Commission), hosted a luncheon for Theobald Smith at Trinity Hall on the 23rd.

Following a Garden Party at Christ's College, the New Examination Hall was the setting for what Theobald's diary termed a "great dinner at 7 P.M. for men." After this formal banquet, from 10 P.M. until midnight, the Vice-Chancellor and Fellows of the College welcomed the guests and their ladies, who joined the men folk after dining separately, at Pembroke College Hall and Gardens. The ceremonial banquet was organized masterfully, from the menu and seating arrangements to the erudite speeches accompanying the toasts. The high level of renown and learning that prevailed among the delegates and guests added to the luster and fellowship of the occasion. The various distinctions of the forty-four men seated at the long head table with the Chancellor and Vice-Chancellor of Cambridge University were fascinating to unravel, superfluous to envy, and futile to compare. At right angles to the head table and contacting it, were twelve shorter rectangular tables at equidistant intervals, each seating thirty-seven persons (eighteen per side and one at the free end). The total of 512 diners included University of Cambridge representatives not officially listed.

Theobald Smith's German-speaking facility placed him next to Prof. W. Kükenthal, Director of the Zoological Institute, Breslau University, and opposite Hofrat Victor Ebner, Professor of Histology at the University of Vienna. William Erasmus Darwin, the only non-scientist son of Charles Darwin, was seated at the head table just opposite Smith's table. Two of his brothers, Sir George Howard Darwin, professor of astronomy and experimental philosophy at Cambridge for the past twenty-five years, and Major Leonard Darwin, engineer, economist, and President of the Royal Geographical Society, were near the other end of the head table. Charles Darwin's remaining two sons, Francis Darwin, the distinguished botanist and President of the British Association for the Advancement of Science, and Horace Darwin, a civil engineer, occupied seats at tables adjoining Smith's.

Presiding over the ceremonial banquet was the eminent physicist John William Strutt, better known as Lord Rayleigh, a Nobel Laureate for 1904, and an original member of the lately established Order of Merit. Recently he had exchanged the presidency of the Royal Society for Cambridge University's chancellorship. On his right were seated Prince Roland Bonaparte, representing l'Institut de France; Marchese di San Guilano, for the Società Geografica Italiana; the Rt. Hon. A.J. Balfour, statesman, philosopher, former prime minister and the Chancellor's brother-in-law (Lord Rayleigh had married Balfour's sister); and Sir Archibald Geikie, the new President of the Royal Society. To the

Chancellor's left were Graf zu Solms-Laubach, representing the University of Strasburg, Conte Ugo Balzani for the Academia dei Lincei, and the Duke of Northumberland, for the Royal Institution.

Several Britishers knighted for accomplishments in science were sprinkled among the diners, provoking many to wonder why such honors had eluded Darwin himself. Smith was pleased to note that two untitled foreign acquaintances, Svante Arrhenius, Director of the Nobel Institute in Stockholm, and Elie Metchnikoff, Assistant Director of the Pasteur Institute in Paris, were accorded head table status. On the last day, honorary degrees were conferred in the Senate House, and the Rede Lecture was delivered by the eminent geologist Sir Archibald Geikie. A luncheon in Trinity Hall was followed by group photographs, garden parties, and a farewell dinner at the Woodheads.

The only stop on the return journey to London was at Ely to see the cathedral. After three days of "tramping about London & shopping," using the Kingsley Hotel again as headquarters, the Smiths packed two trunks with trophies and dispatched them to Liverpool to await their departure for Boston on August 27. After visiting Hyde Park and Kensington Gardens, they made a short trip to Purley to meet friends, who took Theobald for a walk on the Downs.

Theobald and Lilian headed westward for another four weeks of sightseeing. During a few days at Oxford, they explored the various colleges. Some highlights were a "walk via Marston village across Cherwell by ferry," a trip by Thames steamer to Nuneham Forest, and a band concert one evening in Worcester College Garden. The historic city of Winchester was viewed from the top of St. Giles' Hill, and they inspected the cathedral and boys' boarding school. They admired the noble English gothic style of Salisbury Cathedral, with its 400-foot high octagonal spire. In Exeter, the windows of their hotel room framed the harmoniously detailed beauty of the Cathedral.

For a fortnight, a boarding house in Lynton with a balcony overlooking Bristol Channel served as home base for various excursions. The "order of life" began with a warm bath at 7:30 A.M. and ended with bedtime at 10 o'clock. Breakfast, luncheon, tea and dinner were scheduled at 8:30 A.M., 1, 5, and 7:30 P.M., respectively. The inclusive tariff was seven shillings and sixpence daily per person. Theobald took longer walks usually alone in the morning, while Lilian accompanied him on some of the shorter strolls. Once they rode in a charabanc to Doone Valley and caught a steamer to reach Clovelly via Ilfracombe. In the evenings they alternated in reading aloud a chapter from *Westward Ho!*.

Reluctantly, they left Lynton by coach for Wells, saw the Cathedral and the Bishop's Palace, and devoted an afternoon to Glastonbury and its Abbey. The next two days were spent in visiting Gloucester Cathedral, Chepstow Castle, and the ruins of Tintern Abbey. For two nights, which included their last Sunday in Britain, they put up at the "Green Dragon" in Hereford, where they walked alongside the Wye to the waterworks, and of course visited the Cathedral—an architectural gem. Finally, at Chester, after paying respects to the ancient Cathedral and the city parks, they enjoyed a trip on the Dee to Eccleston Ferry, and a walk on the city's Roman walls. On the 27th, they left for Liverpool, to embark on the R.M.S. *Saxonia*. Despite stiff head winds, the voyage was uneventful. Reaching Boston on August 5, they were greeted at the wharf by their three children and Marshal Fabyan.

Smith's monthly account book noted the entire expenses of the whole trip as $1044.36, including $250 worth of "purchases not needed on journey, of clothing, silverware, pictures, miscs." To Lilian, on her first venture abroad, her husband had been a thoughtful if somewhat restless companion. His frugality was genetic and ineradicable. Neither complained of feeling unrested; for such a kaleidoscopic sightseeing trip was bound to be breathless and fatiguing. For her, the intensive exposure to the glories of ecclesiastical architecture was especially valued. For him, the three days in Cambridge seemed an overflowing source of memorable personal encounters and academic ceremonies in a marvelously distinguished setting. Neither of them sensed the potential awareness, resilience and endurance of the local inhabitants of that history-laden island—a misjudgment that persisted with them until the first World War was almost over.

Smith fully participated in the special events associated with the elaborate ceremonial inauguration of President Lowell, October 5–7, 1909. On the morning of the 5th, he still autopsied a horse at the antitoxin and vaccine laboratory, and from noon until 6:30 was occupied with class work or researches in his department at the Medical School. But into his scrapbook ultimately went Platform Tickets for every scheduled event during the next two days.

At 9:30 A.M. on the 6th, Harvard University representatives and delegates of universities, colleges and learned institutions solemnly marched in procession from Phillips Brooks House to the Platform in University Hall, led by the Band and the Chief Marshal, while alumni and other witnesses to the Inauguration found their seats on the lawn in College Yard. The procession comprised four distinct components, the first three representing in turn the University as an academic Institution—Deans, Professors, Associate Professors, and so forth; the delegates from kindred institutions; and representatives of state and federal governments. The fourth group consisted of eight individual participants, ranging from the Corporation Secretary, the Bursar, and the Librarian, bearing respectively the Seal, the Keys, and the Charter of Harvard University, to the Rt. Rev. William Lawrence, Bishop of Massachusetts, who invoked the final blessing. The last figure was the President-Elect, who walked alone. Near the head of the procession, immediately behind a phalanx of Members of the Corporation, President Emeritus Eliot strode resolutely in similar solitude.

The Exercises in the Yard opened with a Latin choral. A prayer from the Dean of the Faculty of Divinity, followed by a Latin oration, heralded the Induction of President Lowell by the President of the Board of Overseers. Between two chorals, Lowell delivered his Inaugural Address. After honorary degrees were conferred, the proceedings ended with the episcopal blessing. Following luncheon at the Harvard Union, delegates and other guests assembled for another formal procession, this time from Massachusetts to Memorial Hall to attend Exercises organized by the Harvard Alumni Association. The ladies accompanying the delegates were luncheon guests at Radcliffe College in Bertram Hall. Women delegates came only from three women's colleges in the United States—Wellesley, Mount Holyoke, and Bryn Mawr—while 164 institutions, including five other women's colleges, and all thirty-one foreign institutions, were represented by men. Evening festivities included a concert by the Boston Symphony Orchestra, after which Harvard students offered a "Celebration" at the Stadium. Theobald Smith accepted instead an invitation to a banquet tendered by Alexander Agassiz at the Somerset Hotel to members of the National Academy of Sciences.

On October 7, Smith attended in Sanders Theatre the Presentation of Delegates to the Governing Board and Faculties of Harvard University. While the alumni lunched at the Colonial Club as guests of the Harvard Club of Boston, the Delegates and Members of Faculties were invited by President and Mrs. Lowell to a Reception and Luncheon in the Faculty Room at University Hall. Special trolley cars were run from Harvard Square to the Medical School on Longwood Avenue in Boston between 3 and 4 P.M. Theobald Smith showed visitors around his department and turned up for afternoon tea offered by the Faculty of Medicine and the Harvard Medical Alumni Association. The two days of ceremonial events and hospitality culminated in a splendid dinner given that evening at the Harvard Union in honor of the Delegates by the President and Fellows of Harvard College.

Commencement Day at Harvard, June 29, 1910 was a splendid occasion, the heat tempered by a light breeze, the College Yard gay with laughter and song, and many distinguished figures present. Theodore Roosevelt, some fifteen months footloose from the nation's presidency, was now pleased to chair the meeting of the Harvard Alumni Association and attend his 1880 class reunion. Sanders Theatre was filled to capacity with relatives and friends of nearly a thousand new graduates joining the ranks of Harvard's faithful sons. An official salutarian flattered the famous, offering greetings liberally in Latin, and unbent with classical gallantries for the ladies.

The dozen recipients of honorary degrees included Charles Evans Hughes (LL.D.), Governor of New York State and U.S. Supreme Court Justice-designate, "a guardian of our institutions in a tribunal that demands both the learning of the jurist and the wisdom of the statesman;" and John Pierpont Morgan (LL.D.), "public-spirited citizen . . . who . . . twice in times of stress repelled a national danger of financial panic." The honorary doctorates of science were conferred upon Sir John Murray (1841–1914), the British pioneer oceanographer; Theodore William Richards (1868–1928), Harvard's professor of chemistry "who has weighed the atoms in his balance;" and Theobald Smith, "who taught men to seek in insects the source of human plagues" and stood among the great benefactors of mankind.

Pasted into Smith's scrapbook were letters of congratulation from his pastor C.F. Dole, and from Simon Flexner. His diary references to the occasion were completely matter-of-fact and laconic. Immediately before and after Commencement, Smith worked as usual in the laboratory. The month's highlights were recorded thus: 8th. "Read paper at Mass. Med. Soc." 14th - 15th. "Exam. candidates for higher degrees." 20th. "Conference at State Bd. on poliomyelitis." 24th. "Speak at closing Exercises of Girls' Latin school." 25th. "Lve. for Dr. Ernst's summer home at Manomet with Lilian who does the cooking." (Ernst was in Japan; he invited the Smith family to use his place while he was abroad.) 29th. "Harvard Commencement. Receive hon. degree of Doctor of Science."[11]

Theobald's decision to give one of three 10-minute addresses at the Closing Exercises of the Girls' Latin School of Boston on June 24, 1910, a few days before the Harvard Commencement, was influenced probably by the fact that his two daughters had graduated with distinction from this school, and that the headmaster was about to retire. One of the other invited speakers was a future summertime neighbor, Rev. Edward Cummings, Congregational minister and advocate of temperance and world peace. Smith addressed the girls as mature women. He deplored that the college world, which many of them would be entering, "is not free from temptations which tend to frustrate the object for which it was established, and for which you will segregate yourselves under more or less artificial conditions for 4 years."

It is fast becoming a miniature everyday world with its excitement about insane and time-consuming objects. Among your male college friends there is even a tendency to run the college, dictate its policy, and resort to strikes to enforce their wishes . . . You must not try to get an education and life experience at the same time. You need not turn a deaf ear to the great problems of the day, conservation, woman's suffrage, socialism, the tariff, international disarmament : . . Study them if you have time, but do not take sides until you can take a part.

Smith applauded the benefits of an advanced liberal education but realized that the world needed "men and women trained to do something well." Specialization was not incompatible with a liberal education, but to be "useful we must be specialists."

> Specializing has its evil, but it is the price we must pay for organization, cooperation, and the division of labor. If we must pay it, we may as well do it cheerfully and without grumbling. In the end we are all of us narrow specialists when confronted with the intellectual achievements of the whole race . . . The essence of our intellectual existence is to look into the future, to anticipate and to prevent.[12]

As his renown spread, Theobald Smith's invitations to participate in ceremonial occasions multiplied. Most of these were gladly declined; but he was upset to be unable to attend a Testimonial dinner on April 2, 1910 at Baltimore commemorating William Welch's election to the presidency of the American Medical Association. He seldom missed a meeting of the Rockefeller Institute's Board of Scientific Directors, however inconveniently timed. (The Board met one snowy Saturday night in midwinter at 8 P.M. at Simon Flexner's apartment and adjourned with business still unfinished at 1 A.M.) Smith attended four meetings of the Board in the spring of 1910, each absorbing about three days. One of these, held during the second weekend of January, was especially memorable. On Sunday the 9th, his Day Card curtly noted: "Visit Institute and see paralyzed monkeys (Poliomyelitis). Arr. home 6:30 P.M."[13]

Theobald Smith had developed a lively interest in the disease misleadingly termed infantile paralysis, and for several years was considered an authority on this malady. He gave talks and informal advice freely; attended a State Health Conference on Poliomyelitis in June 1910; and on July 7, 1910 left for Springfield to study an outbreak on his own initiative: "Drive about town in auto to see cases of the disease until 6 P.M." Next day he inspected the dam and filter beds of the town's water supply—he always suspected these outbreaks to be excretumborne. Simon Flexner used the much greater facilities of the Rockefeller Institute (including the cooperation of Smith's former assistant, Paul Lewis) to extend his investigations of poliomyelitis, with mixed success.

During the year, he also attended a reception and four additional meetings of the Cancer Commission, of which he was a member; and turned up at six evening meetings of the American Academy of Arts and Sciences as a member of its Council. Such punctilious attendance helped to build his reputation as a scientist of conscientious goodwill and broad interests. Besides, he greatly enjoyed the mixed fare available to members of the Academy of Arts and Sciences. At one meeting, for instance, the distinguished astronomer Percival Lowell (elder brother to President Lawrence Lowell of Harvard University) reported on his recent observations of Halley's Comet.[14] One month later, on December 14, 1901, Smith took part in the notable Celebration of the One Thousandth Meeting of the Academy, accompanied by "a substantial Repast," at the University Club, Boston. The menu of bygone dishes commenced with "Baked Indian Whortleberry Pudding."[15]

Theobald Smith's reputation as a competent and scrupulous research scientist, reinforced by the wide range of his publications, led to his frequent serving as expert witness in court cases involving sanitation issues and on bodies investigating various public health hazards. He actually enjoyed the consequent exposures to diverse problems and to distinguished consultants, and did not object to banking the fees.

Smith's familiarity with the bacteriology of water led to his continuous membership on the Charles River Dam Committee since 1903. In 1904, he was an expert witness in the Chicago-St. Louis Drainage Canal dispute. He declined an invitation in 1911 to testify on behalf of New York State in a suit to restrain the State of New Jersey from "discharging into New York Bay a vast quantity of raw sewage."[16] His special interest in air-borne infection led to his appointment in 1904 by the New York City Board of Health to a Commission on Acute Respiratory Infections, along with a distinguished group of physicians and bacteriologists from leading medical schools near New York. In that year also he was nominated to a committee to consider the growing number and complexity of tuberculosis congresses. The unanimous decision to organize a single United States society for the study and prevention of this disease led to the formation of the National Association for the Study and Prevention of Tuberculosis.

In April 1907, Theobald Smith accepted an invitation to join a group of scientific advisers to a university team, led by a zealous professor of chemistry, in researches into the wholesomeness of meat treated with potassium nitrate. The project, subsidized by the industry concerned, ended ultimately, for reasons outside Smith's control, in an out-of-date five-volume treatise. In January 1911, he again joined a group of experts, appointed this time under U.S. governmental auspices to protect the public from the potentially harmful effects of food preservatives and adulterants. The group disbanded for political reasons. Certain details of these involvements are provided for their historic interest.

The American Meat Packers Association supported the researches on meat chemistry instituted at the University of Illinois by Prof. H.S. Grindley and his associates in the Laboratory of Physiological Chemistry, Department of Animal Husbandry. President Edmund J. James of that University was keen to have these experiments extended. They would begin by determining any effects upon human health of the presence of saltpeter in the curing mixture for meats. It was proposed to form a National Commission, composed of "men prominent in the fields of human physiology and medicine and human nutrition," who would devise and review the experimental details, inspect the work as opportunity offered, and approve the conclusions. The University would meet all experimental expenses and costs of attending the Commission's sessions, which were to be held at the Urbana campus, and each member would receive an honorarium of $500 on publication of the findings.

Smith was invited by President James to join Professors J.J. Abel of Johns Hopkins University, R.H. Chittenden of Yale, A.F. Mathews of Chicago and H.S. Grindley on the Commission. The others had met already in New York under Abel's chairmanship. They all felt, wrote Abel, "that your wide knowledge, your experience and ability would be of the utmost assistance to us."[17] They were "guaranteed the most complete independence of action." John Abel, whose parents were of Rhenish origin, was two years older than Theobald Smith. He had procured a Ph.B. degree from the University of Michigan in 1883, and did postgraduate work under Newell Martin at Johns Hopkins University. Currently, he was Professor of Pharmacology and Physiological Chemistry at Johns Hopkins University. Like Smith, he preferred research to classroom teaching and had an international reputation. Smith accepted the invitation, provided his work was "profitable to the cause under investigation and not incompatible with my several other duties here." He added quixotically that in the event of his withdrawal before completing the task, he would "waive all claims to compensation and continue to aid the Commission in all possible ways."[18]

At irregular intervals between May 1907 and January 1917 Smith undertook eight trips, mostly very inconvenient, in connection with the University of Illinois Nutrition Committee. The University was served by the railroad at Champaign and Urbana, but could only be reached from Boston by a tedious train journey through Chicago, sometimes many hours delayed. Besides, the obligations of the Commission proved much more time-consuming than expected, especially for Theobald Smith. During two fairly short periods, he dispatched at least fifty letters (the majority handwritten) to Grindley and other commissioners, and faithfully reviewed reams of experimental protocols and chapters of text sent for his critical appraisal.

The series of meetings began auspiciously enough. On May 9, 1907, Theobald Smith broke away early from the Seventh Triennial Meeting of the Congress of Physicians and Surgeons at Washington and took a train together with John Abel to Champaign, where they were met by Grindley. He conducted them to a lecture by Chittendem on the Urbana campus. That evening, the University of Illinois Faculty hosted a Dinner in honor of the visitors. "Auld Lang Syne" and appropriate College songs were featured.[19] Next morning the Commission met and encouraged Grindley and the University to go ahead with the project.

The Commission's second meeting was held in the Chemistry Building at Urbana again under Abel's chairmanship. Theobald left home the day after Christmas, and had to wait five hours for his train at Indianapolis. During this visit he lunched and supped "at the club where the KNO_3 squad of twenty odd students live."[20] Grindley soon realized that Smith was the only member with a working knowledge of relevant bacteriological techniques and took full advantage of his conscientious goodwill. Smith had developed an interest in fecal anaerobic bacteria and emphasized the importance of noting changes in the intestinal bacterial flora. Unable to find any better applicant, Grindley appointed W.J. MacNeal, in whom he had little confidence, as assistant chief in bacteriology. Smith advised how samples should be collected and offered to go over MacNeal's ideas on procedures with him. By the end of January 1909, Grindley had swamped the non-resident Commissioners by dispatching to each of them all available "Exhibits of the Saltpeter Investigations," alphabetically labelled, A to U.

In the New Year of 1909, Abel inflicted a serious set-back upon the Commission by resigning. Smith was non-committal when asked by James for advice on how to fill the vacancy: "I prefer to leave the matter in the hands of the other members upon whom the extra burden will largely fall if the gap remains unfilled." Chittenden proposed Prof. F.F. Wesbrook, University of Minnesota. Smith acknowledged many years of friendly acquaintanceship with him but questioned the advisability of selecting another person with the specialties of Public Health, Bacteriology and Pathology. However, he wrote to Wesbrook in May 1909, who politely suggested that a clinician be considered. No immediate choice was made.

The next meeting of the Commission was particularly hard to arrange as the three non-resident commissioners had other obligations. Theobald Smith was in the midst of his Lowell lecture series, and President Eliot's retirement was imminent. The group finally settled on May 7–9, 1909, when they held three sessions. After reviewing the data, the commissioners wrote a joint letter to President James, urging prompt and full publication of the work to date, and commending the University for fostering the inquiry. "Rarely had such an extended scientific investigation in the field of nutrition been undertaken."[21]

Fortified by the Commission's letter of endorsement, Grindley now requested the University of Illinois Board of Trustees to grant his Research Laboratory $15,000 to ensure prompt and complete publication of "the results of the nutrition investigation . . . during the past two years." He extolled the accomplishment as "the most extensive, thorough, exhaustive, and scientific investigation upon man ever before made in the world." These studies of the nutrition of twenty-four men controlled for 220 days would be of "inestimable value to the clinician, the physician, the surgeon, the pathologist, the physiologist, the bacteriologist, the biological chemist," as well as to the sciences of human and animal nutrition, public health and sanitation. Grindley almost comically asserted his own claims, adding: "I know positively that this statement is not too strong, nor does it exaggerate the importance or value of this work."[22] His proposition became irresistible to the President and Board when he assured them that on publication of the report the University of Illinois would move to the front rank in scientific work. In July 1909, the Board approved Grindley's application.

At a meeting in May 1910, the entire manuscript of Volume I, including alternative versions of some passages, was placed before the Commission. On many issues a consensus could not be reached. Evidently, far too much was being passed on to the busy external members of the Commission, while Grindley and MacNeal and their laboratory associates were developing divergent viewpoints. However, Grindley thanked Smith "very sincerely for the valuable help and the excellent suggestions which I received from you." The Report's future progress would owe much to the excellent ideas aired at the Commission's meeting.[23] Furthermore, there was general agreement that Dr. David L. Edsall, Professor of Therapeutics and Pharmacology, University of Pennsylvania (soon to become Harvard's Jackson Professor at the Massachusetts General Hospital, and in 1917, its medical dean), should be asked to become the fifth Commission member. In sending a written invitation to Edsall to join them, Theobald Smith stated that practically all the experimental work on the effects of saltpeter on human volunteers was completed and that only one or two more meetings at the University of Illinois were in prospect. Edsall at first declined, but when Smith and Chittenden visited him at his home in Philadelphia, he was persuaded, and faithfully attended future meetings of the Commission.

They all met again at the Hoffman House in New York City on November 5 and 6, 1910. For several weeks beforehand, the four non-resident members had received from Grindley further batches of extensively-revised manuscript material. The meeting discussed at length the application of statistical methods to the mass of accumulated data. Smith (who sometimes set himself calculus conundrums for mental exercise) enjoyed this part of the meeting. He informed Grindley that he had asked B.O. Peirce, the celebrated Harvard mathematician, how best to treat their data. Peirce had thought that success here would depend on "the degree of acquaintance of the mathematician with the biological significance of the data." Grindley proposed that the preparation of Volumes III, IV and V, comprising only experimental findings, could be left to the editor-in-chief.

A fortnight later, a serious breach between himself and MacNeal was exposed by the distribution of two versions of a proposed chapter for Volume II. Exhibit B, prepared by MacNeal, seemed "incomplete and superficial" to

Grindley, whose Exhibit A provided a more thorough study of the data available. At the next meeting at Urbana in February 1911, a conciliatory atmosphere prevailed. Grindley arranged a dinner, which President James attended. A tentative publication schedule was agreed upon, beginning later in 1911 with Volume III. Grindley suddenly fell ill, and before he was restored to working activity in September 1911, three volumes (III, IV and V) of *Studies in Nutrition* had been published or sent to the printer. In all, five volumes eventually appeared, each carrying the clumsy subtitle *An Investigation of the Influence of Saltpeter on the Nutrition and Health of Man with Reference to its Occurrence in Cured Meats*. Volumes III (1911) and IV (1912) cited Henry S. Grindley as author, with various assistants also named. Both volumes proclaimed their contents on the title-page as "The Experimental Data of the Bio-chemical Investigations." Volume V (1912), "The Data of the Physical, Physiological and Bacteriological Observations," appeared under the authorship of Ward J. MacNeal, with four named assistants, after MacNeal apparently had "terminated his services at the University of Illinois" on August 31, 1911.

By early 1913, President James was chafing at the delays. He wrote to Smith: "We are very anxious to close up the work of this Commission as soon as possible and get our final report before the public." Because the scope of the investigation had been enlarged and the work prolonged much beyond the University's expectation, a cheque for $400 (four-fifths of the total due) would be sent to him shortly.[24] The commission last met on January 12–13, 1917, at the McAlpin Hotel, and then disbanded. All four non-resident members and Grindley were present. Their main purpose, "to go over MSS of vol. I of report," resulted at last in the publication of Volume I ("Discussion and Interpretation of the Biochemical Data") of the *Studies*. The authors were Henry S. Grindley and Harold H. Mitchell. The latter had been one of Grindley's assistant authors for Volume IV.

Twelve years elapsed before Volume II was published in 1929. The author was Ward J. MacNeal, with two cited assistants. This final volume appeared about the time when Grindley retired from the University of Illinois with the rank of Professor Emeritus, and twenty years after MacNeal had suddenly left. MacNeal's introduction to this volume stated that the various chapters "were completed prior to August 31, 1911," that the delayed publication was due to "factors beyond the control of any of the authors of this volume," and that an obvious "conflict between the two joint principal authors of this report" concerned not only the "personal viewpoint, methods of presentation and interpretation of scientific data," but sometimes "even accuracy of record of observations."

In vain one may search the literature on the history of meat preservation for references to *Studies in Nutrition (1911–1929)* by Grindley, MacNeal and others.

The reasons seem fairly obvious. First, the mode of preservation was super-seded, and the results therefore rendered superfluous, during the long interval between publication of the statistical data (Vols. III, IV, and V) and their interpre-tation (Vols. I and II). Secondly, a difficult project became unsuccessful through the amateurishness or naivety of its participants—from Grindley's self-praise in claiming the unique importance of the enterprise, and James's ambition to es-tablish his institution in the forefront of biochemical and bacteriological re-search, to the geniality of the arm's-length experts who encouraged progress when they should have called a halt, who endured repeated inconveniences, and were not even mentioned in the final publication. Thirdly, while a minor dispute over the interpretation of certain statistical data might have marred, but not de-stroyed, the usefulness of the work, MacNeal's implication that some observa-tions were inaccurately recorded threw all of them in doubt, and negated what-ever efforts had to be made to publish Volume I.

In some aspects of food chemistry, Grindley had been knowledgeable and pro-ductive. Early in their acquaintanceship, Smith had thanked him for sending a re-print of a paper on roasting meat.[25] During a decade of membership of the Nu-trition Committee, Theobald Smith addressed various groups on topics related to food preservation and published two articles on meat and offal as vehicles of human disease. These publications, together with his editorial in 1898 on the waste and destruction of wholesome meat from tuberculous cattle with minimal lesions,[26] added meat hygiene to his acknowledged fields of authority as microbi-ologist. His address entitled "What Is Diseased Meat, and What Is the Relation to Meat Inspection?", given at the end of April 1909, was presented within three weeks of completing the series of eight Lowell lectures. Reviewed carefully in the *Boston Evening Transcript* of April 30, it was reported as "timely and to the point . . . a masterly discussion."

To Theobald Smith the notion of any kind of waste was philosophically ab-horrent:

> The discovery of waste and its utilization marks many epochs in our material progress. We are everywhere beginning to see waste . . . To discover it means to utilize it. The enlightenment of any nation or community may be measured by its adjustment of means and ends to one another. If there is much waste in attaining a certain end, intelligence is low, for human ends defeat themselves through loss of energy and resources . . . Science furnishes us the insight needed to accurately ad-just means and ends to each other.

Nowadays, some eighty years later, despite all the advances in agronomy, genet-ics and transportation, famine stalks many lands, and protein deficiency is particularly prevalent. More than science is needed to furnish us the insight to "adjust means and ends to each other."

In January 1911, Theobald was asked to replace Christian Herter (who had died the preceding December) on the Referee Board on Food Adulteration as Consultant Scientist to the United States Department of Agriculture. "Drs. Remsen & Chittenden come to persuade me to become a member of the Referee Bd. U.S.," he succinctly recorded.[27] The chairman was Ira Remsen, a distinguished chemist who had succeeded Dr. D. Gilman as President of Johns Hopkins University. The associated experts were J.H. Long, Northwestern University Medical School, R. H. Chittenden, Yale University, and E.A. Taylor, University of Pennsylvania. Chittenden had recommended Theobald Smith as a suitable replacement. Harvard University's President Lowell gave permission, and President Taft approved the appointment, which carried a retainer of $2,000 per annum. Duties were to be "as required by the Secretary of Agriculture." The appointment was described "as showing the desire of the President and Secretary of Agriculture to have questions submitted to the Referee Board investigated in the fullest manner and from various standpoints."[28]

Smith first met his colleagues in Remsen's office at Johns Hopkins University on April 7, 1911 to consider the reported use of sulfur dioxide as a food preservative. On May 10, Smith went to New Haven to review the experiments at Yale for giving foodstuffs containing copper sulfate to dogs, and returned there at the end of June to autopsy six of the experimental animals. This work brought adverse publicity to the Committee. Early in August, a Congressional Committee's investigation provoked this handwritten reassurance from Remsen: "It is all over and nothing at all disagreeable or unpleasant resulted, whatever the papers may say."[29] To Herter's widow Remsen wrote:

> I told the Investigating committee that there is some "malign influence at work tending to undermine and discredit the work of the Board." Afterwards, one of the newspaper men came to me and said "There is a man here who regularly furnishes that stuff to the press. Get the Committee to put him on the stand and ask who pays him." I think I know . . . The Secretary is and always has been most appreciative of our work . . . I told the Committee my skin has become thicker . . . owing to these daily attacks, and perhaps this is to be my chief reward, for a thick skin has its advantages.[30]

Smith contributed a highly specialized section of a report on vegetables greened with sulfate, entitled "Histological Examination of the Tissues of Dogs and Monkeys." This was embodied, along with lengthier sections prepared by other members, in the 461-page monograph published in 1913 as *Report No. 97* of the Department of Agriculture.[31] The Report concluded that copper salts, even in very small quantities, might be injurious to human health. In later activities of the Board, saccharin, sulfur, and alum were among the additives considered.

After March 1914, the annual salary of the consultants was replaced by an allowance of $10.50 per diem "for days actually employed."[32] There was mutual dissatisfaction between the Board and Congress. Remsen suggested, supported by Chittenden, that the Board should submit its collective resignation through him, and that in future endeavors to secure outside expert opinions the Secretary of Agriculture could work through the President of the National Academy of Sciences.[33] Theobald Smith's resignation from the Referee Board was accepted officially as of June 30, 1915.

18

VISITING PROFESSOR
AT BERLIN

The German Exchange Professorships were first proposed at the time of Prince Henry of Prussia's visit to Harvard in the spring of 1902 when German-American enthusiasm was high. They were inaugurated in 1905–06, at which time the Rev. Francis G. Peabody went to Berlin and Wilhelm Ostwald, the chemist, came to Harvard. (Peabody, a pioneer university lecturer in social problems, established a famous Department of Social Ethics in 1906 at Harvard.)

Theobald Smith had indicated his willingness to be considered for the 1910–11 Exchange Professorship, but Hugo Münsterberg was chosen. A note from President Lowell early in 1911 indicated that the time had come for a new list to be submitted to the German Government, and he sincerely hoped that Smith would consent to his name being entered again.[1] In recent months, Smith had felt "used up" and "tired & stale in work of all kinds,"[2] so he informed Lowell in writing that this name could stand, and that the exchange professorship would be extremely stimulating. However, he warned that he would require a preliminary half-year's leave of absence to enable him to "prevent loss of research material here and also prepare for the work abroad."[3] Later that month, Smith again wrote to Lowell, suggesting that his candidacy should be withheld until he knew the specific duties, and had been reassured that members of a professional faculty were eligible. "As to the language I should have no difficulty meeting the requirement you mentioned."[4]

The president's secretary, Jerome D. Greene, informed Smith that the visiting professor received full salary, with a special allowance of $1,200, and customarily gave one advanced course and a second course for a larger number of students, but there was no rule about this. The work usually began shortly after mid-October and extended to about March 1. Whereas the Roosevelt Professorship at Columbia University "frankly avows a semi-diplomatic mission, and is necessarily given to men whose subjects have a pretty broad, if not a popular appeal," Harvard preferred to send first-class scholars in any subject, "provided their teaching would be profitable to a reasonable number of hearers." The chief objective of Prof. T.W. Richards, for example, had been to initiate "about 10 German chemists already holding the Ph.D. into his methods of atomic weight determination."[5]

In March 1911, Geheimrat Dr. Friedrich Schmidt, the Berlin University intermediary, notified President Lowell that although the Exchange Commission would be pleased to accept Professor Charles S. Minot, their first choice was the other nominee, Professor Theobald Smith, whom Geheimrat Prof. Carl Flügge, the Berlin hygienist, would take under his wing. Lowell quoted from Geh. Schmidt's letter (in German) to him, and added: "I am glad you are going, and hope you will enjoy it very much."[6] Smith read the letter with "mingled feelings of delight and misgivings." To make the opportunity "creditable to the University, and a profitable and enjoyable event to me," he must be properly prepared. After a long talk with Prof. T.W. Richards, he felt it impossible to be ready for the *intensive* rather than *extensive* approach to the work, which the Berlin students and staff would anticipate, before March 1912, when he could supplement Flügge's summer session lectures and laboratories. But then he would be obliged to return in August, for he was President of the Section on Bacteriology and Parasitology of the International Congress of Hygiene and Demography, meeting in Washington in September 1912.[7]

Lowell replied that he saw no objection to Smith choosing the summer instead of the winter semester, but he would have to write to the Berlin authorities about it. Meanwhile, the President and Fellows of Harvard College voted Smith leave of absence on full salary for the second half of the academic year 1911–12. As soon as the appointment was announced publicly on March 28, Charles S. Minot sent a congratulatory note: "No one else could represent our School so well and fittingly at Berlin as yourself."[8] Francis G. Peabody wrote him that he was thankful for the University's sake that Smith had accepted the task. His own experience had plainly shown that to commend the exchange professorship to academic opinion in Germany, it must be "detached from loose ideas of international comity and held to severe and elevated standards of scholarship." Two masters, "the love of science and the interests of diplomacy," could not be served. Peabody praised Geheimrat F. Schmidt's trustworthiness and offered his personal help. Before leaving for Berlin, Smith must dine at Peabody's house with "the now rapidly expanding group" of exchange professors, and Professor Kükenthal, the current visiting German professor to Harvard. "We shall all want to give you before your departure a great deal of unnecessary advice."[9] Smith worried that he might fail to convey a fresh viewpoint: "The overshadowing problem is what to bring to our German colleagues which is not a reimportation of their own possessions." He intended to make an "inventory of ideas and concepts which . . . may perhaps give me more courage that I have at present."[10]

Flügge showed pleasurable anticipation as prospective host. At Smith's disposal were "a quiet room looking north, and all the facilities of the Institute, which . . . in some respects are adequate (e.g., about 50 microscopes with oil immersions, etc.)." If necessary, Flügge would share his own summer-semester course of lectures on parasitic diseases, thus ensuring a good audience. He also favored a weekly public lecture in the field of microbiology, to a "presumably very large audience of students from other faculties," and perhaps three to six evening lectures during the semester to more advanced listeners (docents and practitioners) about his personal researches and results.[11]

Schmidt wrote Lowell that the university rector and representatives of the Exchange Commission begged reconsideration of the summer-semester plan. The winter session carried weighty advantages, such as greater attendance at lectures and increased personal contacts between professors. After pondering the matter overnight, Theobald Smith suggested that the wishes of his prospective hosts might be met in part if he left Boston during the Christmas holidays, so that he would have two months of the winter-session in Berlin.[12] On July 3, Schmidt telegraphed that this proposal was acceptable, and wrote also to thank Lowell for cooperating.

Schmidt had managed to insert a provisional statement in the 1912 calendar that Professor Smith would lecture on microbiology during January and February, probably on Mondays from 5–7 P.M. Professor Flügge was still awaiting an answer about his lecture proposals. The delay was due to a severe attack of coliform cystitis, which kept Smith in bed for several days. He now sent a lengthy outline of a course of two lectures weekly during January and February on the host-parasite relationship in microbiology and parasitology.[13] He hoped that such a course might arouse some interest amongst biologists as well as medical men. Flügge acquiesced and extended congratulations on the honorary doctorate awarded Smith by the Medical Faculty of the University of Breslau.

Theobald Smith had been notified recently of this new distinction by letter from Prof. H. Uhthoff, Dean of the Medical Faculty at Breslau.[14] In commemoration of the University's first centenary, celebrated on August 3, 1911, honorary doctorates were conferred upon four Americans: In Theology, Rev. Benjamin W. Bacon of Yale; in Philosophy, Charles W. Eliot, President Emeritus of Harvard; in Law, President Nicholas Murray Butler of Columbia; in Medicine, Prof. Theobald Smith of Harvard. Printed copies of his diploma (of which several were distributed in two scrapbooks) proclaimed the fundamental importance of Smith's prime discoveries—the transmissibility of certain diseases by insects, and the differentiation of human and bovine tuberculosis. A letter from "Camp Rottenweather," signed "Your obedient servant Philip H. Smith," began "Dearest crowned head, Congratulations, congratulations, on the great news."[15] Ehrlich received an honorary doctorate from the University of Breslau in the following year.

Theobald Smith, his wife and three children, aged twenty-one, nineteen, and sixteen years, left New York on December 9 and arrived in Bremen on December 17. The transatlantic journey was uneventful. "Weather good all the way . . . Arr. Bremerhaven 2 A.M. for Berlin traveling all day till 6 P.M."[16] They spent the first two nights in Berlin in a hotel on the Kurfürstendamm and then moved to the nearby Pension Tscheuschner at 112 Kurfürstenstrasse, which became the family headquarters. On the first day, Smith called on Flügge at the Hygienic Institute. He sat through Flügge's lecture and wrote out a notice in German in his own hand, stating that for the next quarter, beginning January 8, 1912, he would lecture publicly on Mondays from 5 to 7 in the Auditorium of the Hygienic Institute, on the relationship between parasitism and disease. The notice was signed "Dr. Theobald Smith, Professor a.d. Harvard Universität, Cambridge, U.S.A."

The whole family witnessed Christmas and New Year celebrations, but Smith himself spent the mornings at the Institute, and sometimes returned to it in the afternoons, between dinner at the Pension from 2 to 3 P.M. and supper at 7:30 P.M. During the first week of January 1912, he worked daily at preparing either his public lectures or the formal Inaugural Address, the *Antrittsrede*. The time and place for the latter was set out in a handwritten letter from Rektor Lenz as Saturday, January 13, 1912, punctually at 12:15 P.M., in the Old Hall of the Royal Friedrich-Wilhelm University. Prinz August Wilhelm would represent the Kaiser. An announcement to this effect was printed and distributed on the 10th to all professors and docents of the university.

At the appointed hour, except for the vacant front row, the lecture hall was "filled to its utmost capacity by students, physicians, and many army officers."[17] Besides Professors Penck, Harting, Hildebrandt, Ostertag, Wassermann and Kisskalt, several Americans were present, including President Edmund J. James of the University of Illinois. Theobald Smith's wife and their two daughters sat in the second row with the Rektor's wife, Frau Professor Lenz. The first row was reserved for Prinz August Wilhelm, who was escorted to his place, along with the lecturer, by Rektor Lenz and Ministry-Director F. Schmidt. Following the Rector's introduction, Theobald Smith took the podium—a "simple, slender man, with a very expressive scholarly head," as a local journalist described him.[18] Several newspaper accounts of the occasion appear in the 1912 scrapbook, with an off-print of the lecture, entitled "Parasitismus und Krankheit," published in a well-known German medical weekly,[19] as previously agreed in correspondence between Smith and its editor. The address was given in fluent but accented German, which some found difficult to follow because of rapid delivery and low voice.

Smith began by praising German contributions to bacteriology, a science which had been initiated by discoveries "made in Germany." He expounded one of his fundamental tenets, that parasitism is a widespread biological phenomenon. The various phases of an infective disease of the host, from the healthy carrier state to the acutely lethal attack, represent different degrees of disturbance in a given host-parasite relationship. In genuine parasitism, there is a mutual adaptation, an equilibrium, between host and parasite in which the latter is the obvious beneficiary, although the host remains undamaged. This equilibrium might be dislocated or shattered by various factors, particularly such trappings of progressive civilization as international travel. According to Koch, the main defensive mechanisms involve suppression or destruction of the parasite, while Pasteur advocated immunization of the host. Chemotherapy was a third possible alternative. Dorothea Smith, then about twenty-one years old, remembered the Prince turning around to ask the girls, "How do you amuse yourselves in Berlin?" The younger daughter Lilian recollected that during the lecture she had a clear view of the wrinkled Hohenzollern neck, encased in a high collar.

Both girls went to school to learn German, and Lilian still spoke it quite well in later life. She remembered, almost romantically, the trumpet motif from *The Flying Dutchman* resounding ahead of Kaiser Wilhelm II, as he was driven three times a day through the Brandenburger Thor, while people stood at attention until he passed. They accompanied their mother on many of the social calls the Frau Professor had to make. Philip also picked up enough German to get around, though his studies at a school for foreigners, and with a private tutor, were curtailed. He found the Berliners boorish, but loved the countryside and enjoyed sightseeing alone. Prof. Ostertag was his social mentor, and his son an occasional companion in the capital, but contacts with them were few. Life became more straightforward when the elder Ostertag persuaded his father that Philip should wear a German suit and square-toed shoes and his cap be replaced by a "derby."

Smith was accustomed to living and working as it were at the periphery of a great university, and the many reciprocal benefits of the exchange professorships included the sense of belonging to a closely integrated community of scholars. Smith made courtesy calls punctiliously upon academic colleagues and was liberal with his visiting cards. University notices were sent to him, such as a black-bordered announcement from Rektor Lenz that Dr. med. Julius Pagel (the distinguished medical historian) had died on January 21, 1912 and would be interred in the Jewish cemetery at Weissensee at noon on February 2. He called at the Kaiser Friedrich Institut für Fortbildungskurse für Ärzte (Institute for Continuing Medical Education) and visited G. Gaffky, Koch's successor as Director of the Institut für Infektionskrankheiten.

Smith took his lecture course seriously and put several hours of preparation into each session. Nevertheless, student attendance was disappointing. The absentee pattern in Berlin differed from that of the Harvard Medical School, where absence from classes was accountable. The course-plan in Germany, with electives (drawn up and printed in 1902)[20] was so intense, that a common corrective was to absent oneself from tedious or redundant components. To the research assistants, to specialists in microbiology and immunology, and to senior workers in related fields, the quietly stimulating, thought-provoking quality of Smith's lectures and demonstrations were commensurate with the exceptional care governing their preparation. Therefore, several instructors were usually present and his research assistants turned up faithfully.

Many distinguished professional men heard his first public address on January 8. Geheimrat Gaffky patronized three of the eight lectures in the winter semester; once he came alone, and on another occasion with Dr. W.P. Dunbar of Hamburg. The lecture course resumed for the summer semester on April 29. Geh. Schmidt had rightly warned of poor student attendance. Despite preparing all day for the first lecture, so few students turned up that Theobald cancelled it. Their attendance did not improve. On June 3, his day card recorded the melancholy news: "Working all day prep,[aring] for lecture but students failed to appear." A few came on the 10th.

Theobald Smith attended the sessions of the Berlin Microbiological Society whenever possible, and on March 7 presented two papers. One described the mechanism and applications of his fermentation tube, and the other illustrated with slides the pathogenesis of generalized *Bacillus abortus* infection in guinea pigs.[21] Cultures of that bacillus produced tubercle-like lesions when injected into these animals, but the infection was seldom fatal. In January 1912, soon after Smith arrived in Berlin, these findings were published by himself and Marshal Fabyan in a German journal.[22] Meanwhile Fabyan had pursued the investigation alone and had prepared a more detailed, illustrated report for an American journal.[23] Two days later, Smith addressed the Anglo-American Medical Club on "Alimentary tuberculosis with special reference to cow's milk."[24] His lectures to such groups were received with enthusiasm.

His connection with the State Board of Health of Massachusetts helped Theobald to build a friendly relationship with the Prussian public health authorities. On May 7 Theobald Smith gave an evening lecture on "American Public Health Work" to the German Society for Public Health, after which he and some members of the Society went to the Heidelberger Restaurant on the Dorotheenstrasse—a favorite meeting place for Americans. A similar "reunion" at the "Heidelberger" followed his lecture two evenings later to the Verein für vergleichende Pathologie (Association for Comparative Pathology) on "Race Formation in Micro-organisms, with Special Reference to Tubercle Bacilli."

Abraham Flexner was in Berlin on a commission from John D. Rockefeller, Jr. to survey prostitution in Europe. His interviews with police and public health officials, as well as acknowledged prostitutes, were conducted with zeal and aplomb. The American edition of his monograph, later translated into French, German, and other languages, appeared in 1914.[25] Smith called on Flexner at the Hotel Adlon, took him to the opening of the Great Berlin Art Exhibition, for which Geh. Schmidt had furnished tickets, and invited him to dinner at the Pension Tsheuschner. They exchanged impressions of the Germans. Smith would have echoed Flexner's appraisal: "One hears—mainly from those who have never been here—that the Germans are a testy, bureaucratic lot; my own experience makes them out courteous, helpful, and most intelligent."[26]

Theobald Smith had been invited by the Kaiser-Wilhelm Society for the Advancement of Science, through the Kultusminister, to participate in an official discussion in January 1912 of the advisability of erecting biological research institutes.[27] Eventually Smith advocated that such a facility should be constructed and that it be under Wassermann's direction. The Society decided to build an Institute for Experimental Therapy. Gaffky hosted a dinner party at the Hotel Bellevue for Wassermann, Smith and Abraham Flexner, to celebrate the occasion. (Theobald's diary simply noted "Dinner at Hotel Bellevue given by Gaffky to Flexner, Wassermann & me.")[28] In 1913, August von Wassermann became director, leaving his position as chief of the Division of Experimental Therapy and Serum Research at the Institute for Infectious Diseases. In acknowledging a personal photograph sent by Smith, Geh. Schmidt expressed his special sense of gratitude for the gesture: "In feeling this, I consider not only the successes of your teaching activity here, but also the good advice which you have given me regarding the Wassermann Institute."[29]

From May 30 to June 1, Theobald Smith attended the meeting of the Freie Vereinigung für Mikrobiologie at the Hygienic Institute. The Association has been cofounded by Rudolf Kraus from Vienna and August von Wassermann. The program was arranged by A. Gärtner of Jena and some fifty titles were listed.[30] Among many transatlantic visitors were Simon Flexner and E.C. Schroeder, who called on Smith beforehand, and brought him up to date on Rockefeller Institute and B.A.I. affairs. Sessions of the meeting were devoted to the cancer problem in man and animals, to epidiascopic demonstrations, and to immunity and chemotherapy in protozoal infections. Of special interest to Theobald Smith among miscellaneous topics were a report by H. Conradi (Halle) on identifying diphtheria bacilli, and papers by R. Kraus (Vienna) on the avidity of diphtheria antitoxin and on the dissolution of tubercle bacilli in the host.

Lange (Dresden) reported on immunity and chemotherapy in trypano-somiasis, W. Kolle (Bern) gave two papers on the effectiveness of organic mer-cury preparations in spirochetal diseases, and P. Uhlenhuth (Strassburg) de-scribed further investigations of rabbit syphilis—all stemming from Ehrlich's work at Frankfurt. From Ehrlich's Institute, K. Shiga reported on the Wasser-mann reaction after Salvarsan treatment, and also on "Kakka" (beri-beri), then still considered possibly infective. Ehrlich himself did not attend and Smith ap-parently did not meet him during that year, even during a brief stop in Frank-furt—a sadly eloquent testimony to the intensity of Ehrlich's preoccupation with his adversaries and his declining health.

Towards the end of March, Smith left for Hamburg to be the guest of Dr. W.P. Dunbar, director of the Hygienic Institute there, whom he had met in 1896.[31] Dunbar had planned a full schedule, which included an evening meeting on the 26th of the Medical Society at his house, followed by a late supper. Among the twenty men present were P. Unna and F. Fülleborn. At Dunbar's Institute, dem-onstrations of algae and numerous fungal and bacterial cultures had been pre-pared. Smith attended a lecture on vaccinia eruptions, and observed vaccine re-moval from calf and rabbit. Fülleborn conducted him over the Tropical Institute, where he met a distinguished group, including S. Prowazek and G. Giemsa. Next day he visited the abattoir, the Pathological College, and the vaccine plant. On the last evening, Dunbar had invited at least fifty people to his home for a "Bierabend."[32] As he was developing a heavy cold, Smith left early next morning for Berlin, promising to deliver some schedule lectures on a return visit.

Theobald Smith returned twice to Hamburg, on June 13 and 19th, to give at Siemens Hall two public lectures on "The Relationship Between the Parasites and the Host in Infectious Diseases," sponsored by the Hamburg Colonial Insti-tute.[33] On the evening before the second lecture, Dunbar arranged a reception at the Hotel Esplanade, with a string quartet playing compositions of Haydn and

Schubert. Smith was guest of honor and addressed the select audience on "The Comparative Organization of American and German Universities." Finally, his memorable trips to Hamburg ended with a flourish on June 20. In the morning, he was taken through the Eppendorf Hospital; discussed with Dunbar in the afternoon the latter's theory that bubonic plague was due to a specific fungus, and his plans to verify it in India; and in the evening gave his concluding lecture at Siemens Hall on the host-parasite relationship, followed by another "Bierabend" at Dunbar's home, lasting until midnight. Then he went back to Berlin for a week of putting things together, in readiness for their final departure from the Pension Tscheuschner; and fulfilling some important farewell obligations—including the Zoo's inhabitants—a big city feature that, whenever available, never failed to attract him. Dunbar had been a thoughtful, generous host. Guests had received elegant printed invitations and program cards to Theobald Smith's lectures. Printed invitations were issued even to the Bierabend of March 29.[34]

A few months after his return to Boston, Theobald Smith forwarded to Simon Flexner at the Rockefeller Institute a copy of Dunbar's outline of a "different theory from that current" on the etiology of bubonic plague. Dunbar had already left for India. He needed 30,000 marks, towards which Hamburg had granted 8,000. "If I were a wealthy man," mused Smith, "I would gamble on just such a courageous enterprise."[35] Flexner replied: "The Dunbar matter interests me very much. It had not been brought to my attention previously, and I have put it among the subjects to come up at the next meeting of the Board."[36] In brief, Dunbar had isolated a previously unidentified fungus from several bubonic plague victims upon their arrival in Hamburg. This fungus, which resembled species known to be associated with spoiled grain, was isolated only from the pus of buboes, and never from cases of pneumonic plague, whose bacterial origin he did not appear to dispute.[37] Apparently Dunbar had been victimized by errors of technique and logic similar to those besetting an earlier generation of microbiologists.

With the coming of spring, the Smith family wanted to get away from Berlin and to see something of Germany outside the capital. They had met graciously their weekly rounds of social obligations, from leaving cards to attending formal dinner parties; and had endured the inescapable propaganda of the imperial entourage. Now they needed a respite, which roughly occupied the month of April, thus intervening between the first of Theobald Smith's visits to Hamburg and the last two trips just before the family's final departure for home. A brief account of that respite is interjected here. On March 24th, the Smith girls went to Dresden, to be joined there by their mother and Philip on April 4. Theobald helped to pack their belongings and retained only one room at the Pension for the rest of April. On April 13th, he boarded a train to be reunited with his family at Weimar—a city that provoked many recollections of an earlier visit. Thence they proceeded together to a pension in Eisenach.

From there, Smith completed and mailed to Chittenden the manuscript of his contribution to the CuSO$_4$ monograph, eventually published in 1913.[38] The girls and Lilian soon became familiar with the houses where Martin Luther stayed in 1498 and where J.S. Bach was born in 1685. Throughout that sunny week, Smith rambled daily to famous viewpoints, either alone or with members of the family; but he devoted several hours daily to reading the literature and preparing for the lectures still to come. They all climbed to the Wartburg, the ancient castle where Luther found refuge while translating the Bible. Before Theobald left for Berlin on the 22nd, an especially long "tramp" with his daughters included another climb up the Wartburg.[39] His own holiday away from Berlin had barely lasted ten days. The family returned to Berlin on May 1. For much of that month, they found frequent relief from the pressures of Berlin by exploring with friends its suburban and adjacent amenities.

The Kaiser had received each year at Court (at his so-called Schleppencour) the American Exchange Professors, along with a few senior academic and administrative representatives of the University of Berlin. The invitation did not include wives. In 1911, the two Exchange Professors were the vain and quick-tempered Hugo Münsterberg of Harvard, still a German citizen, and Alphonso Smith of the University of Virginia, the "Roosevelt Professor." Münsterberg's jealousy was aroused because the Kaiser paid more attention at the Schleppencour to Alphonso Smith. Moreover, Münsterberg had understood from the American Ambassador, the Hon. David J. Hill, that his wife would be received at Court, and she had brought with her an appropriate gown expressly for the occasion. Münsterberg insisted on another Court invitation and Alphonso Smith openly resented this discrimination. A vindictive and unseemly feud developed in the local press, which was magnified by American newspapers.

Following the announcement of Theobald Smith's appointment as the Harvard Exchange Professor for 1911–12, Münsterberg had written to him from Berlin and had airily dismissed the reported quarrels with Alphonso Smith.

> In the whole affair I was entirely passive and was simply the victim of a petty, provincial, jealous colleague who stirred up the American newspaper reporters against me . . . He was disappointed because he was not invited to a certain festivity and got the absurd fancy that I was responsible for it . . . As you will have as companion next year Professor Reinsch of Madison, Wisconsin, who is said to be a very reasonable man, there is no ground for any possible discomfort. But the chief thing is that these court affairs are of no earthly importance here to anyone

who has no special ambitions in that respect . . . German professors do not care for it, and I myself had given no attention to it. There is no need for any American guest to trouble himself with questions of court etiquette or similar rubbish.[40]

Nonetheless, this incident had prompted President Lowell to determine that "Our next representative . . . is not a person to raise any question about etiquette."[41]

Before leaving home, Smith had discussed this situation with previous Harvard Exchange Professors, and with Lilian's concurrence had concluded that wives should not be granted favors denied to the wives of German professors. Accordingly, he informed the new American ambassador, the Hon. John G.A. Leishman, that Mrs. Smith would not attend the Court and that he would prefer not to accept the invitation to the Schleppencour, if it could be arranged without giving offense. Prof. Paul S. Reinsch, a political scientist from the University of Wisconsin, instead of talking the situation over with Theobald Smith, wrote to the Ambassador that any decision made by him and the Court would be agreeable to him.

After some negotiations, Profs. Smith, Reinsch and Edmund James were asked to the Court Ball at 8 P.M. on February 7, 1912. The gilt-edged invitation was prefaced by a typed letter from Kultusminister von Trott zu Solz, advising Smith that he would be "seen" by His Majesty the Emperor and King on that occasion. The simple Royal Evening Meal comprised: Steamed sole./Nesselrode Pudding./Cold duck, Salad./Congress cake with cream./Fruit. All three attended and were presented "at the express direction of the emperor. Mrs. Reinsch was also presented, but Mrs. Smith and Mrs. James did not find it possible to at- tend."[42] The eldest daughter Dorothea recalled her mother's decision not to go to the Ball because American transgressions of Imperial Household protocol were bound to arouse hard feelings among the wives of the few invited German academics.[43] Theobald's day card covering the Court Ball carried the entry: "Hof Ball—Drs. Reinsch, E.J. James and I talk to Emperor William II."[44] The Americans were impressed by the Kaiser's intelligent questions about the Negro problem in the United States.

President James, who was vacationing in Europe with his wife, spent several weeks in Berlin, where two of their children were enrolled in University courses. To a friend in Oregon, he wrote: "I had an interesting time in Berlin. Margaret and I had an invitation from the Emperor to the Court Ball. Margaret felt that she couldn't quite afford the money necessary to get the kind of gown that ought to be worn at such functions, and time was too short for her to get such a gown anyhow, and so she declined, but I went, and had a very fine time. Of course it was an interesting function to see the various crowned heads of Europe tripping the light fantastic with as much gusto and seeming pleasure as the boys and girls at a country fair."

The Smith's social life began almost immediately after their arrival in Berlin. They were invited to a large Christmas Day dinner party organized by the American Consul-General, A.M. Thackara and Mrs. Thackara. Besides these helpful governmental officials, the Amerika-Institut on the Universitätsstrasse strengthened the bonds linking tourists and transplants from the United States. Its Secretary, K.O. Bertling, told Theobald that he hoped the Institute would "become a kind of second home for you in Berlin." Dr. Bertling was also the Secretary of the Harvard Club of Berlin, comprising about twenty Harvard Alumni living in the capital, whose honorary president was by custom the Exchange Professor from Harvard. According to Bertling, "much of the successful development and prestige of the Club has been due to the readiness on the side of the exchange professors to devote some of their time to social intercourse with the younger members.[45] Theobald Smith attended every one of their monthly meetings at the "Heidelberger" during his honorary presidency.

Through the Kultusminister, free tickets were available for many cultural events during the Smiths' stay in Berlin. The season at the Royal Opera House opened with *Madam Butterfly,* which was attended by the Kaiser. Other operas seen by the Smiths included *Cavalleria Rusticana* and *Pagliacci, Der Rosenkavalier, The Magic Flute, Die Königskinder* (Humperdinck), *Das Rheingold, Die Walküre, Lohengrin, Tristan und Isolde,* and *The Flying Dutchman.* They heard orchestral and chamber music concerts at the Königliche Musikschule in Charlottenburg, and an organ recital and a concert at the Gedachtniskirche (Memorial Church). An exhibition of Frederick the Great in Art was viewed at the Royal Academy of Arts. Theobald and Lilian went to hear Fridtjof Nansen, the Polar explorer, speak on "The first discovery of North America through the Norwegians."

Social invitations of various kinds abounded. On January 13, Theobald attended the ninth anniversary of the American Association of Commerce and Trade in Berlin.[46] He and Lilian spent the evening of January 19 at the von Gierke's, where they "met Mrs. Conheim." Two days later, they took Sunday "tea at Miss White's." On the 26th, there was "dinner at Brand's," and on January 27, the Emperor's fifty-third birthday was marked by ceremonies at the University, the key event being an address by Hans Delbrück, famous professor of history at the University of Berlin. Smith was invited by Kulturminister von Trott zu Solz and his wife to a dinner at 4:30 P.M. for about sixty men at their residence on Unter den Linden. Afterwards, they all attended a Gala Command Performance at the Royal Opera House of three scenes from Joseph Lauff's "The Great King" (Frederick the Great), with music by that monarch. This was followed on the 31st by "dinner at Geh. Elster's home very pleasant affair."

Another All-Highest Command Performance, patronized by their Imperial Majesties and numerous aristocracy, was an evening Festival Concert of classical music at the Royal Academy of Music for the benefit of the Pestalozzi Ladies Association, whose good works in aid of musician's impoverished widows and daughters had so depleted its treasury that there was danger the Association would have to end forty years of charitable activities. In February, a masked ball was given at their Pension, and on the 6th they dined with von Wassermann. A "very pleasant afternoon" was spent on Sunday the 11th at Steglitz, on the outskirts of Berlin, where Geheimrath Schmidt had the whole family to dinner at 1:30 P.M. Geh. Reinhardt was also there, as well as Excell. Frau Friedrich Althoff, widow (since 1910) of the distinguished former Director of the Prussian Ministry of Educational and Medical Affairs—Ehrlich's early benefactor.

Theobald was the pre-dinner speaker at a supper-dance of the American Colony of Berlin in the Zoological Garden Restaurant on Washington's Birthday, February 22, 1912, which was sponsored by the Ambassador and the Consul General of the United States.[47] During the remainder of February, the Smiths had private dinner engagements, generally at professors' homes, and often with one or two other professors and their wives as fellow-guests, on the 14th, 17th, 18th, 20th, 21st, 23rd, and 28th. They also attended teas on the 25th at Gross Lichterfelde, at a Frauen Kongress on the 27th, and at the Women's Club on the 29th. There was a small interdenominational American Church in Berlin. The Smiths went there on a Sunday in March and to the Easter Service a few weeks later.[48]

To symbolize their appreciation of the boundless hospitality extended to them, Lilian Smith and Mrs. Reinsch first gave a tea at the American Club to all the Austausch ladies, American and German. Then Reinsch, Smith and their wives offered a large dinner-party at the Hotel Bristol. The selection and placement of sixty-one guests, who received printed invitations for 8 P.M. on May 18, were formidable tasks. A lavish menu was accompanied by several wines, culminating in dry champagne. Theobald Smith welcomed the guests on behalf of both families in a brief speech in German. He thanked them for having so warmly welcomed complete strangers into their family circles. Unfortunately, the "big pond" impeded easy cultivation of this happy relationship, but they dared to hope some of them would visit America. Berlin would be a Mecca, to which they would strive to make another pilgrimage. "Next to the personal influence of your friendship we must not forget the influence of science and art, which this metropolis has offered daily and abundantly for stimulation and enjoyment. The temptation to lay down the work and surrender to these attractions has been very great." He could truthfully "designate the winter months of 1912 as the happiest, most stimulating, and fullest" of his life. He was particularly grateful to Flügge and regretted his absence due to illness. Smith asked his American colleagues to drink to the health of the honored guests, and finally requested the whole assembly to toast the future development of the Exchange Professorships.[49]

The family departed for Switzerland early in June, leaving Theobald Smith to say personal farewells alone. He visited the Institutes of Pathology, Agriculture and Hygiene, not seen by him previously, headed by Professors J. Orth, N. Zuntz and M. Rubner, respectively. Between his two lecturing trips to Hamburg he accepted three successive dinner invitations, the most notable being at Prof. Paszkowsky's home, where other distinguished guests included Excellency Althoff's widow, and a duke.

On the 22nd, Theobald called on Robert v. Ostertag and his colleagues at the Veterinary School, and visited the Gesundheitsamt at Gross Lichterfelde. On the 23rd, he said goodbye to Rektor Lenz, and took tea with Geh. Flügge and his family. His last lecture was on June 24, and he worked on it at the Institute to the last minute. There was a substantial audience, which included many specialists and colleagues. According to a newspaper report, "In extremely stimulating form he discussed the way in which parasites defend themselves against the protective forces of the host attacked by them, and indicated new guidelines for further promising investigations in the field of serum therapy." Wirk. Geh. Oberregierungsrat Elster attended for the Cultus Ministry. Flügge, as director of the Institute, voiced thanks "to the meritorious scientist."[50]

Schmidt took Theobald to lunch at the Adlon on the 25th. The next day was climactic. He bade farewell to Gaffky, von Wassermann, F. Neufeld, M. Hartmann and others at the Robert Koch Institute before proceeding to an emotional evening at a restaurant dinner arranged by Flügge and Institute colleagues. Smith kept the simple but gilt-edged menu card on the back of which his hosts had inserted their signatures—C. Flügge, M. Ficker, J. Schuster, A. Oberstadt, H. Brinkmann, Fr. Kourich, Bruno Heymann, A. Korff-Petersen, and E. Kunoss. Under this column of names, someone had pencilled a couplet, headed "Zur freundlichen Erinnerung" (A Friendly Memento):

> Zwar gilt der Mensch Dir nur wie ein Parasit,
> Doch schatzen wir Dich mehr, wie man hieraus ersieht.
> (Man may appear to you only like a parasite,
> But we esteem you more, as is seen from this.)

The same individuals signed a message of informal greetings and friendly appreciation to Mrs. Theobald Smith on a postcard addressed to her in Switzerland.

During his last days in Berlin, Smith was interviewed by a journalist from the *Berliner Tageblatt* about the differences he had observed between American and

German professors and students. In general, Smith preferred the American pattern of higher education. The American student could be penalized for not attending lectures. He was not status-conscious and summer work enabled poor students to pay their own way. In research, since he was not tied to his professor's "school," independent thought and objective investigation were favored. The American system of inter-collegiate competitive sport was on the whole healthy, and the lack of University sport in Germany unfortunate.

But in the practice of hygiene, Smith thought Germany far ahead of his homeland, where at present this discipline was unsystematically applied. "We waste too much money on unimportant details . . . the layman, who does not understand this business, has a lot to say in it. With you, only the scientific view is important; with us, proper respect for the scientist is still lacking. I suppose that is the result of the all-leveling democracy." Asked if he found fault with anything in the imperial capital, Smith responded humorously: "Berlin would be a very nice city if it had not automobiles. They really ruin one's life—three times I myself have been nearly run over. In no American city would one dare to drive as fast as here."[51]

Smith left Berlin on June 28. Paszkowski came to the train to see him off. He stopped at Dresden for two days, during which time he visited the new abattoir and the vaccine institute under Dr. v. Einsiedel, called on Prof. E. Joest, the comparative pathologist at the Veterinary School, and went to see a suburban sanatorium. At Munich he talked at the Institute of Hygiene with its director, Max V. Gruber, Ehrlich's provocative opponent. While Professor of Hygiene at Vienna, Gruber and his pupil H.E. Durham had discovered and published in separate reports in 1896 the development of specific agglutinins in the blood serum of animals previously inoculated with typhoid or cholera bacilli. A few months later, Ferdinand Widal reported on the diagnostic significance of a raised agglutinin titer against typhoid bacilli in the blood serum of patients with typhoid fever in Paris hospitals. The "Widal reaction" therefore would be termed more justly the "Gruber-Widal" test.

Smith also met Theodor Kitt at the Veterinary School and looked over the Vaccine Institute. After some sightseeing in both Dresden and Munich, he left for Switzerland where he reunited with his family at Gunten. They were soon joined by the Bacons (of the Allyn Bacon publishing firm) with whom they had become friendly in Berlin. In between tramps, excursions and shopping trips, Smith went to Bern, lunching with Koch's former pupil and coworker W. Kolle, Director of the Institute for Infectious Diseases, and with Prof. Bürgli, a pharmacologist. Any unfilled time was used to write up lecture material or to relax by solving mathematical conundrums from Osgood's *Calculus*.

On July 22, the Smiths turned north into Germany again and stayed four days in Heidelberg. Theobald inspected the Institute for Hygiene and the Cancer Institute with their respective directors, Hermann Kossel and Theodor v. Wasielewski. The Kossels took them all by boat up the Neckar River to a restaurant. Hermann Kossel's elder brother Albrecht, Professor of Physiology at Heidelberg, and a Nobel prize winner in 1910 for researches into the biochemistry of the cell nucleus, expressed later his regrets to Smith that he had not been able to join them. The parent Smiths made a side-trip to Oberursel to call on surviving relatives, and brought Franz Kexel and his son to Frankfurt to meet their cousins over supper at the Kaiser Keller. Next day the Smith family took an express steamer down the Rhine to Cologne where they admired the cathedral and the Museum with its Roman relics.

The following five nights were spent in Amsterdam visiting museums and art galleries, the Zoo and the docks. Smith also looked over a vaccine institute. On July 31, Theobald's fifty-third birthday, a steamer took them to Edam and Marken, via canals and the Zuyder Zee. They spent three days at the Hague sightseeing, with short trips to Scheveningen and Delft. Boarding the cross-channel boat at Flushing on August 6, they reached Folkstone early next morning and caught the 9 A.M. train to Canterbury, its streets illuminated for "Cricket Week." After viewing the Cathedral and other antiquities they made an excursion to Tankerton, a small seaside resort.

In London they put up at a boarding-house near the British Museum from August 9–18. On the first day, while Theobald was "working on calculus all morning" and Philip explored London, a foray to a ladies' tailoring establishment on Oxford Street cost Lilian over £18 for costumes for herself and daughters, with an extra coat for Dorothea.[52] Their father introduced them to London experiences such as Sunday Matins at St. Paul's followed by a "walk thro' Lincoln's Inn grounds;" thence on foot from the Museum at South Kensington via the Gardens to Kensington Palace to Westminster Abbey and the Tate Gallery, Hampton Court and Kew Gardens, and the National and Portrait Galleries. Theobald also visited the Local Government Board vaccine plant near the Hendon "Aeroplane grounds," a three-mile walk from the bus stop; the Lister Institute laboratories at Elstree; and the Burroughs Wellcome Laboratories at Herne Hill, where he met O'Brien and Südmerssen, a chemist.[53]

On the 19th, the Smiths interrupted their train journey to Oxford at Windsor, for a glimpse at the State Apartments, St. George's Chapel, and the Long Walk at Eton. They stayed at Oxford until the end of August. The young people were impressed by the grey city of spires, towers and doorways, and its nearby villages and landmarks. The rains flooded the countryside and entry was barred to many practically deserted college buildings and gardens, but Theobald managed to tramp around Magdalen Gardens and Christ Church Meadows, and several other college gardens. He also visited the Bodleian Library; browsed in bookstores; and, braving muddy roads, wandered with both daughters to Beckley via Marston ferry, the river "flooded by rains & greatly broadened." He walked with his wife from Islip to Wood Eaton and back, and returned on foot from a bus trip to Iffley; walked with daughter Lilian to Cumnor Church and to Godstow Nunnery; and with Philip tramped to Water Eaton, punted on the Cherwell and went by train to Blenheim Park and Gardens.

They left Oxford on the 31st for Warwick, a convenient center for excursions to Leamington and Kenilworth, and thence entrained for Liverpool and the S.S. *Laconia* on September 3. Vincent Y. Bowditch and several other Boston physicians were fellow-passengers. The boat arrived in Boston on the 11th. Theobald Smith returned to his laboratories and lunched with Marshal Fabyan on the 13th. Throughout their visit to Europe, whenever opportunity offered, Theobald was ready to conduct or to plan sight-seeing itineraries. This was done methodically, at times almost relentlessly, but as much for the interests of his family as for himself. The womenfolk never needed to be reminded that they were beneficiaries of his very successful visiting professorship. However, they undoubtedly contributed to that success.

Theobald Smith's successor as Exchange Professor at Berlin was Charles Sedgwick Minot, a distinguished anatomist and embryologist, who had invented the automatic rotary microtome. Immediately after learning of his selection in February 1912, he wrote to Smith for information "which will assist me in understanding my duties and fulfilling them efficiently," telling Theobald that "It is a great honor to follow you."[54]

> It is a momentous year at the School. Shattuck, Bradford, Bowen and Putnam have already resigned, Christian has resigned as Dean . . . The Brigham Hospital is progressing steadily in spite of the severe winter. Dr. Rotch had more than half the money necessary to complete his [Children's] hospital. We are living, as you may infer, in a state of fermentation and in an atmosphere of hope.

Minot relayed excerpts from a letter to President Lowell, writing enthusiastically of "the impressions which you and Mrs. Smith had made in Berlin and of the high esteem in which you were held by the University professors."

Minot wrote again to Smith from Berlin in October 1912, reporting that Schmidt was full of praise "of you and your visit." Minot had been shown at the Cultusministerium a copy of the Memorial Edition of Koch's Works, and was told "they would like to send it to you as a memento of your visit, but they were hesitating because Koch had not been quite fair in his treatment of you. I ventured to assure them that nothing of that sort would modify your opinion of Koch's work and . . . I further added that in my belief you would be much gratified by the proposed gift."[55] Minot had timed well his turn in Berlin. Just over two years later, Smith noted on a Day Card with his customary taciturnity: "cold—Dr. C.S. Minot's funeral."[56]

From Boston, the Smiths wrote appreciatively to their Berlin friends, helped by Lilian's thick notebook, kept up to date with the names, addresses and family composition of her husband's professional contacts. Theobald retained a few letters from that happy half-year in Berlin. K.O. Bertling of the Amerika-Institut assured him that his interest in the Amerika-Institut and his personal kindness to its staff would be remembered. "As Secretary of the Harvard Club, I wish to express to you once more our appreciation for what you did for us through your faithfulness as a representative of Harvard University. We shall all miss you."[57] Friedrich Schmidt wrote: "It is very agreeable to find that so much esteem can develop from these international exchanges, where the conditions for understanding are not so simple."

> I always remember gratefully the benefits your activity has brought to our mutual relationship and to German Science. I do not have in mind only the University of Berlin but more particularly consider you one of the founders of the happily progressing Wassermann Institute; because you gave me—and I reiterate this—the confidence to press for its realization.[58]

The warmest tribute was from Carl Flügge: "Your thoughtful, quite way of working and speaking has left on us a most lasting impression. The absolute dependability of your investigations contrasts oddly with the manner in which most etiological questions are treated here. I wish we had you permanently in Germany."[59]

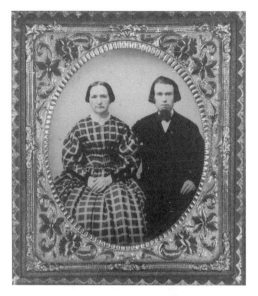
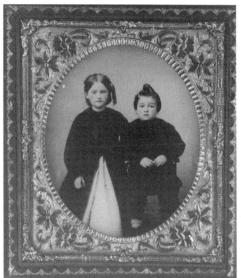
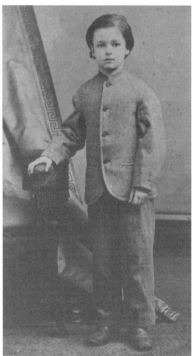
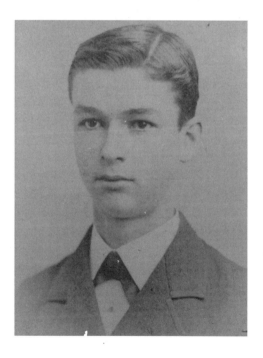

Illustration 1. *Above:* Tintypes of Theresa Kexel Schmitt and Philipp Schmitt, and their children Bertha and Theobald, made probably in Albany about 1864, when the parents were 37 and 35 years old respectively and the children 8 and 5.
Below: Theobald Smith in the 7-to-9 age range (left) and his Albany High School graduation photograph, May 1876 (right).

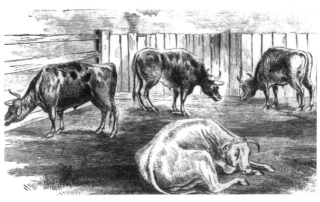

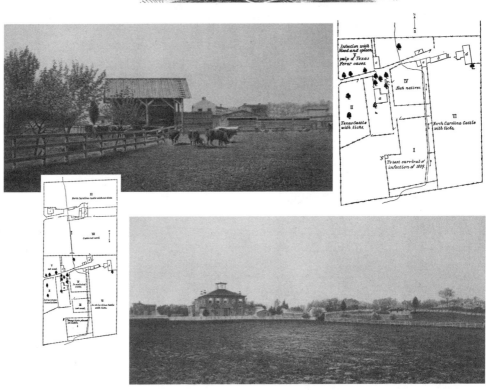

Illustration 2. *Above:* Appearance of bullocks suffering from Texas cattle fever.
Below: The U.S. Department of Agriculture's Veterinary Station, Washington, D.C., about 1884. Accompanying diagrams illustrate the controlled experiments with cattle, both exposed and unexposed to ticks, that Smith carried on in his Texas cattle fever researches.

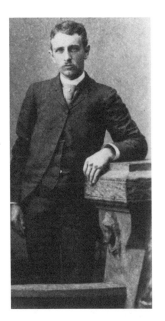

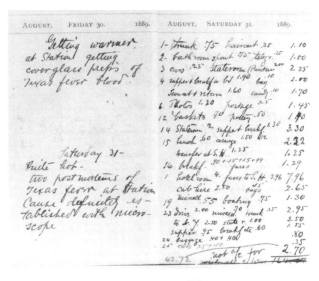

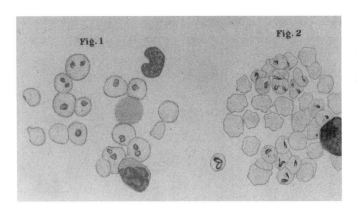

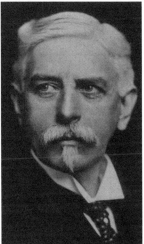

Illustration 3. *Above:* (left) Frederick L. Kilbourne, late 1880s; (right), Double page of Theobald Smith's diary, August 30–31, 1889, recording "Texas fever . . . cause definitely established with microscope." *Below: Pirosoma begeminum* with red corposcles of a Texas fever case, reproduced from plate V of Smith and Kilbourne's Bulletin No. 1 (left); Daniel E. Salmon, depicted in later life (right).

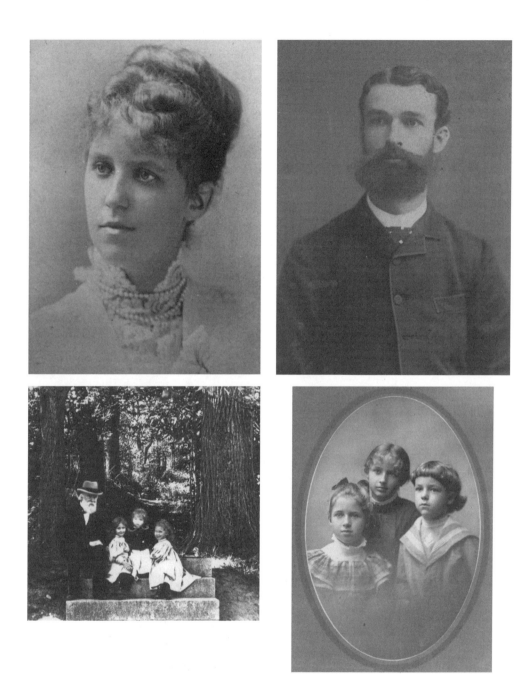

Illustration 4. *Above:* Lilian H. Egleston (left), photographed at about age 30 in 1887, a year before her marriage to Theobald Smith; Studio photograph of Theobald Smith (right), taken in Washington in the late 1880s or early 1890s.
Below: Grandfather Egleston with the Smith children near the Smith home in Jamaica Plain about 1897 (left), showing him with, left to right, Dorothea, Philip and Lilian 2; on the right appear, left to right, Lilian 2, Dorothea and Philip a number of years later.

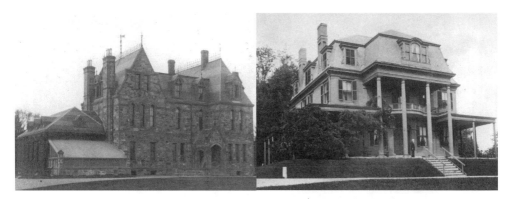

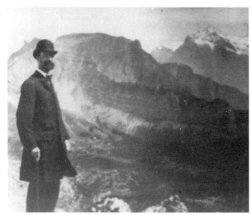

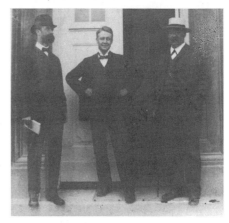

Illustration 5. *Above:* The Bussey Institution (left) in the Jamaica Plain section of West Roxbury, about five miles from Boston, where Theobald Smith carried on his research between 1895 and 1915; the Bussey mansion (right), known as Woodland Hill, where the Smith family lived during the same period. Grandfather Egleston stands at the front.

Below: (left), Theobald Smith viewing a mountain scene in 1903, while on a trip to Montana during the Anaconda suit; (right) Theobald Smith, Theodor Madsen and Svante Arrhenius (left to right) in the doorway of Dr. Madsen's Serum Institute, Copenhagen, 1904.

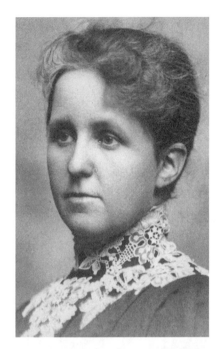
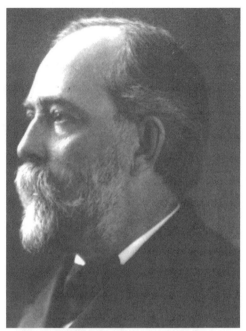

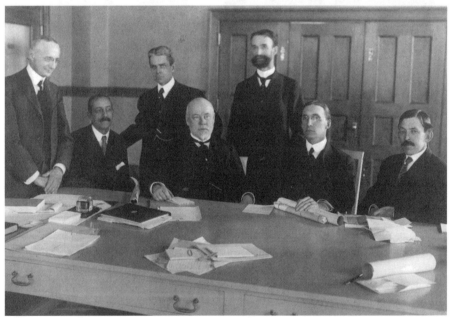

Illustration 6. *Above:* Lilian Egleston Smith, January 1903; (left); Studio portrait of Simon Gage (right), taken in 1906.
Below: The Board of Scientific Directors of the Rockefeller Institute, ca. 1909. Left to right: Simon Flexner (standing), Mitchell Pruden, Emmet Holt (standing), William H. Welch, Theobald Smith (standing), Christian Herter and Herman Biggs.

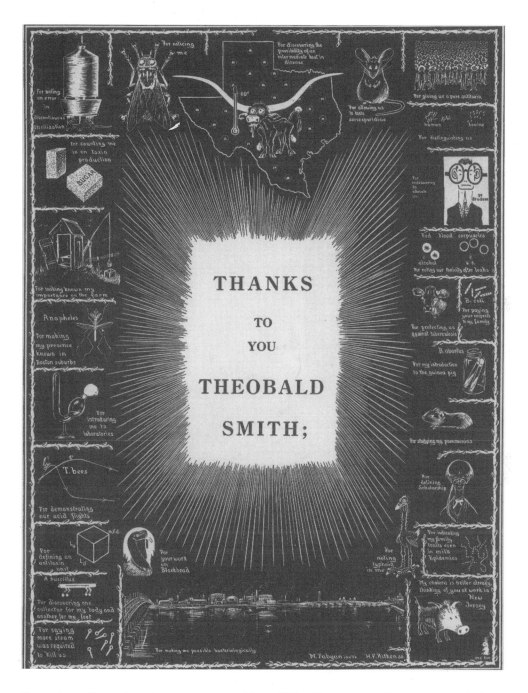

Illustration 7. Souvenir card, commemorating Theobald Smith's many contributions to microbiology. This was prepared by Dr. Marshal Fabyan and given to every participant at the Complimentary Farewell Dinner on June 2, 1915 honoring Smith for his twenty years of service to Harvard prior to his resignation from the University in August following.

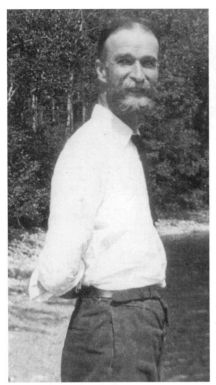
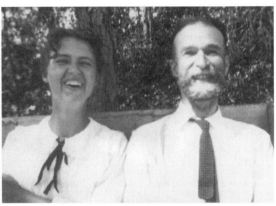
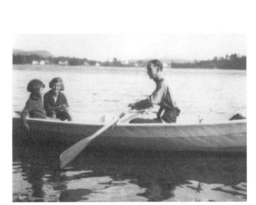
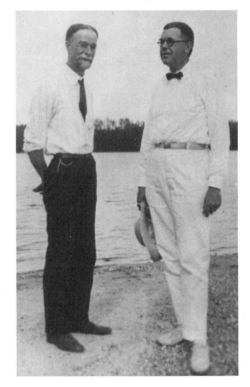

Illustration 8. Scenes of the Smith's life at their Silver Lake, New Hampshire camp:
Above: Theobald Smith (left), late August or early September 1916; daughter Lilian (Lilian 2) with Theobald (right), same period.
Below: Theobald rowing Lilian's (now Mrs. Robert Foerster's) children, September 1929 (left); Theobald Smith and Carl TenBroeck (right), September 1927.

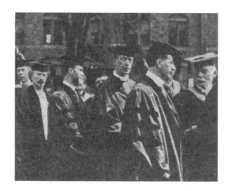
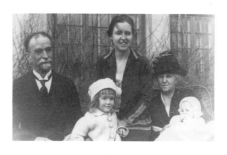

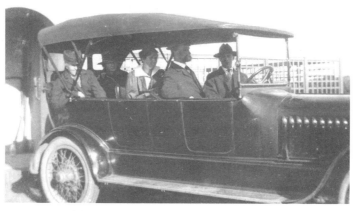

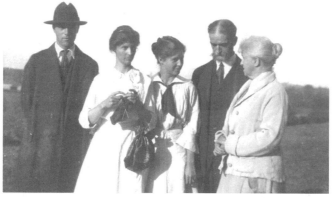

Illustration 9. *Above:* (left), Theobald Smith (third from left) in the academic procession at the time he was awarded an honorary D.SC degree by Yale University on June 20, 1917. Behind him (second from left), looking at the reader, is I. J. Paderewski, the pianist and future prime minister of Poland, with whom he conversed and joked; (right), left to right, Theobald, Lilian 2 and Lilian 1, with Lilian's two daughters. Taken at Larkfields on March 8, 1925.

Below: The Smith family prepared for a tour in their Stanley Steamer automobile, September 1918. Son Philip is at the steering wheel, with his father Theobald beside him, and daughter Lilian directly behind him, in front of (left to right) Lilian 1 and Dorothea. In the scene immediately below appear Philip, Dorothea, Lilian 2, Theobald and Lilian 1, after alighting.

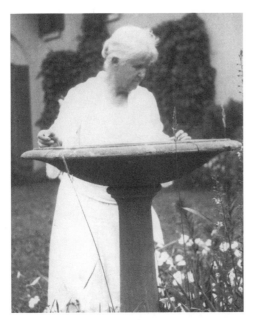

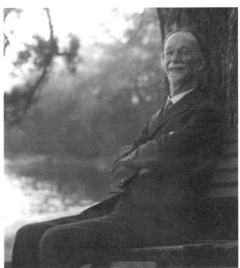

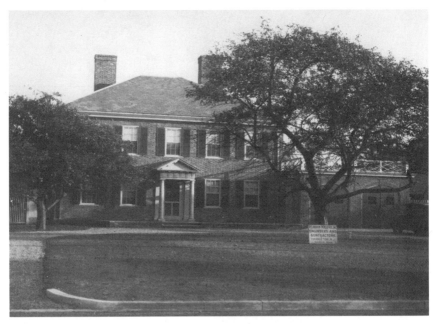

Illustration 10. *Above:* Lilian Smith in the garden at Larkfields, the director's house of the Rockefeller Institute's Department of Animal Pathology in Princeton (left), June 1930; Theobald Smith before a favorite tree at Silver Lake, early 1930s (right).

Below: The Smith's last residence, on Battle Road in Princeton, which they built in 1931–32 and occupied from September 1932.

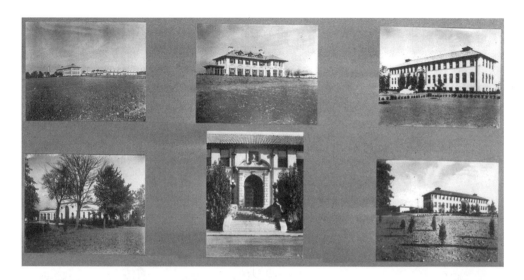

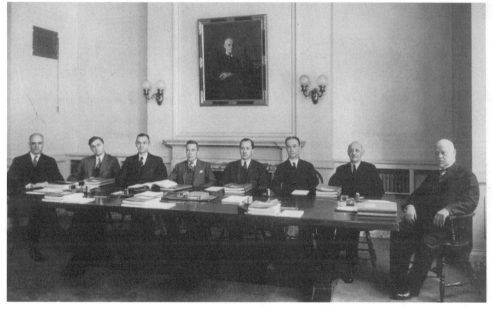

Illustration 11. *Above:* The Rockefeller Institute for Medical Research's Department of Animal Pathology, Princeton, New Jersey, pictured during its early years.
Below: The Board of Scientific Directors of the Rockefeller Institute, 1932. Left to right: Edric B. Smith, Secretary; James B. Conant; Eugene L. Opie; Francis G. Blake; Charles P. Stockard; Theobald Smith; Simon Flexner (without glasses), Director of the Institute and not a member of the Board; William Henry Welch, President.
Courtesy of the American Philosophical Society.

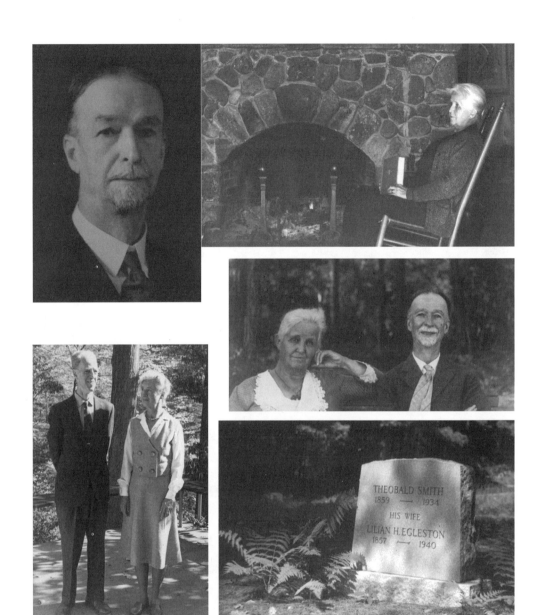

Illustration 12. *Upper left:* Theobald Smith pictured on his seventy-fifth birthday, July 31, 1934;
Upper right: Lilian Egleston Smith before the fireplace of their Silver Lake home, September 7, 1935.
Center: Snapshot of Lilian and Theobald Smith at Silver Lake, summer of 1934.
Lower left: Philip Smith and his sister Lilian Foerster, October 1965.
Lower right: Headstone of Vermont marble erected in the Chocorua Churchyard, following the reburial of Theobald and Lilian Smith's ashes there in the fall of 1967.

19

DISENCHANTMENT WITH HARVARD— ROCKEFELLER INSTITUTE APPOINTMENT

S oon after reaching Boston, Theobald Smith reported to President Lowell, and also to Dr. Walcott at the State House. On September 30 he left for Washington to attend a lengthy meeting of the Organizing Committee of the International Congress of Hygiene and Demography. As president of Section I (Bacteriology and Parasitology), he was guest at a dinner hosted by Surgeon-General George Sternberg in honor of Dr. A.W. Walcott, the Congress President.

At the opening ceremonies on September 23, delegates were welcomed by President Taft. For five days, the Congress held two daily sessions at the Pan-American Building, except for the third afternoon when the Corcoran Gallery was "At Home." Perhaps the most gratifying day was the last, when the morning session on "anaphylaxis"—by which term Otto's "Theobald Smith phenomenon" had become known—was well attended.[1] Smith was in the chair. In the course of occasional lectures, such as that on "Hypersensitiveness to Serum or Anaphylaxis" to the Norfolk District Medical Society, or through participating in the discussion on anaphylaxis before the Otological Society at the Massachusetts General Hospital, he unobtrusively confirmed that he had discovered the reaction. His article on hay fever[2] appeared around this time.

After the Congress, Smith traveled to Albany, where his aging mother resided alone, too decrepit and independent to return to Woodland Hill. Her son-in-law, Arthur Murphy, had died at sixty-three on May 23, 1910, and her grandchildren were dispersed. Theobald located a comfortable boarding house for his mother after discussing the problem with his Albany cousin, Anna Fischer. From meetings in New York, Baltimore, Washington or Ithaca, he returned home habitually via Albany, until her death at eighty-seven on Mary 15, 1914—the last of a hard-working, self-effacing family of four sisters and one brother.

Old routines were resumed. Smith was pleased that as many as ten advanced students enrolled for his two-month course, which entailed a daily morning talk, with afternoon laboratory exercises. Before leaving each day for Harvard Medical School, he dropped in at the Forest Hill laboratory to see that all was in order. If any animal autopsy were necessary, he arrived late at Building E. Usually he reached Huntington Avenue at around 10 A.M., lunched frugally alone in his laboratory (a pint of hot milk or cocoa in a Thermos, "and some bread") and left around 5:30 P.M. for home, where he worked "in evening when not too tired—also a little piano occasionally."[3] He favored Schumann, McDowell, and other Romantics. In January 1913, he was elected "an American corresponding member" of the Helminthological Society of Washington—an honor cordially conveyed by the Society's Secretary, Maurice C. Hall[4] of the Zoological Division of the Bureau of Animal Industry. More than twenty years later, Hall—a parasitologist of no special distinction—wrote an obituary disparaging Smith's discoveries in parasitology.

Theobald's recent stay in Germany brought new obligations. He shepherded and shared hospitality for a dozen *Reisestudien* doctors and attended lectures by and receptions for visiting professors from Berlin. Geheimrat Prof. Eucken, whom he heard lecture in German at Harvard College, came with wife and daughter to dinner at Woodland Hill on Thanksgiving Day. At the end of January 1913, he addressed the Massachusetts Association of Boards of Health on "German Hygiene," and a few days later spoke at the Thursday Evening Club on "Research in Germany and the Kaiser Wilhelm Gesellschaft." None of these undertakings was arduous, yet he felt drained.

One root cause of this stale feeling was the clutter of time-consuming but unstimulating demands. Reluctance to delegate responsibility saddled him with tasks only nominally his. The Antitoxin Laboratory now required just a watchful eye, but he gave it much more. In a nine-week period from the end of December 1912 to the beginning of March 1913, he autopsied two discarded antitoxin horses, several vaccinated calves, and a hog, and dissected numerous chickens. If manufacture of a new product, e.g., typhoid vaccine or meningococcus antiserum, were being considered, Smith consulted experts about appropriate preliminary researches, and edited the wording of the circular of instructions for use.

He had to listen to antivivisection and antivaccination outpourings in the Legislature so that he could refute them better at State House hearings. His dry, unemotional interventions were always thorough and sometimes effective, at least temporarily. He spoke for as long as two hours on one such occasion.[5] Early in 1914, following epidemics of streptococcal sore throat in Massachusetts traced to improperly pasteurized milk, a Milk Bill was introduced in the Legislature and Smith spoke on it.[6] He also tried to acquaint the Legislature with his views on public abattoirs, and on outbreaks of bovine contagious abortion.

According to Curran,[7] Smith was present at an organizational meeting on December 16, 1912 to establish a School of Public Health for the training of health officers. This joint venture, involving Harvard University and the Massachusetts Institute of Technology, was led by Milton Rosenau, Professor of Preventive Medicine and Hygiene at Harvard. Although Smith's diary makes no reference to any meeting on that date, representatives of the two participating organizations did meet and decided to issue jointly a Certificate in Public Health to registrants who satisfactorily completed a one-year course. By the end of September 1913, the first class of eight students was admitted under an Administrative Board composed of William T. Sedgwick as Chairman, George C. Whipple, Harvard's Professor of Sanitary Engineering, as Secretary-Treasurer, and Rosenau as Director. (In the same year, Rosenau found time to launch his well-known textbook, *Preventive Medicine and Hygiene*.) The group of twenty lecturers included Theobald Smith, whose honorarium for eight lectures on the "Relation of Animal Disease to Public Health" was to be $50.[8]

Despite an initial favorable reaction to the founding proposals,[9] their evolution into Harvard's School of Public Health was interrupted repeatedly.[10] In October 1914, another organizational conference was held at the Rockefeller Foundation's General Education Board office in New York City. Harvard was represented by Theobald Smith, Milton Rosenau and George Whipple. Delegates agreed there was need for adequate training facilities for public health personnel, to be achieved by establishing an institute of hygiene affiliated with a university and its medical school. Wickliffe Rose of the Rockefeller Foundation and William Welch of Johns Hopkins University were asked to formulate plans for an ideal institute. Theobald Smith and the other Harvard professors eventually supported the Welch-Rose Report. The Johns Hopkins Institute of Hygiene and Public Health opened in 1918, while Harvard's School of Public Health was launched in 1922. Both institutions were made possible by grants from the Rockefeller Foundation. The initial contribution towards Harvard's School was designated in honor of Henry Pickering Walcott.

In 1909, Theobald Smith had been appointed "to supervise instruction in tropical diseases" in the Harvard Medical School, but did little about it. The Corporation, wishing to offer more formal teaching in this field, appointed a Professor of Tropical Medicine on January 13, 1913, for a five-year period. Richard Pearson Strong, around forty years old, had done well as Professor of Tropical Medicine at the University of the Philippines, Manilla. Smith noted on the last day of 1912: "Interview with Dr. Strong about new dept." Strong wanted his department to have the status of a School, and vainly sought financial aid to that end from the Rockefeller Foundation. His expansionist aims provoked arguments, not only at Rockefeller headquarters, but also among the Harvard Medical School Faculty. In these discussions, Smith played no definable role. A Day Card entry for June 1, 1914, simply recorded: "'Full professors' discuss tropical medicine."

In 1922, the Department of Tropical Medicine was incorporated in the Harvard School of Public Health. When Strong retired in 1938, the association between the Departments of Tropical Medicine and Comparative Pathology grew closer, and they merged. E. W. Tyzzer, Theobald Smith's successor, consequently held the double title, "George Fabyan Professor of Comparative Pathology and Professor of Tropical medicine." Tyzzer's retirement in 1942 was followed by the appointment of René J. Dubos, who returned to the Rockefeller foundation after two years because Harvard would not regard tropical medicine studies as wholly post-graduate.[11]

Smith was overburdened with Harvard committee work. He had duties on Examination Committees for the D.P.H. and Ph.D. degrees, the Cancer Committee, the Visiting Committee to the Bussey Institution (under Dr. Carroll Dunham's chairmanship), and prolonged Faculty meetings, sometimes at Cambridge, on such questions as revising the requirements for admission to the Medical School. Travel to other cities also wasted time. During April and May 1913, various journeys to New York, New Haven, Washington and Philadelphia kept him from his laboratory for twenty-seven days. The Remsen Board still functioned, while his recent election to the Advisory Council of the Phipps Institute also entailed several trips a year. A pleasant interruption was the selection of a silver wedding present for his wife with their daughters' advice; and giving an afternoon tea to mark the anniversary on May 18.

The anomalous daily consumption of time in getting from his Forest Hills laboratory to the Harvard Medical School was good-humoredly mentioned by Theobald Smith himself during his visiting professorship. At a Farewell Dinner convened for the Harvard Club in Berlin by P.V. Bacon, the club's appreciation was expressed of Smith's faithful attendance at every meeting. The guest responded that "the gratitude should be all on his side, as he might truthfully say that not for years had he felt so much in touch with Harvard as during the winter in Berlin. The . . . reasons for this seemingly paradoxical statement was that his laboratory work lay at Forest Hills, quite outside the University."[12]

Theobald Smith's children, especially his daughters, suggested that the main cause of his unsettled state after returning from Berlin was President Lowell's lack of sympathy towards their father's work. But although Lawrence Lowell differed from Charles Eliot scholastically and in personality, he plainly respected Smith's national reputation and international fame. One year after the new president's inauguration, Harvard's honorary D.Sc. degree was conferred upon Smith. Lowell allowed him to accept the salaried position on the U.S. Referee Board in January 1911. He also urged Theobald Smith's candidacy for the visiting professorship in Berlin and praised his successful tenure of this post.

Lowell's sister, Mrs. Elizabeth Putnam, after hearing Smith's plans for enlarging his department's activities, and his comments on the Milk Bill before the Legislation, donated a sum for use at his discretion. The gift, Smith assured the president, would enable him to employ a girl as "laboratory servant" at $30-$40 monthly, thus releasing a trained *Diener* for other work. This temporary arrangement would be very helpful until the department had adopted "a definite field of teaching and research." Smith added that the "farm plan" of course needed a permanent and continuing subsidy. To which the President replied cautiously: "The farm I agree would cost something to buy and to run. Possibly the Massachusetts Society for Promoting Agriculture might help."[13] Mrs. Putnam was more optimistic. Her answer to his letter of explanatory thanks was indeed encouraging: "Do not let the thought of the *future* interfere with your getting the most effective *present* help, for I have no doubt whatever that the money will be forthcoming . . . Such work as yours must not be handicapped by lack of a little money."[14]

When in 1915 Theobald Smith disclosed his intention to resign, President Lowell was regretful. He sincerely endorsed the tributes paid at the Farewell Dinner in June 1915 and helped to burnish Smith's image long after he departed. In 1920, the Corporation awarded the Flattery Prize to Theobald Smith and invited him to give the 1920 Cutter Lectures on Preventive Medicine and Hygiene. Despite all these friendly overtures, Smith was liable to react defensively or aggressively in President Lowell's office. By contrast, his relationship with President Eliot was unique. Eliot had a scientist's training and his analytic mind foresaw the inevitable benefits to public health of such advances as sanitary water and milk supplies, the suppression of insect vectors through the drainage of swamps and marshes, and the control of animal diseases. He anticipated and proclaimed the gospel of preventive medicine. Moreover, Eliot thought Theobald Smith embodied the qualities of the ideal scientist—modest, zealous, thoroughly informed about his special field, and eager to expand and distribute knowledge of it. The two men maintained life-long attitudes of close yet formal esteem. There was no such bond with Lowell.

Theobald Smith knew that his renown rested upon scientific research accomplishments. His instructional talents were more suited to the advanced student or assistant than to the average preclinical registrant for whom the Harvard Medical School program was designed. President Eliot had understood, encouraged and harnessed his special characteristics. Similar insight and tolerance could hardly be expected of a successor anxious to avoid the appearance of favoritism. Still, four years after Lowell's inauguration, Smith worried over his teaching duties. In 1913, he started going over his lectures and laboratory exercises for the course a full month beforehand.

Since his European successes, Theobald Smith's self-confidence had increased, although the core of skepticism and protest in his character was no less tough and resolute. But however much he deplored the curricular rigidities of the Medical School, lack of presidential support dimmed the prospect of remedy. To avoid Faculty disputes, he thought of launching various research projects which would absorb most of his time. Some weeks after returning from Berlin, he set about "considering problems for rest of yr."[15] Enough unpremeditated projects arose to keep him and his assistants fully occupied for two or three years.

Smith had planned to investigate a microorganism then known as *Bacillus abortus* Bang, which he and Marshal Fabyan had been among the first in North America to study. In December 1909, abortion products were received from a valuable local dairy herd. A small bacillus was isolated, whose cultural properties resembled those of strains yielded by other herds in Massachusetts and two strains authenticated elsewhere. The growth requirements and pathogenic effects of this bacillus when injected into guinea-pigs were outlined in January 1912 by Smith and Fabyan[16]—the last account of Theobald Smith's North American work to be published in a German journal. A footnote initialled by Smith recalled that seventeen years before, when he and his assistant E.C. Schroeder were surveying milk at the Bureau of Animal Industry for the presence of tubercle bacilli, one guinea-pig, sacrificed three months after injection of a centrifuged sample, had generalized, non-tuberculous inflammatory nodules, with a greatly enlarged spleen. The changes were indistinguishable from those associated with infection by *Bacillus abortus* Bang.[17]

Fabyan sent an expanded version of that report to Smith in Berlin for correction and approval before submitting it to an American journal.[18] After his chief's return, Fabyan published under his supervision two additional short papers. The first recorded that miscellaneous laboratory animals (guinea-pigs, rabbits, white mice, wild house mice, two pigeons, two monkeys and one rat) tolerated an injection of *B. abortus* culture without apparent illness, and readily yielded this organism from splenic tissue, many weeks—in one guinea-pig, sixty-seven weeks —after the injection.[19] Smith knew that to establish the relationship between *B. abortus* Bang and bovine contagious abortion would entail the use of several cows as test animals. He tried out his culture by inoculating a single calf on July 21, 1911. No further tests were conducted. Even rumors of experiments on bovine contagious abortion caused a furor in the Bussey Farm vicinity. Such investigations were deemed unacceptable in the Harvard domain.

Fabyan's second paper reported three further examples of "inoculation disease of guinea-pigs" due to *B. abortus*. One case came from Smith's unpublished notes on his 1893 survey of Washington milk supplies. In two recent instances also, the guinea-pig method yielded *B. abortus* when direct culture failed. Of twelve milk samples from a scrupulously-kept herd, two were positive; one from a cow that aborted late in pregnancy, while the other animal had calved normally eleven months before, since which time its milk had been potentially infective.[20]

Smith had observed seasonally recurrent epizootics of fatal guinea-pig pneumonia since 1899.[21] Until late in May 1913, he was kept at work most afternoons by an epizootic in the colony. He concluded that this was due to either or both of the following dissimilar microorganisms. 1. *Bacillus bronchisepticus,* currently known as *Bordetella bronchiseptica,* a minute motile bacillus, closely related to the non-motile *Bordetella pertussis,* the causal agent of whooping cough. This microorganism, readily obtained from the bronchi of guinea-pigs with diseased lungs, was also often found attached to the cilia of the respiratory tract in healthy guinea-pigs. 2. *Pneumococcus.* In and after 1908, Smith had identified the *pneumococcus* as a cause of infection in various guinea-pig organs, and isolated it from consolidated lungs already damaged by concurrent *B. bronchisepticus.* The possibilities were raised that pneumococci might be carried by apparently healthy guinea-pigs, or serve as primary cause of pneumonia in that species. Differences in virulence of the parasite, and pregnancy or fatty infiltration in lungs and liver of the host, were postulated as predisposing factors. Theobald reported the results to the Boston Society of Medical Sciences in December 1913,[22] which published them later that month.[23] Incidentally, he had recently been elected president of that Society.[24]

The pneumococcus cultures were transferred regularly, and Smith conducted intermittent studies in this field until the end of 1914. On December 8, he recorded "working on g.p. pneumonia;" and for the period December 28–30, the sole notation was "Pneumococcus etc all day in lab." He accepted McGowan's claim (1910) that *B. bronchisepticus* was the causal agent of canine distemper.[25] However, in 1928 Laidlaw and Dunkin clearly demonstrated that the disease had a specific viral etiology, with *B. bronchisepticus* a secondary invader.[26] The situation was analogous to hog cholera and swine influenza—with specific viruses as inciting agents and particular bacilli as complicating factors.

In May 1913, Smith was called upon to investigate two severe outbreaks of milk-borne tonsillitis or septic sore throat in communities near Boston. (His Day Card of the 22nd recorded, "Lunch at Brigham's Hosp. guest of Dr. Cushing; Working on milk epid. cults. from Canton, Mass.")[27] On the 28th, he went "To Canton in auto with Rosenau and Richardson to inspect pasteurizer of F.—whose milk caused epidemic."[28] Between then and July 1914, Smith received specimens from four smaller outbreaks in Massachusetts and one in New York State. He also obtained cultures which had been isolated previously from epidemics in Boston (1911), Chicago (1912) and Baltimore (1912).

For about one and a half years, more than sixty streptococcal isolates from human and bovine sources were subjected to detailed analysis by Theobald Smith and his assistant, J. Howard Brown, in the Department of Comparative Pathology at the Harvard Medical School. Cultures were isolated and maintained on horse blood agar. The authors' description and nomenclature of and forms of hemolysis around colonies on blood agar plates are still routinely used. The quantitative capacity of each strain to ferment various carbohydrates in one week of incubation at 36°C, and its milk-coagulating properties, were determined. Agglutinogenic relationships were verified by means of immunized rabbit sera. Pathogenicity for man of a given strain was tested by intravenously injecting a rabbit with 1 cc. of a twenty-four hour bouillon culture. Whereas bovine strains were non-pathogenic, virulent human strains either killed the rabbit or caused suppurative lesions in kidneys, peritoneum or joints. Smith and Brown's report was presented to the Boston Society of Medical Sciences on November 17, with subsequent publication in Harold Ernst's *Journal of Medical Research.*[29]

Howard Brown, like his mentor, was a meticulous investigator. The more precise their personal observations of such inconstant cultural properties as colonial size and morphology, or the extent and type of hemolysis, the harder it became to differentiate between truly heterologous strains and homologous strains showing slight natural variations. Also, observed bacteriological facts did not always fit hypotheses based on epidemiological conjectures. Rebecca Lancefield's system of streptococcus type classification could have solved the problem in short order, but that lay some twenty years ahead.[30] Their essential conclusion, confirmed repeatedly by others, was that in milk-borne outbreaks of streptococcal sore throat, the pathogenic bacteria are of human origin. The milker conveys a virulent strain (now Lancefield's group A) through traumatized teats to the udder, setting up a mastitis. The milk is polluted with pathogenic streptococci, and can be rendered safe for human consumption only by boiling or proper pasteurization. Milk from cows with mastitis due to other (bovine) types of streptococci is usually innocuous.

Theobald Smith attended several conferences on infantile paralysis called by the State Board of Health during the period 1909 to 1911, and talked informally about it to professional and other groups. Early in 1910, at the Rockefeller Institute, Simon Flexner demonstrated to the Scientific Directors[31] the *rhesus* monkeys which he and Paul Lewis had inoculated intraventricularly with Berkefeld filtrates of spinal cord suspensions from fatal cases. Paralysis could be induced serially in these animals. Flexner had searched thoroughly for bacterial causes in 1907 and 1909, with no more success than Smith had experienced in similar intermittent quests. The determination by Flexner and Lewis[32] of a transmissible viral etiology directed Smith's inquiries toward natural reservoirs of the virus and possible vectors: "Closing up poliomyelitis work," he succinctly noted.[33] Were certain domestic animals an ultimate source of the human infection? Could water supplies or flies serve as transmitting agents?

By November 1912, Smith and Carl TenBroeck, a twenty-six-year-old third year Harvard medical student, had nearly completed an unsuccessful search for a filter-passing agent in the spinal cords of domestic animals and ground-up stable flies. The investigation was funded by about a dozen private contributors. On the title page of the final report, TenBroeck appeared as sole author, with Theobald Smith responsible merely for an "Introductory Note."[34] However, the textual demarcation is vague. Probably Smith planned the research and edited the whole report. More than half of the animals reported were tested for poliomyelitis before TenBroeck even began work. The article appeared as part of a larger work, "Infantile Paralysis in Massachusetts, 1907–1912," in the forty-eighth *Annual Report* (for 1913) of the State Board of Health.

Thirty animals were selected for infectivity tests. About one-half of these already showed paralysis, while thirteen had been associated with cases of human poliomyelitis. Animals which did not die within a few days after arrival at the laboratory were killed. Berkefeld filtrates were prepared from their nasal mucosa or from a saline suspension of spinal cord ground in sterile sand. Around 5 cc. of the filtrate under test was injected into the lateral ventricle of an anesthetized monkey, sometimes supplemented by about 30 cc. of filtrate injected intraperitoneally. The tissues of nine cats, seven fowls, four swine, four rats, three horses, two cows and one dog were tested. Two batches of stable-flies (nineteen and twenty-two insects, respectively) were likewise ground up in saline, and the filtrates injected into the cerebral ventricles and abdominal cavity of monkeys. None of these monkeys developed paralysis or other evidence of poliomyelitis, though a few died following the inocula. By contrast, two monkeys, injected intraventricularly with a spinal cord filtrate from a child who died

of poliomyelitis, developed paralysis and their spinal cords showed typical pathological changes.[35]

While Theobald Smith sponsored only this single polio project, Simon
Flexner and his assistant Paul Lewis had reported so many observations on the
transmission of poliomyelitis to monkeys that Landsteiner and Popper's earlier
discovery from Vienna[36] was apt to be overlooked. Flexner's researches, moreover, were not restricted to the question of transmission alone. In 1911, for example, he and Paul Clark had reported that the house fly might be a virus source
for at least forty-eight hours after feeding on the spinal cord of a recently para-
lysed monkey; and in 1913 they showed that a dog's fatal paralysis simulating polio was not necessarily due to that disease.

Flexner assigned the task of growing the virus in an artificial medium to his
protégé Noguchi, who claimed to have grown the causal agent of syphilis,
Treponema pallidum, using a medium and a means of establishing anaerobiosis in
peptone bouillon first described by Theobald Smith.[37] Noguchi now set about
growing similarly the poliomyelitis virus. Flexner was sufficiently confident of
Noguchi's success to assume the senior authorship of the ensuing reports,[38] naming the "globoid bodies" (a bacterial contaminant) as the cause of the poliomyelitis transmitted to monkeys by the supernatant culture. Flexner apparently was
unaware that true viruses demand living cells to parasitize before multiplication;
but Smith's anaerobic medium contained small pieces of kidney or other live organ tissue from freshly-killed laboratory animals, which may have furnished
enough viable cells in his experiments for the virus to invade, proliferate, and
transmit poliomyelitis to monkeys.

About the same time (and again using Smith's chopped kidney medium),
Noguchi also contended that he managed to grow the rabies virus. Just before
departing for the annual meeting of the German Society of Naturalists and Physicians (Deutsche Gesellschaft der Naturforscher und Ärzte), to be held in Vienna in September 1913, where he was an invited guest lecturer, Noguchi was
advised by a somewhat skeptical Flexner to show his specimens to Theobald
Smith. Smith recorded the occasion in an entirely unimpressed fashion:
"Noguchi shows me his cults. of rabies virus 10–12 A.M. H.M.S. [Harvard Medical School]. Walk through Arboretum to & fro reading . . . early to bed."[39] Smith
wrote to Flexner that "the organism he has found is certainly suggestive," but
that perhaps Noguchi had "cultivated from the kidney of rabbits some rare parasite or that the organism is a difficultly growing, heavily capsulated coccus. Only
the one doing the work can determine how far he has eliminated such possibilities by repetitions." Flexner thanked Smith for his help. He had not thought of
the kidney tissue as a possible source of the organism. Noguchi "was so anxious
to make a guarded preliminary publication that I consented to his doing so," after

changing the body, title, and emphasis of the article.[40] Flexner thought Noguchi thus had "safeguard himself," until he could give undivided attention to the question on his return to New York. Noguchi's brief note appeared in the *Journal of Experimental Medicine,*[41] but he did not resume these studies.

Carl TenBroeck graduated from the University of Illinois in 1908, and in 1910 interrupted his medical studies at Harvard to work in Christian Herter's laboratory. After a few months of research, which led to a single publication by himself, he returned to Boston, because of Herter's increasing invalidism and death. He was hired by Smith for part-time work before the latter left for Europe. In according him full authorship of the poliomyelitis paper, Theobald Smith was even more generous than with Marshal Fabyan over the *B. abortus* reports. In Fabyan's case, the favor was to an unpaid assistant, whose father was Smith's benefactor. TenBroeck visited the Smith household with exceptional frequency. (For example, Smith recorded in 1912, "Mr. TenBroeck takes supper with us at home.")[42] The Day Card entries indicate the approximate date of his graduation. He was plain "Mr." when he came for dinner on March 30, 1913, whereas the man who stayed from 3 to 9 P.M. on July 6, 1913, was "Dr. TenBroeck." The new young doctor was unmarried, and the Smiths had two eligible daughters. In December, a "coming-out tea" was arranged for them, and their father thought the occasion "a great success."[43]

TenBroeck was keen on the younger daughter, Lilian; but she had another suitor, Robert F. Foerster, an instructor in Economics at Harvard. About three years elapsed before "Lilian 2nd" married Foerster, who first joined the family at a porch supper on a Sunday in June 1913.[44] Lilian resembled her mother in looks, did well in English at Radcliffe, and could provoke her somber father to smile or even to laugh. The other two children looked more like Theobald; but whereas Dorothea was somewhat of a bluestocking, Philip found dancing and automobiles more fascinating than books. At the Radcliffe Commencement in June 1913, Dorothea received *summa cum laude* for Chemistry, in which subject her father had coached her. The Day Card for May 12, 1914 noted, "Both daughters initiated into Phi Beta Kappa." By contrast, the diary for June 12 recorded "Closing Exercises for Philip at Roxbury Latin School, gets by without any honors or distinctions." Yet Theobald was determined that his son should go to Harvard. "Town with Phil—deposit for him, college money 900."[45]

TenBroeck also assisted in another of his chief's more fruitful fields of research—the so-called "paratyphoid group" of bacilli. V.A. Moore, Smith's former assistant and successor at the B.A.I., isolated and described in detail an organism that he named *Bacterium sanguinarium*. Similar strains were isolated by Smith in 1894, and again in 1901, from fowl epizootics near Providence, Rhode Island, as reported by Cooper Curtice.[46] The bacterium, now known as *Salmo-*

nella gallinarum, differed from others of this genus in normally being non-motile. A related subtype, *S. pullorum,* the cause of "white diarrhea" in chicks, has been implicated occasionally in human attacks of bacterial food poisoning traced to chicken salad.

In the first of a series of three papers by himself and TenBroeck, published in July 1915, *S. gallinarum* and *S. pullorum* cultures were compared in biochemical and agglutinogenic properties with strains of typhoid and dysentery bacilli, and with the so-called "hog-cholera bacillus."[47] The *gallinarum* and *pullorum* cultures reacted distinctively, but showed kinship with human typhoid cultures. The authors, alluding to the somatic and flagellar agglutinins investigated by Smith and Reagh in 1903, postulated that the inability of the non-motile species to absorb all agglutinins from a human typhoid antiserum was due to the residual (unabsorbed) flagellar component.

The second article reported the pathogenic effects upon various laboratory animal species of heat-stable, filtrable endotoxin produced in twenty-five day cultures of *S. gallinarum.*[48] Rabbits were particularly susceptible to the lethal effects of such culture filtrates injected intravenously. Their "death within two hours is in many respects like an anaphylactic shock." The third paper illustrated the close relationship between *S. gallinarum* and *S. pullorum.*[49] Despite the extraordinary complexity of the *Salmonella* genus revealed since then, current knowledge of *S. gallinarum* and *S. pullorum* has not greatly advanced in the past seven decades. Smith read an early report on this work, entitled "A Paratyphoid Bacillus (from Fowls) and Its Toxins," to the twenty-eighth Annual Meeting of the Association of American Physicians, held that year in Washington jointly with a triennial meeting of the Congress of American Physicians and Surgeons, May 6–9, 1914.

Theobald Smith not only enjoyed unraveling these complexities in the privacy of his own laboratory, with or without a trusted assistant, but also derived satisfaction from reporting his observations to a suitable audience—his favorite being perhaps the Association of American Physicians, which met annually in Washington. The membership, with a few notable exceptions such as Welch, Flexner, and Prudden, was not expected to grasp the details of his expositions, but to follow their drift and accept his conclusions. Nowadays, the means for imparting new super-specialized knowledge in medical microbiology to practicing physicians and the paramedical professions have to be completely different: Smith would not have been either comfortable with or supportive of current arrangements.[50] The banquet at the New Willard Hotel on May 7 was to be followed by more "papers till 11 p.m." Theobald Smith shared a table with Frank Billings of Chicago, George Dock of St. Louis, Hun, Northrup, and two representatives of the Rockefeller Institute, Mitchell Prudden and Simon Flexner.[51]

In the afternoon of the 8th, the National Tuberculosis Association's program began and continued next morning; but Smith and Paul Lewis broke away in time to reach the Phipps Institute in Philadelphia for a luncheon meeting of its Advisory Council. Mr. Phipps was present at the lunch and attended the dedicatory exercises on the roof of a new building endowed by him, as well as a dinner for about 100 guests. Smith spoke at the dinner. He was a charter member of the Council and his name was listed immediately after Welch's, followed by Simon Flexner, Hermann L. Biggs, Lawrason Brown, Gideon Wells, and seven other names.[52] Smith returned to Boston on May 11, too tired to begin fresh experiments before leaving again for New Haven, where the Remsen Referee Board met for the last time before its unexpected disbandment.

Since his return from Europe, Smith's scant time for research had been apportioned among fortuitous, unplanned, local investigations. A promising long-term project was the mysterious turkey disease which he had first encountered at the Rhode Island Experimental Station at Kingston in August 1894. That preliminary inquiry had been reported promptly to the Secretary of Agriculture, the Hon. J. Stirling Morton, but did not appear in print until 1896.[53] Just before Smith left the Bureau of Animal Industry he described the pathology and other features of this disease, which he termed protozoal infectious entero-hepatitis of turkeys. His more detailed account was published in 1895 as B.A.I. Bulletin No. 8.[54] Presuming an analogy with human amebic dysentery, Smith designated the protozoan *Amoeba meleagridis n.sp.*, but gave no derivation for the specific term. In Greek mythology, the Meleagrides, sisters of the hero Meleager, wept unceasingly after their brother's untimely death, until changed by Artemis into guinea-hens (turkeys), and transferred to another island. The true nature of the parasite, the geographic distribution and mode of spread of the disease, and the means of controlling it—apart from the liberal use of antiseptics—remained elusive.

In 1908, Cole and Bradley at the Rhode Island Experiment Station concluded that *Amoeba meleagridis* was probably the schizont stage of *Coccidium cuniculi*. A Station bulletin of 132 pages and eleven plates with evidence supporting this claim was not published for two and a half years.[55] Smith denounced it as adding "nothing whatever . . . to existing knowledge." In a lengthy letter to the editor of *Science,* he scornfully dismissed Cole and Bradley's claim as "merely an inference or hypothesis,"[56] contending that they had failed to recognize a double infection prevailing at their Station. Recently, he had autopsied young turkeys, the majority dead from blackhead, without finding a single coccidium, while various workers had described avian coccidiosis with no liver involvement. Incidentally, Smith's authoritative experience with coccidiosis[57] entitled him to point out that the designation *Coccidium cuniculi* should be reserved for the agent of rabbit coccidiosis—a very unlikely avian parasite.

This letter was at least four times as long as the "special article" in which Cole and Bradley made their original claim. Smith deplored "the publication of premature, undigested, controversial statements . . . years before the appearance in print of the actual work on which such statements are presumably based." To avoid any misunderstanding of his motive, he disarmed critics by admitting that his earlier work on *Amoeba meleagridis* was tentative and incomplete. Final determination of the protozoan's nature and life cycle, and the mode of infection, might require "years of experimental breeding and rearing [of turkeys] in carefully guarded territories."[58] The letter was quite atypical for never again did Smith so strongly denounce the work of others, or so openly acknowledge gaps in his own investigations. It served also as goad to resume researches on turkey hepato-colitis whenever circumstances permitted.

Since the accommodation and supervision available at the Harvard Medical School was inadequate for turkeys, Smith decided to rear his own. Behind the mansion at Woodland Hill, he constructed a high-wired enclosure about twenty feet square, on grassland preserved free from domesticated birds for at least eighteen years. On May 13, 1913, he recorded, "Start incubation in cellar with 36 turkey eggs."[59] The eggs were hatched in a gas-heated incubator and brooder, while the poults found shelter and roosting at night in a shed within the enclosure. Smith favored white Holland turkeys and eventually grew very fond of his tame flock. On fine summer evenings, after a long day at the laboratory, he would take a kitchen chair into their enclosure and chatter to them, while they flutter about, landing or climbing on his lap and shoulders.

The problems they were intended to solve proved very intricate, and these 1913 experimental results had little significance because only five of thirty-six disinfected eggs hatched and three of the poults died soon. Special attentions were lavished upon the two survivors, which became pets. He noted on Day Cards throughout 1913: "Working all Sunday AM setting up brooder for turkeys" (June 8); "Tending to two little turkeys" (June 29); "Take turkeys to walk" (August 12); "Turkeys out scratching among leaves" (November 2); "Rather raw [weather]—my ♀ turkey stolen last night" (Christmas Day); "Killed ♀ turkey & ex[amined] thoroughly—no more left now." (December 27). This sad march of events was accompanied by evening relaxations; either compensational, such as "reading some turkey literature," and "working chiefly on turkey disease," or consolatory—strumming Schumann's *Noveletten*, tackling conundrums in calculus, or reading Goethe's *Dichtung und Wahrheit*. About four months before their untimely end, the birds received on two consecutive days a twice-daily dose of chopped cecum from infected turkeys. One victim appeared healthy when stolen; the other at autopsy was uninfected.

In the spring of 1914, Smith launched another venture. Of nineteen turkeys raised as before, five were killed by a rat and three others were discarded or died of intercurrent disease. None of those eight showed any post mortem abnormality. The eleven survivors were penned in an enclosure with nine bronze turkeys from an infected flock, thus being exposed to air-borne or alimentary infections for a variable number of weeks before they were sacrificed and autopsied. All but one of the bronze turkeys showed heavy infection with *A. meleagridis,* whereas only one white survivor was infected. The negative experimental findings of 1913–14 suggested that *A. meleagridis* is "poorly adapted to its young host," and that invasion of the walls of ceca and liver is not conducive "to the discharge of parasites for passage to another host"—in fact, the parasites lie "buried within the host lesions."

Smith's inconclusive results opened several alternative pathogenetic mechanisms for this puzzling host-parasite interaction. He suggested "The disease may represent a kind of aberrant parasitism, the true host being some other species. Or the parasite may undergo its normal development in the contents of the ceca and the invasion of the tissues may be abnormal. Or there may be still other stages and an intermediate host."[60] The true explanation was unfolded through prolonged experimentation carried out elsewhere by Smith and his associates.

One late summer evening in 1913, Simon Flexner received a telephone call from Hermann Biggs, chief medical officer of the New York City Health Department, and a fellow-director of the Rockefeller Institute. Biggs was a close friend and medical adviser of the family of James Jerome Hill (1835–1916), a railroad magnate, whose northern line penetrated farm lands of the West. He relayed an offer of $25,000 or more if Flexner would begin the study of hog cholera, which was devastating the farmers of Hill's railroad territory. Flexner deferred acceptance of the offer since "he was not the person to make the investigation,"[61] but he undertook to look into the problem.

The next meeting of the Scientific Directors, on October 11, included a visit to the Rockefeller Institute's "Biological Farm" at the village of Clyde, just outside New Brunswick, New Jersey, "to plan development." The Corporation of the Institute had met at the Whitehall Club, Battery Park, on the previous day, and Smith had dined with the Flexners that evening; but neither Hill nor hog cholera are mentioned in Smith's diary or Day Cards. Members of the Board of Scientific Directors who resided in New York City became an Executive Committee under Mitchell Prudden's chairmanship to deal with urgent problems. At the next meeting of the Executive committee, Flexner reported on a conference with Hill, who had repeated the offer made through Biggs. The Executive referred the matter to a special committee comprising Flexner and Smith.[62]

Flexner promptly proposed to Smith a visit to Boston on October 28 for a talk about hog cholera. He enclosed a letter from Paul Ehrlich, enthusiastically praising Noguchi, who on October 1 had "demonstrated his numerous outstanding preparations, with the greatest applause from the assembled physicians of Frankfurt. I said a few words at the end congratulating Noguchi on his discoveries and described briefly the wonderful development of the Rockefeller Institute under your direction. The Congress of Physicians thereupon suggested that a congratulatory telegram be sent to you also." Ehrlich thought Flexner and "the magnanimous founder" should be very happy with the course of events. Because Flexner knew "how to collect at the Institute the best-qualified heads of the whole world,"[63] further accomplishments could be anticipated. Smith commented that the letter "was a very fine and just tribute to the work of the Institute, and it is consoling to have a few very appreciative spirits among us whose words have weight." He would gladly see Flexner as suggested.[64]

Although quite interested in Hill's proposition, Smith expounded his conviction that studies of the host-parasite relationship in animals illuminated many problems of human infection. Flexner certainly knew Theobald Smith's concern with animal pathology, but had not realized how extensively his interests were focused upon this field. He was impressed by Smith's enthusiasm, and on returning to New York added these words to his note of thanks: "Perhaps there will be something more to be said about the subject before long," adding, "I wish to tell you . . . how much light I got on the question of animal disease from your exposition."[65] Smith replied: "I have pondered a great deal over the information which you brought from New York City, and I hope that it may lead to something of substantial benefit in the direction of the public welfare."

Hill's offer and Smith's reaction confirmed Flexner's inclination to establish a department of animal pathology at the Rockefeller Institute. Uncertainties about the standards and efficiency of the biological farm near New Brunswick, upon which the Institute depended for its supply of laboratory animals, had induced Flexner on several occasions to conduct Theobald Smith over the farm. This anxiety had been aggravated by the increasing demand for antimeningococcus serum, and by the growing political influence of antivivisectionists. Moreover, present arrangements were ill-adapted to any researches into, for example, bovine tuberculosis, Bang's disease, or rabies. Hill's crusade against hog cholera and Smith's willingness to reactivate his interest in that disease reinforced Flexner's natural expansionist tendencies. A few years before (1910), he had stretched the bounds of medical research to justify recommending the appointment of Jacques Loeb to the Institute Staff to head a department of experimental biology.[66] Inclusion of a department of animal pathology within the Rockefeller Institute for Medical Research seemed entirely appropriate, not only to Flexner but also to the Rockefellers and their Trustees.

From the beginning, opinions on such proposals were sought and reactions were carefully weighed. At an Executive Committee meeting in November 1913, Flexner reported on his conference with Theobald Smith "regarding the study of hog cholera and the establishment of a department of animal pathology in the Institute." The Committee voted against "undertaking the study of animal diseases upon a gift or pledge of $25,000;" but favored requesting Smith to suggest the essential machinery involved in the study of animal diseases.[67] Some confusion developed because animal "pathology" became displaced temporarily by animal "diseases," but Smith's own preference for the former eventually won acceptance.

In mid-December, Smith met with the Committee in Prudden's New York apartment at 160 West 59th Street. On hand for consideration at the January 7, 1914 meeting of the Executive Committee was a five-page typed letter, addressed by Theobald Smith to Prudden as chairman. The opening paragraph drew attention to the dual nature of the project: "In order to combine two objects, the organization of a department in animal pathology and the study of a definite disease or group of allied diseases, the plant might be built and the staff organized with reference to the study of infectious swine diseases." Among miscellaneous basic requirements were isolation pens, a large incinerator, an incubator, a specialized library, and ample acreage. "The department should be geographically more or less independent of the territory and buildings planned for the use of the now existing departments of the Institute." For each domestic animal species whose diseases would be under study, Smith estimated a requisite staff of fifteen, from department head to farm hands, with "clerks or stenographers to be engaged as needed." Among more distant objectives, he listed studies of nutritional disturbances, and the diseases of fishes, field rodents and insect pests. Mentioned also were causes to which he was long devoted—the promotion of rural hygiene, the training of volunteer workers in animal pathology, and the establishment of a high-class journal of comparative pathology.[68]

Three days later, the Board of Scientific Directors (including Smith) advised Flexner to confer with the Trustees about establishing a Department of Animal Pathology. In Smith's temporary absence, Welch voiced the prevailing opinion that this step should "be conditioned on Dr. Smith's willingness to assume its direction."[69] The go-between in the negotiations was to be the Business Manager of the Rockefeller Institute, Henry James, Jr. (son of the philosopher, William James, and nephew of the novelist, Henry James, Sr.), who talked with Smith in mid-January, and again two weeks later, at Harvard Medical School.[70] At the next month's Executive Committee meeting, James reported that the Trustees not only favored establishment of the department, but were ready to "move forward with the matter independently of any support from Mr. James J. Hill; further, that Dr. Theobald Smith had been asked to prepare a preliminary budget for current expenses."[71]

As usual in fiscal matters, Smith curbed any flights of fancy, and was very economical. On March 6 he was still "typewriting on An. Pathology div. of Rock. Inst.," but the report would be available for the Manager to present a few days later to the Executive Committee. He outlined some building plans, and estimated a start-up budget of $30,000 to $35,000, including salaries. The Committee voted that if the Trustees authorized the Department, the Manager should invite Theobald Smith "to organize and assume the direction of the Department of Animal Diseases in the Institute," with the rank of member of the Institute, and the title of Director of the Department of Animal Diseases. The appointment would take effect on July 1, 1914, or as soon thereafter as suited Smith. A salary of $10,000 was mooted, but on that point the excerpts from the Minutes were left blank.[72] At this juncture Theobald's wife perhaps became aware of the threatened upheaval, for a family legend holds that on learning something of his plans, she asked him about the future salary—only to be told that he had not inquired. The Trustees had yet to make a formal offer.

On March 20, 1914, The Board of Trustees met at its headquarters, 26 Broadway, New York. After Simon Flexner had enlarged upon the recommendations of the Board of Scientific Directors, it was resolved by the Trustees that Flexner, Henry James, Jr. and their Secretary, Starr Murphy, should constitute a committee to secure the enabling legislation, provided the estimated costs of $127,000 for the land and buildings, and $46,000 for salaries and annual maintenance could be financed.[73] The directorship of the Department was settled shortly afterward at a separate meeting of the Trustees. As Theobald Smith was sole candidate for the post, and unanimously endorsed by the Executive Committee of the Board of Scientific Directors, the main problems were concerned with his salary and pension. in settling a salary, Welch's reflection should be borne in mind that "no one gives up a Harvard professorship."[74] As regards pension, Theobald Smith himself had expressed already certain apprehensions to the Executive Committee of the Scientific Directors, probably through Henry James. He now asked if he could be credited with five years of service for pension purposes; and whether, in the event of disability or death before the full benefits of his retiring allowance were reaped, his widow and dependent minor children would be entitled to no less than if he had remained as Professor at the Harvard Medical School. These requests seemed more consistent with his customary prudence than the impractical detachment from financial matters which family legend attributes to him.

The Executive Committee recommended that the Rules Governing the Institute's Retiring Allowances should be adjusted according to Smith's own proposal. The Board of Trustees accepted all of the recommendations, and instructed Henry James to invite Theobald Smith to become Director of the Department of Animal Diseases in the Institute at the annual salary of $10,000. James was also asked to convey the Trustees' resolution that "the Institute agree with Dr. Smith, in case he accepts the appointment," that the Rules Governing Retiring Allowance should be adjusted to meet his requests.[75]

Before these decisions could have reached Smith officially, there was news of a further philanthropy, sealing his future. John D. Rockefeller had added another million dollars to the general endowment of the Rockefeller Institute for Medical Research, earmarked for the organization of a "department for the study of animal diseases." Smith celebrated the occasion by recording on his Day Card: "Announcement of gift to establish Dept. An. Path. Rockefeller Inst. lab all day —miscell. work."[76] The brevity of this comment did not measure the confused state of mind revealed in the letter he wrote that same day to Flexner, expressing his "appreciation of Mr. Rockefeller's confidence in the institution he has founded and nurtured" by a further endowment, but which left him "somewhat dazed."

Evidently aware of some fiscal details of the Executive Committee's recommendations to the Board of Trustees, Theobald Smith now mildly decried their generosity. The plan took "such a big sum for the salary of the head of the department that the balance of the income seems much shrunken. However that is a criticism that comes with poor grace from a candidate." As regards pension, a man in his position "should get his standing as it was at the place from which he retired: Anything beyond would be unfair. A young man would of course come in under the regular pension scheme." He was confronted not only by the honor and confidence shown, but also by "the painful uprooting of my family. I have not yet seriously talked with them, for they are very fond of their present home and their many friends." And he expressed the hope "that my possible candidacy may be kept among ourselves . . . as long as possible." They had to get their balance and meet the crisis in their lives. This was "the most important proposition that I have had to face."[77]

The next day, a press release announced that the Rockefeller Institute "will shortly organize a department for the study of animal diseases," and that to promote research in this field, Mr. John D. Rockefeller had given it an additional endowment of $1,000,000. The staffing of the new department was not mentioned. The release stated that the Institute had also been pledged $50,000 by

Mr. James J. Hill, to aid studies of hog cholera. Hill, who had increased his pledge by letter of January 20, 1914 to Biggs, was pleased to be named.

After talking the matter over with his family, and brooding overnight on "real and imaginary difficulties," Smith wrote Flexner a longer personal letter, beset with hesitancies. Reasons for lack of confidence in being able to handle the undertaking included doubts whether he, as head, could be "cognizant of all details" of the operation, or could stand the heat of midsummer. Besides, the foundations for animal pathology were very weak, and few were working "to broaden and strengthen this foundation. The pressure for practical results is too great."

> The question of residence is a difficult one. At present my family would I think find themselves totally lost in an ordinary business community and Princeton seems the only alternative. There is a good train service from there to New Brunswick and in good weather an automobile would probably not be too tiring and give the desired outdoor life . . . Eventually I should prefer a nearby farm but I cannot induce my family to take up this kind of existence.

Smith proposed, tentatively and unofficially, a two-year trial for the Rockefeller Institute and himself, with the first year-and-a-half "largely taken up with organization and formulating lines of work." Admittedly President Lowell might not consider any request for two years' leave-of-absence. He would not negotiate his Harvard relationship "until you feel satisfied that the details of the situation are cleared up, so far as the Institute is concerned."[78]

Meanwhile, in a letter which crossed with Smith's latest two, Simon Flexner brought news of progress, and also indicated that he expected the department of animal pathology to be a closely linked component of his New York Institute. Flexner was a punctilious correspondent and therefore had to write many trivial notes; but his important letters, which reflected his character and sustained his successful directorship, often showed touches of both benevolent thoughtfulness and implicit authoritarianism. To this particular recipient they customarily began "Dear Dr. Smith" and ended "Yours sincerely, Simon Flexner." The formality was reciprocated. They never resorted to first names. The first three paragraphs of Flexner's letter went thus:

> Mr. James has written you the splendid news of the gift of Mr. Rockefeller of the endowment for the department of animal pathology. The provision will be enough to permit of a full development of the plan that you submitted.
>
> It has, as you know, been understood throughout that you would become the head of the new department. Without that assurance the department would not have been recommended by the director or created by the trustees.
>
> I am very happy over the prospect of having you in New York and closely asso-

ciated with the actual work of the Institute; and since the new department really provides for your own special field and for your personal direction of the work within it, I am especially gratified.

Flexner stressed his own key position with the Trustees by referring to their settlement of the salary at $10,000 per annum, and their approval of the pension provisions. After the Trustees had met again soon to adopt suitable resolutions, a formal invitation to join the staff of the Institute would be presented. Meanwhile, he would "be happy to come to Boston or to have you come here," to discuss any point. The letter closed "I need not add that we will all welcome your family to the environs of New York."[79]

As Smith had foreseen, the family recoiled from any suggestion of moving even to the suburbs of the metropolis. The children now had grown-up preoccupations, but their mother's situation was different. Lilian loved her way of life at Woodland Hill. She had attuned household activities to her husband's work and welfare, yet developed her own resourceful personality and illuminated the bounds of womankind. At the end of May, for example, while Theobald dined at the Harvard Club with officers of the Society for Tropical Medicine, she was hostess at a gigantic women's tea party. "Anti-suffrage tea at our house, 257 guest."[80] There was scant comfort in reflecting that in just over one year neither the setting nor the guests would be available. Further, Lilian spurned all ideas of her husband working in or adjacent to the Institute. From the outset, Smith's plans for properly isolated animal quarters and laboratories were clearly incompatible with Flexner's more restricted initial vision of a neighboring fiefdom. When the other members of the Executive Committee adopted Smith's viewpoint, Flexner deftly envisaged governing a satellite division by remote control.

Flexner's reply to Smith's two letters was kind and soothing. Flexner fully understood "the doubts and perplexities" besetting him. James would deliver copies of the resolutions of the Board of Trustees and bring him up to date on practical developments. "We shall all wish to make the transition to the Institute as easy as reassuring to you and your family as possible." From the beginning, Smith could so arrange his staff that he could "break the work for good periods in the summer, and, as you will have no teaching obligations, for periods in the winter, too. We shall be jealous of your health and strength and shall wish to see them protected and conserved in every way." Flexner had also considered "the new work being in New Jersey and I have conceived of a plan that I believe will in some degree mitigate the (scientific) isolation." He offered to come to Boston on April 9 to go over any points. Everybody concerned would hold in confidence "the invitation extended to you by the Directors and Trustees."[81]

This letter dissipated Smith's last doubts. The die was cast, and Henry Walcott should be the first to know his intentions. "P.M. visit Dr. Walcott at Cambridge and discuss my going to Rockefeller Institute."[82] In accepting Flexner's reassurances, Smith mentioned this interview. "I have received the formal invitation of the Directors, have seen Mr. James, and had a long talk with Dr. Walcott of the Corporation. He begged me to postpone any formal answer to the Directors until Tuesday [April 7]. Both he and President Eliot have been like a father to me and it was a trying task to tell him. but I see no retreat now and the delay will not change the situation." Within the next few days, he would seek President Lowell's permission to remain on the faculty for the 1914–15 academic year, without teaching duties, so that he could write up completed researches and also plan for the new department.[83] Smith revisited Walcott later that day, but with his mind already settled: "Discuss with Dr. Walcott my going to New Jersey."[84]

On April 7, Theobald Smith went over to Cambridge to see President Lowell, who neither tried to dissuade him from accepting the Institute's offer nor favored the prolonged leave-of-absence proposal. Smith was asked to submit a date of resignation and a plan of work for the interim. On the 8th, he entrained for New York, and next morning went to the Rockefeller Institute for "lunch with Messrs Gates & Murphy & Green etc accepting invitation to form new dept. of institute."[85] "Green," was Jerome D. Greene, former Secretary to the Harvard Corporation, and now attached to the personal staff of John D. Rockefeller, Jr. Greene proved an invaluable Trustee of the Rockefeller Institute. The "etc" in Smith's Day Card entry presumably covered Simon Flexner, Henry James, Jr., and any others at the luncheon. On the same day, at a meeting of the Committee of Scientific Directors, "a letter for informal acceptance of the position of Director in charge of the Department of Animal diseases was presented by the Manager [James]."[86] After a quiet Easter at home, Smith wrote his formal "acceptance of directorship of the new dept. animal pathology."[87] Flexner recalled nearly thirty years later, "There was great rejoicing when, on April 16, 1914, Smith accepted. The ideal director had been secured."[88]

A week after their interview, Smith wrote to President Lowell. The letter coolly outlined how Smith proposed to spend the ensuing year at Harvard. It sought no favor, conveyed no regret, expressed no appreciation. His usual courses had been announced for the coming year. With one assistant's help he would "carry through the necessary work and finish certain MSS," and perhaps complete some researches.

I hope to get a little of the sabbatical year I had originally planned to apply for, even if only in fragments. I shall give at least half my time to the Medical School work and the other half to rest and plans for the new work.

Whatever financial arrangements are made by the Corporation for this year will be satisfactory to me. I shall look to the Institute to make up any deficiency.[89]

Walcott hoped to enlist Corporation colleagues to exert last-minute persuasion to shake Smith's resolve. At a meeting between himself, Smith and the president on April 17, Lowell agreed to see Smith again, after the next meeting of the College Fellows. Major H.L. Higginson, one of Harvard's wealthy benefactors, scrawled an urgent message to Smith, asking him to telephone whether he had time for a brief talk. If the chat transpired, it was fruitless. Other friends of Harvard voiced sympathetic regrets. Carroll Dunham wrote rather sententiously to Lowell, "Although I feel sure that Dr. Smith suffers real grief at the prospect of severing his connection with Harvard, it seems to me that his devotion to duty, the comparatively few years of full working power to which he can reasonably look forward, and the extraordinarily favorable conditions offered him for advancing knowledge and organizing *wissenschaftliche Forschung* in his great subject, unite to oblige him to accept this new responsibility."[90] Lowell replied that after three talks with Smith about his going to the Rockefeller Institute, "the gift of J.J. Hill of $50,000 for the investigation of Hog Cholera turned the stream and was followed by a very large appropriation by the Rockefeller Institute for the study of animal diseases; so much that we could not possibly compete for it." Though he felt Smith would like to continue that work at Harvard, there was "no hope of turning this research in our direction."[91]

Finally, Charles Eliot sent a heart-warming benediction: "Dr. Walcott and I talked over your leaving the Medical School a few days ago, and although we were both of us very, very sorry to have you leave Harvard, we agreed that the offer of the Rockefeller Institute was one which you, as a devoted servant of science & humanity, could not well decline." Eliot unintentionally made his blessing more poignant by driving home the Woodland Hill issue. "It comforts me that you need not leave your present residence before July 1, 1915; because your family, which cannot be so well off in New Jersey or New York as it is in Forest Hills, will have a respite."[92]

At their meeting on April 17, President Lowell had commented to Theobald Smith upon exclusion of the proposed Rockefeller animal "experiment station" from New Jersey. A Bill authorizing establishment of the new department of animal pathology, sponsored by State Senator Colgate, had been passed on April 13 by both houses of the Legislature unanimously; but antivivisectionists persuaded Governor Fiedler to veto it. The governor was sensitive to the lobbying of this group of zealots, who had stirred up trouble previously over the Institute's animal farm at Clyde. Lowell requested Smith to keep him informed of developments, and to ensure that he would be consulted before any public announcements were released regarding the directorship. A few days later, from Washington, where he was attending meetings of the National Academy of Sciences, Smith affirmed these undertakings: "I did not write earlier because the Board members all felt that if the new plant was not to be in N.J., it would be in N.Y. near the Institute buildings. There was however no special fear or apprehension that legislation would not be favorable next year. The announcement as to the directorship will not be made without consultation with you (by Mr. James, Jr.)."[93] When he revisited Lowell on May 5, the president reported that the Fellows were in accord with the plan outlined by Smith. They agreed amicably that the resignation should take effect as of July 31, 1915.

The Board of Scientific Directors of the Rockefeller Institute passed two resolutions: 1. "That in addition to the necessary facilities for the scientific work, the Department of Animal pathology should be situated in a community in which its Staff will find congenial association." 2. "That owing to the many advantages in situation and accessibility of our present facilities at Clyde, or in some other place in the general region between Princeton and New Brunswick . . . every effort should be made to secure legislative action favorable to our work before renewed research is made for a site for a farm and special laboratories in New York State."[94]

At this same meeting, Smith's formal written acceptance of the directorship was approved for transmission to the Trustees, coupled with the recommendation that the Department's official designation be Animal Pathology. Smith also "expressed a desire to have it recorded that work on hog cholera be interpreted to mean a study of all the acute infectious diseases of swine."[95] However, the Board of Trustees tactfully recollected that their new venture owed its inception to Hill, though his initial offer was rejected as inadequate, while even the $50,000 was greatly overshadowed by the Rockefeller endowment. Hill could be a bad-tempered despot. His nicknames ranged from "Empire Builder" to "One-Eyed Old Sonofabitch." He might angrily resent any down-playing of his generosity. Press releases about the new department therefore usually mentioned him. He died in May 1916, before the buildings at Princeton were ready for hog cholera research. His son and other relatives refused to honor the pledge.[96]

Early in May, Smith reminded Flexner that Henry James should warn him when the public announcement would be made. "I may be able to escape the penny newspaper reporters by a short vacation."[97] The appointment became public on May 18, at a time when Smith was resting at home. His Day Card noted, "Resting after the troubles & sorrows of last week . . . Newspapers announce my going to Rockefeller Institute."[98] On May 14, he had been summoned to Albany as his mother had become very feeble and was in a private nursing-home. He saw to her comfort and went back to Boston, but she died early on the 15th. Theobald returned at once to Albany, Lilian taking a later train. They attended his mother's funeral service at the Chapel of Our Lady of Angels, with burial in the local cemetery on May 17, 1914—their 26th wedding anniversary.[99]

Flexner always took special care that Institute publicity for the general scientist should be tasteful and accurate. Mitchell Prudden put together a "quite charmingly done"[100] tribute to Theobald Smith for *Science;*[101] a few days later, the medical profession was briefly informed that Professor Theobald Smith of the Harvard Medical School had "accepted the position of director to the new department of animal pathology at the Rockefeller Institute for Medical Research."[102]

Still undecided was the date of Smith's resignation from his State Board of Health obligations. Walcott revealed his own intention of leaving that year. He was seventy-six years old and had chaired the Board of Health for twenty-eight years. The Board would be reorganized as a Department of Health, of which the Laboratories would constitute one among several divisions. Smith wished to minimize his involvement in such reforms and resigned all his public health laboratory duties as of July 31, 1914. To Walcott he suggested interim arrangements which could "run at least for another year." Herbert R. Brown "has business sense and can act promptly under pressure," and was capable of taking charge of the commercial production and administrative aspects of the laboratory. He should be acting-director, with a salary of $2,500. Dr. A.T. Reagh could manage vaccine preparation and the venereal disease work for a salary of $2,000. Smith himself would be "ready to confer with and advise these men as heretofore," as long as he lived so close to the laboratory.[103] His proposals were implemented. When Theobald Smith finally left for full-time duties under Rockefeller Institute auspices, his part-time activities as State Pathologist and as Director of the Antitoxin and Vaccine Laboratory were taken over for about five years by his colleague M.J. Rosenau.

The State board of Health received Smith's resignation "with the deepest regret" and recorded "its appreciation of the great services he has rendered to the Commonwealth by extensive knowledge, unselfish devotion and clear judgement. These services have been rendered at a salary wholly inadequate and which has represented in no way their value to the community. Dr. Smith's reputation as one of the real leaders in the scientific medicine of his time has been of the greatest value to the Board."[104]

Theobald Smith stayed with the Gages in January 1914, between visiting his mother and the other Albany relatives on the 7th, and a meeting of the Scientific

Directors in New York on the 10th. At Cornell, he lectured on vaccines before a Conference of State Veterinarians. Early in April, he wrote to the Gages: "I know you would like to hear a continuation of the story that began last January."

> As you have read, the dept. of an. diseases is established & endowed with 1 million. I am offered the directorship, which makes the dept. a *coordinate* part of the Institute, the others being the Institute laboratories and the hospital. I shall accept, for my dept. here has been running down badly because I do not constantly kick and advertise. Everybody thinks I'm happy and rolling in facilities. It's very trying to leave the old friends like President Eliot and others—but—.[105]

In a letter written to Gage in August of 1915, Theobald confirmed his decision, telling Gage, "Whenever I think the whole situation over again, I cannot but think the move is in the right direction."[106] On Christmas Eve, 1914, Smith wrote to Gage, confirming the death from cancer of their mutual friend C.A. Minot. "There are only two or three men in our faculty left who were on hand when I became a member in 1896. Now I am going. It seems trying to leave, but matters were not going well and I did not care simply to draw my salary and do nothing."[107] By the late summer of 1915, shortly before his departure for Princeton, his grievances were more pointed. "My dept. was in a bad shape, physically and financially. New 'schools' were being organized to the detriment of the old ones. Salary for a single assistant had to be dug out of gifts & income, not to mention many other difficulties. Moreover, we could not have remained in our home indefinitely in any case."[108]

Gage was Smith's sole apparent confidant for written explanations of his resignation from Harvard. Those rationalizations hardly inculpate the University. Most universities, and especially the medical schools, were and are highly competitive *milieux,* where the aggressive "constantly kick and advertise." For several years, he was disaffected at Harvard. His restlessness persisted until temporarily relieved by the Visiting Professorship to Berlin. Now a generous offer had come from an organization representing almost inexhaustible opportunities for medical research. Theobald Smith accepted their offer. About sixteen months later, he surrendered his tenancy of Woodland Hill—"our dear old home where the children grew up"[109]—thus severing the last link with Harvard. In glancing back to some turning-point in their life, few will admit to having made the wrong decision. Theobald Smith's vision, courage and pride quashed any impulse to question his own judgement.

20

FAREWELL HARVARD AND
JAMAICA PLAIN

The news that Theobald Smith would be leaving Harvard for the Rockefeller Institute for Medical Research brought him many messages of appreciation and encouragement. He was surprised at the number of well-wishers. Fulsome articles appeared in the press. *Harper's Monthly Magazine* described him as "unquestionably the greatest living American scientist, and one of the greatest scientists of this or any other time . . . the founder of one of the most fascinating branches of bacteriology,"[1] ranking him with other North American contributors to medical science, such as Morton, Beaumont, O.W. Holmes and Walter Reed. *The World's Work* devoted an article to the "romance" of unlocking the mysteries of Texas cattle fever, wrongly claiming that Theobald Smith foresaw from the outset "some basis for the agricultural superstition" associating Texas fever with the cattle tick.[2] These articles, torn from the magazines, went into the scrapbook.

Now that the end of his University duties was in prospect, Smith seemed to shoulder his full share almost eagerly. He faithfully attended faculty and committee meetings; prepared and delivered addresses with special care and conviction to graduate students, as well as to professional and lay groups; and tidied up his research projects with dispatch and efficiency. These were short-term, incidental projects. He suppressed temporarily the longing to engage in some research undertaking that would be difficult to solve and fundamental in significance. He spent whole days at the Medical School participating in oral examinations of second-year students. At the end of September he started the usual painstaking lectures and laboratory exercises for students enrolled in his fourth-year optional course.

He faithfully kept his obligations whether long-made or unforeseen. On November 6, 1914, an organizational meeting of the twenty-man Commission for the Investigation of Bovine Tuberculosis was held in the Executive Chamber at Albany, with Governor M.H. Glynn presiding. Theobald Smith was elected chairman of the Commission, and Dr. L.R. Williams (New York Commissioner of Health) nominated secretary. Four further meetings were held in Albany during the winter of 1914–15. Also during November were Founder's Day Exercises at the Peter Bent Brigham Hospital on the 12th; three joint papers with J.H. Brown or TenBroeck at the monthly meeting of the Boston Society of Medical Sciences, on the 17th; a Complimentary Dinner on the 18th at the Copley Plaza Hotel to celebrate Major Henry Lee Higginson's eightieth birthday; and the Dedication of the Forsyth Dental Infirmary for Children on the 24th. On the 23rd he attended the funeral of his friend C.S. Minot.

He was often the guest of honor or chief speaker at luncheons, such as the 1:30 P.M. "dinners" of the Massachusetts Agricultural Club. His long and close association with bovine tuberculosis made him a ready target for the program committees of miscellaneous groups connected with the cattle industry in search of a speaker with specialized and unbiased information about this disease and its relationship to human "consumption." Thus, within a period of a few weeks in 1914, he accepted invitations to address the Sixth Annual Conference of State Veterinarians at the New York State Veterinary College, Ithaca; the Boston Society of Medical Sciences; the Gurnsey (*sic*) Club; and the Grange at Framingham.

But of course he did not wish to be known as a narrow specialist. Indeed, having unshackled himself from an organization of highly specialized educationists, Theobald Smith seems to have resolved that he could speak authoritatively on almost any topic within the bounds of public health. In roughly the same time frame, he addressed the Boylston Society after dinner at the Harvard Club, on *vaccines;* the Bug Club at the Copley Square Hotel, on *Medical Versus Sanitary Science;* the Legislature's Agricultural Committee at the State House on the *Milk Bill,* followed next day by an attempt to hold the attention of the same Committee on *Public Abattoirs* ("too crowded"); and two addresses to the Women's Municipal League, the first on an unspecified topic ("I talk"), and the other, six weeks later, on *Cleanliness.* The plasticity of these unpublished speeches is evident from comparing the printed invitation to interested "men and women in Waban" to hear an address by the "leading authority on malaria and infantile paralysis in this part of the country" on "Some Considerations Important to the Public Health," in the vestry of the Union Church,[3] with Smith's own curt reference: "Go to Waban & speak on malaria, church parlor."[4]

Until an active start could be made on plans for the new department at the Rockefeller Institute, Theobald Smith judiciously banked his fires, while cultivating the art of adaptation to environment which he had learned to establish during his visiting professorship in Europe. He spent an afternoon inspecting a leather mill with Austin Peters for anthrax hazards,[5] and traveled to Woods Hole to attend the inaugural exercises for the New Laboratory Building at the Marine biological Laboratory.[6] He served as one of three "foreign microbiologists" (the others being A. Calmette of Lille and A. Gaffky of Berlin), along with Danish representatives, in nominating the 1914 Prizewinner of the Emil Christian Hansen Fund. The Hansen Prize (a Gold Medal and a monetary award) was unanimously awarded to Jules Bordet of Brussels for his work on the whooping cough bacillus, on the microbe of avian diphtheria, and on the phenomenon of alexin-fixation. Smith proposed Hideyo Noguchi as alternate: "his work on the cultivation of spirochaetes and the microbe of poliomyelitis is not excelled by any of recent years."[7]

Miscellaneous undertakings included three trips to New York on Rockefeller Institute business; meetings of the American Academy of Arts and Sciences; the Annual meeting of the National Academy of Sciences in Washington (the retiring president, Ira Remsen, being guest of honor at the Dinner); an invitation to dinner from former President Eliot; and the commencement of his new course of eight lectures on "Animal Diseases and the Public Health" for the combined Harvard-M.I.T. School of Public Health. He faithfully attended meetings of the Thursday Evening Club, as well as of the Eliot Club, whose membership had grown surprisingly to 200 by 1914–15. When free of other engagements, his working day was divided typically into periods of two to three hours each, during which he successively transferred a vast collection of cultures, wrote up his notes on any recent experimental results, and prepared the next address.

Into the scrapbook went every Programme for that season of the Boston Symphony Orchestra. In mid-March, 1914, he heard Paderewski give a rendering of his own *Concerto*.[8] In April 1914, at the National Academy of Sciences meeting in Washington, Smith heard Sir Ernest Rutherford lecture and attended a reception given by Alexander Graham Bell.[9] On October 16 there was a dinner in New York honoring Simon Flexner. This period was not without honors for Theobald Smith himself. In December 1914, he was elected to the Board of Trustees of the Carnegie Institution, and in January 1915, to the presidency of the American Society for Experimental Pathology. At the beginning of March he became an honorary member of the Aesculapian Club of Boston, and in April a member of the American Philosophical Society at Philadelphia.

Theobald Smith delivered the Harvard Fellowship address on December 2 to a distinguished audience.[10] Among many important friends and acquaintances present were the Bishop of Massachusetts (William Lawrence), Major H. Lee Higginson, and Dr. Henry P. Walcott. About two months after Smith's death, Abraham Flexner and his wife called on Lilian Smith and her daughter Dorothea in Princeton. Flexner borrowed from Theobald's widow a reprint of this address, along with a copy of Smith's reflections on a research career written to Dr. E.B. Krumbhaar some twenty years earlier.[11] When returning the documents, Flexner stated they contained much that he would "like to keep close at hand," for he believed that "The address is full of jewels . . . and ought to be reprinted for the benefit of the new generation."[12] His secretary had copied out one particular paragraph of the address, which he would show to some of the younger men, who often wanted assistants for work which to be truly scientific must be gone over and thought out by themselves. Assuming that the present-day scholar was "devoted to the intellectual life," Theobald reflected, in his Fellowship address,

> He does not need to be a hustler, or organizer, or contractor of intellectual labor. The rule of business, not to do anything that some one else can be delegated to do, is not a safe maxim for him. His work, like that of the artist, bears the stamp of his personality. It becomes vitalized and it grows in his hands. It can never be too good for improvement.[13]

Abraham Flexner had considered that paragraph a special "jewel;" but the address was bestrewn with epigrams equally precious and self-revealing.

> A mere display of absorbed knowledge does not make a scholar . . . inactive erudition, often the badge of what has been called culture, is thrown off by him, as ballast from a rising airship . . . To sit in a room, to study, and to think, are the necessary antecedents of the scholar. No wonder that scholarship is distasteful to many who are reaching for its fruits . . . The scholar's rewards will always be small. The distinguished men who have gone before have not been in the habit of thinking of themselves, and this habit should not be encouraged . . . Great discoveries which give a new direction to currents of thought and research are . . . due to the eruption of genius into a closely related field, and the transfer of the previous knowledge there found to his own domain.

Formerly, medical schools "paid but little attention and less respect to the unusually rich field of animal life as a source of information," he pointed out. "Today, every department of medicine fills its available working spaces with animals which are the subject of profound study. The results have revolutionized human medicine within a generation."

Theobald made two references to the European war. Perhaps "human society has been surfeited with the achievements of the mind. The worship of physical force, which has eclipsed scholarly taste and which breaks forth with equal energy on the field of sport and the field of battle, may be due to the very creatures of intellectual labor, the huge machines of industry." The other allusion was aimed directly at the John Harvard Fellows, who had studied "one of the greatest achievements of cooperative activity . . . the commonwealth of cells, called the human body." Identical laws were involved in mankind's biological and social evolution. Medicine was learning to replace the mere treatment of symptoms by the preventable underlying causes or preconditions. Might not the serious student of medicine provide analyses of the "sequences leading to great human catastrophes or diseases of the social organism like the one we are now passing through?"

World War I had begun in Europe. The Sarajevo assassination at the end of June culminated in the guns of August. Smith, like most Americans, was at first unconcerned. Neither diary nor day card mentioned the outbreak of hostilities. But by early December 1914, he considered the calamity appalling. Three times during October he recorded writing letters to Germany, and once noted "Talking much about European war."[14] In November, he contributed to the German Relief Fund, and on Christmas Eve wrote to Gage that he had sent "letters in German to my friends now shut in by England as no other language would pass muster."

Immunology—Dead or Alive?

The American Association of Immunologists was originally composed solely of men who had worked with Almroth Wright. A.P. Hitchens persuaded the Association to broaden its membership qualifications, and to include a subscription to the proposed new *Journal of Immunology* in the annual dues. Before the first volume was published by the Williams and Wilkins Company in 1916, Arthur F. Coca, the journal's founder and for many years its Managing Editor, canvassed prominent American scientists, to estimate the demand for such a journal. Their responses ranged from William Welch's unconditional approval to Theobald Smith's purported warning: "immunology is dead."[15] This dictum should be critically examined, for it conflicts with Smith's record of progressive researches on immunological problems, and with his charter subscription to the new journal, officially receipted by Coca.

Arthur F. Coca retired as editor-in-chief of the *Journal of Immunology* in 1951.

He was succeeded by Geoffrey Edsall, who gave way to John Y. Sugg in 1954. Neither Sugg nor his successor knew of any evidence (other than Coca's account) that Theobald Smith ever made that statement. In his inaugural address, "What is Immunology?"[16] Edsall sought to interpret the alleged dictum, but said nothing about the paucity of archival material. Smith's published researches established classic milestones in immunology, from his 1886 report on heat-killed vaccine protecting pigeons against hog cholera bacilli,[17] to the discovery of the non-identity of flagellar and somatic agglutinogens in microorganisms of the paratyphoid group in 1903,[18] the "Theobald Smith phenomenon" of acute serum anaphylaxis in 1906,[19] the passive transfer of immunity to diphtheria toxin from the immunized, lactating guinea pig to its offspring in 1907,[20] and the active immunity induced by mixtures of diphtheria toxin and antitoxin in 1909.[21] Still to come, beginning in 1922, were his important papers on the protective action of colostrum in new-born calves.[22]

These pioneer reports, which often led to novel or accelerated use of biological products as preventive agents, were interspersed with philosophical reviews of immunological problems that also broadened the intelligent application of the measures available, as, for example, his 1906 statement that "all immunization is a confession that the parasite has broken through barriers and has come to stay."[23] In 1910, his critical evaluation of Almroth Wright's vaccine therapy helped to curb unbridled resort to stock and autogenous bacterial vaccines for therapeutic purposes. Animal experiments indicated that immunity and susceptibility were purely relative terms. But the most effective prophylactics against animal infections could not be safely used on the human subject, for whom "methods must be so toned down as to fit the weakest and most susceptible. In animal life . . . it is desirable that the weakest be eliminated and that it shall not propagate its kind." Smith closed this address at the Annual Meeting of The Massachusetts Medical Society by warning against repeated assurances that therapeutic "vaccines do no harm." Their administration should be considered experimental, and restricted to persons familiar with immunological principles.[24]

His paper, "An Attempt to Interpret Present-Day Uses of Vaccine," delivered at the Annual Conversational Meeting of the Philadelphia Pathological Society in April 1913, introduced the host-parasite concept into a discussion of the benefits and hazards of vaccination. He deplored the commercialization of vaccines:

> The medical profession should see to it that vaccine therapy does not degenerate into inconsiderate and reckless experiments on human beings, that it does not create false hopes . . . and that it does not originate and end in . . . the desire to exploit the weak and unfortunate . . . The charlatan of today simply flourishes on the harvest sown unknowingly by the profession of a former generation.[25]

These reflections certainly do not manifest the author's rejection of immunology as an orchard of fruitful discovery.

In May 1916 Theobald Smith read a paper entitled "The Underlying Problems of Immunization" to a meeting of the Congress of American Physicians and Surgeons at Washington. Again emphasizing the quantitative aspects of immunity, Smith introduced fresh material into a presentation showing both leadership and restraint. He granted the established efficacy of live vaccines—"it is the coming method, not perhaps in our day." Apart from the investigation of other ways of artificially attenuating homologous microorganisms for use in vaccines, he urged a more diligent search for "naturally attenuated strains." Many years before B.C.G. vaccine was adopted as an immunizing agent for tuberculosis, Smith declared, "The preconception that strains of very low virulence cannot immunize toward highly virulent strains, should not stand in the way of actual trials."

Prophetic insight was illustrated also by enthusiasm for studies of partial antigens. "To discover some one ingredient of a micro-organism which can prevent infection with the micro-organism itself would rank with the subtlest discoveries in biochemistry, for it would at the same time eliminate from the vaccine substances which are injurious and without any useful antigenic properties."[26] Theobald Smith evidently found no dearth of problems in immunology worthy of thoughtful experimentation in 1916. Five years later, in his second Pasteur Lecture, entitled "Theories of Susceptibility and Resistance in Relation to Methods of Artificial Immunization," given before the Institute of Medicine of Chicago, he further demonstrated the significance of immunology as a science whose practical purpose was helping "to keep parasitism within safe limits."[27]

Nothing here suggests that Theobald Smith would seriously write or utter the words that Immunology was "dead." Instead, surely he would rather have endorsed this definition, published about half a century after his death: "Immunology is not only the most rapidly developing area of biomedical research but one that holds out the greatest promise of major advances in the prevention and treatment of a wide range of diseases."[28]

Farewell Dinner to Theobald Smith

Late in 1914, a few key members of the Harvard Medical School formed a committee at the instigation of Marshal Fabyan to plan a suitable tribute to Theobald Smith, whose retirement the following summer would end twenty years of service to Harvard University. During November and December 1914, the committee met three times in Dr. Harvey Cushing's office at the Peter Bent Brigham Hospital. Cushing himself, M.J. Rosenau, R.P. Strong and Marshal Fabyan attended every meeting. Also present initially were H. Ernst, R. Hunt and J.L.

Brewer. The decision was to extend a Complimentary Dinner to Theobald Smith at the Harvard Club, Boston, the basic subscription being $5; and if possible to commission a distinguished local sculptor, Bela Pratt, to make a suitable bas-relief for presentation to the Harvard Medical School. Reductions of the sculpture were to be distributed to all subscribers of $10 or more. By common consent Fabyan controlled all arrangements from the outset, and the outstanding success of the Dinner was due mainly to the organizational skills and zealous loyalty of this unpaid Assistant.

Fabyan kept notes at these meetings, not as minutes, but as reminders. "See Mrs. Smith about size and men to ask . . . find when Societies meet." "Dr. R. suggests the Wives be invited." "Dr. C. to see Lowell and Higginson . . . Noted men to be written to at once: Lowell, Welch, Flexner, Shattuck, Walcott." "Letter for bas-relief approved." "No ladies."[29] Eventually, some ladies (including Mrs. Theobald Smith and daughters) heard the speeches from seats near the entrance. In consultation with President Lowell and Theobald Smith himself, April 17 was selected as the date for the Dinner. Fabyan extended the invitation to Lilian Smith to listen to the speeches in a letter which also told of Bela Pratt's commission, and inquired whether any of the reductions should be sent to European friends. The first of several sittings in Pratt's studio occurred on January 2, 1915. Lilian Smith replied from Woodland Hill:

> Of course, I am dying to see the bas-relief, even though I know the feeling Mr. Pratt has about having it seen by friends. You and I should be able to know even better than he if it is really like Theobald. I am most grateful that you could plan to have us in for the speech-making. If it proves possible, I hope Mrs. Fabyan will feel like coming in.
>
> How you are putting yourself into this dinner! Be sure that I know how much it means and how little perfunctory there is about it. To my husband I am sure it will become a very precious and valued memory as time goes on and he looks back on his twenty years in Boston, and I like to think how your friendship will always make you a large part of the memory, since all these years have been passed so closely in touch with you and yours.[30]

The Farewell Dinner, planned for April 17, 1915, in Harvard Hall, had to be postponed because the guest of honor fell ill. For several months, Smith had suffered sacroiliac discomfort, but the affliction grew more acute in the new year. On January 12 he sought professional advice from Dr. Elliott G. Brackett, an orthopedic specialist, who traced the source of the pain to a sacroiliac ligament, and prescribed a leather corset to be fitted over the affected joint. This brought temporary relief, but a spate of extracurricular activities within the new few weeks aggravated the condition and left the disability worse than ever.

Nevertheless, he talked to the Thursday Evening club on "raising healthy animals" (January 21), and two nights later turned up at the Tavern Club for a dinner in his honor, given by some young doctors, the "Extensor Communis Club." In the second half of January, he kept at least three dental appointments, and also sat several times for his profile at Bela Pratt's studio. Before the end of February, he made numerous train journeys to New York on Rockefeller Institute business; to Princeton, to examine possible building sites with Prudden; to Albany, for meetings of the Bovine Tuberculosis Committee; to Washington, to confer at the Department of Agriculture on foot-and-mouth disease; to Chicago, to go over the Stockyards and try to appease George Fabyan's urgent clamor for advice on various animal ailments; to Champaign, Illinois, to lunch at the University with President James and attend a late afternoon reception at a meeting of bacteriologists; to Cambridge, to see Prof. F.G. Peabody, then Harvard University's Emeritus Professor of Social Ethics (in whose department Robert Foerster held the rank of Instructor) "about a future possible son-in-law;" to Elizabeth, New Jersey, to take dinner with the Eglestons; and to Silver Lake, New Hampshire, to inspect the new "camp" buried in a foot of snow.

On one occasion at the end of January 1915, in Albany he attended a murder trial sitting behind his old high school friend, George Addington, who presided as judge. He had met Judge Addington and other friends and companions of his high school days, such as Montignani, now a lawyer, and Whish, during a short visit to his mother at Albany in September 1909. (Montignani settled the estates of Theobald's father and mother.) On another visit (February 25), Smith looked over the family's former home at 54 Alexander Street, and also the prospective buyer, before reluctantly executing a "deed for sale." He did not forget to visit his parents' graves.

On March 4, Smith returned to Dr. Brackett about his "lame joint." His jottings about it remained on the whole calm and objective: "Lying on couch to ease my sacro-iliac pain" (March 8); "Can't sit on a/c of sciatic back . . . massage of my back by Herbert R. Brown" (March 19); "Joints much worse this A.M. Lying down much of time. Kneel to eat meals" (March 21); "lying on bed all day, getting up for 2–3 min. only, taking 6 gr aspirin per day" (March 26). Lilian's engagement to Dr. Foerster was announced in the *Boston Transcript* of March 27. Next day he stoically penned: "In bed. Engagement of Lilian and Robert celebrated down stairs. Many friends. Many roses." His subsequent diary entries read: "In bed. Use crutch & cane to bathroom but pain in rt hip very severe and not bearable; Taken to Dr. Dodds in ambulance & thoroughly x-rayed. Put under ether & rt. leg manipulated. Much nausea & vomiting" (April 5); "Drs. Brackett, Broughton, TenBroeck and Brackett's assistant put me in plaster jacket extending to rt knee" (April 9); "Lilian takes care of me . . . sciatica calming down"

(April 11); "This was to have been the night of the 150-men dinner to me at Harv. Club" (April 17); "Have not looked out of window to ground for 2 weeks" (April 18). "Pain evidently disappearing" (April 22).

He slowly improved in May, reclining for hours on a couch, reading, writing, or receiving visitors, when not being encased in or cut out from a plaster jacket. At last, allowed to put his foot gently on the floor, he managed to get around gingerly by "sliding along with crutches on weak leg." He still practiced walking when Nurse Doyle left two days before the Dinner. On June 2, he lay down until 5. That evening, Dr. A.N. Broughton kindly drove him in his car to the Harvard Club. "Day of Dinner . . . Driven to Harvard Club in auto by Dr. Broughton— 175–200 guests. See Scrapbook."[31]

At their meeting on May 10, 1915, the President and Fellows of Harvard College officially voted to express to Theobald Smith "their deep appreciation of his devoted and skilled service to the University for so many years and of his important contributions to the knowledge and prevention of disease." His resignation, to take effect August 31, 1915, was accepted with regret. These sentiments were formally conveyed and gratefully received. However, Theobald found much more moving the speeches and spontaneous remarks at the Farewell Dinner.

Marshal Fabyan arranged the seating for more than 180 guests at twenty-three small tables with twenty persons at the head table, where Theobald Smith sat as centerpiece, uncomfortably propped in a high chair, flanked by President Lawrence Lowell, who was toastmaster, and Charles W. Eliot. This situation prompted Smith to ask pardon, at the close of his speech of thanks, "for sitting in an arm-chair all evening at a higher level than the two Presidents of Harvard University." He endured with characteristic modesty the greetings and plaudits of the assembly, and flattering speeches from well-known persons, each given a ten-minute time limit by Fabyan. These speakers were introduced in turn by Lowell: "the beloved physician," Frederick C. Shattuck; the Baltimore malariologist, William S. Thayer; the "robber," Simon Flexner; "the father of the modern Harvard Medical School," Charles W. Eliot; and "the great wise man of medicine," William H. Welch. The Dean of Harvard's Faculty of Medicine, E.H. Bradford, also spoke a few words. He wished "the torch bearer . . . all health and all prosperity . . . We Harvard men look forward to his coming new work as something which will illumine the whole world."[32]

At this juncture, the bas-relief of Theobald Smith by Bela Pratt, who sat at the head table, would have been unveiled, but the work was unfinished because of the subject's illness. Eventually it would be presented to the Medical School, said Lowell, to stand as "a memorial of what he did, and what he was to us." Two further sittings six months later left Pratt dissatisfied with the likeness and he asked

Smith to send him a photograph, taken in the same position.[33] When the tablet was finished late in 1916, it was placed on the stairway fronting Smith's laboratory in Building E. Here it remained for some fifty years, until removed to Thomas H. Weller's Department of Comparative Pathology and Tropical Medicine in Harvard's new School of Public Health building.

Before calling on the guest of honor, Lowell mentioned the dozens of telegrams and scores of letters of regret, praise and goodwill, and cited a few. All had been directed to Marshal Fabyan's home address. Among those who telegraphed were President Schurman and Simon Gage of Cornell—the latter's wife was seriously ill; E.O. Jordan of Chicago; T.C. Janeway and W.G. MacCallum of Johns Hopkins; President Edmund James, University of Illinois; Chancellor D. Starr Jordan of Stanford; George Whipple, Hooper Foundation, San Francisco; and E.L. Trudeau (dead within a few months). Some lived far afield, e.g., Manila (Bartlett), Milan (Belfanti), Tokyo (Kitasato) and Copenhagen (Madsen). From the Pasteur Institute in Paris a joint letter had been signed by Roux and Metchnikoff, while Laveran wrote separately. A tribute from Ronald Ross has been cited previously.[34] From Hamburg, W.P. Dunbar added warm recollections of the Jamaica Plain setting—"its quietness, its old trees, the quaint and comfortable house."

Ehrlich recalled his "good fortune, eleven years ago, to meet you personally in Boston, and to pass those pleasant hours in your laboratory and your home . . . From my heart I wish you good health and good luck for your brain and its work. Rest assured that many in Germany besides myself are filled with appreciation of your influence on learning."[35] Ehrlich's own health had failed and death came soon afterward.

From war-bound Europe came pathetic salutations from other German friends. For example, Fülleborn wrote to Fabyan: "Since the Fatherland has need of me, I am a regimental surgeon at the front in France. Possibly when the war is over, I may clasp hands again with Professor Smith . . . Pray forgive the pencil, there is nothing else here, and I must send my letter unsealed." Gärtner of Jena defined Smith to Fabyan as "a first-class man of learning and the most amiable colleague I ever met." He began his letter, "You are right, it is not possible, in this terrible war obtruded upon Germany, to join you at dinner in honor of Professor Theobald Smith," and ended with "Three cheers for our dear friend Theobald Smith, three cheers for the science whose high priest he is." W. Kolle, formerly of Berne, wrote from Lille, "For the past six months I am in the field and have passed through many dangers and privations, working with our victorious and wonderfully brave army." Until the Germans manifested "frightfulness" in their first use of poison gas in April and May 1915, many Britishers tended to regard the war as a kind of sport.

From Oxford, Sir William Osler reassured Fabyan early in January that he would be delighted to send a brief message for the Theobald Smith dinner: "I am awfully sorry that you are losing him in Boston," and adding, "All is going well here. It is a slow job, but we will come out all right in the end."[36] Americans had lost their complacency when the "Lusitania" was sunk early in May. The revulsions that followed this act matured slowly, but meanwhile promoted assistance just within the bounds of official neutrality. In that spirit, the Harvard Unit of the American Ambulance Hospital was established at Neuilly, then a suburb of Paris, staffed by distinguished medical professionals, including Harvey Cushing as surgeon-in-chief and director of the Unit, who was therefore unable to attend the function honoring Theobald Smith.[37]

Invited by Lowell to speak without rising from his chair, Theobald Smith remarked that his life and work had been "particularly influenced by personalities." For his Washington success he was indebted chiefly to Professor Welch. The present occasion derived from the liberality and friendly interest of George Francis Fabyan, who had endowed the chair of Comparative Pathology. Two men, President Emeritus Eliot and Dr. Henry P. Walcott, "through their unfailing kindness, their personal friendship, the confidence they placed in me, and the absolute academic freedom to do or not to do with which they surrounded me, did more than any other persons to make possible what little success I have attained." Smith took the opportunity to emphasize publicly how much Harvard University had done for the State, in money and lives saved and illness aborted, through its sponsorship of diphtheria antitoxin production. He closed by thanking them all for coming, some from distant points, and especially "the committee, which has endeavored to deliver me up to you before and failed, and which has had great trouble in doing so this evening."[38] These events were duly chronicled in the *Boston Medical and Surgical Journal*.[39] Theobald Smith's entry for the day's event was very dry: "Dinner given me at Harvard Club."[40]

Every participant at the Complimentary Dinner received a souvenir card measuring about 25 by 19 cm., and inscribed "Thanks to you, Theobald Smith," on a central white rectangle, from which light irradiated into the surrounding darkness. In the margins was drawn a sequence of twenty-six vignettes, each aptly subtitled, representing Smith's contributions to microbiology, immunology, and public health. For example, below a sleek mouse appeared a swollen-headed bespectacled student, captioned respectively "For studying my pneumonias," and "For defining Scholarship." Under the student, long-chained streptococci cavorted near the inscription "For indicating my family traits even in milk epidemics." So it went, all the way around the source of illumination. The card, designed by M. Fabyan, was professionally executed by H.P. Aitken, a medical illustrator.[41] Fabyan assembled and had bound in leather all the formal speeches, with the Menu Card and copies of the telegrams and letters received from absentee friends. This volume was presented to Theobald Smith as a memento of the occasion.

In notes received by Fabyan after the dinner, W.S. Halsted thanked him for "the Theobald Smith anapogram. It was a happy idea to refer in Alice in Wonderland fashion, and represent so graphically that even a surgeon can understand, the contributions of this remarkable and lovable man."[42] Sir William Osler congratulated him for his originality. "That is a delightful group of pictorial thanks to our friend Theobald Smith . . . How pleased he must have been, and all the guests. I hear it was a great occasion and worthy of the man."[43] The psychiatrist William Noyes, one of the Smith family's closest friends, sent an illustrated note to Fabyan next morning: "It was a howling success all right. There was nothing but praise for the way it was managed." Underneath was a hurriedly-sketched illustration, a take-off on the central feature of the card, "Thanks to you, Marshal Fabyan."[44] The son of Dr. A. Van Derveer (Professor of Surgery in Theobald Smith's time as a student at the Albany Medical College, who later became its Dean) was "glad to know that the souvenir of the dinner is to be in the nature of a bas-relief of Dr. Smith, for there are many of us in Albany who think that the sun rises and sets in him, since he is a graduate of our own little Medical School, which, sad to say, is undergoing a rigid reorganization that some of us are very worried about."[45]

The octogenarian Major Henry Lee Higginson scrawled a note to the late George Francis Fabyan's second son, Francis Wright—not present at the Dinner. Higginson (1834–1919) a generous benefactor of Harvard and Fellow of the Corporation since 1893, was head of the prosperous banking and brokerage firm of Lee Higginson & Co., with which firm Theobald Smith had deposited $3,000.00 "for investment" a few months before this Dinner.

> I did not see you last night and had but a word with Dr. Fabyan. The management, which was his—the arrangement of seats, speeches and all was very, very good . . . and it is no easy matter. Sitting between Dr. Welch and Flexner, I was in clover—and Theobald Smith's speech was charming—so modest, so gentle, so appreciative of others. Your father's face was constantly before me . . . the kind of man who makes our country high-spirited, high-minded, and valuable to the world.
>
> I always remember his coming into our office and saying, "Henry, I am going upstairs with this cheque ($100,000) to help research—my father was a doctor and I wish to do this thing." And again later his bringing another cheque to make the gift "ample" . . . The evening was a tribute to your father.[46]

And he also told in his letter, "As for Dr. Smith, nothing is too good for him."

The philanthropist's eldest son, George Fabyan of Chicago, attended the Dinner. He had prospered from the meat-packing industry, in whose social circles he was known as "Colonel" Fabyan. George waited a fortnight before expressing his puzzlement and concern in a letter to President Lowell.[47] His father certainly would not have wished him to criticize the College administration. But he claimed to know Theobald Smith better than anyone outside the Smith family; and allowing for a sympathetic listener's exaggerations and improvisations, the basic features of his explanation for the imminent departure could have come only from Smith himself.

> Professor Smith with a knowledge of all microbes and bugs, living in a house not connected with a sewer, not convenient to his laboratory, requiring an hour on the street car in the morning, an hour to return at night, or 20% of his time out of a 10-hour day, devoted to waiting for street cars and riding in them. His department situated on four floors of the Medical Building, 17 ft. between floors, an elevator provided, but no money to hire an operator, making it necessary for him to climb the stairs. In the winter, the heating plant which supplies heat for the building and the hospital, the capacity of the plant insufficient, the hospital has the heat and in cold weather, Dr. Smith's quarters are almost uninhabitable—I have seen him there huddled up in a coat . . . and the students likewise. Dr. Smith made excuses, the students did not.
>
> There were many facilities which Dr. Smith wanted and needed, which were denied to him . . . all of which appeared to be within the possibilities of the casual observer. Dr. Smith's efforts on the turkeys in his backyard were pitiful. He tried to get along without the necessary facilities and make something else do. The result was the turkeys were stolen and the experiment lost. Some few inexpensive buildings at the Bussey would have enabled him to accomplish some important work. These were not only vetoed, but those which he had . . . were taken away from him as being unsightly, and not corresponding with Mr. Sargent's view of the Arboretum, until one begins to wonder whether the Bussey Institution is going to be the Arnold Arboretum . . . and is told that it is considered the part of wisdom not to antagonize Mr. Sargent . . . it would seem that only about 50% of Dr. Smith's time was secured by his work, the other 50% being spent on the street cars, climbing up and down stairs, and doing work which assistants could have accomplished equally as well.

"Dr. Smith . . . goes to the Rockefeller Institute," Fabyan told Lowell, "because he will have the facilities . . . furnished without vexatious delays." With the Rockefeller Institute he would have "the opportunity . . . of making his time count nearer 100%."

After two weeks, Lowell sent an unruffled reply. Professor Theobald Smith lacked some equipment for work that he would like to do and "ought to have a large farm, with a number of assistants; but we have not had the means of supplying him with that."

> The fact that Dr. Smith lived a long way from the Medical School where his chief work of late years was done, was not essential. He could have lived elsewhere, and I suppose he started in Jamaica Plain because he was near the Bussey. On the other hand I do not understand why his Department should have covered four floors in the Medical School . . . and still less do I understand why his quarters should have been uncomfortable from lack of heat. The case of the turkeys was certainly pitiful and I feel that we—the authorities of the University—were to blame for not appreciating the danger of those birds being stolen.
>
> I am much obliged to you for your letter, and if you will bring to my attention any cases of other professors . . . who are not contented with their opportunities for research, I will do what I can to help them, though . . . the resources of the University are very limited.[48]

Fabyan answered that the University's resources were bound to be limited, "as long as it continues to spread out in so many different directions. Theobald Smith will undoubtedly have a greater field and a broader scope with Rockefeller. He has gone from Harvard, and I thought that the facts that were presented might be the means of preventing others from leaving. The pigeon hole is responsible for many failures in commercial life."[49] Lowell again thanked Fabyan. "We need to be reminded this way constantly, even things that we know about. Smith spoke to me about some of his difficulties—said he needed a diener and I procured some money for that purpose; but he never spoke to me about the turkeys until after one of them had been stolen. If he had, perhaps we could have made some arrangement for protecting them. I suspect he did not realize the danger of theft."[50]

George then quoted some provocative remarks received meanwhile from his brother Marshal: The President's "job is chiefly one of looking pleasant, and trying to locate cash to meet constantly increasing debts."[51] Lowell's curt rebuttal ended the correspondence: "Your brother . . . appears to have got things wrong . . . It is not my business to beg for money, and I do not propose to do so."[52]

In June 1915, Theresa Smith's bequest of $1,800 to each of her granddaughters was paid. While they quietly celebrated, Robert Foerster happily brought his mother to Woodland Hill to meet them all. Lilian and Foerster married at Princeton a year later, on June 5, 1916, amongst "many flowers and some friends." As for Theobald, Dr. Brackett allowed him to get up for only a few hours daily, with walking restricted and requiring two canes. When lying down, he studied calculus, or kept busy "writing turkey report."[53] This report, although published after he had moved to New Jersey, carefully acknowledged help received from the Massachusetts Society for Promoting Agriculture.[54] Smith still wore the leather jacket into the summer and complained to Gage, "I am gradually getting my muscles back after the three months confinement. My back, however still grumbles when I try to work out-of-doors a little."[55] He missed the Radcliffe College Commencement on June 23 in Sanders Theatre when his daughter Lilian graduated in History, *magna cum laude.*[56]

Both daughters did well at Radcliffe. Dorothea hoped for medical training, but her father discouraged that ambition. Intermittent illnesses and severe underlying diabetes hampered her professional career as a microbiologist, despite a thoroughly deserved Ph.D. Philip's First Year (1914–1915) Report was pasted faithfully into scrapbook No. 5 opposite the newspaper notice of the resignation of his father from the Fabyan Professorship.[57] Despite being graded C for three courses, D for two courses, and E (failed) in a Physics course, Philip eventually got an A.B. from Harvard. He stayed away following the dismal first year, but was persuaded to resume his studies, and graduated with a major in German from Harvard in 1919.

Theobald Smith had arranged an extension of the rental-lease on Woodland Hill until the end of September, but the task ahead was daunting. For his wife the uprooting had developed from unwelcome prospect into devastating reality. The selection of furnishings suitable for their new summer home at Silver Lake was, however, a relatively simple process, and she left for there on July 19 to attend to it. His more difficult task was to discriminate between worthwhile and unwanted manuscript notes, reprints and correspondence. Early in July, Theobald began "tearing up" papers and letters; and when Lilian went to Silver Lake, he stayed behind at Woodland Hill with TenBroeck, ostensibly to finish the job. They took their meals at the "Bussey Mess," which had been set up in the former residence of the horticulturalist B.H. Watson. In a few days Smith left for Silver Lake with his microscope and slides of turkey tissues, and TenBroeck remained as caretaker at Woodland Hill.

Theobald Smith spent nearly two months at Silver Lake. Typical Day Card entries show him doing several hours of work daily, reviewing microscope slides and also beginning to row again, as well as "cutting wood, a little sawing—reading Far fr. Madding Crowd."[58] He took only one trip to Princeton via Boston and New York, inspecting "farm houses."

On September 21, Dorothea accompanied her mother to Boston to pack household goods, while Theobald remained a few days in their increasingly chilly summer home. On the 29th, he arrived in Boston, just before the extended lease on Woodland Hill expired. His train had passed his wife's headed in the opposite direction. In their old home, professional packers were still at work. Theobald visited them daily, lending a hand with papers and letters until the job was finished on October 6. He boarded and slept at the "Bussey Mess," where he and TenBroeck usually took lunch with staff members of the reconstituted Bussey Institution, which now included Professors W.E. Castle (Animal Genetics), E.M. East (Plant Genetics), and I.W. Bailey (Plant Anatomy).

Prof. Bailey, interviewed by the author half a century later, recalled the repugnance with which he and his messmates, particularly the graduate students, heard Theobald Smith and Carl TenBroeck express pro-German views and sentiments. Since the European war erupted, Smith contributed regularly to German relief drives and seemed to prefer the bellicose persecution-complex prevalent in that country to the lackadaisical tenacity of the British—whom he considered too sloppy to be on the winning side.[59] Smith associated with Hugo Münsterberg, the philosopher-poet, described as "one of the most brilliant Harvard professors of his time," who nevertheless "had quite as many foes as friends." Münsterberg retained German citizenship after twenty years at Harvard and courted publicity through propaganda, yet Harvard University and President Lowell left Münsterberg "absolute freedom of speech."[60] He died suddenly in December 1916, a few months before the United States entered World War I.

Carl TenBroeck, about to leave Harvard as Smith's chief associate, changed his views when the United States entered the war in April 1917 and joined the U.S. Army soon after. His chief continued to deplore the follies of mankind, and to mourn the loss of his Teutonic contacts, but gamely apostasized. He fulfilled an American patriot's obligation to invest in Liberty Loans. Scrapbook No. 5 contains a color-printed certificate, signed by representatives of The Princeton Bank and Trust Company, testifying that Theobald Smith had subscribed to the Third Liberty Loan, and that in consequence his name and address would be placed on the Treasury Department's Roll of Honor. This document offered the naive assurance of having "no intrinsic value, but it is evidence of the patriotism on the part of the holder, who gave financial support to the Government in the War of the United States with Germany. Dated at Princeton, May 8, 1918."

On October 9, Lilian Smith fell down the stairs at their summer home and broke her right upper arm. Next day, she was sent to Boston in the train's baggage car, and thence taken by ambulance to Faulkner Hospital. An X-ray showed a fractured neck of the right humerus.[61] On the 11th, Theobald twice visited his wife in the hospital. He walked through the Arboretum for the last time on that "beautiful day," before catching a steamer to New York. Next morning, he went on alone to Princeton. His wife stayed three weeks in hospital. The arm mended very slowly and remained an encumbrance for several months.

The Summer Camp at Silver Lake, New Hampshire

Until he was past fifty, Theobald Smith's vacations were haphazard and short. Then, after methodically trying out various regions as possible sites for a summer home, he built his own large "cabin" at Silver Lake, New Hampshire. In mid-September of 1909 he was invited by William Noyes to stay at their lake side camp near Naples, Maine, at the southern end of the narrow Long Lake. Next summer, when Harold Ernst and his wife visited Japan, Ernst offered occupancy of his summer home at Manomet to the Smith family if Theobald would assume editorship of the *Journal of Medical Research* during his absence. Manomet was a small place on Cape Cod Bay, about forty miles from Boston. From late June until early September, at least two members of the Smith family safeguarded the villa, enjoying the coastal setting and the sea breeze. Smith commuted, seldom staying longer than a short weekend. His fifty-first birthday fell on a Sunday, so it was spent at Manomet. He rowed, walked, studied the fauna, read medical reprints, and watched many warships maneuver off-shore.

Early in July 1911 there was a heat wave. Philip had been packed off for two months at a boys' camp at North Belgrade, Maine. The girls had to do the chores in a large and maidless household: "No servants since June 1, and none in sight," was recorded on Labor Day, September 4, when Theobald interrupted his day's labor at the laboratory to see them off for a short visit to friends at New Harbor, Maine. On September 6, Smith set out for New Hampshire to inspect a house for sale near Silver Lake. This was the name both of a small village some two miles east of Chocorua and of the adjoining lake, about two miles long north and south and one mile across at its maximum width. On this occasion, as on several later visits, he stayed at Silver Lake House, an inn with guest rooms. He was much impressed with the locality, but did not buy the property. A fellow-passenger on the Boston train was Rev. Edward Cummings, temperance advocate and father of the future poet and pacifist "e.e. cummings." With his wife and son, cummings had established a lakeshore home. He offered to show Smith some building sites around the lake from his motorboat, and a date was arranged about two weeks ahead.

On September 16, Theobald and Lilian made a brief excursion to "The Ark" at Jaffrey, in the southwest corner of New Hampshire. They explored neighboring pastures and brooks as alternative settings for a summer camp, and satisfied themselves of Silver Lake's advantages. Before the end of the month, Theobald Smith twice briefly revisited Silver Lake. He explored building sites from the Cummings's motor boat, took lunch with the owner, and was introduced by him to neighboring farmers. He also rowed alone around the lake and observed how Prof. H.L. Warren, an architect and landscaping expert, planned his house on the bluff. Finally he inspected some of the lots in greater detail, and noted more "nice sites" when walking toward Chocorua. During the summer of 1912, until the end of September, the Smith family went sightseeing in western Europe and England, after Theobald completed his visiting professorship at Berlin. There was no chance to explore further the question of a "summer camp" until the following summer.

Then, late in June 1913, Simon Flexner wrote to Smith for advice on a technical question. Flexner had reported recently on the favorable results of treating 1,300 cases of epidemic meningitis with antiserum, and on "accidents" associated with subdural injections of the serum. He sought Smith's comments on the allegation that these were due to phenol, tricresol, or other preservative present in the serum.[62] Flexner then inquired if Smith had "ever penetrated into this region of the White Mountains, where hills and water are so charmingly combined. I should like to encourage you and Mrs. Smith to make a trial sometime." In his reply, Smith named chloroform as an apparently innocuous preservative in serum. He added that indeed he had spent a few days in that region some years ago. "I was interested in several places at Silver Lake that can be reached by a good smart walk from Chocorua, and I may go up there again before the summer closes to see whether there is anything we might use for a summer camp."[63]

About a month later, the Smiths rented a cottage on the shore of Long Lake, Maine, near their 1909 holiday site. For a fortnight Theobald rowed, tramped, wrote letters, fetched groceries and mail, visited a haunted house, and loafed. He also inspected a lot for sale. Then they went by train through North Conway to Madison, and made Silver Lake House their headquarters for the next three nights. The Cummings family welcomed them warmly, treating them as future good neighbors; they invited them to dinner, drove them by auto to Conway, accompanied them on inspections of buildings sites, and on one occasion at least entertained them until nightfall when "L2" went "canoeing in moonlight with Mr. Cummings etc."[64] The Smith family returned to Boston in favor of the Silver Lake district. When the Rev. Cummings next preached at a nearby church, the Smiths attended and invited him and his wife to dinner at Woodland Hill.

For the next two or three weeks in the fall of 1913, Theobald Smith was extremely busy. When he was not otherwise engaged, a typical Day Card entry would read: "Lab all day as usual, studying till 10.30 P.M."[65] But at last, on October 17, he made up his mind to act: "L've at 12.50 with Phil for Silver Lake— Buy shoreland fr. Mr. N.K. Forrest for $1600." The long and narrow lot, twelve acres in all, bordered by a strip of tangled undergrowth and young trees, mostly pines and fir, broadened enough at its north end for a large dwelling, with accessory ice- and pump-houses.

Using twelve-foot stakes and a level, Theobald drew a primitive contour map of his new domain, thereby locating the construction site that entailed the least landscape disturbance and the fewest tree fall. The large size and high quality of the structure built on that chosen site reflected the knowledge that in vacating Woodland Hill, the whole family would "plunge into the unknown." Every member of it, especially Lilian, by now accustomed to one or two servants, surely deserved compensation for losing a share of that oversized mansion. In addition, Simon Flexner had given assurances in April of "no teaching obligations," of good summer breaks, and of concern to protect his colleague's "health and strength." What better recourse from city heat and humidity than a summer cooled by lake waters, in which the children could swim and sail, and he could row whenever the spirit moved, where he could study microscopic preparations at leisure, with his own beach and woodlot adjacent, and sleep upstairs in a porch open to the sky and fresh mountain air?

On May 10, 1914, when the Rev. and Mrs. Edward Cummings took tea at Woodland Hill, they offered to rent their cottage, "Wyannet," to the Smiths, if family members should want to stay at Silver Lake until their own camp was habitable. The Cummings were enlarging their establishment, and a comfortable annex would be available for them. The offer was accepted, although none of the Smiths could get away before the last ten days in June, when "both Lilians and Phil" went up to Silver Lake. The two younger ones started tidying up the cluttered foreshore, and made a preliminary survey for the critical route through the woods to the village highway—a route that should be aesthetically attractive, as well as smooth, level and direct, involving a minimum of rock removal, shrub displacement and tree felling.

While Theobald Smith issued final approvals, his wife should be credited for most of the general layout and the floor plans of their summer house. Toward the end of July, all the three Smith siblings, accompanied by Susan Hopkins, their mother's friend from Williamstown, and Jock, a stray terrier who had adopted the family at Jamaica Plain, went up to "Wyannet." On the 31st, three letters of congratulation reached Theobald on his fifty-fifth birthday. Lilian-2 wrote the most. Early in August, the Smith youngsters were joined by their parents and Nellie, the servant. J.H. Brown, research assistant on streptococcal types,[66] occupied the Woodland Hill mansion with his family for the next eight weeks. Theobald stayed at Silver Lake until the end of September. About one hour daily was set aside by Philip's father for tutoring him in plane geometry. There were unavoidable interruptions—many of them unwelcome visitors. Among welcome visitors were the Bacons—friends of Berlin days, who in September brought Philip from Cambridge in their automobile, and returned him. The young people thrived on fun and games—tennis, boating, and swimming—

while their elders looked forward to friendly gossip and simple picnics on the beach or in the woods.

The Cummings and Smiths negotiated a mutual aid pact whereby in any emergency either party would summon the other by gunshot. During that summer, on learning of his acceptance as a freshman at Harvard, Philip excitedly fired a shot into the air from the Smith "point." The Cummings family responded promptly by racing across the lake in a canoe, the Reverend paddling ferociously amidship, Estlin in the bow with the other paddle, and his mother peering apprehensively from the stern. Philip greeted them rather sheepishly on the beach. Only Estlin was amused.[67]

Theobald began work on their point of lakeshore land by "slashing shrubs & small trees" to clear a roadway through the woods. His Day Card entry for Sunday, August 9, read: "laying out house on point. Call by Cummings. Towed over to meet Flexners. Quiet afternoon, all go to our beach for supper." On the 22nd, they walked over seven miles to visit the Flexners. Carl TenBroeck came as an invited guest for a week of trail-cutting in mid-September. By then, a well had been dug, and good water found at nineteen feet down. Three men were hired to work on the road; N.K. Forrest (the vendor of the lake side lot) had been instructed where Theobald's stock of discarded railroad ties were to go as steps; and the house plans, on which so many hours had been spent by both Theobald and his wife, were completed. On September 24, they had a bonfire on the beach, followed by a bathing party; on the 25th the plans were completed, and the contract for building the house given to a local carpenter, Mark E. Nickerson. Next day, September 26, Wyannet was closed and the Smiths returned to Boston. On October 1, Smith finished "typewriting contract for house at Silver Lake." As a first instalment on the contract he paid Nickerson $1,000. By the time Gage was informed at Christmas 1914 that the camp was "up & shingled,"[68] another $1,000 had been paid.

Theobald briefly revisited the site in October and December, while Lilian went there on November 17, staying at the village inn. At the time of his last visit, work had stopped for the winter; but the huge wooden camp stood firm on its concrete piers, the railroad ties were in place as entrance steps, the windows installed, and the shingles stained. On returning to Boston, he recorded, "All closed in now. Lake partly skimmed over, traces of snow—walking along Cummings side of lake in morning."[69] Nickerson apparently received another $1,300 in dwindling installments. His total therefore came to $3,300. The final payment of $100, made in July 1915, was entered in Smith's monthly accounts as "Silver Lake house contract completed." When adding in all the extras, from shingle stain to plumbing and cesspool, the total cost of constructing the camp, including the pumphouse and ice-house, was about $5,000.

Downstairs was a combined dining-and-living room area of about 30 by 35 feet, with an attached kitchen. A large stone fireplace, built from rocks found on the property, was centered at one end of this room. Enclosed at opposite corners were Theobald's study and a small spare bedroom. Upstairs were five bedrooms, three of which had adjacent sleeping porches. Theobald's bedroom, with space for a desk as well as a single bed, abutted a large corner sleeping porch. His wife's bedroom adjoined his, occupying the other corner. The remaining two corners were to become sleeping porches, each with an attached bedroom. The bathroom and a small bedroom without porch completed the upstairs layout. The cellar was used for stacking firewood and stowing boats—the sailing canoe and a flat-bottomed rowing skiff.

The house looked bleak and uncomfortably large: no furniture or fixtures, leaking rain, and liable to swarm with insects. Some of the deficiencies were remedied in 1915, when Lilian went to Silver Lake in mid-July with both daughters. Theobald followed on the 21st. Phil joined the family for part of August, while his "chum," Foster Damon, stayed a week. These two, together with Estlin Cummings, made a handsome trio. TenBroeck and Robert Foerster both lent a hand at Silver Lake for a week each in September. When Theobald Smith arrived in Princeton on October 12, his summer camp, though still unfinished, stood solid, ample and inhabitable on twelve acres of lake side real estate. The total cost was under $7,000.

21

THE CHOICE OF PRINCETON—
IMPROVISATIONS AND EXPEDIENTS

The slow unfolding of events, and the eventual choice of a site near Princeton for the new Rockefeller Department of Animal Pathology, mockingly echoed George Fabyan's allegations. During the long struggle for proper quarters and staff, Smith often craved a few days for quiet reflection—with no striving to make his time count "nearer 100 percent;" and only too frequently those "facilities . . . furnished without vexatious delays" were illusory. The early years of turmoil, critical decisions and inescapable anxieties, of handicapped efforts to create an outstanding department of animal pathology, have been too little appreciated. The meticulous and far-sighted planning of the Princeton department, with its ready expansibility in research laboratories and animal quarters, the staff accommodations at walking distance from the work place, and the securing of harmonious relations with the neighboring University, were due largely to the versatility, enterprise, and self-effacing capacity of Theobald Smith.

The Boards of Trustees and of Scientific Directors of the Rockefeller Institute did not anticipate the range of problems entailed by the Institute's decision to launch this new department. Among the more urgent, interdependent questions were the site, size, and type of buildings to erect; the source, qualifications, and accommodation for staff; and the funds available for constructional and general budgetary purposes. The Directors could not have been expected to foresee that Theobald Smith's temporary physical disabilities would curb and even cripple his participation in crucial plans bearing on these problems, thus adding to delays or uncertainties. Still less was it predictable that far worse hindrances would be unleashed by the vagaries and tragedies of an intensifying war.

The Rockefeller Institute for Medical Research from the beginning drew no clear line between human and animal disorders. "Indeed, by appointing America's most successful investigator of animal pathology, Theobald Smith, as one of its charter members, the Board of Directors . . . had inescapably accepted the principle that human pathology cannot well be studied apart from that of lower creatures"—that "pathologists and bacteriologists draw no lines between human ailments and those of animals."[1] Smith himself had championed the even broader doctrine that the study of diseased conditions should be viewed as a branch of biology. The Institution's acceptance of those principles did not, however, simplify the task of the director of a new department of animal pathology who wished to avoid its being mistaken for the veterinary division of the Institute. The study of a disease in animals in place of, or supplementary to, its direct study in humans, has been accepted in medical research since the earliest days of Pasteur and Koch. But the demarcation between this practice and veterinary medicine may not always be clear-cut. In view of Theobald Smith's hypersensitivity to some veterinary types, it is not surprising that this area should be among the sources of minor irritation that inevitably developed between the Princeton division and its New York headquarters.

At the postponed Testimonial Dinner, the guest of honor, still partially crippled by sciatica, expressed concern that he might have only a few years of useful service to offer the new employer. Soon after the Dinner, he thanked Simon Flexner "for coming to Boston and helping to make the farewell a success . . . How to live up to the idealized portraiture will be a task hardly to be met in the brief span ahead of me."[2] He was doubly anxious to begin, especially since Flexner had notified him recently that the Governor of New Jersey had signed the amended Bill "legalizing animal experimentation under modern conditions in New Jersey. We can now proceed with our plans."[3] Governor James F. Fielder had vetoed the original Bill—passed by the Legislative Assembly in 1914—under pressure from the Bill's opponents. The counter-arguments of Welch, Flexner and Smith himself—all three experienced in dealing effectively with antivivisectionists—were reinforced by the efforts of Princeton University's eminent Professor of Biology, Edwin G. Conklin, who had assured Smith in June 1914 that he planned to discuss soon with Henry James "the possibility of getting a liberal Bill through the legislature allowing animal experimentation in this state. We are as much interested in this matter as you and shall be very glad to do anything possible to accomplish this result."[4]

For Simon Flexner, the 1914–16 period was especially memorable. The gift of one million dollars to permit establishment of the Rockefeller Institute's Department of Animal Pathology was announced at the end of March. Within three months Flexner informed Smith that "Mr. Rockefeller has just made a gift to the Institute of something more than $2,500,000."[5] That sum was to cover the construction and maintenance costs of a second laboratory building at the Institute's New York property, besides a much larger power house, improved animal quarters and internal changes in the original laboratories. It also included the purchase of land to the west of the existing boundary. By good fortune, sound judgment, effective supervision, and general pushfulness, the objectives were all met before wartime shortages seriously intervened. Flexner himself was increasingly busy and often away from the Institute during this expansion, but he liked to verify progress—in the large. More exacting tasks, such as close inspections of workmanship and checking blueprints, were left to Henry James and his managerial staff, pursuant to Flexner's stated view, "I have rather used others to do finely detailed things."[6]

News of important developments affecting the Institute usually spread among staff members well before the official press releases, which were arranged by Simon Flexner and the Business Manager. Particularly large endowments for specific purposes, for example the Hospital, might be more formally celebrated. On such occasions, Flexner appeared as it were from the wings to pay brief tribute to the generosity and farsightedness of their benefactors, and to the wisdom of the Trustees. (Especially generous donations were also felicitously acknowledged in writing by Welch.) The Board of Scientific Directors debated and approved the allocation of funds for important projects, but operating decisions and disbursements were left to Flexner, who was granted amply leeway. As the enterprise expanded, his rights of leadership grew. During his directorship, $60 million from Rockefeller sources passed through Flexner's hands for the Institute's buildings and research activities.[7]

Karl Landsteiner, when gazing at a portrait of Simon Flexner on one occasion, referred to him as "Caligula;" but this was not fair, for Flexner was no cruel despot.[8] Indeed, he had neither the physique nor the temperament for browbeating of any kind. Threats and hectoring were as foreign to his style as wheedling, cajolery or flattery. Not that he lacked emotions. He was far warmer-hearted than he appeared to be—an important attribute of many successful leaders. Yet anyone whose behavior in Flexner's view threatened the interests of the Institute (e.g., Paul de Kruif) might find himself confronting a cool demeanor, ruthless logic, and inexorable judgment. Flexner occasionally lapsed into bouts of aloofness, but these were often counterbalanced by his forbearance and leniency towards such members of the Institute staff as Hideyo Noguchi and Alexis Carrel. At times, he revealed concern for a very junior employee by some act of personal kindness.

In mid-October 1914, a Dinner was held at Delmonico's Restaurant in New York honoring Simon Flexner on the tenth anniversary of the opening of the laboratories of the Rockefeller Institute for Medical Research. In his speech of thanks, the guest of honor confessed that on arrival in Baltimore in 1890, with a fresh M.D. from the University of Louisville Medical School, he was "unformed, inexperienced, ambitious, over-strenuous, and inconsiderate."[9] At that time, he was also ill-educated. Simon Flexner had come a long way in twenty-four years. He never sought to hide or dress up his ancestry. He was the fifth of a family of seven consecutive sons and two daughters, the offspring of impoverished but industrious German-speaking Jewish immigrants. His younger brother, Abraham, likewise achieved high distinction.

Flexner rightly credited much of the success of the Institute's first decade to his wife Helen, who brought about "a true expansion of his personality," and to William Henry Welch, his sponsor. Just before this period began, when Simon Flexner was past forty, he had married the thirty-two-year-old Helen Whitall Thomas, his opposite in temperament and upbringing—a literate, intelligent, highly sensitive member of prosperous, feminist, Quaker stock. She introduced him to a new world of humane letters and the arts, while he strengthened her purposes, provoked a more realistic appreciation of life, and aroused her ambition to further his "powers to the utmost in the cause of science."[10] Through his marriage, Flexner became related to such well-known figures as President Carey Thomas of Bryn Mawr; Bertrand Russell, the philosopher-mathematician-pacifist; and Bernard Berenson, the authority on Italian painting and Renaissance art.

In the last twenty years of his working life, Theobald Smith was ultimately responsible to Simon Flexner. Although the directorship of the embryo Institute probably would have gone to Smith if he had so chosen, it soon became evident that Welch's second nominee was more suitably cast to lead an expanding Institution. Notwithstanding certain shared background features, their temperaments were quite different. Their mutual respect stemmed from high perceptiveness, tolerant judgment, and good manners. Both came of poor, thrifty families that lacked learning but honored it; both realized their very inadequate professional training in medicine; and both married intelligent women who did their utmost to further their husbands' scientific careers.

But whereas Smith was reticent, over-modest and self-sufficient, with few relatives or close friends, Flexner was talkative, at times ebullient, ambitious, with a host of supportive friends and acquaintances, and a ramifying network of relatives. Smith remained distant and formal, even with "Professor and Mrs. Gage," his closest confidants. Occasionally he began with "Dear Friends" in letters to the Gages, whereas Flexner often sent his "love" and signed himself "yours affectionately" in letters to his chief mentor, William Welch. During World War I, Smith's sympathies were as pro-German as Flexner's were jingoistically American. Neither man was physically robust and each tended to coddle himself; yet at night Smith slept soundly, and at his own command, while Flexner's worries often kept him awake.

Although Flexner sincerely admired Smith's scientific productivity, streaks of criticism sometimes appeared in his written allusions. Following Noguchi's death in West Africa in 1928, he reflected: "Theobald Smith is a deeper mind, more general and philosophic. He pursues a subject wonderfully, but impresses me as less an explorer than Noguchi. It is hard for me to imagine N. missing anaphylaxis in the guinea pig and turning the crude phenomenon over to Ehrlich as Smith did."[11] Yet Flexner himself had not followed up a pioneer anaphylactic observation involving rabbits, made by him in 1894.[12] Again, in a letter sent within a few months of Theobald Smith's death, concerning unordered reprints for a recent paper, Flexner commented: "Dr. Smith had a marvelous way of reincorporating (reusing) fundamental ideas prepared for different occasions. If he did not see fit to have reprints, it was, I feel, because he had used the ideas before and was merely presenting them in fresh form for a particular audience."[13] Fundamental ideas turned up rarely in Flexner's own researches. "For Flexner, to reach any result was to publish."[14] Some unverifiable results were the consequence of this haste.

Smith's publications, on the other hand, were not only of very high average quality, but their total was nearly double Flexner's—308 to 159. Worldwide recognition of Theobald Smith as America's leading microbiologist derived mainly from the conjunction of quality and quantity in his published output. Flexner coveted renown in laboratory circles that would match his reputation as administrator, but he lacked the time and opportunity, the patience and discrimination to sustain the effort; whereas Smith, though uncomfortable with administrative duties, resolutely tackled every obstacle, including some better left to others. To compensate for his disdain for the "finely detailed things," Flexner held an active interest in the psychology of human relationships. Perhaps this helped to keep the Institute's staff from excessive rivalry without curbing individual enterprise. If details were needed, he availed himself of the Manager's propensity for inserting a probing finger in every handy pie.

Henry James, Jr. had succeeded Jerome K. Greene in 1912 as supervisor of the Institute's financial affairs. Greene resigned the comprehensive position of "General Manager" to assume more direct responsibility for the Rockefeller philanthropies. James was appointed simply as "Manager," while his successors carried the more specific rank of "Business Manager." Corner[15] has drawn attention to the Institute's good fortune in the widely-recognized "high character and abilities" of its successive business managers. Ambitious and industrious, James was also highly intelligent, literate, and of unquestioned probity and discretion. "Harry," as he was known to his family and close friends, was the eldest son of William James, the Harvard philosopher, and his wife Alice, and the senior nephew of Henry James, the novelist. His literary talents, evident in his clear, venturesome and usually decisive letters to Theobald Smith while in the army in 1917, were recognized early by his uncle, whose sole literary executor he became in 1916. In 1930, he published a Pulitzer prize-winning biography of President Charles W. Eliot of Harvard, from which University he had graduated in 1899.[16]

In 1917, when thirty-eight years old, he married a wealthy New York socialite, whose family inhabited an enormous mansion. Peyton Rous knew Harry well and relayed waggish tales of pre-war receptions at which guests were greeted in a pillared hall lined with footmen. The pompous William James supposedly once shook the hand of the nearest well-dressed flunkey, patted his back as though he were a long-lost friend and exclaimed, "My dear fellow, how are you?" Harry rebelled against all this, and got divorced. His second marriage was very happy.[17] He cultivated the ability to respond effectively to almost any request, large or small. Restlessness took him to Europe for several months in 1914–15, and in 1917 he resigned to join the U.S. Army, serving at first in the ranks. Like Greene, he demonstrated a continuing interest in the affairs of the Rockefeller Institute by playing an active role on its Board of Trustees.

The Manager focused early upon the question of the new department's location. The Trustees, who had responded generously to every personal fiscal issue raised by Smith, also noted his adamant objection to housing the department in or near New York city, or an "ordinary business community." Smith had declared Princeton "the only alternative." However, the Scientific Directors and the Trustees were now undecided whether or not to upgrade the Rockefeller Institute Farm at the village of Clyde, near New Brunswick. If their decision were affirmative, a suitable location for the new department might be found somewhere between Princeton and New Brunswick. But if the Governor and Legislature of New Jersey proved unstable in their attitudes toward animal experimentation, a site near the metropolis in New York State might be necessary.

Shortly after the June 1913 meeting of the Scientific Directors, Henry James wrote to remind Smith that he planned to visit England and continental Europe that summer in order to become better informed "about animal arrangements, because no one else here is giving much attention to them," and careful heed would have to be paid to the matter in developing the Farm. The Executive Committee had canvassed the possibility of a change that spring, and "are now of the opinion (which I hold very strongly myself) that we should consider our present Farm as a permanency." They were there to stay, and with a promising Superintendent could make much greater use of the Farm, especially if they did not delay the needed new buildings and improvements. James therefore proposed visiting "the farm and animal quarters of the Pasteur Institute, the Lister Institute, the Board of Health in Berlin" and any other places or individuals Smith would advise him to see.[18] In reply, Smith added to James's list the State Serum Institute in Vienna and the Institute for Infectious Diseases in Berlin.[19] James returned from Europe with his natural zeal reinforced by a measure of acquired expertness in the field of laboratory animal care and accommodation.

Even before Theobald Smith had committed himself formally to the Rockefeller Institute in April 1914, the Manager wrote about a new record-keeping system for guinea-pigs which he had worked out. The animal handler supposedly would turn in a daily report, using the new forms, to the Superintendent. Cages were of three kinds—"breeding cages in each of which is a boar and three or four sows. Brooders, in which the sows have their litter . . . one sow and litter in each. Pens, in which the weaned stock is kept. The animals in these pens are not marked, and from them are taken the animals . . . to be shipped to the Institute." The system had not yet been tested, and criticisms would be welcomed.[20]

James followed this shortly with a sketch of his own version of the reconstructed Farm, redrawn to scale by Charles Coolidge, of the architectural firm, Messrs. Shepley, Ruton and Coolidge. They had designed the buildings of the Rockefeller Institute in New York and the new Harvard Medical School. James did not regard his proposed floor arrangement as final. "The placing of doors, etc. had got to be carefully considered: exact shapes and sizes of stalls also. Mr. Coolidge's office is now engaged in further work on these sketches . . . The rooms marked No. 1 and No. 2 are intended to be farrowing rooms."[21] Soon after Smith's appointment to the Rockefeller Institute, the future of the Farm was considered. Smith and James were asked to make recommendations. Before going on to Clyde, they went over the B.A.I. Experiment Station on the outskirts of Washington. Smith also spent an extra night in New York in order to meet Mr. Coolidge to discuss animal quarters at the Clyde Farm.[22]

That year's Annual Meeting of the National Academy of Sciences at Washington on April 21–23, 1914 was of special interest to Theobald Smith. The retiring president of the Academy and guest of honor at the Annual Banquet was Ira Remson, former chairman of the now defunct Referee Board. Brig. General William Crawford Gorgas, and his arch-rival, Col. George Washington Goethals, were presented with Medals for "Eminence in the Application of Science to the Public Warfare." On the 21st and 23rd, Sir Ernest Rutherford inaugurated the W.E. Hales public lectures by discussing "The Constitution of Matter and the Evolution of the Elements." These seemed relatively simple problems then. Smith's comment on the first lecture is typically unrevealing, but suggests that Rutherford's exposition of Matter was very over-simplified: "Rutherford lecture on atoms. Electrons."[23] On the 21st, Smith also attended Alexander Graham Bell's late-night reception at his home.[24]

In the afternoon of April 23, Smith and James left for Princeton, putting up at the Inn. Next morning, after exploring the neighborhood on foot, they motored to New Brunswick and thoroughly inspected the Farm. Smith was unimpressed by New Brunswick as a setting for his future department and skeptical about the adaptability of the Rockefeller Farm to the Institute's future needs, even with extensive renovation and expansion. But he made no hasty judgment, informing James that he wished to spend another whole day at New Brunswick and Princeton.

The Scientific Directors met on June 13. Although Governor Fielder seemed likely to sign the revised Bill due to come before the New Jersey Legislature that winter, it appeared prudent to survey possible sites in the State of New York readily accessible to the Rockefeller Institute. Next morning, Flexner, Smith, James and Greene set out to prospect an area in Westchester County, on the east bank of the Hudson between Croton and Ossining. They motored about, looking for suitable estates on which they might locate the new department, but found nothing; so after lunch they dispersed.[25]

The future locations of the Farm and the new department remained undecided. Obviously they should be at least close neighbors, and it was agreed that a veterinarian would be appointed and temporarily headquartered at the Farm to meet the needs at both places. In June, Smith received a telegram and a letter from James. "A committee meeting will be called tomorrow as to location of Farm. Very much desire an expression of your opinion as to relative desirability of locations in Westchester County or New Jersey. If New Jersey seems to you more desirable than New York would you consider Princeton or New Brunswick the preferable neighborhood." The letter was only slightly more expansive. They were "trying to forecast a rather ambiguous future" for the Farm, and they required Smith's opinion.[26]

Smith's hastily telegraphed an indefinite reply that somehow reached its garbled addressee—Mrs. Henry James, Jr., Orck Fellow Institute." Although insufficiently investigated, New Brunswick was preferable to Westchester, which would present the problems of an isolated community. Smith's follow-up letter was slightly more conclusive. "I think that on the whole the New Jersey plan is still the best." The Board had already stressed the advantages of topographical association with an institution of higher education (such as Princeton University or Rutgers College at New Brunswick) which the Westchester

County sites lacked. "In New Jersey the environment is distinctly rural or agricultural, and apparently free from the untoward influences of the proximity of a great city." Besides, the soil was probably better in New Jersey. (Surely a farmer, especially one associated with scientists, should be able to feed his own livestock.)

Theobald Smith expressed on this occasion no strong preference for Clyde, the Princeton area, or any other locality. "It is the remainder of the staff whose interests we must carefully consider. The influence of either educational institution in N.J. would be very valuable in maintaining ideals of a broader outlook than our work will supply." Two points mentioned in the letter struck the committee members as decisively favoring the Princeton location. First, the department would still be near enough, in case of need, to the State Agricultural College stationed at New Brunswick, in close association with Rutgers. Secondly, the proximity of the large Walker-Gordon Dairy farm to Princeton was "a desideratum not to be neglected . . . they will probably have much material for our use. The problem of udder infection in which I have become interested in connection with our tonsillitis epidemics could be studied nowhere better."[27]

Shepley, Rutan and Coolidge estimated the cost of Farm improvements at about $77,000. This included several additional two-storied structures—an administration building, a stock barn, a small animal house, and an antitoxin stable—as well as a power house, dog kennels, a monkey house, and extensive fencing. Larger boilers and electric lifting in the power house would be an extra $5,000. In other words, high quality animal quarters would cost around $80,000[28]—a jolting figure. Theobald Smith was worried already because the $1 million Rockefeller endowment had to pay for land and buildings, leaving only the balance for operating budget. "It is true that we have Mr. Hill's money. But we must start other problems at the same time." They needed a large budget, which might entail considering "whether to put up shacks or expensive permanent buildings at the outset" for the staff, and "improvised temporary buildings for animals." In the unlikely event of another Executive Committee meeting that summer, "this important question should be settled for the next few years."[29]

A Committee of the Trustees was authorized to buy land in New Jersey, near Princeton or New Brunswick, for the Department of Animal Pathology of the Rockefeller Institute.[30] The Manager's next letter showed how radically the future of the Farm had altered within a few months. Although they should "keep on trying to find a good veterinarian" to be put to work at the Farm temporarily, they would otherwise "get on from hand to mouth as we have done for the last few months."

Meanwhile the availability and price of land between Princeton Junction and Princeton was being discreetly investigated on behalf of the Rockefeller

Trustees. James suggested that in August, Smith should "look the ground over both at Princeton and at New Brunswick more thoroughly" than heretofore.[31] Smith replied: "Shall be ready to come to Princeton whenever the need arises. My family insists on going to Madison [the station nearest to Silver Lake on the Boston and Maine Railway] during August, so I can lie in wait up there."[32] On August 3, a Monday, after much fussing around—reading and destroying old letters, running errands in Boston, inviting TenBroeck to dinner, lunching at the Medical School with J.H. Brown, his latest research collaborator—Theobald set out for Silver Lake with his wife and Nellie the servant. The Brown family moved into the house at Woodland Hill.

At the end of August he moved to Boston for two busy days at the Harvard Medical School. Thence he traveled to New York with Henry James, en route to inspect possible land purchases around Princeton and New Brunswick. Near Princeton, a 300-acre tract owned by two sisters named Gray was for sale. Soon after returning to Silver Lake on September 6, Smith received from James a geological map of New Jersey on which he had located the Gray Farm. (Later on, when the Gray property was finally purchased, Smith requested a somewhat more detailed sketch for study, with contour lines roughly drawn in.)

Nothing was yet settled with the Gray sisters when James suddenly left New York for Belgium. Smith was annoyed to read of his departure in the evening paper *before* receiving the news in a hurried letter of the same date.

> I have been asked to go abroad as a member of a Commission to inform the Rockefeller Foundation how it had best spend money in European Relief Work. I may be gone three months. I am very sorry indeed to interrupt the work in which I have been so much interested in here with reference to the development of the new department, and other things, but the decision is one which I did not find possible to refuse, so I am off.

The land question would be settled very shortly. He suggested engaging a sanitary engineer to survey the land topographically, with particular regard to water supply and sewage disposal. The detailed arrangement of the buildings and their final planning would be troublesome, but "I can't help thinking that I shall be back by then." Nonetheless, he added, "I was very much pleased that we have secured this very desirable location for the new department at the Institute." His own relatively minor suggestions, in Coolidge's hands, would not be taken up until Smith had worked out his own views of the most important buildings, those for the isolation of animals, and the laboratory.[33]

When Theobald Smith's appointment with the Rockefeller Institute was ratified, Flexner had offered personally to clarify any still obscure or uninviting points. But Smith appeared to have become more resilient and light-hearted about the move. The map sent by Henry James showed the New Jersey roads, making that State seem nearer and distances less formidable. There would be no need to feel isolated scientifically, for New York would be close.

> The break will be perhaps more trying for my family for a time, but they are beginning to train for it already. As to your visit to Boston . . . Mrs. Smith is waiting for the Arboretum grass paths to dry up a little and the spring beauties to unfold before insisting on a visit from you and Mrs. Flexner. From here you can visit friends in Boston or hide in the Arboretum among the trees and shrubs.[34]

The Flexners spent the last weekend of May (23rd to 25th) at Woodland Hill. The time passed happily. On the Sunday, the Dean of the Bussey Institution, William Morton Wheeler, a distinguished entomologist, accompanied by his wife, motored the Flexners and the Smiths through towns and countryside westward of Boston: "Flexners, Wheelers & us out motoring in morning, clear weather— Wellesley, Weston, Newton, Waltham. Cushing at tea."[35] Lilian lent Simon a recent newspaper editorial[36] decrying Governor Walsh's proposal "to abolish the entire administrative machinery of the public health service of the Commonwealth and substitute therefore a new model of his own construction." This was sent back promptly with a characteristic note of thanks:

> I like exceedingly the spirit as well as the facts of the editorial. May I add that we had a delightful visit with you and your family. I should not wish to have missed the opportunity and coming just at the period when we did, we were able to enjoy the charm and beauty of your rare surroundings . . . In a few days you will receive the little book on Mexico which I spoke about. It is understood that it is not to be returned.[37]

Although war clouds darkened over Europe, prospects for the Rockefeller Institute had never seemed brighter. One month after the visit to Woodland Hill, Flexner informed Theobald Smith about the $2–1/2$ million gift for expansion of the Institute in New York.[38] Flexner wrote again on December 7 to Smith that suitable land for his department had been secured and the initial payment made. This property comprised about 340 acres, purchased for just over $70,000 by Jerome D. Greene on behalf of the Rockefeller Institute's Board of Trustees. According to Corner, the claim is not quite correct that when Theobald Smith became director of the department, as of July 1, 1914, "The Institute had already bought a tract of land near Princeton."[39]

Jerome Greene, the ostensible purchaser, conducted negotiations through Walter B. Howe, a real estate and insurance broker of Princeton, and J.V.B. Wicoff, of Wicoff and Lanning, counsellors-at-Law, of Trenton. An adjacent tract of about eighty-three acres, known as the Simon Van Dyke Farm, came on the market early in 1915. This area, on higher ground overlooking Lake Carnegie, stretched in a southeasterly direction to the Princeton and New Brunswick Turnpike, where it became contiguous to and in alignment with the half mile wide property already purchased. The full length of the entire rectangular property would be about one and one half miles. Flexner was against further acquisitions, and Jerome Greene only posed searching questions respecting its future usefulness. Some Directors favored the additional purchase.

The issue was settled by a Night Letter from Theobald Smith . . . THINK BEST TO BUY EXTRA LAND WILL MAKE COMPACT RECTANGLE OF ENTIRE PROPERTY . . . SORRY JAMES NOT HERE TO MAKE THOROUGH INVESTIGATION. The message came from Jamaica Plain, to which Theobald had just returned from Chicago. He was now "in bed with grippe probably for a day or two." In Flexner's absence, the telegram was sent to Prudden, who had accompanied Theobald Smith to Princeton after the mid-January meeting of the Scientific Directors to inspect the original Gray estate from the standpoint of building sites. About three weeks later, Greene telegraphed Simon Flexner in Florida: WE HAVE JUST VOTED TO PURCHASE ADDITIONAL LAND AS RECOMMENDED.[40] The price was $22,000. Problems involving a few tenanted houses and occasional crop-bearing fields were settled through negotiations. By September 1915, the Rockefeller Institute had bought full title to the "compact rectangle" of some 425 acres and several houses free of all encumbrances, for little more than $100,000. This ample estate was increased later to about 800 acres.

The requested survey was conducted and a scale map of the area drawn by C.S. Sincerbeaux, a civil engineer of Princeton. A rough plan appeared in the April issue of the *Princeton Press,* whose editor had inquired about the Rockefeller Institute's local intentions.[41] This illustrated that the tract adjoined the northern length of the Walker-Gordon Milk Farms, and was crossed by the Trenton and New Brunswick Turnpike. The westerly side of the rectangle abutted on and overlooked the Delaware and Raritan Canal and Lake Carnegie. About two miles beyond its southwest corner was Plainsboro Station, on the main line of the Pennsylvania Railroad, to which the Institute had arranged a right-of-way across Walker-Gordon territory. Nassau Hall of Princeton University was about two miles west of the laboratory building site, while by road the town center was some three miles away.

In November 1914, Theobald Smith had written to Flexner, "I see from the Transcript that you are going to do some work on Foot and Mouth Disease. It might be well to collect some lymph from fresh vesicle, seal it in full tubes and freeze it up. It may remain alive in this way for a year or longer." Although Smith suspected that the disease had "permanently gotten away from control," the Government would withhold permission to experiment as long as there was any hope of stamping it out—the position adopted during the eastern epidemic about ten years before.[42]

Flexner replied that even if the Department of Agriculture still disallowed animal experiments with the virus, he saw no reason why they should object to test-tube experiments. When Smith had his "bomb-proof" stalls, Flexner hoped he would "feel secure in taking up just such a subject as this."

> It seems to me a great pity that in this country . . . study of so important a disease
> . . . should be rendered impossible by the lack of safe and adequate facilities. The
> problem coming just at this time . . . is very welcome, since it bears so directly on
> the new department and perhaps on the manner of completing your units.[43]

Theobald Smith wrote from Boston, "We are not properly equipped for such important and delicate work, and the possible escape of the infection might create a great deal of trouble since so many men are engaged hereabouts in raising fancy stock. With your experience and equipment, I should think it might be of great interest to you to see what can be done towards the cultivation of this virus. I do not see why you should not succeed."[44]

In February 1915, Smith journeyed to Chicago in response to clamorous pleas for his advice about the control of foot-and-mouth disease, which was epizootic on many cattle farms around Elgin, near Chicago. The federal Department of Agriculture's policy (approved and applied by the B.A.I.) of destroying infected animals was ruining the farmers. The Kane County Farmer's Improvement Association, led by Colonel George Fabyan of Chicago, and others such as the President of the Illinois State Board of Agriculture, had petitioned President Lowell to urge Smith to respond to their appeal, Fabyan informing Lowell that "The conditions around Elgin on account of the hoof-and-mouth disease are intolerable."[45]

Fabyan also requested Simon Flexner to sanction Smith's assistance. Smith wrote to Flexner explaining the pressure he was under to provide "some outside assistance," and urging that the general policy involved should be thoroughly talked over. He presumed that "the Institute is expected to be of service to the public, at the same time this service should not . . . interfere with the real object of the new department—namely, investigation and the obtaining of results."[46] The whole problem was freely discussed at the meeting of the Rockefeller Institute's Scientific Directors on Saturday, January 16. On returning to Boston, Smith wrote to Fabyan: "It was though best to find out the attitude of the Department of Agriculture towards my visit."

The temporary absence of Secretary Houston from Washington made it impossible to determine the desirability of holding a conference in Chicago, with all interested parties present. "Though disliking this trip, I should be most ready to do anything in my power to assist you and others interested in clearing up this most trying situation . . . I do not, however, wish to take the position of a partisan engaged by one party as their expert to combat the position of the other." He had been troubled by simultaneous requests from several organizations, which raised doubts as to what he was invited to do. "Especially your telegram to Dr. Flexner requesting that other invitations be ignored left me still more uncertain."[47]

Having received suitable reassurances, Theobald Smith went to Washington on Monday, February 1, to confer with U.S. Department of Agriculture officials on foot-and-mouth disease. He left that afternoon for Chicago, where George Fabyan took charge and put him up at the Chicago Club. Next morning, after visiting the stockyard, they motored to Geneva (a few miles south of Elgin, in Kane County), to review the general situation and control measures with U.G. Houck of the B.A.I. On the 3rd, Smith and Fabyan went by train to Champaign to visit the state university, anticipated about three weeks before by an editorial in the *Chicago Herald,* headlined "FAMOUS HARVARD MEDICAL EXPERT CALLED TO SAVE ILLINOIS HERDS."[48] Immediately after the visit, the *Herald* proclaimed "HARVARD SAVANT PRESENTS PLAN TO END PLAGUE."[49]

Smith's Day Card indicated only that he lunched with President James, met Profs. Davenport, Mumford and Harding, attended a reception for bacteriologists at Harding's home from 5 to 6 P.M., and returned the same night to the Chicago Club with Fabyan. However, according to a staff correspondent for the *Chicago Herald,* Smith proposed a comprehensive plan at an afternoon conference at Urbana with President James, Dean of Agriculture, Davenport, and Professors (of Animal Industry) Mumford and Harding. This plan met with the approval of the "university authorities"—presumably the spontaneous approbation of the president, the dean of agriculture, and the two professors of animal industry.

Smith envisaged the establishment of a veterinary school of the highest standards at the state university, with first-class diagnostic and research laboratories operating at the Union Stock Yard in Chicago, as well as at Urbana. The state of Illinois, harboring the world's greatest cattle market, had abundant working material for research into the earliest stages of such scourges as hog cholera, bovine tuberculosis, and foot-and-mouth disease threatening the nation's livestock. The "horse doctor" would be abolished; graduates of the school would be as expert in ailments of chickens as in those of horses and cattle. Within a year, the institution would save twenty times its costs of inauguration and maintenance, and Illinois could become the nation's advisor on livestock diseases. But despite Theobald's pleadings, a College of Veterinary Medicine did not begin instruction at the University of Illinois, Urbana, until 1948.

For epizootics of hoof-and-mouth disease, Smith was opposed to the "slaughter-all" policy. Slaughter was justifiable only if very few herds were infected, "but when the disease has spread to 16 states and threatens to sweep the country, it is time to think of the great economic waste of slaughtering thousands of cattle, hogs, and sheep that are only exposed. This meat is just as good as that of the animal not exposed. Were I a butcher I would prove its safety to the public by serving the first chunk of it at my own dinner table."[50] Admittedly, serum-therapy was too expensive for field use, but spontaneous recoveries did occur and the residual carrier state was by no means inevitable. As a public health safeguard, pasteurization of all marketable milk products was of course essential. Quarantine measures should be reserved for thoroughbreds—he was scheduled next morning to inspect a prize herd of 700 animals at the Hawthorne race track, in which the disease had been allowed to run its course.

Theobald Smith returned with Fabyan to the Chicago Club. On the final day, after inspecting a great many pure-bred show cattle quarantined at the race track, and lunching at the stockyards with representatives of the meat packers, he was motored around the city before finding refuge in his Pullman compartment. He reached Boston thoroughly exhausted. The 2,000-mile trip had aggravated his physical discomfort and given him a heavy, febrile cold. In the following week he recorded several days of small accomplishment, spent in bed, culminating in the pathetic entry, "Get up & do a little work on lab plans etc. feel very wretched."[51]

Contributing to his unhappiness was the realization that he had been unable to offer the Kane County cattle farmers any better advice about controlling foot-and-mouth disease than was available more than twelve years before, when he wrote an editorial on this malady.[52] Despite wide acclaim as the leading North American microbiologist, renowned for pioneer studies of animal diseases, Smith could not amplify significantly the 1898 report of Löffler and Frosch.[53] Even now he was merely designing "bomb-proof" isolation quarters for animals at Princeton as a prerequisite to progress in such fields. However, the *Country Gentleman* asserted in an editorial:

> Even the men most carefully trained in the diagnosis of animal diseases find difficulty in recognizing so dangerous a malady as foot-and-mouth disease . . . An ignorant practitioner . . . not only fails to recognize dangerous diseases, but he spreads them from farm to farm . . . Dr. Smith would abolish the "horse doctors" and eliminate politics in favor of efficiency—both of which are more easily said than done. The quacks and inefficients can be cut out when the substitutes are ready, but politics is a hard thorn to extract.[54]

In March 1915, the Report of the New York Commission for the Investigation of Bovine Tuberculosis was published.[55] Recognizing that "few states in this country or in Europe are now as far in the rear as New York" in legislation "against the menace of diseased milk," the New York *Evening Globe* reported,[56] a bill was submitted to the Joint Committee on Agriculture of the New York State Legislature at Albany. The bill represented "the best thought of a commission well qualified for the work and headed by a man, Dr. Theobald Smith, recognized throughout the world as an authority on the subject." It was at no point "harshly coercive." Although the commission recommended state-wide compulsory pasteurization of all market milk as a public health measure (for which the State Health Department already had ample powers of enforcement), the bill before the Committee on Agriculture was concerned chiefly to put "a premium on sound cattle" and their products. To this end, it sought approval of two measures—the confidential tuberculin-testing of all dairy cattle; and pasteurization of skimmed milk and whey (from cheese factories) with which calves were fed.

The bill was rejected. As a *Globe* editorial afterwards commented,[57] its passage "was opposed by the ignorant farmers, who resent as intrusion every effort to give them the benefits of scientific research."

> The master of the State Grange . . . scenting danger to be the farmer who rejoices in untrammelled freedom to run his cows, sick or well, to suit himself, had no difficulty in persuading [the] committee that Dr. Smith did not know what he was talking about and that men like the master of the grange were far better advisers and had the interest of the public more closely at heart. Lest any member of the committee might be susceptible to argument and enlightenment the job of killing the bill was completed before the report of the commission upon which the bill was based had been printed.

The newspaper accounts of Smith's vision of a new type of professional veterinarian, who would play a leading role in the conquest of foot-and-mouth disease and other animal plagues, followed by his Commission's recommendations for the control of bovine tuberculosis, set the stage for a third public announcement involving him. In April it was reported that an institute for animal disease research would be established on land adjacent to Princeton University. Extravagant headlines went with such textual inaccuracies as Dr. *Leopold* Smith. The *Boston Transcript* grabbed attention with "MILLION FOR RESEARCH," followed by four lesser captions: "New Jersey to Have Its Own Pasteur Institute. A Comprehensive Study of Animal Disease. Dr. Smith of Harvard Is to Be in Charge. Rockefeller Foundation Provides the Funds." Governor Fielder had "signed an act of the Legislature empowering the Rockefeller Foundation to organize this bureau, which will be one of the most important institutions for the study of biological and medical science in America . . . and it is likely to become one of the greatest laboratories for the study of comparative pathology in the world." Although not directly connected with Princeton University, the development would "greatly affect the future of the University and will add an immediate stimulus to her work in biology. It is already evident that there will be a most cordial cooperation between the two laboratories."[58]

Since the department's future locale had now been disclosed, Smith felt especially obliged to make progress by collaborating with Charles Coolidge. Whenever possible, he spent several hours a day on the building designs. To reduce painful cramps and tenderness in his back and legs, many of the preliminary plans were drawn as he lay on a couch or bed. As the task grew increasingly complex and more painful, the cheerful load-sharing interventions of Henry James were sorely missed. His adaptability to various fields of activity was almost legendary.

By contrast, Theobald Smith was viewed by many of his medical school colleagues, and by the Harvard administration, as a monomanic research scientist dedicated to microbiology and public health, with a peculiar concern for diseases of animals. Even now, one of his urgent objectives seemed to be the resolution of certain mysteries about an epizootic turkey disease. He had requested the Assistant Manager to look into the prices of incubators and brooders for turkey eggs. Yet here he was, gravely handicapped physically, struggling with problems that required the talents of an accountant, architect and structural engineer, estate agent, landscapist and agriculturist, as well as electrician, librarian and employment counsellor. The financial uncertainties about the enterprise troubled him but could only be settled by Simon Flexner, who was either temporarily indisposed, inaccessible, or away. Beginning in August 1915, for instance, Flexner went with William Welch on a visit of several months to Japan, Korea and China as fellow members of the China Medical Board.

Smith meanwhile faced a range of technical questions, some relatively easy to settle, such as the form of electric current delivered to the Princeton area; whereas others, such as the most suitable ventilation arrangements, were very controversial. Again, though he could order suitable journals for the future departmental library with confidence, a specific kind of knowledge was required to locate successfully the toilet facilities for the new buildings. As a result, Theobald was greatly relieved when he was informed by E.B. Smith in mid-March, "We hear that Mr. James has been cabled to come home at once and that he is either in London or on the sea."[59]

At the beginning of April, the Assistant Manager wrote "Mr. James is back again." Henry James came to Woodland Hill on April 13, and again for two days at the end of the month. His return relieved Theobald Smith temporarily of the crushing weight of minor questions and offered him a chance to deal with several major problems. A small staff had been recruited, with duties still indefinite.

The new department was due to begin operating later that year, yet its buildings would not be ready. Moreover, beginning in October, the director would require some residence for himself and family in or near Princeton.

After the Princeton site had been selected for his future department, Theobald Smith focused his interest on that area as a setting for his family's living quarters. Even while New Brunswick was still under consideration for the Rockefeller development, Smith thought Princeton a preferable place to reside. In reply to a request for advice, Prof. E.G. Conklin, the distinguished evolutionist (whom he had met at Woods Hole) replied: "You would find no more beautiful nor delightful place of residence in this country . . . My colleagues and myself would count it great good fortune to have you as a resident of our town, for we should then have a chance to see you occasionally and to learn something of your work." He named two local estate agents and assured Smith of "a hearty welcome and pleasant association."[60]

Throughout the first six months of 1915, Theobald Smith was too preoccupied and disabled for systematic house-hunting. He tackled the tedious job of sorting and packing his books and papers, and tearing up unwanted letters. Material to be preserved, along with furniture not needed at Woodland Hill, was sent to Silver Lake, where at least two members of his family stayed during that summer. Lilian made a short excursion at the end of June, and returned to Boston with a one-year renewable lease on 42 Cleveland Lane.[61] The house belonged to H.J. Ford, Professor of Politics and Government, who had obtained leave of absence from the University in order to write some books.

Besides going over his personal belongings at home, Smith had to deal with the more detailed plans and specifications now demanded by the architects. The animal isolation quarters were of unique design, while the laboratory accommodation and equipment for staff members, some of them already appointed, presented seemingly kaleidoscopic problems. If the new department was to begin work in the fall, some temporary space would have to be found. Smith turned to Conklin. "Owing to delays in getting plans into final shape, our laboratory building and accessory stables etc. will not be ready until early spring." The remodelling of one of the farmhouses on the estate, and the use of others for storage purposes, had been discussed. But perhaps "Princeton University might have some spare rooms to let. We would rather pay rent than try to fit up farmhouses . . . We could get along in a building adapted for *any* laboratory work, provided we had running water, gas and electricity . . . We would provide our own furniture, apparatus and Diener."[62]

Conklin replied that in his own department one small (10 x 24 feet) research room, "with excellent north light," would be vacant for next year. Several rooms in their Vivarium had water, gas and electricity, and could be made temporarily available. These rooms contained various types of animal cages, including aquaria, which could be moved if in the way. Conklin suggested that Smith should look over these possibilities in the near future. "If you think that you could get on with the private room in our main building and some or all of the Vivarium rooms we shall be delighted to have you take them and to feel that you are for the time being one of us."[63] Smith wasted no time in accepting. Henry James promptly offered to pay rental for the rooms. Conklin felt sure the university authorities would decline to take payment, but he would write to President J.G. Hibben about the situation. The Dean of Arts and Science, H.B. Fine, and through him the Chairman of the Committee on Grounds and buildings, both agreed "that we must of course extend every courtesy to Professor Theobald Smith and his associates."

Considerable correspondence ensued between Conklin and Smith during the next seven weeks, in which the former offered alternative accommodations—four rooms in the basement of Guyot Hall, headquarters of the Department of Biology. In his next visit to Princeton, Smith found these basement rooms in the main building more suitable for his purposes than those in the Vivarium. But it troubled him that this accommodation was sought for part-time usage only, for a work program as yet unsettled. "Should we be hampered in spite of all that you are ready to do for us, the rooms we ask for might not be utilized with that intensity which your coworkers would exercise, and therefore it would seem as if we were appropriating what we are not using intensively . . . We could probably get along very well" with three basement rooms (one of these shared with Conklin), and one animal room in the Vivarium. "An additional room would be an enormous help, especially for the depositing of certain books and for carrying on miscellaneous work." During their stay in Guyot Hall, he and his colleagues would refrain from working with any organisms dangerous to man.[64]

A later note, conveying appreciation of Conklin's very generous reaction, mentioned the two staff members who would use these borrowed quarters in the coming year. On September 1, Werner Marchand, a parasitologist, would begin a mosquito survey centered on the Rockefeller land. Smith's associate, TenBroeck, would look through the new quarters on or about September 15—or he could wait until Conklin was back from Woods Hole. As for Smith himself, "I shall probably not go to Princeton until later, possibly early October, as my family must be moved."[65] Lilian was laid up with her broken arm, so he set out for Princeton alone on October 12. The Nassau Inn provided lodging until the 14th, by which time enough furnishings were uncrated and distributed at 42 Cleveland Lane for his temporary sole occupancy.

22

GROWING PAINS—

WARTIME FRUSTRATIONS

During the next few days, Smith unpacked everything at 42 Cleveland Lane, from personal books to "kitchen and pantry goods." With a black lad's assistance, he also uncrated and distributed various items in the assigned space in Guyot Hall, about one mile away. At first he prepared his own breakfast and dined at the Nassau Inn, but when his proposed membership at the Nassau Club became effective later that month, he took meals there. On October 25, he brought Dorothea to Princeton. She was convalescing from one of a series of physical ailments which impeded and eventually halted her promising career as a microbiologist. With the black boy's help, they rearranged the furniture in the house. But several attempts to hire household maids proved futile.

Within a few weeks of his arrival, Theobald Smith had explored the Graduate School with TenBroeck and shepherded his skeleton staff into their respective rooms, attended two biology seminars, and established a semblance of his former routine—attending to correspondence, examining microscopic slides of diseased turkey and swine tissues, and "working on lectures." He lunched with Henry James at the Faculty Club, enjoyed a piano concert in the University's McCosh Hall, and took Dorothea to the Harvard-Princeton football game. On November 8, his wife at last came from Boston with their younger daughter. Dr. Fauver, a Princeton physician, visited daily to manipulate and dress Lilian's crippled arm. Its active mobility was not fully restored for nearly a year.

Theobald Smith welcomed the social, cultural and educational opportunities of the special relationship and the proximity to Princeton University. President and Mrs. J.G. Hibben, Dean (of Science) H.B. Fine, as well as many senior Faculty members, plied him and Lilian with dinner invitations. Others extending hospitality included William Paton, author of travel books; representatives of the department's neighbors, St. Joseph's Seminary and the Walker-Gordon Dairy Farms; and Mayor and Mrs. McClellen of Princeton. He heard Thomas Hunt Morgan lecture on *Evolution,* Jacques Loeb on *Instincts,* and Ira Remsen on *Liebig.* He listened to expositions on the *Philosophy of War* and on the *Causes of War.* There were luncheon talks at the Nassau Club, such as those by Prof. Crampton on *Samoa, Guiana, etc.,* by Col. Tillman on *The West in '69,* and by an unidentified pundit on *Simplified Spelling.* There was also music. The Philadelphia and the New York Philharmonic Orchestras provided Symphony concerts; the Kneisel and other string quartets performed regularly; and there were plenty of instrumental and vocal soloists.

Smith's reciprocal gesture was modest and somewhat tardy. He deferred addressing a Nassau Club luncheon group on *The Rockefeller Institute for Medical Research* until March 22, 1916. Two days later, he added praise of other medical research institutes and eulogized Koch, and presented the revised version as a dinner speech at the Phipps Institute in Philadelphia, to commemorate Koch's announced discovery, thirty-four years before, of the tubercle bacillus. Thereafter, his references to "working on lectures" became frequent and related to more ambitious undertakings. Shortly after Lilian joined him at 42 Cleveland Lane he noted, "Accept invitation to give Herter and Mellon lectures."[1]

These and other honors that came to Theobald Smith during those early Princeton years brought additional luster indirectly to the adjacent University. A local periodical, saluting the new Department's proximity, published illustrations of its Laboratory Building and of the novel-featured Isolation Building for animals. After quoting Conklin approvingly, an editorial proceeded:

> President Wilson once declared that his ideal for the future development of Princeton was that it should become a great university not by the addition of new schools of law, medicine and engineering, but rather by the development here of schools and institutes dealing with the fundamental sciences underlying the technical courses in those subjects. The establishment of an independent department of the Rockefeller Institute here is a long step towards the realization of that fine ideal.[2]

The issue contained a short review by Simon Flexner of the future Department of Animal Pathology, emphasizing that it was an integral and not independent unit of the Rockefeller Institute for Medical Research, and affirming that "It is the aim of the Institute in this department, as in those already organized in New York, to study fundamental biological and medical problems."[3] This article likewise foresaw mutual benefits—"a congenial and stimulating atmosphere"—resulting from proximity of "the Institute's new department" to the University. Apart from its research activities, the department would look after "the serum horses and other animals . . . hitherto kept at Clyde, near New Brunswick." The article ended by naming the departmental staff so far appointed. Besides Theobald Smith as Director, two men were cited, viz. Carl TenBroeck, A.B., M.D., Associate, and Werner Marchand, Ph.D., Assistant.

The relationship between the Smiths and TenBroeck was mutually advantageous. Robust and thirty-five years younger than his chief, TenBroeck could be useful in many ways—on field expeditions, as caretaker for their house at Woodland Hill, or as handyman around the Silver Lakes property. Although Theobald Smith never called him "Carl," his wife Lilian often did. One of her 1916 letters to her husband from Silver Lake indicated that she had not asked "Dr. T.B. . . . to write about you," because Theobald had been so "good about writing that I've not needed information from outside, but I am glad to have someone in Princeton who would write me if there were any reason."[4]

His chief's renown protected and furthered TenBroeck's own career and ultimately determined his succession to the directorship. Rockefeller philanthropy contributed to almost every stage of his close postgraduate association with Theobald Smith. Even before TenBroeck had completed his M.D. requirements, Smith's dependence on him was noticeable. For instance, in March 1913, Smith wrote to Simon Flexner: "He seems to have based his determination to stay mainly on two facts. He knew that I should be practically without any trained assistant next fall if he went. Secondly, he felt that he might broaden out a little so as to be better prepared for the unknown problems awaiting him if the opportunity came to him another year."[5]

Early in 1914, TenBroeck was awarded a $1,700 Rockefeller Traveling Fellowship to Europe; but by August it was foreseeable that he probably would be unable to use it, so Smith suggested an alternative: "What do you think of recommending him for an appointment at $1,500 next year to do research here or to assist in any other way to get our Department under sail?"[6] This appointment was arranged, and TenBroeck was delegated to visit western Experiment Stations for ideas bearing on the Rockefeller Institute's plans for its Department of Animal Pathology. Starting out on May 1, 1915, he headed southwest to Knoxville, before turning northwesterly to "Iowa and working towards Minn. & N. Dakota."[7] Hence his absence from Theobald Smith's Complimentary Dinner on June 2.

Werner Marchand was associated with the Department of Animal Pathology because of a letter sent by Theobald Smith to Simon Flexner in May 1915. Prof.

Wheeler had mentioned a temporary worker at the Bussey Institution "who might be a promising candidate for our parasitologist. He is the son of Prof. Felix Marchand of Leipzig. He had a very good training, including zoology, botany and entomology. Besides, he is a very good draughtsman."[8] Marchand assembled his credentials for Flexner's next visit to Boston and was hired despite his German citizenship, poor physique, and professional unadaptability. Although Flexner later described him as "gentle and well-disposed," Marchand did little to enhance the department's prestige.

His first assignment—a survey of mosquito species in the Princeton area—was intended mainly as a test of his entomological talent. When malaria was said not to exist locally, the survey was extended to biting flies in general; but in this field he lacked background and proficiency. During Smith's absence at Silver Lake in August 1916, Marchand made four trips to Philadelphia to examine the literature on biting flies and then submitted an expense account to his chief. Henry James covered this unauthorized expenditure but advised that a notice should be posted in the departmental library stating that book loans were to be requested only through the Institute's librarian. Theobald Smith wished his staff to take part in the biology Seminar for graduate students in Guyot Hall. Smith himself lectured on *turkey blackhead* in mid-November 1915; a month later (to "Conklin's class") on *diphtheria;* and in February 1916 on *infection and parasitism.*[9] In the New Year, TenBroeck dealt with *anaphylaxis,* followed by Marchand on *butterfly variations.* A second seminar by Marchand was concerned with his very confusing personal theory of *evolution.*

When the United States declared war on Germany in April 1917, Werner Marchand automatically became an enemy alien; but he had an American wife and went on working. Early in 1918, Theobald Smith regretfully informed Simon Flexner that he could not recommend Marchand's reappointment; for his sole scientific interest was in problems that "threw light on the evolutionary relation between plants and animals" and he was "quite innocent of any knowledge of pathology." Further, summertime asthma hampered his working capacity during a season of maximum potential usefulness.

> He is an indefatigable collector of data . . . If he could only get some position in a museum . . . he would be very productive in the normal direction of his tastes and temperament . . . The only suggestion . . . is to vote him another year's salary and send him to the Bussey Institute, where he thinks the atmosphere for his work is just right . . . He is probably ineligible for work in the Bureau of Entomology as he is not a citizen.[10]

Werner's departure from Princeton was quietly secured.

Rhoda Erdmann, also a German citizen, lame, pushful, and demanding, caused much more trouble. She was a mature researcher, who came to the United States chiefly to learn certain techniques at American expense and consistently published in German periodicals in the years immediately before and after World War I. Papers by herself alone, or in collaboration with L.L. Woodruff, appeared regularly in American journals during the period 1914–1919. Several articles were on *Paramecium,* others on sarcosporidiosis. She also described a new culture medium for Protozoa.

In April 1914, soon after Smith accepted the invitation to form the Rockefeller Institute's new Department of Animal Pathology, Dr. Erdmann inquired of Simon Flexner whether she could pursue tissue culture studies at the Institute instead of renewing her annual $1,000 Fellowship at Yale under Prof. Ross G. Harrison. Flexner referred her application to Theobald Smith, who favored renewal of her fellowship, because he himself might be away during the second half-year. "Harrison tells me she is somewhat anspruchsvoll [presumptuous] about apparatus, keeping 4 microscopes going all the time. Our dept. has no apochr. outfit except the one I am using." If he could "see her at work in her own atmosphere," he would have a better idea of her wants and needs. As this could not be managed, at Smith's suggestion she visited him in Boston on April 30. Following the interview, Smith wrote to Flexner: "I have no doubt we can take care of Dr. Erdmann."

Flexner offered to send microscopes and other apparatus (even an apochromatic outfit) for her use—"to supply trypanosome material" which she had requested—and to let her work in New York pending Smith's return from his trip abroad. "I do not wish to press her on you and I am a little inclined to think from what you say that she may be unpleasantly strenuous. On the other hand, if you would like to make some such arrangement as that and if she should fall in with it, I am sure that it could be brought about."[11] Two days later Flexner changed his mind and urged that action upon Dr. Erdmann's request be deferred for a year.[12] It was agreed that Miss Erdmann should apply for renewal of her Fellowship at Yale, and she was so advised by Henry James, Jr. on May 9, 1914.

In April 1915, Smith wrote to Flexner weighing the pros and cons of Rhoda Erdmann's appointment as parasitologist in his department. "For a year or two she might be in our way instead of a help. If she could be taken care of a while longer, I would surely have material enough for her provided she is still pliable enough to accept problems from another. She might be allowed to go her own way and some other one appointed later to take the problems arising out of our work."[13] Flexner replied that it was doubtful if Dr. Erdmann were willing or able "to adapt herself to problems not strictly her own. Would it not therefore be better to start out fresh with a parasitologist who would be primarily and immediately interested in your problems? Just where such a person is to be found, I do not know."[14]

Flexner's caution now seemed to challenge Smith's irresolution: "I have no doubt that she would eventually be led to do the work that grew out of the new department's problems voluntarily and perhaps with great interest. This would take time, however, and should not be a forcing process. In the meantime, it is simply a question of means. We must have a parasitologist in any case."[15] Rhoda Erdmann was interviewed by Flexner and Smith at the Rockefeller Institute on March 31, 1916, following which Henry James sent her an offer of a fellowship in the Rockefeller institute, dating from July 1, 1916.[16] This was tenable in the new department at Princeton when laboratory space became available there in the autumn of 1916.

The official expectation had been that the new department of the Rockefeller Institute would begin to operate from its Princeton quarters in the "fall" of 1916. As that season drew near, the projected date of the move was estimated at "between middle of September and the first of October."[17] Actually, Smith noted in his diary for October 31, "First full day in lab. of new plant;" yet when Rhoda Erdmann visited Princeton on November 11, her room was not yet ready. She inquired, through James, if she should stay for the present in New Haven. Theobald Smith wrote, "By all means advise Dr. Erdmann to stay in New Haven . . . we shall be ready for her by the 1st [December], since the electric lights are now only being placed and we shall want the refrigeration started before she gets here."[18]

Erdmann was still at Yale early in February 1917, when she produced an abundantly illustrated manuscript on the behavior of chicken bone marrow in plasma medium, which she allegedly had submitted to the *Journal of Experimental Medicine* with Flexner's encouragement. When Theobald Smith first looked over the manuscript, he angrily disputed Flexner's proposal to charge his annual appropriation for the many plates. "The whole thing is so new to me that I shall have to think it over a few days to adjust myself to it." If the Institute intended to foot any part of the bills, they should be shared with the New Haven laboratory. The work was "of her own doing and its crediting to this department does not interest me in the least." In future, he would attempt to avoid similar difficulties "by carefully prescribing the kind of work to be done. This may be impossible in her case and we are again brought to an impasse."[19] The issue was resolved when the *Journal of Anatomy* agreed to publish the article, with the plates, for $235; and Smith informed Flexner that if Erdmann could prevail upon Prof. Harrison to contribute one-half of that sum, he would settle the issue by paying the other half.[20] In due course, the article appeared.[21]

Rhoda Erdmann arrived at the Princeton department shortly before the official declaration of war by the United States against Germany on April 6, 1917. Her belligerently uncooperative behavior soon became so obnoxious that Smith firmly reminded Flexner not to renew her appointment at Princeton from July 1, 1917. The outcome was the decision by a subcommittee of the Board of Scientific Directors, relayed in a letter to Dr. Erdmann from Theobald Smith, that the Rockefeller Institute would grant her $2,000 for the ensuing year "to take up your work in the Osborn Zoological laboratory under Professor Harrison," with whom Smith had conferred four weeks beforehand. Harrison "would provide suitable space and apparatus," but current expenses of the work would have to be met from the grant. The Board would not supply apparatus or pay for supplies. The rooms she now occupied must be vacated by July 15. At least part of her time would have to be devoted to "protozoology in its bearing on animal pathology. The subject of sarcosporidiosis, which you are now working upon is acceptable," although coccidiosis in birds would be preferable to the Department.[22] Flexner approved the letter. "I am really very much relieved that she is not to continue with you. I had a delightful glimpse of your family and cottage at Silver Lake a few days ago."[23] From Silver Lake, Lilian also expressed relief: "On the whole, I am glad that Dr. Erdmann is leaving. There is no sense in your being loaded down by such an unadaptable person."[24]

A department of animal pathology must have ready access to adequate veterinary services. Henry James had undertaken to recruit a suitably qualified person, with immediate responsibility for the care and supervision of the Institute's farm at Clyde (including Alexis Carrel's dog colony). But he sensed he was getting out of his depth here and asked Theobald Smith, still in Boston, to define the prospective veterinarian's chief duties. Smith responded that "The veterinarian you are looking for should be trained in handling animals . . . he should be a handy man."[25] Besides being used to handling animals, he should know how to collect and bring them uninfected to the Station. "He should be able to do a certain amount of surgery, obstetrics, [and] to take care of horses' teeth and feet. If we need research veterinarians we will have to choose them later and with much care."

Additional comments revealed Smith's familiarity with more mundane aspects of animal care. For instance, "we can use meat for dogs, and send it to the Institute for bouillon. Here at Forest Hills, the employees are quite willing to take the veal from our vaccine calves home." Refrigeration of carcasses was important, for if not nearly covered with ice, "they are frequently so bloated in the morning as to interfere with autopsy. This occurs also in winter." Again, he wondered whether New Jersey laws permitted electrocution as a means of killing animals. "Shooting or killing with a blow causes small hemorrhages besides destroying the brain." James concluded that worthwhile candidates would be sent on for an interview: "You are a much better judge of qualifications, and I think it would be fairer to the candidate to let him talk to you. He would learn things about his work from you which I might not be able to tell him."[26]

According to James, the first promising applicant had a good family background, seemed soundly motivated, was physically robust, and pleasant in appearance and manner. He was Ralph B. Little, a recent graduate of the University of Pennsylvania Veterinary School. James had emphasized that "for a year or more he would have to devote most of his time to the present farm, which is by no means in the best of condition, and where he would have little or no association with scientific work." The salary quoted was $1,500 a year, with house rent worth another $300. Little was willing to accept the job, but matters were left open until both Smith and Flexner had interviewed and approved him.[27] By late October, Little had been appointed and settled in at the farm. Smith proposed (with hog cholera researches in mind) that he should "start on a small scale to raise pigs. Better now than later. He will learn to handle large numbers successfully . . . I expect to have him raise turkeys for me in the spring so that my experiments will not be delayed."[28] In Boston, Theobald Smith had sorted his collection of reprints. He wrote to Flexner, "I am having my pamphlets catalogued for shipment as soon as a place is ready. There are about 6000, mostly on animal diseases, which I have selected. I am also packing a large collection of agricultural pamphlets and books to go to Dr. Little until the station is moved."[29]

Early in the new year, Prof. F.C. Winkler of Rutgers University, who was also Animal Husbandman at the affiliated Stage College of Agriculture, wrote to Theobald Smith in response to Little's request for the estimated costs of raising a small herd of pigs. Winkler was pleased they were "taking up investigative work with hog cholera" and promised the Experiment Station's full cooperation. At the Station, fifteen acres were set aside for swine researches, mostly into nutritional problems.[30] Smith wrote appreciatively to Winkler. "Our problem is to have on hand . . . a stock of animals as free from infection and parasitism as possible, so that when we come to experiment we may not be misled in our interpretations. The question of special breed is not of much importance until we come . . . to determine their resistance to disease."[31] The gist of this principle was repeated to Little. "Very frequently the high-class, high-bred animals are more diseased than common stock . . . in the case of poultry Dr. Rous may have some special breed which he would prefer. He has been studying chicken tumors for a number of years, and probably uses a great many animals."[32] In a follow-up note to Little, Smith estimated that $700 would "probably take care of the entire experiment until October."[33] This amount was granted by the Board at its meeting in January 1915.

At the beginning of his long association with the Rockefeller Institute (1914–1950), Ralph Little was apt to be impetuous and careless, lacking in judgement, and attracted by clandestine money-making ventures. Early in 1915, Theobald Smith requested him to procure a few turkey eggs. As the farm also needed an incubator, Little ordered 160 turkey eggs, to fit into a large incubator which he had located. Smith complained to James: "What curious ratiocination led him to contract for 160 eggs! It shows the need of close personal oversight . . . Little should also have known that a 160-egg incubator is based on hen's egg size."[34] Smith wrote repeatedly to James about disposing of the Clyde property, and the future of the employees there, including Little, in whom he lacked confidence.

By the end of June 1916, the proposed abolition of the animal farm was an issue of such import that Simon Flexner accompanied Theobald Smith and James to the Farm one afternoon. Their decision to close it down led Smith to make a more thorough visit alone next day: "Motored to New Brunswick farm & back, spending all day at farm, making notes on pens, dissecting turkey, g.p.'s & mice."[35] Final transfers extended over several weeks, but most of them took three days at the beginning of July 1916.[36] The Day Card entry for July 3 read, "Working chiefly on N. Brunswick farm, moving all day." The two subsequent days were spent "working all day," and "ditto, moving," respectively.

That decisive move did not eliminate all the laboratory animal difficulties. In August 1916, Smith reported: "The problem of the mice is again coming up and I fear that we are now in the grip of another epidemic."[37] Little was not necessarily to blame for that. However, to be seen pocketing a fee for setting the broken leg of a neighbor's turkey was different. Though a strict disciplinarian, Theobald Smith found it distasteful in later life to rebuke a delinquent employee; so he asked James "to tell him nicely but quickly that miscellaneous practice must stop." Again, one of Flexner's horses died unexpectedly at Princeton and was autopsied by Smith, who suspected mercury poisoning and took specimens for analysis. Little used tablets of corrosive sublimate "in profusion . . . to wash his hands when using leaky syringes," although warned repeatedly to cease the habit.[38]

But Little stayed on. Flexner worried whether the Institute could meet increasing demands from war-torn Europe for meningococcus and pneumococcus antisera, which necessitated an expanded stabling capacity and a strong staff for procuring, handling, immunizing and bleeding horses. This was no time to dismiss a veterinarian who was genuinely fond of animals, got on well with his human associates, and was cheerful and candid. Two years later, Little "fell on his head and had a severe concussion."[39] From this accident he also recovered, to engage for many years in useful routine duties and cooperative researches, including some with Theobald Smith himself. In February 1965, when he was interviewed in retirement, Little and his wife owned an antique store in Princeton. He died suddenly of a heart attack about six months later.

In April 1915, Theobald Smith wrote to Simon Flexner and the Executive Committee outlining the research approaches into which their commitment to J.J. Hill could be divided. Each division would require direction from a specialist. Four qualified staff members would be needed for these hog cholera researches alone—a bacteriologist and immunologist, a second bacteriologist, a parasitologist, and a veterinary clinician. He advised Flexner that "The kind of men to look for . . . will . . . be conditioned largely by the hog chol. work we have agreed to take up."[40]

Just before Christmas 1915, Theobald went to New York to discuss the new department's finances, first with fellow Scientific Directors of the Institute, then at 26 Broadway with Trustees Gates, Greene and Murphy. Smith supplemented his verbal outline of the situation by a written statement, requested by Starr J. Murphy, "to aid him in submitting the Institute's needs in connection with the Princeton development to the Trustees of the Foundation."[41] In this memorandum, hog cholera researches came first, "placed in the foreground by Mr. Hill's gift." Although plans had been pared down twice already, the total costs of current proposals would far exceed the estimated $50,000 of two years before. Soon after that estimate was made, the U.S. Department of Agriculture appropriated $500,000 for this purpose. Besides, many states now sponsored similar activities through their own Agricultural Experiment Stations. So the scope of the Rockefeller Institute projects perforce expanded.

Smith's memoranda projected that the Department of Animal Pathology's present plans envisaged a three- or four-pronged approach. Each experiment "must be housed in an isolation ward of one of the animal hospitals, so that the virus cannot be carried to any other ward." For a year or more the Department's entire energy might be directed toward this disease. Eventually hog cholera researches could still involve as much as three-quarters of the budgetary outlay. "Only by a cooperative, concerted effort . . . may we hope to discover any features, rectify present information and improve methods of dealing with this malady in practice." However, he noted, to devote all the Department's energies to a single disease would be shortsighted. After a few years there might have been little progress beyond the limits of current knowledge of hog cholera. Hence the desirability of taking up at the start several other diseases. This arrangement would also enable the staff to keep fully occupied if the hog cholera researches should lag. Separate space was therefore reserved for differently affected animals. Smith's plans for stables and laboratory equipment also allowed for unpredictable emergencies, such as those previously encountered by the Institute— dysentery, or epidemic pneumonia.

Since the Department's anticipated researches related almost wholly to infective diseases, from which valuable food-producing animals mostly suffered, their investigation demanded costly isolation units, screened against flies, mosquitoes, and vermin. The budget allowed only for small-scale studies of those nutritional disturbances which were especially relevant to both agricultural economics and problems of human disease. The memorandum made clear Theobald Smith's prime resolve to meet the hog-cholera stipulation of James Hill.

Soon after the pre-Christmas meeting of the Board of Trustees, Henry James reported that "the trustees of the Foundation" had voted an additional one million dollars towards the endowment of the Department at Princeton. This made the Department of Animal Pathology independent of the Hill money, as James was quick to point out.

> The action is so generous that after these last months of squeezing and compressing I feel a bit like a barrel from which the hoops have suddenly been knocked off. I hope that if you have the same feeling it will not affect you unpleasantly. It is really a very ample provision and I have no doubt that . . . as soon as the work begins we shall find it necessary to plan and to do things not yet foreseen.[42]

The new donation from the founder at first only seemed to accentuate Smith's intentions to re-enter the fray against hog cholera. In February 1916, he recorded, "All day at lab working over old swine disease notes;" and six weeks later, "lab all day working on hog col."[43] In March, he informed Flexner that he expected an application for a fellowship from a young veterinarian from the Iowa Experiment Station at Ames who was "doing very good work on hog cholera."[44] This was Ernest W. Smillie, granted a fellowship in July. Smillie began working with Smith on turkey blackhead.

By then, however, all intimations of a major attack upon hog cholera had ceased. James Jerome Hill died suddenly on May 20, 1916, and his pledge of $50,000 for hog cholera research was repudiated by Louis Hill, his son. The news officially reached Theobald Smith several weeks later, when James sent him a copy of a letter from the younger Hill. James undertook to inform the Trustees through Starr Murphy. He supposed they would spurn laying any claim against the Hill estate. The Trustees would "want to know whether, in case you do not make a study of hog cholera, any other provision for the support of the department during the next year or two will be necessary."[45]

Although this turn of events must have shocked Theobald Smith, the default was unmentioned in diary, day cards, or any personal document. He had mulled over so many unsettled problems. Was the virus a single entity? To what extent did secondary bacterial agents affect symptomatology, or alter morbidity and mortality rates? Were inciting agents important in establishing this host-parasite relationship? How could serum therapy or prophylaxis be improved? What protection could be expected from active immunization through a vaccine? Not only Smith, but the whole Board of Scientific Directors of the Rockefeller Institute apparently ceased to ponder such questions about hog cholera. References to hog cholera researches merely disappeared from the Department of Animal Pathology's program. Individual researches in that field were by no means banned, but any integrated assault on hog cholera was tacitly ruled out. This changed attitude had little to do with the loss of anticipated funds. Hill's grant was a timely stimulant, but obviously would have proved inadequate for any sustained attack on the broad front delineated by Theobald Smith.

The short summary of these events in Corner's *History* seems unfair to Smith. "Apparently Theobald Smith, always careful in money matters, preferred not to call for payment of the pledge until he was ready to begin his investigation, and when Hill died after a brief illness in May 1916 the gift lapsed." In other words, Corner alleged that Smith over-cautiously interpreted the Department's preparedness for hog cholera investigations, and was directly responsible for the failure to request an earlier redemption of Hill's pledge. Neither implication seems warranted.

There is abundant evidence that Smith's program for hog cholera research was the Department's earliest and chief commitment, and that his plans were fully supported by the Scientific Directors and the Trustees; that Smith prepared himself for directing the research campaign; that he arranged for the training of a veterinarian in pig-raising, and for a sufficient stock of pigs to be bred for the first six months of experimentation; and that Hill died at least five months before the laboratory building and the animal isolation quarters were ready for occupancy. Furthermore, James Hill's latest undertaking, addressed to H.M. Biggs, clearly expected the Institute to commence the work shortly after payments began. "I am ready to give, as may be required, the sum of $50,000.00 to be devoted to establishing a remedy for hog cholera and whenever the Rockefeller Institute is ready to take up this work, I will arrange to make the payments as may be called for through Mr. . . . who will always be readily reached."[46] Had it appeared prudent or desirable to request that Hill's payments be collected in advance, then Biggs, Welch, or Simon Flexner, as fellow-members of the Board of Scientific Directors, or the Secretary of the Board of Trustees, all of whom received Smith's frequent progress reports, could have taken the initiative more fittingly than Smith himself.

Theobald Smith's lectures, always scrupulously prepared, would have been livelier if he had been less painstaking, and permitted himself an occasional spontaneity. But reading from a text gratified a sense of detachment from the audience. Besides, preparation of a single lecture sometimes required weeks of intermittent attention, both at the lab and in evening hours and Sundays at home—time too precious to be whimsically thrown away. Even for the biology graduate seminar on turkey blackhead in Guyot Hall in mid-November, which surely called for an informal discussion or talk, he wrote out a "paper."

He first specifically mentioned his future Herter lectures at the end of November 1915, when he recorded on a Day Card, "Work on Herter lectures."[47] Thereafter, despite many other obligations competing for his attention, the hours devoted to "working on lectures" seemed to multiply. He often had several topics in mind, usually for delivery, though not always for publication. The climactic week for the Herter and other lectures was to be May 10–17, 1916; but even in less hectic periods his lecturing and social engagements were demanding, the more so because most of them entailed a train journey to and from New York. For instance, at the end of April 1916, Theobald had commitments in that city for three successive days. On the 27th, he was invited by the Trustees of the Carnegie Institute to attend an afternoon celebration of the Twentieth Founder's Day.[48] On the 28th, before a staff meeting at the Rockefeller Institute, he presented a paper (unpublished) on "The Topography of Pneumonic Lesions in Certain Mammals."[49] Next day Smith attended the Supper at Sherry's,[50] "tendered by the Harvey Society in honor of William Welch, who had addressed the Society a few days before on the topic of "Medical Education in the United States."[51]

Although Smith and Welch greatly admired each other, in character they were opposite. Many people envied Welch's facility at discoursing authoritatively on almost any topic, and shared his obvious enjoyment of the adulation evoked by his erudition and eloquence. The Flexners have revealed[52] that Welch was not above stuffing himself with encyclopedic data in advance of some occasion, to be regurgitated when he had steered the conversation adroitly in the right direction. Although Theobald Smith never resorted to such devices, he gladly joined the 130 guests at the Supper honoring Welch.

On May 10, Smith participated in Washington in a symposium on "Immunization and Its Practical Applications," arranged as part of the Tenth Meeting of the Congress of American Physicians and Surgeons. His contribution was entitled "The underlying Problems of Immunization."[53] Fellow speakers were Ludwig Hektoen of Chicago, on "Vaccine Therapy," and William H. Park of New York on "Serum Therapy." The symposium was to be followed by a discussion, in which Frank Billings of Chicago, Rufus Cole and Thomas W. Hastings of New York, and Theodore C. Janeway of Baltimore were leading participants.[54] On Thursday, May 11, Smith left for Baltimore, where he delivered the three Herter Lectures during the next four-day period (11th, 12th and 15th). Two dinners were given in his honor—the first by his host, John J. Abel at his home on the 12th, and the other by Welch at the Maryland Club on Sunday the 14th. On the Saturday he made a side-trip to Philadelphia to attend a Council Meeting of the Phipps Institute.

The purpose of the Herter Memorial lectureship was "to promote a more intimate knowledge of the researches of foreign investigators in the realm of medical science." Four of the earlier lectures, beginning with Paul Ehrlich, had been distinguished pathologists or physiologists from German universities, and the others were from the United Kingdom; but there was no bar to opening the lectureship to "leaders in medical research in this country." A committee comprised of Drs. Welch, Abel, and Janeway had decided that wartime and other conditions made it expedient for an American to deliver the Ninth Course of Herter Lectures; and further, that Theobald Smith should be accorded that responsibility. Smith's chosen theme was "The Relation of Infections and Immunizing Processes to the General Phenomenon of Parasitism." These three lectures were not published and manuscripts pertaining to them have disappeared. Their general content can only be surmised from their respective titles. I. Aberrant Parasitism in its Bearing upon Disease. II. Adaptation of Parasites to the Natural Defenses of the Host. III. Immunity and Parasitism. The lectures were "illustrated by lantern slides and specimens."[55] For several months, until mid-February 1917 at least, Theobald Smith intermittently tried to put his Herter lectures into publishable form; but when the United States entered the war on April 6, he became too distracted with other problems. Nevertheless, the principles laid down in his Herter Lectures gathered substance and strength for nearly seventeen years, until brought to life again in the Vanuxem Lectures. These in turn were transformed in a terminal effort into one of the classics of science, *Parasitism and Disease*.[56]

Although Smith often seemed older than his years, during that week in May 1916 he proved remarkably tough. He spent the night of the 15th at home, took an evening train on the 16th to Pittsburgh, and next day, at the Mellon Institute for Industrial Research,[57] delivered a lecture on natural and acquired resistance to tuberculosis, staying overnight at the home of R.B. Mellon. He left by train for Princeton on the morning of the 18th. Although this concentration of lectures had drained his energy, they fortified his finances. The house rent ($100) was substantially higher than he had been paying Harvard for Woodland Hill. The Mellon Lecture fee was $200, and the Herter Lectures yielded $1,000.[58]

On May 20, Simon Gage had his sixty-fifth birthday. That night, at Cornell University, a Dinner in his honor was to be held, which also would memorialize the presentation of the "Fund for the Simon Henry Gage Fellowship in Animal Biology." Theobald Smith was to be among the seven scheduled speakers but decided that an immediate trip to Ithaca would be overtaxing. He explained his predicament to Gage, who promptly responded that it would seem "wicked to

urge you to come in the face of all which you must do. I care more for your expressions of confidence and affection than for all the formal occasions." He
would like Smith to "write a little letter to be read Sat. Eve." and invited him to
Ithaca when the pressure was less. "I know how to run the Ford now, and we will
see some of the wonderful places around Ithaca, and feel the soothing touch of
mother Nature, and let the restfulness and strength which she gives us fully enter our souls."[59]

Smith put together a short statement, titled "Professor Gage: the Friend," that
was read out at the Dinner by the Toastmaster. Beforehand, B.F. Kingsbury, J.H.
Comstock, and A.T. Kerry extolled Gage's qualities as Scientist, Student, and
Colleague, respectively; and G.S. Hopkins' tribute to Gage as Teacher came afterward. In two sentences Smith summarized his debt to his old friend: "Professor Gage as a personality had a great influence in my life. It was he who was
largely responsible for turning me towards biology." And in a clumsily-worded
but penetrating passage, Smith condemned the disdainful teacher who fails to
convey warmth and enthusiasm to the ordinary student—an astonishing feat of
self-criticism. "With insistence on productivity in research as the sole indicator
of the teacher's value, there is apt to be lost the unselfish out-going of the
teacher's best to his students," he observed. "Unless the scholarly productivity
we are looking for is associated with and intimately linked with the teacher's
work as such, the teacher himself looks upon teaching as a secondary performance, and his efforts become directed to finding out with how little contact
with students he can get on."[60] In responding to the evening's spate of tributes,
Gage revealed that he had once wanted to be a physician. "I . . . came to this university to get the best possible foundation in science .. but at that time (1873) biological knowledge was just coming into full appreciation, and the teachers
were few; so I became a teacher."[61]

Gage had been a lonely widower for nearly eight months. His wife, Susanna
Phelps Gage, had died suddenly on October 5, 1915 of a cerebral hemorrhage,
following a lovely automobile drive alongside Cayuga Lake into the sunset, and a
demonstration by her son, Henry Phelps Gage, of his newly invented daylight
glass, with its valuable qualities for microscopy. To Mrs. Gage, a scientist in her
own right, was dedicated the December 1916 number of the *Journal of Comparative Neurology*. Theobald Smith, who knew the family so well, was thanked by
Gage for the comforting "pressure of a friendly hand," in a gallant account of
their last weekend together.[62]

Neither the Scientific Directors, nor the Board of Trustees of the Rockefeller
Institute for Medical Research, to whom Theobald Smith faithfully reported
progress at Princeton, seemed to realize how deeply he longed to return to laboratory research. In particular, he had suspended his promising studies of the

turkey blackhead disease, now a widespread epizootic, devastating a formerly flourishing industry. He was also eager to look into various disease problems troubling the neighboring Walker-Gordon dairy farm. If any of Smith's fellow directors (Welch and Prudden, for instance) were disquieted on his account, this was allayed by the resolute efficiency and attention to detail with which, despite obvious constitutional frailties, he tackled all sorts of physical problems. The ingenuity that once governed the fashioning of simple apparatus to meet special needs was transformed into coping with the missing or the unwanted building supply. The laborers around the place might refer to him as "Old Whiskers" or "Nosy Parker," but to those who dispensed Rockefeller funds, "Dr. Smith" stood for probity, versatility, and thrift.

Despite the irksome administrative duties and improvised work space, Theobald Smith made up his mind to resume researches into turkey blackhead. The project began about six weeks after he took up residence in Princeton. Turkey eggs were obtained from farms near New Brunswick: "lab all day—family drive to New Brunswick in Farm car for turkey eggs. Philip chauffeur"[63]—a Ford had been purchased for the Department's use. And he noted six weeks later that "carpenters build small turkey shelter outside Guyot Hall."[64] The eggs were brought carefully to the laboratory, washed with disinfectant and incubated. Twice daily they were turned. After culling, forty-one eggs yielded twenty-three vigorous offspring, which were transferred to a brooder in the sheltered back porch of Smith's rented home, under his personal care. Fourteen days after the hatching, the brooder and its poults were conveyed to a wire-screened, rainproof shelter that had been erected on the lawn adjacent to Guyot Hall. When one month old, the poults were released into a screened enclosure about 1/8 acre in extent. By night, and when it rained heavily, they were locked in the shelter. Theobald pampered the poults, which remained gratifyingly free of disease and deformity for at least six weeks after hatching.

By July 19, when Theobald turned up at Silver Lake, he had confirmed or discovered certain points about turkey blackhead: 1. The disease was not transmitted through the egg. 2. Well-fed and carefully-tended poults could be reared in complete health for at least twelve weeks after hatching, despite environmental changes. 3. The suggestion that other poultry might convey the parasite was ruled out for one brand of domestic fowl. Turkey poults exposed for one month to yearling White Leghorn hens remained healthy. 4. Blackhead developed in a group of poults exposed to an infected turkey on non-infected ground. 5. The blackhead agent was seldom transmitted by infected turkeys that were either young, or in the early acute stage of the disease: it was probably carried and shed by the older survivors. Smith recognized that lack of cultural methods, and uncertainties of exposure to the parasite under field conditions, weakened the conclusions drawn from these experiments. However, his resources would be strengthened by the assistance of E.W. Smillie, who would take charge of the turkeys and would help to follow up his director's observation on the makeshift poultry run: "Sparrows and songbirds visited the grounds daily."[65]

With Smillie's assistance, Theobald Smith now set about retesting Hadley's 1910 assertion that the causal parasite of turkey blackhead, first described and designated *Amoeba meleagridis* by himself in 1894, was merely a stage in the life cycle of the avian coccidium, *Eimeria avium,* disseminated by various bird species. Smith opposed this hypothesis, but since sparrows frequently appeared in the unprotected yard of his turkey poults, he and Smillie investigated whether such birds played any part in the situation. They trapped or shot fifty-four apparently healthy sparrows in the turkey yard during the latter half of 1916. All the birds were adult, mostly from the University campus, but some from the new Department buildings on the other side of Princeton. Practically all sparrows caught in the summer and fall showed sexual stages of coccidia present in scrapings of duodenal mucosa. However, rectal contents or fecal cultures revealed the parasite in the form of a two-spored oocyst, unlike the four-spored *Eimeria avium* described by Hadley.

These findings, which disclosed a need for further study of avian coccidiosis, account both for Smith's unfulfilled wish to impose that field of research upon Rhoda Erdmann, and his resolve to obtain a trained parasitologist for his departmental staff. H.W. Graybill, a veterinarian with several years' experience at the B.A.I. and at George Washington University, was recruited late in 1916. Not until 1920 did Smith and Graybill together elucidate the complex epizootology and pathogenesis of turkey blackhead. Meanwhile, during December 1916, Smith wrote up the studies made by himself and Smillie. The resulting two papers were submitted early in January 1917 for publication, and they both appeared two months later.[66]

By mid-November 1916, after much "Mechanics pounding & scraping everywhere, gas fitters, steam fitters, plasterers, telephone people, painters, linoleum layers, etc.,"[67] the laboratory building for the Department of Animal Pathology was at last nearing completion. A few of the rooms were already occupied so that the loaned space in the basement of Guyot Hall might be vacated before the University year opened for the Fall Term. Although general occupancy of the building was not yet possible, on November 8 Theobald Smith and his wife led a party of eight or nine staff members, including recently-appointed *Dieners* and stenographers, aboard a motor bus, to the new workplace and grounds—a trip of venturesome exploration for many of them. Whenever an assigned room became habitable, office equipment or laboratory apparatus was transferred from storage to the new quarters. Smith carefully packed his books and currently-used paraphernalia, retaining one room in Guyot Hall for their storage until it too became redundant. He capped the arrangement with Princeton University by writing a note of cordial thanks to Conklin and his Biological Department colleagues for their kindly accommodation of himself, TenBroeck, and Marchand.

The new buildings were about three miles east of the Princeton post office. Theobald Smith generally commuted by bus, but occasionally used his bicycle, or even hired a taxi. He rejected the privilege of being driven in the departmental Ford car, and once reputedly rebuked TenBroeck for rustling up a horse-drawn sleigh to take him home during a snowstorm.[68] An alternative route was by train. This entailed tramping along the Trenton and New Brunswick Turnpike to or from Penn's Neck, a small stop on the Pennsylvania Railroad branch line from Princeton Junction to Princeton. On special occasions, such as Christmas Eve, when Phil had returned from Harvard and his sisters were at home, he would take them in the family Ford to pick up their father from the lab. Theobald recorded such happenings as if he enjoyed them.

The distance from town quickened the argument for a Director's House on the Institute's Princeton estate. The continuing increase in wartime demands for horse antisera, which already necessitated enlargement of the stables near the new Laboratory, called for yet more construction. To the triple objective presented at the end of 1916—the completion of the Laboratory building, the increased accommodation for horses, and the situation and construction of the Director's House—Smith devoted his main efforts for the next several months, without overlooking the need to fill gaps in his staff with trained and compatible personnel. In these tasks he anticipated the continuing strength and resourcefulness of Henry James, and he hoped for an *alter ego* kind of help from a newly chosen secretary.

On October 13, 1916, Theobald Smith went to New York to interview prospective employees at the Rockefeller Institute. As his personal secretary, he hired Nathaniel Shaw, a plausible, would-be Man Friday, who in less than two years of service developed a genuine regard for Smith's character and accomplishments. More than twenty years later—five years after Theobald's death—Philip Smith asked Shaw (already afflicted with ultimately fatal Parkinsonism) to type out some reminiscences that might throw light on "what made father tick." In those days, according to Shaw's memoir, there was much "swank and glitter about the Institute." Smith was pointed out to him arriving on foot, mounting the outer steps:

A slight, slender, quick-moving gent in a black overcoat, wearing a black slouch hat, whiskered, inclined toward the stately, and carrying a green felt bag. Long before he arrived, I could see that he was greatly respected by the underlings about the Institute. They watched his approach with an absorbed interest. They liked it that he didn't roll up in a handsome automobile—nor even in a taxi.[69]

A few days later, Shaw went down to Princeton. He and Smith were driven out to the buildings over a very bumpy road, one holding a balance, the other a microscope. The main laboratories were in a terrible muddle. After depositing their instruments, the pair walked around, identifying pipes and testing taps. As Shaw remembered,

> He tried a spigot marked Compressed Air and got a steam of water against his chest. This seemed to me very funny; but I tittered alone. He marched on and I followed, listing with a pad and pencil the matters to be attended to . . . With about fifty such notes in my pockets, we called it a day. There was some difficulty about getting the automobile in which we were driven out from Princeton. The workmen departed and left us there with a watchman.[70]

Similar annoyances pestered Smith for weeks. One day he told Shaw a story about a visitor to Wassermann, who had become head of the Kaiser Wilhelm Institute in Berlin. After conducting his guest over the building, Wassermann had said, "Now you see why I can no longer do the research work that I used to enjoy when I lived in a slum area with six guinea-pigs. Running this complexity leaves me no time and saps my energy." Smith also resented that others could divert one's hard-won experience into responsibility for aggrandizing some establishment. The greater the experience, the larger and more diversified grew the responsibility—for the conscientious. "Of course," he added, "everyone talks about 'chances of advancement.' But what they mean by 'advancement' is less work for a higher salary. I will never encourage such aspirations." Neither would he foster extravagance nor tolerate any kind of waste. Smith's innate simplicity resisted elaborate and costly apparatus, so that as an administrator he often disapproved of his junior colleagues' requisitions. "This wasn't understood, and didn't sit well. It appeared niggardly. But he wasn't thinking of how it would appear. He pointed out to me . . . that often when a man couldn't see his next step, he sat down and wrote out a few requisitions . . . some of them fantastic . . . Dr. Smith would hold back his initials."[71]

Shaw clearly treasured these recollections of his chief. Their touches of novelty and unexpectedness, despite their verisimiliitude, were like unposed snapshots. The director was seldom informal with "underlings," and when he did unbend, the occasion became legendary. For example, he once went to a movie that greatly impressed him. Next day he recounted its highlights to a dumfounded clerk in the chemical storeroom, and then to the lady librarian. In essence, *The Last Laugh* depicted the fate of a handsomely uniformed doorman of a Berlin hotel who eventually lost his job through superannuation. Finding life unbearable without his uniform, he stole it from the hotel. Shaw felt the doorman's obsession with masculine plumage was so unlike Smith himself that the movie's appeal lay in the affinity of opposites.

In Guyot Hall, Theobald kept up his Harvard custom of lunching alone in his laboratory; a Thermos bottle of cocoa or tea sufficed, with a few crackers or a slice of bread or cake, sometimes supplemented by an orange or banana. An unavoidably robust lunch was liable to downgrade his supper, as shown by these jottings during a 1916 visit to Boston: "About town having bank books verified—to Med. School for specimens—lunch with Dr. Broughton—writing on lectures—sup on peanuts & chocolate . . . Have been taking little more than 2 meals per day—feel good."[72]

However, when the laboratory building opened and the departmental staff enlarged, they tried out one of Simon Flexner's favorite notions—that a better team spirit prevailed if social barriers were lowered during lunch. Smith duly played his part, though at irregular intervals and rather against the grain. He would munch through a couple of sandwiches, listening to the arguments while seated around a bare table in an otherwise unused room. He once ended a discussion of the world's woes by interjecting, "The country isn't being run by philosophers"—adding with a grin, "fortunately." A trend toward excessive familiarity would be brought up short by his muttered modification of some old saw. "The proof of a pudding is in the eating thereof" was especially baffling to miscreants.

His collection of fancy-colored academic hoods of honorary doctorates, awarded by American and European universities, was displayed once for Shaw's opinion about whether neckties or something useful could be made of such good material. Particularly memorable was the Yale D.Sc. episode. Early in June 1916, Smith accepted the Yale Corporation's offer of an honorary degree on their Commencement Day, June 21. On that day, having forgotten the invitation, he read a Princeton newspaper account of the award purportedly made to him. He sent a contrite note to the Yale authorities, "Trusting that you will pardon the first blunder of this kind which I am guilty of."[73] Smith received his degree a year later, by when the country was at war. May 1916 had been overcrowded with lectures, and was followed understandably by a month of confusion over other kinds of calendar commitments, since on June 5, 1916, Theobald Smith's daughter Lilian was married to Robert Foerster. And on June 8, Washington University at St. Louis conferred on Smith an honorary L.L.D. degree.

The postponement of his Yale award brought an unexpected compensation.

When finally receiving his Yale degree, Smith walked in the procession with I. J. Paderewski, the famous pianist and future Prime Minister of Poland (Illustration 9). They chatted and exchanged jokes (in German) and during the ceremony sat together. According to Shaw's somewhat garbled account, in the garden his chief later confided: "At college I used to play the organ. Above all things, I wanted to be a musician. But I was a failure at it. Then I tried to be a physician . . . a teacher . . . a laboratory worker. And now at last they have made me into an administrator—for which I have no capacity to speak of. Yet . . . just because I got my dates mixed up last year, I have walked beside Paderewski and have spoken with him. He was very pleasant with me."[74] The Day Card for June 20, 1917 simply noted: "Receive degree of Sc.D. sit next to Paderewski."

Four days previously, Smith had been awarded an honorary Sc.D. degree from Princeton University. The ambassadors of several Allied Nations also received honorary doctorates. In response to a request from Dean of the Graduate School A.F. West, who was to present him for the degree, Smith had summarized his life work, beginning in 1883, as "A study of the causes of infective diseases and a search of means for their control." West presented him as "an unwearied student of the causes of infectious disease . . . It is to him that the world owes two discoveries . . . of capital importance for human health—the demonstration that tuberculosis in man and the domestic animals is not the same, and the proof that insects may be the necessary and only carriers of certain diseases—thus becoming the forerunner of discoverers of the control of typhus, malaria, yellow fever and other insect-borne plagues. For this many owe him their health, and even their lives, and all men their gratitude."

Lilian left early that morning for Silver Lake.[75] Nathaniel Shaw moved into the Cleveland Lane house and kept Smith company for the next two weeks. When Shaw's vacation began, J. Howard Brown came from Boston with his wife and child and stayed with Smith in the house for a few weeks while one of the estate cottages was refinished for them. The appointment of Brown (who had collaborated with Smith at Harvard on streptococcal classification) greatly strengthened the Princeton staff. Soon after the Brown family left "for their new home" on August 14, Shaw returned to help Smith pack books and other goods. Lilian's efforts to get their rental lease extended had failed, so the Smiths had arranged to board at the Peacock Inn from the beginning of October until the Director's House was ready. At this juncture, Philip arrived on a short visit from Boston, needing treatment for poison ivy blisters on hands, wrists and ankles. He became friendly with Shaw. In September, when the rest of the family was at Silver Lake, they stayed on in the house, enjoying the expensive but somewhat dried-out cigars salvaged by Theobald Smith from meetings in New York. Their friendship lasted for many years. Shaw appears now and again as the "Deacon" in Philip Smith's book, *Perennial Harvest* (1948).

Shaw's "memoir" of Theobald Smith drifted into a disjointed miscellany of recollections, few of which seem sufficiently novel or revealing to cite. He noted that a touch of Smith's fingers could calm frightened rabbits or guinea-pigs. Smith's persistent concern for detail might be exasperating until one realized (as Henry James once pointed out to Shaw) that the experimental results could be ruined by the slightest procedural deviation. One of Theobald Smith's favorite descriptive phrases for his researches was "fumbling along the periphery of the unknown." He might work on a problem for twenty years, only to conclude "The facts seem to indicate." His habits, Shaw felt, stemmed from acts of Will. The same resolute, unexploitable Will that governed his capacity to start prompt sleep at bedtime despite the day's worries, and to lie down for ten minutes' rest during the day, likewise controlled his scrupulous dedication to proper experimental performance. "He would never give a haphazard opinion, like the rest of us. The differentiation between appearances and fact had been built up into such a structure that the human being who had built it and lived therein was scarcely ever visible, never intending to be personally impressive."

> There was . . . some resentment of the careless extravagance and efflorescence of rough-shod American ways. He was strong enough to convey that attitude to those about him. It shut him off from life the way it was lived . . . from the easy availabilities. He was respected and admired, but because of the austerity and devotion to work, remained always aloof.[76]

Joseph Needham has cited a motto: "*Laboratorium est oratorium*—the place where we work is a shrine of prayer." Shaw's independent insight defined Theobald Smith's concentration on the job before him as "something like the effect of a religion—a constant awareness of an unattainable felicity—beneath the glow of which one is able to dismiss all nonsense."[77] Near the end of his memoir, Shaw referred twice to his "private quandary," probably meaning his homosexuality. Some months after the events recorded here, he was found allegedly compromised with a stable-boy by TenBroeck, who summarily dismissed them both, supposedly without the prior knowledge of Theobald Smith, who had promoted Shaw recently to the rank of Superintendent. Shaw's abrupt departure is confirmed by Smith's Day Card for July 3, 1918: "Mr. Shaw stays with us overnight to leave tomorrow"—presumably early next morning, for the TenBroecks lunched with the Smiths. It was a "very quiet 4th." Smith's Diary for July 3 merely reported: "Nath. Shaw supt. leaves Institute." In a letter to Henry James, devoted to Princeton developments, Prudden simply stated "Shaw has had to leave, leaving the director a bit handicapped."[78] Shaw joined the Army and served overseas. On May 20, 1919, returning from France, he called on the Smiths at Princeton—"merely a matter of paying my respects before I doffed my uniform."[79]

Although there was nothing surreptitious about Henry James, Jr.'s departure from the Princeton scene, it seems also to have been unexpected. From the outset, James was closely involved in the new Department's building and staffing plans, and did his utmost to secure its successful operation. "Spend much time at new buildings with Mr. James, & discussing force,"[80] was a typical jotting by Smith a few weeks before the "force" moved in. During the last months of the Rockefeller Institute's building program near Princeton, James averaged two half-day visits each week to the construction sites or for discussions with Theobald Smith. The latter would sorely miss these meetings. James' talents ranged from his impeccable sense of propriety in the formalities, to an emollient capacity in the rough-and-tumble of fulfilling building contracts in wartime. The value of his services to the start of the new Department can hardly be exaggerated.

In January 1916, Smith acceded to James' request for a formal summary of a personal collection of nearly 200 journals and annual reports, 200 volumes of studies from various laboratories, about 4,500 reprints, and some 400 pamphlets on agricultural subjects, transferred to the library of the Department of Animal Pathology. Shortly afterward, the Board of Scientific Directors recorded its "grateful sense of the importance of this gift to the library of the new department and of Dr. Smith's generosity in making this gift." The Librarian was instructed to mark each item appropriately. Correspondence between the two men often listed the oversights, mistakes, or plain stupidities discovered by one of them on his own latest tour.

By the end of 1916, these litanies related chiefly to the hurriedly designed quarters for "serum horses." In one such letter, Smith noted that the refrigerator in the power house had been supplied with shelves instead of ceiling hooks. "Inasmuch as this room will be used chiefly for hanging up large chunks of meat from horses, hooks in the ceiling should have been arranged rather than shelves. Just what can be done about this now I do not know." The writer proceeded: "Is it for us to clean the sinks in the animal buildings which have not yet been cleaned of the debris resulting from the building operations, or should this be done by the contractor? These sinks will soon be in use."[81]

As 1917 ended, James' name appeared less frequently; but he remained on the job until his apparently abrupt departure. Theobald's Day Cards at this time read: "Jan 5, 1918. James lunches with us at home. Jan. 11. Confer with Mr. James. Jan. 30. Conferences with Mr. James. Feb. 13. Mr. James to leave the Institute. Feb. 14. Exec. Com. meets at Dr. Prudden's at 4.30. Mr. James' last meeting." Henry James, Jr., had joined the United States Army (the Military Police) and without seeking a commission, according to Peyton Rous.[82] After the war, James was appointed chief executive officer of Teacher's Insurance and Annuity Association. From 1929 until his death in 1947, he was an active member of the Rockefeller Institute's Board of Trustees.

The situation and type of residence for the Director of the Department of Animal Pathology presented some critical problems. There were obvious pros and cons to living in the town of Princeton, though the car he had decided to buy would minimize the disadvantage of distance. Theobald Smith himself raised the issue at a meeting of the Scientific Directors in New York in April 1916. The Board voted that Smith should consider the location of a residence for the Director and for the other staff members of the Department, and report to the Executive Committee for its appropriate action. A few days later, Smith wrote to Henry James: "My family is ready to state that we shall live in the Institute grounds if the house is provided."

> I shall be better off near the plant. As I must expect to be called away . . . proximity to the laboratories will enable me to make up mornings and evenings and keep my work going in this way. Being near the work I shall be better able to inspect at any time what is going on. Mrs. Smith thinks she might help in concentrating her interests on the general welfare and social side.[83]

He suggested $1,500 to $1,800 for annual rental, garage included. If the Institute were to be responsible for gas, electricity, garbage and waste removal, and repairs, another $100 to $150 per annum should be added. An early decision ought to be made, because favorable opportunities for house purchases in town were scarce, and the final lease on their present quarters would expire at the end of September 1917. "If we leave the borough we shall put up with the 'refrigerator' we are now in for another year."

James assured Smith that he would "sound the Trustees at the earliest opportunity." He understood that Smith's decision would be simplified if he "knew what possibilities existed in the direction of the Institute's land;" but any offers from the Trustees should "in no wise constrain your choice of a place to live."[84] The matter was further discussed on June 2 at the next Executive Committee meeting, which voted in favor of a residence for the Director of the Department of Animal Pathology "on the grounds of the Institute." The resolution was to be conveyed to the Board of Trustees for the necessary authorizations.

Early in August 1916, James sought the Board of Trustees' approval for the Coolidge architectural firm to estimate the cost of constructing a house for the Director on the Rockefeller property near Princeton. Everything would have to be settled and the building started by November 1916 if Theobald Smith and his family were to "move into residence by the autumn of 1917," when the lease would expire on his present rented house.[85] At the Annual Meeting of the Trustees, held in New York on October 30, the Director's house was agreeably located and financially secured.

Theobald and Lilian Smith meanwhile had selected an attractive site within a mile of the main working plant—a treed mound, in the so-called "West Plot," overlooking the Delaware and Raritan Canal and Lake Carnegie to the southwest. A large field that lent itself to strip contour farming sloped down to the canal. Various other staff dwellings were scattered around the westerly side of the Trenton and New Brunswick Turnpike, some extensively renovated and already occupied. The laboratories, horse stables, animal isolation quarters, and power plant were all clustered in the "East Plot." By judicious roadwork and some skilled reconstruction (including a Smith-devised State-supervised underpass beneath the Turnpike) a serviceable road system eventually linked all the staff houses with the main plant, and also with the town and with Princeton Junction on the Pennsylvania Railroad. Coolidge approved the site. Its outlook, accessibility, natural drainage, and landscaping potential, were all good. Drawings and estimates were submitted and approved promptly, and the chances seemed bright that the Director's house would be ready by October 1, 1917. But holdups then began, lengthened, and multiplied. The family prepared to board at the Peacock Inn annex after expiry of the lease on 42 Cleveland Lane.

On June 8, 1917, despite "feeling quite used up," and after a night of "palpitating heart," Smith presided at the Alumni Association of Albany Medical College Annual Meeting, and that afternoon addressed forty-two members of the Graduating Class on "The Significance of Laboratory Research in Medical Education."[86] On July 14, Philip drove him in the family Ford to Silver Lake. After dealing with especially unpleasant swarms of mosquitoes, he relaxed for nearly three weeks, returning to Princeton on August 4. Taking meals at the Nassau Club, Theobald attended to urgent laboratory problems, and sorted books for packing and storage before returning to Silver Lake for another short visit, from September 5 to 18. His return to Princeton two days ahead of his wife and daughter Dorothea allowed him to put laboratory affairs in order before they all repacked their household goods for storage.

For six days they packed dishes, books, papers, and their own furnishing and the children's possessions. These belongings were dispatched to various places of storage around the estate. Thus four loads went to a "storage house," another four to a "warehouse;" several loads were sent to the "dog kennels," and one load to Peacock Inn "to live with." The piano and unpackable furniture were transported "early to kennels" (where Carrel's dogs were handsomely billeted). On October 3, the house was finally vacated.[87] During the ensuing confusion, Smith hurriedly composed a report for the Rockefeller Boards of Trustees and of Scientific Directors, which held their Annual Meetings in New York on October 18–19, 1917.

On October 28, almost a month after the previously anticipated date for moving into the new house, Smith recorded "Director's house building." Now that the foundation of the structure were laid, and growth above ground level was visible, Smith and family members visited more frequently. But the rewards of patience came slowly. In January 1918, a letter to Gage ruefully described their situation: "We are now in a boarding house (since Oct.) and expect to move into a Director's house not far from the Institute buildings whenever it is completed."

> Aye, there's the rub. The Govt. first commandeered our roof tiles and then our carpenters. The second batch of tiles came after 3 mos. delay. Now for the radiators, which are probably in some cantonment . . . Personally I do not mind. We are sheltered and the temp. in our rooms not below 60° today.[88]

It had been nine months since America had entered the Great War, an event which Theobald referred to in his letter as "the debacle of our 19th Century civilization, which you or I shall not see restored or replaced;" and another ten months would lie ahead—with the last six of them demanding hard fighting and many casualties by American troops—before the four-years of bloodletting finally came to an end.

On May 13, 1918, Theobald and Philip began "sleeping in new house," and on the 20th the rest of the family moved in. An inclusive rental of $125.00 monthly became operative in June 1918. As there were no servants, the noon and evening meals were taken at Peacock Inn. Lilian longed to be in the new house, which she had helped to plan. In July 1917, Theobald had relayed to Silver Lake some queries about wall and floor coverings. Nearly nine months later, Lilian and Dorothea had to select "patterns and tints" all over again from a very contracted range of choices. The house was much larger than their needs. The first floor comprised a reception room, a living room, library, and a huge dining room. On the second floors were five bedrooms, with two large sleeping porches, and three bathrooms. The housekeeper had a separate apartment of three rooms and a bath. A two-car garage and two tennis courts were adjacent.

Early in September 1918, Simon Flexner "spent an afternoon at Princeton. Dr. Smith looks tired. Mrs. Smith was rather grouchy, because I suppose the Doctor had had no vacation. He promised to go off for two weeks . . . We talked his work over for a couple of hours."

Then I went with him to the new house. I must confess my conscience is not wholly clear on that rather extravagant domicile. I should fear rather Mr. Gates' sharp eye on it. The Smiths are merely camping in it, which probably does not help her temper, as there is no sign of servant about. I can't suppress the notion that H.J. was building himself a monument![89]

Several weeks after, in his review of Institute affairs for Henry James, Prudden commented in kindly fashion: "The Theobald Smiths haven't yet got settled in their stately mansion because nobody can get help any more, and so I believe they are sort of camping out still."[90] The servant problem at the Director's house was never properly resolved, though Lilian was well liked by the community. Most people know her best as the flower gardener and landscapist around the house. She was particularly fond of the prospect toward the lake. Early in February 1918, she had visited the site with Theobald. They were pleased to find "work going on; plastering; bathroom work."[91] But what had thrilled Lilian most was the unforgettable sight and sound of meadow-larks soaring from the intervening slope. Their greeting determined her name, "Larkfields," for the Director's house. Fifteen years later, after she and Theobald had vacated the residence, meadow-larks (singing farewell) formed also the theme of the porcelain memento which Simon Flexner presented to Lilian Smith.

23

ADMINISTRATIVE TENSIONS— RESEARCH STARVATION

Theobald Smith was profoundly distressed by the extension of the European conflict into World War I. The loss of life, sacrifice of health, wastage of human heritage and destruction of civilized amenities were the antithesis of all that he had upheld. Most of the leading universities in the United States were at first very tolerant toward Germany. President Lowell of Harvard allowed Prof. Hugo Münsterberg to stay on the faculty, despite his almost seditious propaganda. On the other hand, Lowell made no apology to the prospective 1915 exchange professor from Berlin, who had protested the publication of an undergraduate satirical poem, *Gott mit Uns,* in a college periodical. Lowell became the leading spirit of the League to Enforce Peace, and later strongly supported the League of Nations. One of Smith's correspondents even claimed that President Lowell was sympathetic to the proposal to induce "half a dozen (or more) Harvard doctors . . . to go as a medical unit to Germany." Did Smith think sufficient personnel might be willing to go; and if so, would he extend the invitation? No reply has been found. Any analogy imagined between this proposal and the Harvard unit established earlier at Neuilly under Harvey Cushing was not in tune with the changed American attitudes about the outcome of the war.

Theobald Smith accepted an invitation to join the Committee on War Prohibition, of which President Emeritus C.W. Eliot, was a Vice-President. He found himself grouped with familiar names, such as Roger Babson, Drs. Haven Emerson and R.C. Cabot, Surgeon-General Gorgas, Major Henry Lee Higginson, and psychiatrist William Allen White.[1] As the situation grew more critical, other organizations sprang up, some with quite ludicrous proposals. For example, the Emergency Peace Federation invited Theobald Smith to join a delegation of 200 that would take a special train leaving New York at midnight for Washington on February 11, 1917, the eve of Lincoln's birthday. After joining a Washington contingent at the Raleigh Hotel, the total assemblage planned "to ask Congress not to declare war without giving the people an opportunity to speak through referendum."[2]

Smith could not believe that the country of origin of Bach and Wagner, Koch and Ehrlich—a country that had shown him genuine friendship only a few years before—could produce this merciless ferocity, this "frightfulness." Moreover, his own genes were undeniably German. So he relayed Manifestoes on Peace with covering letters to friends and acquaintances, urging them to sign the documents and transmit them to their Congressman. The responses were discouraging. A colleague in the Nutrition Laboratory of the Carnegie Institution of Washington tersely accounted for his inaction: "I feel as if practically all our measures are so futile and . . . so subject to all sorts of gross misinterpretations that I question if signing anything under heaven will do any good." Desperately, Smith wrote to his own congressman: "I am taking the last opportunity to assert the rights and privileges of citizenship by expressing to you my conviction that some other way than an aggressive war should be found to lead us and the world out of present difficulties. I hope that Congress and the President may find this way."[3]

Theobald Smith's sentiments during the early part of the war were not merely pacifistic but also pro-German. In a letter to Geheimrat Gaffky at Hannover, written a few months after the outbreak of hostilities, he complained (in German) that his plan to spend a few months in Germany in 1915 was now "self-evidently wrecked." As Gaffky's guest at the Institut für Infektionskrankheiten in January 1912, when he met so many excellent persons, he had not suspected that this calamity would befall them all so soon. "But the courage and dedication of the German people will finally bring victory."[4]

To Prof. H. Kossel at Heidelberg, Smith wrote in October 1914: "I suppose it is unnecessary to tell you how deeply the news of the war has moved us. We fear that the great, well-constructed edifice of German science will suffer from the heavy sacrifices. We often think of our many German friends and of their fate in these days . . . Unfortunately the mood here is very anti-German, but we hope that soon a better understanding will break through."[5] Kossel replied promptly and appreciatively: "We Germans are very grateful for any sign of sympathy, particularly when it comes from men who know Germany well, and therefore can judge best the severe injustice done to our people through the slandering lies of opponents . . . We rely on our friends abroad to retain their friendly concern for us, not to despair of us, and to help us later to tear apart the tissue of lies."[6]

Smith had also written at the end of October 1914 to Medizinalrat D. Weber of the Reichsgesundheitsamt, now an Army staff doctor in the field near Malmedy. Weber answered:

Heartfelt thanks for supporting Germany . . . You are right, the Germans must have been slandered very much in the American press. You speak about distorted reports on Louvain and Rheims. The Belgians and French alone are guilty of the damage. Or were we to let our soldiers be shot down, with our hands in our lap, when the enemy used for defense purposes historical buildings which we also view and treat with respect?[7]

In the early stages of World War I, German academics proved highly suscepti-ble to casuistic arguments justifying pillage and slaughter. Geheimrat Friedrich Schmidt wrote to Smith, three weeks after Germany marched into Belgium: "You know our peace-loving German people and our cultural strivings . . . Our Kaiser grasped the sword only after he had attempted everything for the preser-vation of peace, and he only anticipated the well-prepared attack. Further, the German nation stands behind him with unanimous enthusiasm . . . An army which with God fights for Kaiser and Fatherland, cannot fail."[8] Smith replied in mid-October from Forest Hills:

It is hardly possible to give you any conception of the emotional turmoil we went through when we received the news of the declaration of war. Even now every day is upsetting, and we talk of nothing else . . . Fortunately, sympathy from other countries is not needed for union of the German people, and we hope that will-ingness to sacrifice and unity eventually bears rich fruit, and soon will bring "peace with honor."[9]

During June and July of 1916 and 1917, when Theobald mostly stayed in Princeton, Lilian wrote at least twice weekly from Silver Lake. The flow of her lively gossip about the latest anti-mosquito measure, the antics of their children, and the comings and goings of neighbors was liable to interruption by allusions to the war. She had been "using kerosene on our Masurian Lakes." (The Masurian Lake region of northeast Poland, then in East Prussia, was the scene of several battles fought between German and Russian armies from August 1914 to Febru-ary 1915, won by the Germans.) She blamed President Wilson for allowing the country to drift into war—"I cannot forgive Mr. Wilson for his mismanagement of the question"[10]—and dreaded the militaristic reports of the newspapers. She reported that Philip had declared recently: "There isn't one man in a thousand who can see that there are two sides to a question. *Dad can,* and he is about the only one, and I admire him for it, lots!"

Two weeks later, Lilian rejoiced that the German submarine *Deutschland* had arrived safely on July 9 in Baltimore harbor. "Isn't the *Deutschland*'s coming a pretty fine piece of work! We put all our German flags on the supper table to celebrate this peaceful victory & manful exploit. How proud & happy the Germans here must be!"[11] Once war was declared, her letters avoided expressing such pro-German sentiments. Instead, she became increasingly involved in movements for international peace and happier human relationships. Meanwhile, Lilian's stance led to her being circularized by certain organizations as a German-American, as well as by numerous societies advocating peace and democracy. She sent Theobald a circular favoring a "German Republic." "I don't know why they thought me a German-American—I am a *friend* of Germany."[12]

A close sympathizer at Silver Lake was their friend and neighbor, Rev. Edward Cummings, whose name graced the letterhead of the World Peace Foundation as General Secretary. The Board of Trustees, which included A. Lawrence Lowell, proclaimed lofty aims: "The foundation supports the efforts of the United States government and the Allies to win the war and set up an international organization which will guarantee permanent peace with justice, and so make the world safe for democracy and civilization."[13] Such objectives served as foundation for the League of Nations.

Theobald Smith's pro-German attitude continued until early 1917. He made no comment on the notorious "Appeal to the Civilized World," proclaiming the innocence of their peace-loving fatherland and signed by ninety-three German "intellectuals," including Paul Ehrlich. Contributions to various relief agencies—all German—were recorded almost monthly. Beginning with $5 to the Relief Fund in November 1914, similar amounts were donated to Widows, the Information Service, Babies, War Relief, and the Milk Fund. Widows and Orphans got $25.00. At the eleventh hour, Smith donated $20 to an American organization, the Emergency Peace Foundation.

The diary for March and April 1917 concealed his profound chagrin, his deep personal sorrow and disappointment, as the United State officially entered the war on April 6. Since Germany had declared itself an enemy, repudiated its foreign debts, and boasted of destructive accomplishments and murderous intentions, his patriotic allegiance was reversed. His pro-German utterances ceased, he contributed generously ($25 and $50) to the American Red Cross; invested in several Liberty Bonds of $500 each; and accepted without demur the entirely unsought (and generally unknown) promotion to Major in the Medical Reserve Corps of the United States Army.

Family legend holds that Theobald Smith resigned his commission in the Army Medical Corps—date uncertain. The facts are:

1. He had been appointed First Lieutenant in the Medical Reserve Corps of the United States Army, effective July 5, 1908. President Theodore Roosevelt, who signed the document, declared that he reposed "special trust and confidence in the Patriotism, Valor, Fidelity and Abilities of Theobald Smith . . . This commission to continue in force during the pleasure of the President of the United States for the time being."[14]

2. On September 24, 1915, Theobald Smith wrote to the Surgeon General, submitting his resignation as First Lieutenant in the U.S. Army Medical Corps. The resignation was rejected. The Surgeon General's representative was directed to state that in case of necessity, "you can be of more use to the Department in the vicinity of your home than at any other point." No copy of Smith's letter of resignation has been found.

3. A few days after Congress declared war against Germany, Theobald Smith was commissioned a Major in the Medical Corps of the United States Army.[15] Preserved along with the certificate is a scroll headed "The Association of Military Surgeons of the United States," proclaiming that "Major Theobald Smith, Medical Reserve Corps, United States Army, has been elected to date from the 1st day of January, AD 1921, an active member of the Association, and is entitled to all the privileges and benefits thereof." The document was dispatched eight months after Smith's election to these entitlements.[16]

4. At the end of March 1923, the Adjutant General's office notified Major Theobald Smith that he had been mistakenly assigned a serial number some ten months before. At that time, his commission as Major, Medical Officer's Reserve Corps, had terminated "by reason of the expiration of the five-year period for which it was issued." The Adjutant General's office noted that "Your patriotic action in placing yourself at the disposal of the Government during the World War is appreciated" and "regretted that the law . . . does not permit of your reappointment."[17]

Theobald Smith was therefore a commissioned officer in the U.S. Army Medical Reserve Corps for nearly fourteen years, from July 5, 1908 to April 10, 1922. Throughout the First World War, he held the rank of Major in the Medical Reserve Corps. When that Commission finally expired, he was nearly sixty-three years old.

Besides Theobald Smith, other scientists of the Rockefeller Institute, some of them now American citizens, were linked elsewhere genetically. The Institute's two great biologists, Samuel Meltzer and Jacques Loeb, were (like Simon Flexner) of German-Jewish ancestry. A visionary streak led Meltzer to found a society of physicians, "Fraternitas Medicorum," dedicated to the maintenance of international amity. The society flowered exuberantly until the United States went to war with Germany, when it withered and died. Loeb, the mechanistic philosopher, ascribed a warmongering society to the ambitions of narrow-minded politicians, who stimulated the superstitions, ignorance, and primitive promptings of the mob mind. His celebrated address on "Biology and War"[18] postulated the peacemaking benefits of scientific logic applied to the causes of international tension.

Simon Flexner's reactions were different. Initially, he provided self-effacing leadership for the Institute's earliest contribution to the Allies' war effort—an increased supply of horse antisera for the treatment of cerebrospinal meningitis and bacterial pneumonia. In due course, the Institute undertook many projects for the War Department, so that in August 1917 its two main components were designated U.S. Auxiliary Hospital No. 1 and U.S. Auxiliary Laboratory No. 1. Most of the already commissioned officers took to uniform, and others applied for commissions. Only a few, like Peyton Rous, remained civilian.

Flexner began his Army life as a Major, but was promoted soon to Lieutenant-Colonel, thus acquiring a double authority over the officer-scientists at the Institute. Eventually, his advisory duties took him away so frequently from New York that he picked the wise, kindly, unflappable Mitchell Prudden as substitute. "In my absence," Flexner wrote to Theobald Smith, "Dr. Prudden will be in charge of the Institute office . . . the things you formerly brought to my attention [should] now be brought to his. He expects to be at the Institute daily from October."[19] Subsequently, Prudden whimsically outlined the local situation in a letter to Henry James, whose choice of "privacy" rank in the Army tickled his fancy: "While Simon Flexner is away . . . I am serving as ballast to keep the good ship Science on an even keel."[20] He would sacrifice a good portion of his "Institute salary to see you come to attention and salute on all the frequent appropriate occasions. But perhaps ere this you are the salutee." Prudden told James that he had been "hanging around this place forenoons ever since you left . . . Colonel Flexner is the Chief, with an adjutant to keep all soldiers' records and transmit orders to various subordinate officers scattered about loose . . . Nearly all of our leading lights have now gone over to the military."

Actually the only full Colonel closely attached to the Rockefeller Institute was William Welch, who insisted on wearing military uniform despite a considerable paunch. At the War Department, he was very influential and much consulted by Surgeon General William Gorgas. It was Welch who first suggested that the Institute laboratory be organized under Flexner, to be called upon for "expert advice whenever needed."[21] Smith refused to don the uniform to which he was entitled and banned military attire for the staff, despite the powerful examples of Welch and Flexner. Smith mistrusted the military mind, and would not risk the armed forces seizing control over the department of animal pathology.

The demand mounted for horse antisera of various kinds. Responsibility for their production was transferred to the fledgling department of animal pathology at Princeton, where the project was supervised admirably by J. Howard Brown. Theobald Smith, though involved only remotely, kept aware of developments, and wrote to Flexner or Prudden about any hitch. Smillie and Little became skilled at procuring horses in a very competitive market. In caring for and injecting the animals, the two veterinarians had different approaches, Smillie being gentle, Little notoriously the opposite. They also conducted all horse autopsies, and helped with the serum assays in Brown's laboratory. Marion L. Orcutt was Brown's efficient laboratory assistant.[22]

Initially, with production confined to pneumococcal and meningococcal antiserum, three types of each antigen were prepared in the laboratories of Rufus Cole and Simon Flexner, respectively. Anti-dysentery serum was distributed later, mainly at Flexner's instigation. The Scientific Directors also endorsed "gas gangrene" antitoxin. In 1917, C.G. Bull and Ida Pritchett had identified at the Rockefeller Institute the nature and role of the toxins produced by certain cultures of *Clostridium perfringens,* and prepared horse antisera of prophylactic and therapeutic value.[23] This gas-producing bacillus (known formerly as *Clostridium welchii* because it was first isolated in 1892 by Welch and Nuttall)[24] was liable to contaminate war wounds owing to its presence in normal soil. Without specific treatment the resulting gas gangrene often caused loss of limb or life.

The various antigens for immunization of the horses, prepared in the New York laboratories, were shipped by train and picked up at Princeton Junction. Live animals were often exchanged by the same route. That these arrangements so seldom went awry was a remarkable tribute to the alertness and dedication of all concerned. However, until serum production was supervised by Howard Brown, this function was a frequent source of irritation between the Princeton division and the New York headquarters. Early in 1917, Smith displayed exasperation about the non-arrival of antigens for the horses: "We have to send a machine into Princeton Junction to bring them in from the train. This is the fourth time that we have sent for them when they either failed to appear or else came on a later train. It seems to me that they should be here when they are announced to be here."[25] Flexner apologized.

At the peak of wartime operations some sixty horses were undergoing immunization, housed in a well-kept barn with adjacent paddock. After the war, the

Health Departments of the City of New York and of the State of New York at Albany gladly purchased the surplus horses. Provision of specific antisera was seldom acknowledged as a vital contribution to the Allied war effort. However, a message of appreciation from the British Admiralty for "the valuable results obtained from the use of Doctor Simon Flexner's Antimeningococcus Serum for cases of cerebrospinal fever in his Majesty's Navy during the War" was passed on to Flexner and Theobald Smith.[26] Prudden wondered how to respond to a letter which had referred to "My Lords Commissioners" and closed with the declaration, "I am, Sir, your obedient Servant."

Meanwhile, the main Institute (the War Department's Auxiliary Laboratory No. 1) conducted courses in the bacteriology, clinical chemistry, and techniques in pathology for medical officers and technicians. Flexner gave the total enrollments in these courses as 422, 107, and 40, respectively. Each month, the U.S. Army sent twenty to forty men and women for instruction to Lieut.-Col. Flexner and his distinguished staff of military and civilian scientists.[27]

Flexner had another statistic. When the United States entered the war, the Rockefeller Foundation financed the construction and maintenance of a fifty-bed War Demonstration Hospital on the Institute grounds. The Hospital consisted of two twenty-five bed wards and an operating pavilion, with quarters for personnel—in all, sixteen portable wooden structures—erected in only six weeks. At the outset, patients were civilians, but in due course wounded American soldiers replaced them. An investigational unit, headed by Dr. Alexis Carrel, comprised four French military surgeons and a number of medical officers, bacteriologists, and biochemists assigned by the United States Army for a fortnightly course in the Carrel-Dakin method of wound treatment. Flexner reported a total of 735 registrants in the twenty-one month period ending March 1919.[28]

These courses aroused controversy. A leading challenger was Arthur Dean Bevan, Director of General Surgery in the office of Surgeon General Gorgas. Bevan had been head surgeon at Rush Medical College for the past ten years, and was the current president of the American Medical Association. He had canvassed other expert opinions, and of course visited the Demonstration Hospital and read Carrel's recently published book, *The Treatment of Infected Wounds*.[29] He reached the conclusion that "Carrel's part of the work is not scientific and cannot be accepted." Bevan conveyed specific criticisms, with proposals for an objective appraisal of the method, in a lengthy letter to William H. Welch, whose deep interest in the sound "organisation of the medical department for this war, and . . . in the success of the Rockefeller Institute," was fully recognized.

> The Carrel treatment cannot and should not be accepted at this time as a demonstrated truth . . . The very exaggerated claims that have gotten into our medical

journals and even into the lay press should be discouraged by those who are in a position to control the situation, and the mistake of fathering a piece of half-baked work should be avoided both by the Rockefeller Institute and the medical service of the government.[30]

Bevan gave Welch permission to use this document as he saw fit. A reply would be welcomed. None has been found. Welch handed the letter to Abraham Flexner, presumably to avoid being himself the messenger of bad tidings to Simon, who coldly acknowledged the receipt: "Abe handed me Dr. Bevan's letter to you regarding the Carrel-Dakin technique . . . There is no doubt that Bevan does not understand either the technique or Carrel's point of view . . . I have not shown the letter to Carrel." The hospital was running well, yet he defended the enterprise lamely. "There are patients enough, although the wounds are not strictly 'war wounds' or like them, except now and then. But the available material suffices to show the points of the general method. As far as one can tell, the class is satisfied."[31]

Carrel's close association with the Rockefeller Institute dated from 1906, when granted a Fellowship by the Institute, until his reluctant retirement in 1939, as detailed in Simon Flexner's "Diary."[32] His skill at vascular anastomoses, and his daring experimentalism, mostly using dogs, presaged advances in human arterial grafting, organ transplantation, and thoracic surgery. In 1912, the first Nobel Prize awarded in North America went to Carrel for his work on "vascular suturing and in the grafting of blood vessels and organs." The Rockefeller Institute raised his rank to Research Member, entrusted him with direction of the Department of Experimental Surgery, and allotted generous space and budget.

Carrel was holidaying in France at the beginning of August 1914; and as he had retained French citizenship, he was promptly mobilized and sent to the Hotel-Dieu at Lyon, where the need for better treatment of lacerated war wounds caught his attention. Through Henry James, he negotiated a grant from the Rockefeller Foundation for conversion of a luxury hotel at Compiègne into a hospital laboratory, where he was soon joined by Henry Dakin, an able chemist. Simon Flexner had persuaded Dakin (a former associate of Christian Herter) to collaborate with Carrel. The surgeon and the chemist together developed the Carrel-Dakin method of irrigating wounds with buffered sodium hypochlorite solution, and the procedure was standardized by the autumn of 1916. This was the technique taught in the War Demonstration Hospital put up so hurriedly in New York in 1917.

Carrel returned to France in the spring of 1918 to find his method being superseded. Nevertheless, the Institute greeted his arrival back in New York after the Armistice by expanding his facilities. In January 1920, Theobald Smith (and inferentially, other Scientific Directors) took over the responsibility for the re-furbished Department: "Quarterly meeting of Directors. Lunch with Staff. In-spect Carrel's new floor and dog house."[33] The unsightly wooden shacks still crowded the southwest corner of the grounds nearly a year after the Armistice: "I expect to come in on Tuesday re the War Demonstration Hospital."[34] On Prudden's advice, Smith charged the Department of Experimental Surgery for having to "open the Kennels at Princeton to care for eighteen dogs which the Carrel improvements have legacied upon him."[35]

Carrel's postwar activities were mostly in the field of tissue culture, whose application to studies of cancer had stimulated him previously. Later, he made extravagant claims about the culture of whole organs, which aroused much pub-licity, especially when Charles A. Lindbergh, the famous aviator-engineer, vol-unteered his collaboration in developing a perfusion pump, with *The Culture of Organs* appearing in 1938 under their joint authorship.[36] Three years before, in the year of Flexner's retirement as director of the Institute, and a few months following Theobald Smith's death, Carrel alone had published his shallow, pre-tentious credo, *Man the Unknown*.[37] This pseudoscientific work, streaked with bigotry, mysticism and plain nonsense, had a fleeting popularity; but it shocked many scientific colleagues who had long been offended by his in-house egocentricities and showmanship.

Flexner, who had risked his reputation by fostering some of Carrel's costly projects—the semi-secret "mousery" is probably the worst of such extrava-ganzas[38]—was finally disillusioned. He wrote in his "Diary," after a stormy inter-view with Carrel: "In the later years, he did not strike a new vein. It may, I think, be doubted whether he was gifted with many ideas."[39] That Carrel never doubted his own superiority was underlined by his final emigration from the United States to France early in 1941, having denounced the Rockefeller Insti-tute publicly, and his acceptance of the title "Regent" of the Fondation Française pour l'Étude des Problèmes Humains,[40] bestowed by Marshal Petain, which, in time, evoked the comment, "Dr. Carrel's politics have very little to do with his scientific achievement."[41]

As a charter member of the scientific directorate of the Rockefeller Institute, Theobald Smith shared responsibility with other members of the Board, espe-cially Chairman William Welch, for not advising Simon Flexner to be cautious in supporting Carrel's activities. But Smith, while both observant and reflective, was known to be mistrustful of any form of advertisement for scientific accom-plishment; whereas Flexner, while disavowing any desire for personal credit, was always eager to please the non-scientific Board of Trustees, including the Rockefellers, by demonstrating good returns upon their investments. In the Carrel situation, Welch and Flexner in a sense conspired to defy the skeptics, while Smith (who would have been familiar with Almroth Wright's wartime work on the damaging effects of antiseptics upon the polymorphonuclear leucocytes of the blood and tissues) preferred not to risk an unseemly struggle if Flexner should prove obdurate.

Flexner neither wanted nor intended to relinquish any important power as director of the Rockefeller Institute for Medical Research. A letter dated early in September 1918 from Flexner to Prudden raised a score of numbered issues. They ranged from very precise statements, such as "The foundation has appropriated $33,302 for war work," and "the Institute will, of course, wish to be fully identified with the drug [Tryparsamide] and its manufacture," to suggestions for improving the situation at the "Farm," i.e., the Department of Animal Pathology. Jones was "itching to go to Peru"—which he soon did—to investigate a fatal disease on the sheep farms. Other young men in the Department were "restive." TenBroeck would soon be commissioned, while Little and Smillie would "prefer being in the service and assigned to Princeton." Theobald Smith wanted Smillie to move into one of the houses on the estate "to help him out in running the place." The young man he had as clerk and who had been doing well has been called to camp.[42] The "young man" was presumably Nathanial Shaw.

Prudden seldom interfered with Flexner's decisions. He considered his own main function was to lessen the day's burdens for anyone in trouble, to lighten the prevailing mood for everyone, and to keep the director posted on developments. In October 1918, he chaffed Flexner about "your conferences and your hobnobbings with nobility and gentry, and your possible tastes of war."[43] The influenza, to whose outbreak Smith had referred in his Day Card of September 24 ("Severe influenza epidemic in U.S. esp. Boston") had struck New York. "The place looks rather comical," reported Prudden, "with masked creatures flitting about here and there, and the handicap of absentees is considerable, but thus far we have been able to hustle along without too much rattle in the machinery." The annual meeting of the Boards of Trustees and Scientific Directors had been uneventful, with "Welch recuperating from the grippe at Atlantic City, Theobald Smith thinking it wise not to leave the relative security of Princeton, and yourself flitting about Heaven knows where, so that Biggs, Holt and I kept the standard of the Directors floating as best we could." To cope with the influenza situation they had "established a sort of public health visiting nurse on a good salary."

In response to Flexner's earlier communication that "some kind of superintendent will have to be found for Smith,"[44] Prudden had visited Princeton, where "one reads still upon the lintels of their door post *La vie comme c'est amère* [Life, how bitter it is]." Prudden no doubt did his best to sweeten the motto. Finally, he informed Flexner, the director "doesn't want a superintendent just now. The new house is about done."[45]

Early in 1919, Theobald Smith changed his mind about Smillie becoming Superintendent. In one of several letters to Prudden regarding the Department's current problems, he expressed a desire to have Smillie assume this position. Prudden transmitted the letters to Flexner, who approved the various proposals, adding these comments to the question of the Superintendency. He had recently conversed with Dorothea Smith. "Obviously Dr. Smith is suffering from overwork and nervous strain and his family are deeply concerned about him."

> They are even considering sending him to Baltimore: If Smillie can be used as Superintendent for a couple of years it would give Dr. Smith the relief at once he needs, would help our new business Manager to get his feet before having to tackle the Princeton business problem, and would add to the happiness of the Smith family, an important item. Let's put it through immediately if you approve.[46]

During Prudden's visit to the Farm in the fall of 1918, Smillie (who had always been completely deaf in one ear) expressed the intention of getting his low military classification raised. Prudden flattened this idea by asserting that whereas the Army could teach Smillie in a year or two to shoot someone, it would take much longer to train a substitute for his Princeton department duties. Smillie had worked with Smith, at first,

> in space provided in the Biology Building at Princeton University. Dr. Smith was then working on blackhead in turkeys. Whenever a bird died, I did the initial autopsy and passed it on to him for more detailed study. In the new building, I had my lab. next door to Dr. Smith . . . He had a tremendous stock culture collection, which filled one large refrigerator. Cultures had to be transferred regularly. For many months, before entrusting me with this task, he would watch over me to make sure that I did things right. Cultures of tetanus bacilli caused him special anxiety. He stood for long periods observing my precautions against bubbling of the loop contents when I flamed them. He was a strict disciplinarian and very meticulous; and this gave me the finest training a young man could possibly have.[47]

Smillie was always amazed at the scope of Smith's knowledge. "He was the greatest man I have ever known. He came to Princeton undoubtedly intending to leave his influence there, but it may well be that he was happier at Forest Hills."

Theobald Smith eventually gave way to pressure from Flexner and Prudden, and offered the Superintendentship of the Farm to E. W. Smillie at a salary of $2,500, commencing the second half of February 1919. "It seems to us," wrote Prudden to Smith on February 15, "that you might be entirely relieved of the work of the farm and a whole lot of other things which are so burdensome, and he can consult with you as much or as little as you may determine. There is plenty of money for this." Smith gradually delegated the routine supervision and did not interfere. Smillie made a big success of the job. According to Smillie,

> The Director usually arrived at the Laboratory around 8 A.M., well before the buses brought the staff at 8.30. He walked to and from his house, always briskly, and left for home generally around 4 P.M. There he had a comfortable office, completely sheltered from noise and distraction. In the early years of the Princeton Division, the younger staff were invited regularly into the Director's house, where he would play the piano for an hour or so, mostly classical music. These evenings left a wonderful impression on the young people, and "Mrs. Smith—a sweet lady—insisted on keeping up these occasions as long as possible. Dr. Smith did not like parties as such, but did enjoy the "musicales."[48]

The Princeton Division of the Rockefeller Institute was a complete unit totally independent of the adjacent University and City. Smillie remembered that "I kept records of everything that went in and out of the Farm."[49]

> We had our own powerhouse and water supply, while coal was trucked in from Pennsylvania. There were separate crews for the powerhouse, grounds, and animal care. It was my job to see to all that sort of thing. Every day, including Sundays, Dr. Smith would come and talk over any problems. Then he would work in his laboratory, mostly looking down his microscope, until 11 A.M. After that, he would interview senior people in his office about their projects, or go on a round of inspection.

Of the total estate, 600 acres were developed into a producing Farm by a foreman and five men (100 acres per man). They harvested and sold thousands of tons of alfalfa to the Walker-Gordon Dairies. The woods also were regarded as models of reforestation. The Farm was cited by the New Jersey Experiment Station as one of the best in the State. The revenues, amounting to around $75,000 per annum, went directly to the New York headquarters of the Institute, which seldom questioned budgetary submissions from the Princeton Division.

After Theobald Smith had discussed with each scientist the financial requirements of his own project for the coming year, the budget for the whole Division was worked out in consultation with Smillie. Smith frequently censured the extravagant demands of other Divisions, especially the Hospital, prophesying "They will be sorry! The time will come when the money won't be there for them!" Some scientists on his staff complained that their work was handicapped by his thrifty foibles—his obsession with curbing waste—which imposed irritating restrictions and gave straightforward regulations a legendary twist. A favorite example was the instruction to the storekeeper not to issue new electric light bulbs until the "burn-outs" were returned. Said Smillie: "In those days light bulbs cost more than they do today. Some persons would unscrew old bulbs from the socket and take them home, and then ask the stores for new ones. This was plain theft."

Smith inspired a kind of awe, which Smillie illustrated by another anecdote. Smillie was dressing a painful open sore (of pneumococcal origin) on a horse's fetlock, with Little and stable hands helping, when the animal stamped on Smillie's foot, causing him to swear lustily. During such convivial disturbances, it was customary for someone in the group to greet their imaginary chief. So when Little looked up and said "Good morning, Dr. Smith!" Smillie went on swearing. On this occasion, Theobald Smith was indeed watching. Great was the relief when he slowly turned and walked away, with a trace of a smile. Smith never mentioned the incident.[50]

Many stories were told of Smith's troubles with the economics of owning and operating an automobile, but Smillie preferred to stress Smith's thoughtful generosity, exemplified by one unforgettable episode.

> I owed a local doctor $75, and could not afford to pay him. A friend took me to the Princeton-Yale football match, where we encountered this doctor, who taunted me with managing to watch football while unwilling to pay anything toward his bill. The story got around to Dr. Smith, who offered to loan me the $75, on condition that I immediately paid the doctor, but should never use his services again . . ."If you can't pay me back, find an opportunity of doing something similar for another."[51]

Smith's plans for expanding the department were set back by the enlistment of two associates, Carl TenBroeck[52] and Paul Howe. The Howes got to know the Smiths at Silver Lake. For three months in the summer of 1916 they kept Theobald company at 42 Cleveland Lane while Lilian tended the lakeside encampment. At the end of September, Paul Howe resumed his assistant professorship of biochemistry at Columbia University. In 1917, he accepted an appointment in Smith's department, but within a few months was granted leave of absence to serve in the Sanitary Corps of the U.S. Army. Demobilized in 1919, he returned to his former position in the Rockefeller fold.

TenBroeck in April 1917 married Mrs. Paul Howe's sister Janet. He joined the Medical Corps of the U.S. Army in the fall of 1918, and was posted to the base hospital at Camp Upton, New York. A letter to his long-time mentor pictured the daily routine in the camp's bacteriology laboratory. The 2,000-bed hospital was served by over 100 doctors, mainly country practitioners eager for this post-graduate training. When a wave of influenza swept through the camp, the laboratory overflowed with respiratory tract specimens, which were searched for hemolytic streptococci, pneumococci (to be typed), and the "influenza bacillus." Fifty autopsies were done in eight days. Procedures were now more varied. TenBroeck had persuaded his commanding officer that one carefully-performed autopsy a day would be more instructive.[53] Ten months after TenBroeck returned to his former duties in May 1919, he was offered and accepted an associate professorship of bacteriology at Peking Union Medical College, the Rockefeller Foundation's most ambitious project (through the China Medical Board) for promoting Western Medicine in China. The TenBroecks left for China on June 26, 1920.

Both Welch and Simon Flexner had been members of the China Medical Board's second commission, sent out in 1915 by the Rockefeller Foundation. It recommended that Peking Union Medical College, founded by the London Missionary Society, be converted into a modern medical school, with hospital, laboratories, nursing school and well-trained faculty.[54] Some fine new buildings were erected already. TenBroeck was fairly representative of the faculty-recruits in standards. Letters to his former chief during that initial year in Peking bewailed the lack of laboratory supplies and the inefficiency of assistants, the language barrier, and the passivity of students. On the other hand, he and Janet found the staff congenial, the nursemaids devoted to his small son, Carlon, their home comfortable, and the passing scene of unusual interest.[55]

TenBroeck saw potential but elusive scope for animal pathology in China. The farmers had no large herds, and it was "common practice to sell an animal for food as soon as it becomes sick. They even eat animals that die from various diseases." Rinderpest, pleuropneumonia and *Rotlauf* were apparently common.[56] He launched a small-scale research project—the isolation of tetanus cultures from the stools of hospital patients. Tetanus was a common disease in China. He also "started a problem in immunity," but had to stop when the stock of guinea pigs ran low.[57]

TenBroeck had heard rumors that Theobald Smith would be among those invited to attend the upcoming dedication ceremonies for the Medical College's new buildings. He hoped Smith would accept, "for we want very much to see you here. Plan to stay as long as possible and you will of course be our guests. There are hundreds of fascinating things to see here and the weather is wonderful until early December."[58] Smith replied from Silver Lake: "I regret that we are not going to China as you thought we were. The journey is expensive and my presence here is necessary while the department is still in an immature state of physical development. The scientific output has not been very brilliant during the past year, and the department needs some new blood infused into it."[59]

John D. Rockefeller, Jr., took his wife and daughter, accompanied by William Welch, across the continent by private railway car en route to the dedication exercises in Peking.[60] TenBroeck sent Theobald an "Opening" Program. "It was inspiring in many ways and we were sorry that you and Mrs. S. were not here to add to it. Dr. Welch was quite put out about you not being invited.[61] Mr. Rockefeller made a very good impression, as he was very keen and very cordial and simple. Having the Trustees here was quite a good thing as they were better able to appreciate some of our problems, and were more liberal in the budget than they had planned to be . . . Am making no definite plans for the future but think now that I will not accept a reappointment."[62]

Simon Gage switched his enthusiasm from bicycle tours to forays in his Ford automobile at least three years before Theobald Smith had mastered the art of driving a car. In the summer of 1915, Gage had mentioned the pleasure he and his wife had found in drives through the countryside. Smith gloomily replied: "There are many playthings which seem nice until the burden of playing with them undoes us. We shall have to use one sooner or later in N.H., but I dread the added trouble & responsibilities. Around Boston they are so numerous that it seems hardly safe to run one."[63] By early 1918, however, Theobald was finally giving in: "I must learn to drive a car . . . and the prospect is not gilded."[64]

Although Smith himself still could not drive, he bought a Ford in Boston in June 1916, thus easing pressures from Philip, who had developed a passion for automobiles. The vehicle was seldom used for family purposes, and remained mostly in Philip's custody in Cambridge, where Robert and Lilian, also had access to it. For flying visits between Boston and Princeton, a car was indispensable. In the summer of 1916, Lilian Smith was initiated into the art of driving a Ford, presumably by Philip. She wrote to Theobald: "Yesterday . . . I took my first lesson in driving and I think I shall be a slow pupil."[65] That forecast was correct.

In July 1917, Philip drove his father in the Ford from Boston to Silver Lake.[66] By now, Philip had a motorcycle, which provided fun and excitement. Two of his friends came to grief on it. According to his mother, the accident was wholly the fault of an automobile driver, who "is glad to settle. The machine is being thoroughly repaired and will be better than before the smash . . . How glad Philip will be to see and talk with you! . . . In these days, boys need to talk with their fathers!"[67]

About six weeks later, in January 1918, Philip purchased in Boston on his father's behalf a 7-passenger Stanley Steamer with a special aluminum body, slightly used by the company's president, but reduced to nearly half-price, at $1,525. These cars were notoriously temperamental; and although their top speed was moderate, they accelerated very rapidly. Philip delivered the Stanley Steamer one early morning (2–3 A.M.) in mid-April. For two days previously, Theobald Smith had studied books on the Stanley car. On the first test drive the boiler gave out. Philip had to drive the vehicle (under low pressure) to the nearest agency at Newark. A few days later, he returned to Cambridge.[68] Minor repairs and installations of the new boiler took until the end of May, when Theobald obtained a driver's auto permit at Trenton, and two weeks later a full-blown driver's license.[69]

Allegedly, as soon as Theobald Smith settled in the driver's seat of the Stanley Steamer, it would careen around corners on two wheels. He eventually learned to curb the monster, after spending most of a weekend under it, trying to match the maze of pipes with the manufacturer's line drawings, until he understood its operation. But he always needed to be reminded well before reaching an intended stop. Once he indignantly rammed a car from behind. The only family outing enjoyed in the Stanley was in September 1918 when the Smiths took friends to the seashore at Long Beach, New Jersey, fifty miles away.[70] Repairs were frequent, costly, and usually long delayed. The simpler jobs were attempted at home, e.g., stuffing and packing the steam boxes and tightening the joints because of steam leaks. The results were often unsatisfactory and, on one occasion, a half-day wasted: "Spent 4 hrs starting auto very little time at lab."[71] In April 1919, ten months after the driver's license was procured, the Stanley Steamer was sold for $1,400 cash to a New York newspaper editor. The old Ford remained headquartered at Cambridge or Boston, whence Philip was always ready to drive it almost anywhere.

Theobald Smith returned to Princeton at the beginning of September 1919, after his customary summer at Silver Lake. Philip now had a job in New York, but visited home at weekends, and applauded his father's purchase of a new Ford sedan. In about a week, Theobald was using the car independently. He is said to have jacked up the car by the hubs at the end of the day to spare the tires, and to have saved gasoline by turning off the engine at the crest of hills, descents being punctuated by backfires. On cold winter nights, the radiator would be drained so that no antifreeze need be used. Before a start, the radiator was refilled with warm water, and the journey began with three hood covers, which were successively removed until the engine was thoroughly heated. His wife expostulated in vain that this ritual was unnecessary and somewhat ridiculous.[72] Eventually the driver's eccentricities were modified, and Theobald found the car very useful for short trips, though he never used it for long-distance travel. About three years after its purchase, he sold the car to an employee in the powerhouse and bought a new Ford sedan.

Philip faced many personal wartime and early postwar difficulties. Soon after he arrived at Silver Lake in June 1917, his knee and ankle were swollen and bandaged, and he was exempted from military service. He tried unsuccessfully to enlist as a dispatch rider in the Motor-Cycle Division, and to enroll as a mechanic at the Naval Aviation School in Washington, D.C. During the summer of

1918, he made munitions on the night shift at the Watertown Arsenal. He maintained a firm friendship with e.e. cummings, the poet, his fun-loving fellow-undergraduate. He and Estlin were both very good dancers and greatly enjoyed this innocent form of social mixing. The latter was a conscientious objector and at one stage of the war supposedly sheltered himself from the law in a treehouse. Estlin's mother prepared his meals, hauled up by rope.[73]

Philip's parents welcomed him almost every weekend at Princeton. During the summer of 1919 he did not visit Silver Lake, but resumed weekend trips to Princeton in September—before long in company with Dorothy Davis—until exceptionally severe winter weather supervened. Icy rutted roads and snowdrifts then made motoring impossible and traffic was confined to sleighs. Influenza again swept the community, the Rockefeller Institute in New York being badly stricken. At Princeton, Smillie became very ill, and the staff stayed at home. The Director's house was shut in by drifts. Early in March, Theobald and Lilian celebrated the thaw by attending a Kreisler concert, spending the night at the Peacock Inn. Then, on March 29, as the snow melted and the ice left Carnegie Lake and the fleeting spring was imminent, Theobald recorded: "Philip married in rectory of N.Y. Cathedral to Dorothy Davis. Lilian & I & Dorothea present."[74]

Dorothy's father, Arthur P. Davis, headed the Reclamation Service for the Northwestern United States and was involved in the building of the Boulder Dam. Dorothy had grown accustomed to socialite circles and enjoyed patrician ways. But she followed Philip's lead, from New Haven (where they temporarily lived) to Princeton; then to New York, or Philadelphia, wherever Phil found or sought work; and back again to Princeton. Early in 1922, a Day Card noted: "Phil & Dorothy have been in this house since June 28. Start today to N.Y. to find job & a home."[75]

Theobald and Lilian Smith's children grew up in spacious surroundings amongst a quiet, well-ordered, and cultured society, such as was provided by the Woodland Hill mansion, or later, by their summer "camp" at Silver Lake. This place was described by Prudden in one of his informal reports to Flexner: "I ran over one afternoon to see Theobald, and found him and the family apparently in good spirits and enjoying, as well they may, their castle by the inland sea."[76] The Director's House that slowly took shape in 1917–18 on the Rockefeller Institute farm estate also seemed overlarge, particularly in the eyes of many New Yorkers. The structure afforded ample privacy to five or six adults, working or sleeping, with guest room, and quarters for housekeeper and one or two live-in maids. The space was indeed excessive, since the whole family was rarely at home together, visitors seldom stayed overnight, and suitable servants were very difficult to find.

By the time the Director's House was at last ready for occupancy, daughter Dorothea—a graduate scientist of Radcliffe but a cardiac invalid—was only intermittently at home; and Philip had returned for a final year at Harvard. The other daughter, Lilian, also a graduate of Radcliffe, who had married Robert Franz Foerster in June 1916, when he was assistant professor of social ethics at Harvard University, now resided in Cambridge. Foerster had been Director of the Social Research Council of Boston (1911–13) and was currently a member of a special committee on Social Insurance of the Boston Chamber of Commerce. In 1919, he published the standard text in its field, *Italian Emigration of our Times.* He became professor of economics at Princeton University in 1922.

Philip doted on Robert (who was more than a decade older), and they all made good company for Lilian Smith. One of her June 1916 letters from Silver Lake to "Theo," who stayed behind at Princeton, started by complaining about mosquitoes, but ended by praising Robert.

> The netting does not keep them out, they can wriggle through . . . Last night Robert says he killed about fifty & toward morning he sat by Lilian's bed killing them so that she might sleep. Such devotion! . . . Robert & Philip have great fun together—one hears roars of laughter and really Robert is . . . good for our boy in many ways. Philip calls his new brother a "peach."[77]

Daughter Lilian was particularly fond of the Silver Lake camp. She joined her mother and sister there in 1917, and in 1918 the Foersters and also Dorothea and Philip soon went up to Silver Lake, while the sweltering parents moved into the new Director's House. In the fall, the Foersters stayed with them in Princeton for six months, until the end of March 1919, when they left for Cambridge.[78]

During his prolonged absence from Harvard, Robert was in Johns Hopkins Hospital for three weeks, under investigation for insomnia, followed by another three weeks of convalescence at Atlantic City. Early in June 1919, on the third anniversary of her wedding day, Lilian had a miscarriage in the Boston Lying-In Hospital. Her mother rushed to bring consolation. The Foersters' first child (Lilian Egleston) arrived in the spring of 1922. Theobald was too preoccupied to mention his grandchild until she arrived in mid-May by train at Princeton Junction with an impressive entourage: "Lilian,, the baby, also nurse Miss McIsaacs, & Robt come fr. Boston P.M. to live here for a time."[79] Robert returned to Boston next day to tidy up affairs before rejoining his family four weeks later for the rest of the summer. His new appointment dated from August 1, 1922. On October 9, Lilian & Robert headed for their apartment in Princeton, leaving the baby in custody of her grandmother. Soon after, the grandfather recorded,

"Drive L & Robt. & the baby with all her paraphernalia to 24 Bayard Lane. Baby with us continuously since May 15, now goes to her own home."[80]

Theobald was generous with his children, all of whom received cash donations from their father throughout this period. Lilian Foerster, for instance was given $250 by him in May 1919, while Phil was subsidized repeatedly. Moreover, he assumed (and recorded) all the substantial costs of their holidays at Silver Lake. Smith's thrifty ways allowed him to be generous, as noted before, with causes he found especially worthy. In 1920, Harvard University launched an Endowment fund-raising campaign. He transferred to this Fund the honorarium of $500 which accompanied the award of the Flattery Gold Medal. A pencilled draft of his acknowledgement of that distinction ended thus: "It seems fitting that the money value of the Prize should go back to the University to swell by a little the Endowment Fund for the better compensation of its teachers. I am therefore enclosing its equivalent."[81] In 1922, Theobald Smith donated $100 to a similar campaign for Radcliffe College.

The Director's House was too big for an unaided housewife to keep tidy. For the first few months, Lilian managed with a cleaning woman two days a week plus intermittent help. Beginning in September, "Nellie" stayed for nearly a year, including the summer of 1919 at Silver Lake. When she left, for a few weeks they were alone again. In mid-October 1919, a woman with a toddler started duties as cook. Within the next month, a miscellany of guests included Mrs. Noyes for several days; George Dreyer, professor of pathology at Oxford, for a visit to the lab; Mrs. Mann for a long week-end; Jerome Greene and his wife for luncheon; Dr. K.F. Meyer (a possible employee of the Rockefeller Institute), for dinner and supper; and Howard Egleston (not seen for years), for dinner. They managed another kind of guest during the harsh winter and the renewed influenza breakout of early 1920. "Lab all day. Much sickness among Inst. people for a week due to influenza. Richard Gelhoff lab helper just recovered in our house fr. flu."[82] Theobald Smith got to the lab in a horse-drawn sleigh driven by Little, and stayed there most days for a thermos-style lunch.

Their second long-term cook lasted for nearly a year, including the summer of 1920 at Silver Lake; but she left with her child at the beginning of October, and for a time they made do with a rapid succession of cooks, practically all of them with infants. Occasionally, they were alone in the house. One Day Card, dated two months after the last cook had gone, noted: "Living for some time, since Oct. 1, without any servants. Dorothea away since Oct. 28 at Stockbridge Sanitarium. Mother cooks & we eat in the kitchen with Shawn for company."[83] (Dorothea stayed several months at Dr. Riggs' Sanitarium, learning to adjust her life-style to the realities of a weakened heart and diabetes.)

After further disappointments over potential servants from cities as far away as Boston, the Smiths advanced the fee for a German girl from Breslau. Her arrival was delayed until the end of November 1921, by which time Theobald had sent for another girl from Breslau, who turned up four months after the first. The girls got along very well together. They also left together, without notice, one night in mid-October.[84] Lilian and daughter went to New York to remedy the deficiency. Dorothea returned with "a Jamaica (colored) girl & 2 yr old child for servant."[85]

Lilian was determined to avoid being again left indefinitely without household help. She resolved too that the Director's House would be much more than a comfortable refuge from big city life for her married daughter and son and their spouses. The whole estate acquired beauty and dignity when Mrs. Farrand, a professional landscapist, brightened it up with lawns and flowering shrubs, while Lilian herself continually added deft touches to the flora around the house. As for the spacious interior of the actual residence, Lilian made the large dining and reception areas on the ground floor more purposeful by opening them up for evenings of music and conversation, and for afternoon tea parties, attended by staff wives and families. Occasionally the Board of Scientific Directors met here over a substantial lunch, with the senior staff of the Department. Lilian still enjoyed the family gatherings at Thanksgiving, when her brother Melville drove over with his wife and daughter from Elizabeth. And Theobald joined in the fun when guests began to assemble at the Smiths' House early in May to watch the annual boat races between Princeton and rival university crews. By 1922, this was a recognized vantage point—"Boat race this afternoon; 2 carloads of Atwoods come & take tea."[86]

Theobald Smith seldom felt or looked relaxed. For many years he had questioned his suitability for the present job. His first anxiety had been not to disturb the equilibrium of family life at Woodland Hill, and he had quailed at the mere thought of Princeton's summer heat. Besides, to work out the operating details of a new department would be overtaxing—his familiar argument in comparable circumstances. He foresaw and mastered the special problem of strengthening the fundamentals of animal pathology without yielding to pressures for practical aid to farmers and veterinarians. Again, he cooperated admirably in transferring much of the administrative load to Smillie. Yet, instead of looking forward to the occupancy of the Director's House, in 1918 he had gloomily forecast: "I am not going into it with any zest, knowing it will only be for a short time, for the job is getting too heavy for me . . . Perhaps . . . the work will lighten up and a real research atmosphere can be lived in for a little while."[87] His directorate of the Princeton department lasted another eleven years, and he worked five years beyond that. Many of the seventy reports and addresses published in those sixteen years were of first-rate importance.

By nature a pessimist, Smith was subject to hypochondriacal spells, and in Flexner's estimation was apt to be downright negativistic. That the two men clashed so seldom testifies to their far-sightedness and self-control. With the end of the war, there were two particular sources of disagreement—the recruitment of new staff, and the appropriate public relations of a medical research institution. Smith was very cautious about new staff. "A serious task to select new candidates or reject them," he confided to Gage. "I wish I were more of a 'Prussian' at times."[88] Whether he considered a recent graduate to be trained on the job (E.W. Smillie) or an already trained specialist to fill a particular gap in his own research team (H.W. Graybill), or an established worker seeking facilities to pursue an inseparably attached objective (Rhoda Erdmann), the process was painfully slow. Flexner's quicker judgements were not necessarily more fallible.

The other source of friction was more complex. It was difficult to persuade Smith that the Princeton department should be officially opened, and exhibited to an invited group, with appropriate hospitality, on some stipulated occasion. The problem was surmounted through a conjunction of circumstances to be outlined shortly. A related fact was that nearly three years after the Department of Animal Pathology began operating in its new quarters, Mr. John D. Rockefeller, Jr., was moved to remark when shown a photograph of the new complex that "Particularly interesting is the picture of the buildings at Princeton, which I have never seen."[89]

Flexner was accustomed to responding very promptly to any request from the Rockefeller family and considered Theobald Smith's aloofness a solecism needing immediate action. Smith merely commented: "I hope that Mr. Rockefeller may see this end of the Institute soon. However, the cleaning up is going along and he will see a more attractive place as the days go by."[90] Not until April 27, 1922 did Theobald Smith send his invitation to Mr. Rockefeller, who finally drove down with his wife on a showery day in May 1923 to look over the estate. The visit was recorded phlegmatically: "Spent most of day entertaining Mr and Mrs John D. Rockefeller Jr. We drive about the Institute grounds & take lunch at our house. Guest leave at 2:30 P.M. for New York via their car."[91]

Flexner had a long memory, but seldom nourished a lasting grudge. His prerogatives as Director of the Rockefeller Institute included the final say on salary ranges and increments. During and immediately after the war there were two kinds of increases—general bonuses, granted annually to all employees, subject to the approval of the Scientific Directors and the Trustees; and individual supplements, assigned personally by Flexner. Theobald Smith received the general bonuses of 15, 10, and 15 percent, respectively, for the years 1916, 1917 and 1918. In addition, he got a personal note from Flexner about an extra $2,000 per annum, apart from his basic salary of $10,000, "projected to cover the period of January 1, 1920 to June 30, 1922. I am venturing to add that this under-standing between us be of a confidential nature."[92] Flexner knew well the charm and the healing virtues of magnanimity.

This was the most disagreeable period of Smith's life. He felt trapped in a snare which to some extent he had set. Without model to follow, and with no qualified assistant, he was responsible for quickly establishing a large community on 800 acres of partly developed land for the laboratory investigation of un-solved questions in veterinary pathology. He had not expected to be rendered al-most helpless periodically, for several weeks or months, by bouts of sacroiliac disease. Also unforeseeable was the multiplied burden imposed by wartime con-ditions, which brought the certainty that nothing, from bricks and mortar to microscopes and manpower, should ever arrive on time or as anticipated.

Smith proved to be a good improvisator; but he could not conceal his greatest longing—for the opportunity to be alone in his own laboratory, preparing to unravel some short tangled fiber in Nature's limitless skein. This agony of unfulfillment is revealed in the jottings which sprinkle his Day Cards, particu-larly in 1916–17. "Working on lab notes to find problems most of day," he re-corded early in December 1916. "Miscellaneous thinking on problems P.M." was the entry for April 6, 1917, the day congress declared war on Germany. He was driven by the reflection he voiced in 1920, that "a living research dies under de-lay and must be born again . . . to be brought to full development."[93]

24

LECTURES DE PROFUNDIS—
RESEARCHES ON
BOVINE CONTAGIOUS ABORTION

During the last lean years 1916–17, Smith's bibliography comprised three accounts of early experimental findings on turkey blackhead.[1] His four other publications of this period were in essence more philosophical than experimental.[2] Smith foresaw that the type and number of published items would increase conspicuously after the second half of 1918 and he let Flexner know that he found the lure of the laboratory irresistible—confiding to him that "The attractions of the work are too great in the laboratory" and assuring him that "Certain things are left undone which will receive attention here at home."[3] Between September 1918 and the end of 1921, of nineteen reports (six collaborative), sixteen were of recent findings in Smith's own laboratory. The other three consisted of in-depth analyses of research in animal pathology; of the interrelations between heredity, environment, and parasitism in zymotic (infective) diseases; and of susceptibility to infection and artificial immunization. The highlights of these latter reviews will be depicted after the development of a temporary rift between Simon Flexner and Theobald Smith has been outlined.

As Flexner's war-time duties diminished and finally ceased, he began to appraise more critically the domain whose full-time direction he now resumed. He was perturbed by Smith's ultraconservative program for future development, as well as by other weaknesses in the new department at Princeton, and he set about rectifying some of the deficiencies. When Flexner realized that staff recruitment for the Department of Animal Pathology was determined by factors largely beyond his control, relations with Theobald Smith reverted to a state of wary mutual respect—with one notable exception, just before Smith was due to retire as Director of the Princeton division.

Meanwhile, they shared similar views on many questions, e.g., on the discouraging record of women in research. For example, Flexner agreed "that it would be an advantage if you found a man for the position. I think the question of how far women will go in research is still so open that one cannot predict what the future will disclose. My own experience with women is not particularly encouraging up to the present time." In Baltimore recently he had reviewed with Welch and others the quarter-century during which the Johns Hopkins Medical School had "turned out women along with men." They could point only to Dr. Florence R. Sabin "as having distinguished herself."[4] Smith replied: "with us women's work is perhaps even more restricted than in your laboratory because of the necessity of outdoor and stable work with large animals. We have three women here now . . . quite enough for the time." Then he carried his restrictions further—too far perhaps for Simon Flexner's taste—"We do not wish to have this department either feminized or veterinized, and will have to exercise due caution in appointments." This forthright declaration was followed by a remarkably clear-sighted analysis of their staffing problems: "Our people have little or no outlook for better positions, owing to the character of the work, unless they are unusual. The result is that they stick indefinitely and tend to fossilize the department. During the war we had no choice but to maintain the status quo."[5]

To Flexner, Smith seemed too little concerned about public relations. The delay in showing Mr. and Mrs. Rockefeller over the developing estate was accentuated by his discouraging response to repeated requests for formal opening of the Princeton division. Flexner began by quoting one importunate sightseer. "Mr. Ivy Lee is very eager to have the formal opening that he spoke of. I do not see how it could well be arranged before the Spring, do you?"[6] As a full year passed without apparent plans for any such occasion, Flexner wrote to Prudden: "Apropos of the corporation meeting, it was decreed at the last one that there should be some exercises at the Department of Animal Pathology. First, they were postponed from the spring until the autumn, and then passed over *in silence*. As none of the Trustees has seen the Department, I think it a pity that Dr. Smith has not done something by way of carrying forward their wishes . . . and this especially in view of the impending economic stresses to which the Trustees must very soon be exposed."[7]

Flexner's indignation was unfair to Theobald Smith. The initial oblique reference to a formal opening had been acknowledged promptly. "Concerning Mr. Ivy Lee's suggestion," Smith wrote, "I am of your opinion that it would be difficult to do anything without taking a great deal of time which is needed to get the Institute started now that our war work is over."[8] Again, upon receiving the Trustees' renewed proposal, Smith sent Prudden a lengthy "preliminary statement," listing some of the obstacles. These ranged from shortages of seating space during the exercises and the poor accommodation in Princeton for those wishing to stay overnight, to the inconvenient train schedules to and from Princeton Junction, the catering uncertainties, and the deplorable state of the local roads.[9] Although Smith left little doubt on his own feelings—he would "be disappointed if much time had to be taken from the actual work of the laboratory"—he neither ignored nor vetoed the Board's request. Instead, he summarized the many difficulties of the alternative.

Invitations to the State Governor and the Secretary of Agriculture, for instance, had been discussed: "I should prefer to have scientific men do the speaking," commented Smith, "men who know their subject and can present it well." The program of speeches would be "the most difficult thing to provide." He envisaged three short addresses on certain inter-relationships—animal pathology to general pathology and to medicine—"our work to agriculture and the food problems"; animal diseases and human diseases; and a fourth address on "the practical aspects of animal pathology, including a discussion of biological products, and the stand the Institute should take against the new quackery in such products."[10] However, the Board of Trustees decided not to press for the troublesome alternative.

Flexner had an early opportunity to get his own way without obvious offense to Theobald Smith. The National Academy of Sciences was to hold its annual meeting at Princeton University on November 16 and 17, 1920. Flexner invited all Academy members and their wives to inspect the Department of Animal Pathology and to take luncheon on the 16th as guests of the Rockefeller Institute. Flexner sent a sample letter of invitation to Prudden, emphasizing that this meeting was a substitute for the unavoidably postponed exercises:

> On no other occasion is it likely that so many distinguished scientific men would be available to visit the Department of the Institute as this meeting of the Academy affords. It is Dr. Smith's hope as well as my own that you may be able to be present on this occasion . . . An invitation is also going to our Trustees and we are all very eager to have all those who have not seen the Department visit it . . . Somehow, they must be shown the place and made to feel its importance.[11]

Train schedules would be sent them and the "Department motor" would meet the trains at Princeton Junction.

Heavy rain on the 16th discouraged outside exploration, but scientific interchanges were plentiful. (Lilian, in a new dress, was a charming hostess at the luncheon. She and Theobald assisted President and Mrs. Walcott in receiving members of the Academy and their wives and other guests at Tea.) Prudden's next letter to Smith ended with words of praise: "Your party was a great success. Everybody seemed to be most enthusiastic."[12] He accepted without demur the luncheon bill for nearly $600.00, which Smith sent him, along with the Academy's official thanks to the Department.

The afternoon session of the 17th had opened with a short paper by Theobald Smith, titled "Biological Aspects of the Process of Infection." Smith considered this "only a fragment," intended to illustrate the analogy between the irritative effects produced in blackhead by roundworm (*Heterakis*) ova in the cecum of chickens and turkeys, and other forms of injury, in starting the parasitic cycle.[13] The "fragment" was incorporated in the 1920 reports by Smith and Graybill[14] on the epidemiology of blackhead. Graybill left the Department in 1924, having greatly assisted Smith in establishing this subsidiary factor in the transmission of the causal agent of turkey blackhead. Although E.E. Tyzzer, Smith's successor at Harvard, subsequently found that the roundworm played more than a passive role in the spread of blackhead, the turkey breeding industry already profited from the fundamental findings of Smith and Graybill, that turkey poults should be kept apart from chickens and from soil infected with *Heterakis.*

Flexner was not at the Princeton meeting but soon afterwards indicated to Welch his intention to tackle other weaknesses in the Princeton division. "I was very much interested in your suggestion regarding animal pathology," he wrote, "and I shall look into the work of Gowen . . . I believe with you that a good deal can be done with the Department of Animal Pathology, but I rather think that we—you, Prudden and I—will have to take the initiative."[15] John W. Gowen, an able young biometrician, assisted Raymond Pearl at the Maine State Agricultural Station at Orono, where they conducted long-term animal breeding studies. Gowen had also benefited from early training in genetics under T.H. Morgan at Columbia University, and had a sound grasp of basic Mendelian mechanisms. Flexner wanted Gowen to become the biometrician and geneticist in the Department of Animal Pathology, with a roving commission to attach his disciplines to suitable projects.

Smith successfully fought this proposal until 1926, when Flexner—who had arranged meanwhile that Raymond Pearl should receive an annual grant from the Rockefeller Institute, beginning in 1921—appointed Gowen an associate member of the Department of Animal Pathology. Gowen's main departmental assignment was to study the inheritability of high milk production and its possible correlation with certain physical properties of the dam and sire. The work was to be done at Orono under John Gowen's supervision. During the later stages of his employment in the Department (at the end of which he was appointed to an Iowa university professorship of genetics), Gowen's scientific interests were focused—to Flexner's chagrin—upon fruit flies rather than cattle.

When Flexner sought in general to broaden the outlook and scope of the Department of Animal Pathology, Smith again reacted negatively. The latter viewed the possible diversion of funds to newfangled subspecialties, jeopardizing a thorough investigation of the many unsolved but more familiar problems bearing on the infectious diseases of domestic animals. Nonetheless, if this restrictive policy came insupportable, it was overridden. For instance, when John H. Northrop threatened to resign from the Rockefeller Institute because he detested New York City as a workplace, Flexner personally secured suitable accommodation for this distinguished biochemist and his research team in the main laboratory building of the Princeton division. Similarly, when Normal B. Stoll, the helminthologist, joined the department, Smith at first begrudged the space committed by Flexner, but later acknowledged Stoll's deserved repute.

The Department once failed to recruit a bacteriologist with specialist training because Theobald Smith seemed to prefer overloading his own hands. Before demobilization of the American Expeditionary Force was completed, Colonel Welch had advised J.F. Huddleson, a young expert on bovine contagious abortion, formerly at Michigan Agricultural College, of a pending vacancy at the Rockefeller Institute's Department of Animal Pathology at Princeton. Nothing came of Huddleson's inquiry.[16] An earlier letter from Smith to Flexner perhaps encouraged the inaction: "Just now I need a *good* bacteriologist to push the abortion work, but we have enough of them on the staff . . . I can manage the work myself, provided I neglect administrative duties more or less for a while . . . Only a highly experienced man can make headway in it alone. I have the main data in hand and all that is necessary is someone to work out external details."[17]

Another type of difficulty arose when Flexner attempted to secure a more senior appointee to the Princeton department. An aggressive Swiss veterinarian, Karl F. Meyer (D.V.M. Zürich), had applied to spend a sabbatical year in the Department of Animal Pathology. He was seeking the best opportunity for his future career. He hoped to settle in California. Favorably impressed by Meyer and eager to capture his allegiance, Flexner expostulated that most of the intellectual wealth and resources of the United States lay within 500 miles of New York. In California, an able scientist might get lost in the desert or drowned in the Pacific.[18]

Meyer greatly admired Smith and always spoke of him respectfully. They had first met in Boston in 1911, sharing a particular interest in the pathology and bacteriology of bovine contagious abortion. Smith now resented what he interpreted as Flexner's negotiations behind his back, and sought an explanation: "I am interested to know whether . . . you invited Dr. Meyer to come down here permanently or, as he had expected, for a sabbatical year, because . . . it is rather important that I should know exactly where we stand . . . He is more or less undecided because he may get a much better offer in California and possibly become Head of the Hooper Foundation."[19]

Flexner replied a week later that he favored a generous offer being made to Meyer for a permanent appointment in the Department of Animal pathology. Further, he hoped that the Scientific Directors at the October meeting "may act not only with reference to Dr. Meyer but also specifically with reference to the nutrition problem . . . Would it be worth while to invite the two or three leading animal nutrition experts . . . to come to Princeton for a conference?"[20] Smith had resisted any attempt to implant a senior nutritionist in his department and no doubt Flexner's next assurance was intended to be placatory. "My feeling is that your approach to the subject will be quite different from theirs and I should naturally wish to follow your lead and take a new rather than an old direction of work." The Scientific Directors perhaps found this avowal clumsy and insincere. At any rate, no action with taken about the proposed conference on nutrition. Karl Meyer went ahead on his own.

Flexner's imagination, despite his general shrewdness, could not foresee how far Karl Friedrich Meyer would go during a long lifetime of service to public health in the San Francisco Bay area and beyond. Meyer contributed with characteristic gusto and panache to a wide diversity of diseases, such as brucellosis, botulism, mussel poisoning, psittacosis, and Western equine encephalomyelitis. Productive enthusiasm also illuminated his hobbies—color photography, philately, and such peculiar pursuits as "disinfected mail."[21] Yet his self-assertiveness and love of limelight made him incompatible in any subordinate role, and Smith was wise to question his suitability.

These examples portray some of Simon Flexner's methods of strengthening perceived weaknesses in one component of the Institute. However, when he wanted to be tough and emphatic, he conveyed that impression unmistakably, although his letters to Theobald Smith seldom displayed impatience. For the most part, besides being a good administrator, Flexner was a kindly, modest man. He sometimes felt the need to emphasize his modesty. In a letter to Welch, he eloquently and sincerely disavowed personal credit for the Rockefeller Institute's accomplishments, and sought to dissuade Welch from implying otherwise, saying, "I am not to be elevated through your more than personal kindness beyond my fellows."[22]

On January 20, 1922, the Board of Scientific Directors was to host an afternoon party (4 to 6 P.M.) at the Cosmopolitan Club in New York, to commemorate the twentieth anniversary of the founding of the Rockefeller Institute for Medical Research. Both Theobald and Lilian attended that party and enjoyed it since musical entertainment was provided.[23] Flexner took delight in these occasions, and usually instigated them; they boosted morale. This time, John D. Rockefeller, Jr., would make a ten-minute speech and it was hoped that Welch would do likewise. Flexner asked a favor—"that my name figure as little as may be in any reference you may think it well to make to the growth and accomplishments of the Rockefeller Institute." An explanation followed.

> The Institute is the product of cooperation on a large scale—Scientific Directors, Trustees, and Scientific Staff—and such success as it has achieved is the work of all, and in respect to the scientific product itself, of the group of scientific workers as a whole . . . Through physical connection and a common scientific ideal, a group of men has been assembled to work out their own ideas . . . in a harmonious and helpful way.[24]

Again, when Flexner was notified of election to Foreign Membership in The Royal Society, his typical modesty was displayed. "I cannot pretend to have deserved the honor," he wrote, "which I take as a tribute rather to the work of the Rockefeller Institute than to that of myself, but I am grateful to the members of the Society for the distinction they have conferred upon me."[25]

Lectures and Trophies

Although he yearned for his own laboratory, and for time to work in it, Smith had sufficient unpublished data, as well as firm opinions, for several addresses. Like Robert Koch, he grew to disdain personal involvement in didactic lectures to medical students, apparently preferring the role of *preceptor mundi*. The audience was sometimes small and apt to dwindle. The delivery could be dry and the array of facts very formidable; but at his best, Theobald Smith was a matchless lecturer. Listeners were as fascinated by his profound sincerity and self-confidence as by the skillful buttressing of unfamiliar doctrines with crucial experimental findings and occasional aphorisms. Many hours of concentrated and specific preparation were devoted to most of his addresses, but the flow of useful ideas about a coming lecture might continue even while he "rested"—he once recorded, "resting and thinking about a lecture"[26]—in this instance between several dental appointments.

In the early days at Princeton, before being overwhelmed by constructional and administrative details, Smith recklessly committed himself to delivering five special lectures between May 10 and 17, 1916. The first address, due on May 10 at Washington, entitled "The Underlying Problems of Immunization,"[27] introduced a symposium on the "Causation of Etiology of Infectious and Parasitic Diseases," organized by him on behalf of the Tenth Triennial Congress of Physicians and Surgeons.[28] On May 11, 12, and 15, he gave a series of three Herter Lectures, dealing with various aspects of immunity, which remained unpublished. Finally, on May 17, he delivered the second Mellon Lecture at the University of Pittsburgh, on "Certain Aspects of Acquired Resistance to Tuberculosis, and their Bearing on Preventive Measures."[29]

For a whole year after that intensive effort, Smith undertook no formal lecturing. Then, early in June 1917, with "palpitating heart in night," and "feeling quite used up,"[30] he went to Albany, where on June 8 he presided at the annual meeting of the Alumni of the Albany Medical College, and later in the day, addressed the eighty-sixth Annual Commencement of the College on "The Significance of Laboratory Research in Medical Education."[31] Smith did not dispute that a direct study of hospitalized patients should be "a dominating part of medical education," but he urged that every medical school should also have an attached research laboratory where the aspiring young doctor could cultivate "the power of original creative thinking." He relentlessly contended that medical progress depended upon laboratory research.

> Without denying that bedside observation has done much to advance our knowledge and that it is indispensable as a cooperating agent with laboratory research to promote analysis of disease processes, yet we may truly say that if all physicians had kept vigil at bedsides during the whole of the nineteenth century, this kind of activity would not, in itself, have brought us any nearer to the great discoveries of that century.[32]

He cited Bagehot's quotation from Pascal, that most of the evils of life were due to man's inability "to sit still in a room." The modern world needed "above all the steadying influence of men accustomed to think . . . to sit still and think, to produce results, and this is in part the training which research imposes . . . Research redeems the individual and makes him an expert." Smith had used the Pascal allusion about two-and-a-half years before, when addressing students at the Harvard Medical School on "Scholarship in Medicine."[33] This duplication of a particular quotation appears unique in his publications, although he was deft at variously embroidering a given theme for different occasions. The repetition here surely signifies endorsement, for Theobald Smith knew very well how to sit still in a room and think, and produce results. He only mourned the dearth of opportunity amidst the pressures of administrative obligations.

When Smith gave this advice, he did not foresee how soon and suddenly his duties would change. The World War ended without mention in his diary; but an outbreak of bovine infectious abortion on the Walker-Gordon farm revolutionized his life, and his day cards became sprinkled with references to hours spent in the laboratory, sometimes just "thinking about problems," examining calves' foetal tissues and cultures. "It takes time to produce good work," he complained to Welch in 1921.[34] By then, there could be no doubt that the eventual harvest again would be novel and illuminating.

Meanwhile, he passively acquired occasional trophies. For example, in October 1919, the President and Fellows of Harvard College invited Theobald Smith to give the 1920 Cutter Lectures on Preventive Medicine and Hygiene. He chose as subject, "Medical Research and the Conservation of Food-Producing Animals." The dates of delivery were October 19 and 20, 1920. These two lectures were given annually in Boston under a bequest from John Clarence Cutter, "free to the medical profession and the press." Smith's Cutter Lectures, like his Lowell and Herter series, remained unpublished. His explanation: "I had hoped to prepare them for publication, but the amount of material was so abundant, and the need of going into veterinary education was so evident, that I put the whole matter aside, hoping one day to perhaps prepare a book on the subject."[35] He stayed at the Shady Hill Square apartment of Robert and Lilian, who attended the lectures. The audience was unenthusiastic. He estimated the attendance for the second lecture at about one-half the original.[36]

In May of that year, he was doubly satisfied to win a high award through Harvard University, and to make a benevolent gesture toward that institution by returning the cash portion of the award. In 1920, Maurice Douglas Flattery instituted a Prize—a beautifully engraved gold medal, and $500 in cash, to be awarded annually "to the person the President and Fellows of Harvard College may adjudge to have made a discovery in any branch of science that would result in the greatest good to humanity in the prevention of disease or conservation of health in the broadest sense."[37] A Committee recommended to the Corporation that the first award be made to Theobald Smith.[38] Theobald promptly donated the $500 to the current fund for improving the salaries of Harvard's professional staff.[39] President Lowell and the Fellows expressed their cordial appreciation and gratitude "for your gift to the Harvard Foundation, which has helped to relieve a very serious financial situation."[40]

On September 21, 1920, Theobald Smith caught an evening train at Philadelphia for Lincoln, Nebraska. He was to give the main address at the dedication of the Animal Pathology and Hygiene Laboratories of the University of Nebraska's College of Agriculture. By now he was thoroughly galvanized into a new phase of research activities. The westward journey was hot and uncomfortable. He arrived at Lincoln around noon of the third day, and that evening addressed the Faculty Club on animal pathology and the Rockefeller Institute for Medical Research. His main address, "The Importance of Research in Animal Pathology to

Agriculture," was delivered at a mid-day luncheon on the 24th. After viewing the local sights, and stopping overnight at Ames, Iowa, in order to visit the Veterinary School, he resumed the administrative grind at Princeton on September 29.[41]

The address at Lincoln began with exposition and analysis of the value of research to any scientific enterprise, particularly as regards prevention. Prolonged research will seldom wipe out plagues, "but it may, by discovering and disseminating new facts . . . prevent them from starting . . . Research . . . must be continuous, not interrupted. It may die out in one direction and grow in another, but continuously alive it must be," he instructed his audience.[42] There was no finality to any single research finding, he believed. "It is a link in a chain, or a strand in a cable." Continuity in research requires the best possible personnel to be sought, given financial security, and left alone with their problems. "The time has come when the genuine research worker should be relieved of all teaching except in his special field."

Smith defined animal pathology as simply "a study of disease," in which the communicable diseases "occupy the center of the stage, as they have done for over forty years, since Pasteur and Koch began work in this field, one with his genius for generalization, the other with his methods to make accurate work possible." Other areas of study would soon command attention. "Unlooked-for trails have led from the study of bacteria into remoter fields of pathology. Only in roundabout, usually unanticipated ways are nature's most important activities laid bare, almost never by a direct frontal attack." Confining his remarks to the field in which he was an acknowledged expert, Theobald Smith illustrated by many examples that animal pathology entailed much more than the "study of all kinds of organisms which may live on or in the body" of their animal host. It must cover also the study of their interrelationships with that host under various conditions, as well as their interactions with one another.

In discussing the importance of immunological and serological procedures among the services for which these buildings were now being dedicated, Smith decried the quackery which threatened the reputation of established vaccines and antisera. "Commercialism moves faster than scientific enquiry" and was apt to make unscrupulous claims. Finally, he urged the need for interstate cooperation, recognizing that some states cannot afford the trained manpower and suitable plants for the study of unusual disease. Neighboring states with similar livestock conditions might agree each to "specialize in a separate branch . . . and thereby produce a group of institutes which taken together . . . would form the complete organization needed."

Alternatively, he visualized the development of a "higher institute . . . manned by the best talent available," with which state institutes would be in close touch, and to which unusual specimens or rare animal diseases might be deferred. He recognized that political considerations made the common-sense advantages of such a plan too idealistic for early implementation. Portions of this address seem as suffused with idealism as were Smith's proposals about superior veterinary education to President James and his agricultural colleagues at the University of Illinois more than five years before. The streaks of pessimism and skepticism now apparent, were due perhaps to the intensity of his struggle to increase opportunities for personal research.

Without comment, Simon Flexner sent reprints of the lecture to Welch and other Scientific Directors. Smith received a lengthy typed letter from his old friend and former President, C.W. Eliot, now in his eighty-seventh year, who had read the address "with great interest."[43] He found the "doctrine about the separation of teaching and research rather discouraging." Surely the best sort of teacher has some "practical acquaintance with research," whereas "if the research man does not teach, he will hardly create a group of disciples and followers." Smith replied on the eve of the New Year, overquoting himself: "I stated that the research man should do teaching in his own field of research and the teacher should do research to keep himself fresh and to be able to have some opinion of his own concerning new research work."[44]

Eliot, in his letter, bewailed the extreme scarcity of research men for preventive medicine, human and animal, but appealed eloquently for the first-rate training of veterinary practitioners, who must deal with ten or more animal species, and upon whom the animal pathologist relied for basic data. He expressed interest in referral centers for complex pathological investigations, and asked, "Have you in mind any means of accomplishing so good a project?" A privately endowed organization was less prone to "political control," he believed. Smith rejoined that in his own experience, the high costs of such institutions could result in a cooperative pooling of interests and establishment of "one good research institute for a group of states."

The Nebraska venture caused a local stir, but Smith's next philosophic address brought him much wider acclaim. He felt on surer ground, for the more distinguished audience included many friends, and the topic had broader professional appeal. Moreover, the organizers (the Association of American Physicians) had suspended their custom of meeting annually in Washington, and chose instead the more glamorous Atlantic City. On Tuesday, June 10, 1921, Smith's day card stated, "Read my paper on Etiology which was well received . . . About 150 men present." At the dinner, he sat between two visitors from England—Dr. Stanley White and Sir Thomas Horder—while other neighbors, Drs. Frank Billings and Henry Hun, reminisced about the Association's early years.[45]

In his address, "Parasitism as a Factor in Disease,"[46] Smith reserved the term "etiology" for *total cause*. He knew the importance of the concept of etiology to modern medicine: "On it is founded all rational progress in prophylaxis and therapy. First to comprehend the cause, then to intercept and suppress it, and thereby to prevent the next step, is the kernel of medical science and practice." He set out to narrow and rectify the post-Kochian misconception that a particular parasite and a given host connote a specific disease, claiming instead that "The forces and conditions controlling disease are a mixture of heredity, environment and parasitism." These factors interact with each other and with the host, reaching a state of unsteady equilibrium, which prevails while the parasite pursues four successive objectives—to enter the host, to multiply therein, to facilitate escape of the progeny, and to promote their re-establishment in a new host.

The early bacteriologists looked to sanitation, through disinfection and isolation, to destroy or dilute the parasite, or at least to minimize its chances of successful transit from the convalescent to a susceptible host. Despite heavy expenditures, these efforts yielded limited benefits. Epidemiology remains a fruitful source of data on the role of non-parasitic factors in the contraction of disease. Problems of specific resistance, or of immunity and susceptibility, are encountered, as well as practical questions of treatment by specific biological agents, when the parasite has "run the gauntlet of the blood, lymph and the phagocytic cellular elements," and multiplies in the host tissues.

Smith postulated two main categories of parasites—the saprophytic or predatory type, in which factors such as heredity and environment are paramount; and the highly parasitic type, in which other factors are of little importance. There are, of course, many intermediate types. He illustrated his theme by examples based on his own work, reinforcing their cogency by pithy epigrams or crisp axioms, such as "Experiments are imitations of Nature with the unknown factors controlled or eliminated;" "the science of one generation becomes the practice of the next;" "Great discoveries are, as a rule, half-truths that must be brought into line by patient after-research."

Smith did not prefix the word "disease" by "zymotic," "infective," or other qualifying adjective. Koch's doctrines were still so recently popularized that the non-parasitic diseases tended to be overlooked. Smith expounded here the concept of parasites to include ultra-microscopic microbes ("viruses" in today's parlance) which might destroy epithelium and thus prepare the way for the saprophytic predatory types of bacteria "which are readily recognized because easily cultured, and therefore regarded as summing up the entire etiology." Since his hog cholera disappointment, Smith had considerable respect for the viruses: he has been falsely accused of indifference to them.

This memorable paper was published first in *Science* and then in the Association's *Transactions*. The most pleasing tribute was from David Fairchild, his old friend from the early days in the top floor of the Department of Agriculture Building. Fairchild wrote: "I can't resist writing to say how keenly I have enjoyed your paper on Parasitism as a Factor in Disease. It is the broadest, clearest presentation which I have ever seen. My mind goes back to 1890 or was it 1892? when you showed me the protozoon parasite in blood from the cattle tick in the old Department Attick here in Washington. I felt sure that you were a great man. I know it now."[47]

Among many plaudits received, those from Prudden gave special satisfaction. The first, dated early in October 1921, finished thus: "I am sending for some extra copies of *Science* which contains your work on Parasitism, of which I hope you will have plenty of reprints. They all tell me it is 'amazing fine'."[48] Later, he asked Smith's consent to Flexner's wish to have the Rockefeller Institute purchase 500 reprints of that "remarkable address," for it "ought to have the widest currency. But don't forget that you are going to make a book of it all sometime."[49]

In March 1920, the Institute of Medicine of Chicago had invited Theobald Smith to give its first Pasteur Lecture, under a generous new endowment. The Institute's membership included the principal practitioners of the Chicago area, as well as such distinguished professors as Hektoen, Jordan, Kendall and Carlson from Chicago, Illinois, and Northwestern universities.[50] Smith responded regretfully: "I shall be unable to accept because I am far behind in present obligations, which I may even be compelled to repudiate because of lack of time. I would also be unable to get together enough material which would be of sufficient importance to deserve the name of a Pasteur Lecture."[51]

Smith was then invited to give the second Pasteur Lecture, and accepted for October 31, 1921, it taking place only four months after his lecture on parasitism. The topic, "Theories of Susceptibility and Resistance in Relation to Methods of Immunization,"[52] was prepared with conspicuous care, one or two hours being assigned to it almost daily for several weeks beforehand. Automobile traffic disturbed his first night's sleep at the University Club. He delivered the lecture next day after dinner at the City Club, whose largest room was filled. Next morning, Jordan hosted a luncheon for the visitor and several colleagues on the University of Chicago campus. After "Long talk with Keyes on immunity,"[53] Smith left for Princeton.

As a symbol of profound respect for Pasteur (whom he never met), Smith began with an epigraphic quotation from Walt Whitman: "It is provided in the essence of things that from any fruition of success, no matter what, shall come forth something to make a greater struggle necessary."[54] This rather inelegant dictum was paraphrased in Smith's opening sentence: "The function of great men seems to be not only to bring revolutionary ideas and concepts into the world before they are due, but vigorously to maintain and defend them in a hostile environment." There was no touch of egocentricity in this. Smith had silent pride in his own accomplishments—so often extolled at honorary degree conferments—but he shrank from any kind of self-advertisement. His tribute to great men was pointed at Pasteur alone. Yet as he modestly fulfilled the two-fold task of reviewing post-Pasteurian developments in preventive inoculation, and of expounding "the complicated biologic machinery underlying immunity," Theobald Smith stood revealed to the spellbound audience as a true and worthy successor.

He attained his self-imposed ends with admirable lucidity, drawing upon his unequalled experience with diphtheria bacilli, vaccinia virus, tubercle bacilli, and "*B. suipestifer* or the hog cholera bacillus." He lacked personal familiarity with the anthrax bacillus, but he commented memorably on Pasteur's famous demonstration at Pouilly-le-Fort some forty years before: "Epoch-making discoveries usually happen through a combination of industry, accident, and the rare capacity to seize on the fleeting apparition of success. So it was with anthrax in the hands of Pasteur. No other vaccine has given such definite results."

Smith's general attitude toward his subject was far from conservative. On sexuality among bacteria, for example, he commented: "The discovery of a series of stages in the sporozoa, involving both vegetative and reproductive processes, makes it probable that the parasitic bacteria may not be without similar, even though rudimentary phases." He was also self-confident, and at times bold, in assigning the roles of natural and acquired immunity in the host's resistance or susceptibility; and he emphasized that such factors might play as significant a part as the inherent virulence or toxigenicity of the parasite, in any infectious process. That doctrine, foreshowed in several of his earlier reports, particularly in his recent lecture on parasitism, constitutes the core of his favorite concept—that infection should be considered a manifestation of the host-parasite relationship. In March 1922, Prudden received two copies of Smith's new lecture. He wrote encouragingly: "It is fine and so full of interesting and important points of view . . . that of course we want more copies . . . We ought . . . to have not less than three hundred copies."[55]

The acclaim accorded these occasional lectures on fundamental principles of infection and immunity helped to restore Smith's equanimity. Moreover, since 1919, his theoretic dissertations had been outnumbered by reports about recent personal researches, mostly on bovine contagious abortion, which had obliged him to spend more time in his laboratory. This factor had contributed much to his greater contentment. The new ventures resulted from proximity to the large

Walker-Gordon dairy establishment, and can be traced to early 1916, when he recorded, "Drive to Walker-Gordon in new Ford. Talk over diseases with Jeffers."[56]

Researches on Contagious Bovine Abortion

The pediatrician Emmett Holt, one of the Scientific Directors of the Rockefeller Institute from its inception until his death in 1924, campaigned in the 1890's to improve the safety of New York infants' milk supply. He learned of a similar quest already launched in Boston by the Walker-Gordon Dairy Company. With the financial and moral support of Christian Herter and a group of New York physicians, this company started a branch at Plainsboro, New Jersey. A Milk Commission approved the Walker-Gordon Company's undertaking to supply "certified" milk to the metropolis and several other cities from its dairy farm at Plainsboro. That location was chosen presumably for its good pasturage and convenient railroad connections; and perhaps because New Jersey had pioneered in sponsoring the certified milk movement in the early 1890's.

Throughout the spring of 1915, Theobald Smith was incapacitated with sacro-iliac disease. His appointment had been announced as director-designate of the new Department of Animal Pathology of the Rockefeller Institute. The future site of the necessary buildings had been revealed recently as a 400-acre estate (later increased to around 800 acres) between Princeton and Plainsboro. One day, as he lay there, confined to bed and corseted, silently deploring his disabilities and ruminating on the prolonged celebration following the official engagement two days before of his daughter Lilian to Robert Foerster ("many visitors, many roses"), Smith himself had a visitor: "G.R. Walker of Walker-Gordon calls."[57] Characteristically, Smith wrote nothing about the duration, purpose or outcome of the encounter. Though it was probably only a courtesy visit, senior representatives of future neighboring organizations had at least met.

Preliminary negotiations about the nature and extent of cooperation between the dairy company and the Institute were left to two men, Theobald Smith and Henry W. Jeffers, manager of the dairy at Plainsboro. Jeffers had little grounding in veterinary medicine, or in the public health aspects of milk production and distribution; but he was shrewd and managed daily to dispose profitably of the output of about 1,000 cows. Until June 1918, the Company apparently hoped for some kind of formal "coalition" with the Department,[58] but the Rockefeller Institute's Board of Scientific Directors deferred action when Smith, in characteristic pernickety fashion, doubted that any formal agreement was then prudent.[59] However, Smith's conferences with Jeffers continued.

By the end of World War I, bovine contagious abortion was rampant at the farm. Smith fully appreciated by now the interdependence of the two institutions. Late in 1920, he sent to Prudden, for his and Flexner's consideration, a five-page report on a "Proposed Cooperation Between the Department of Animal Pathology and the Walker-Gordon Laboratories Company in the Prosecution of Research in Bovine Pathology and Dairy Sanitation."[60] The report was based on "a personal inspection of the plant and a study of pathological material during the past 14 months." Smith grouped the problems under two headings, Pathology and Public Health. Pathology was subdivided into nine categories, one of which outweighed in local importance all the others combined, viz. "Diseases of the foetus and the foetal membranes, including what is popularly known as infectious abortion." These diseases would be studied with reference to types of infectious agents, the ways in which infection is carried, and the means of diagnosis. Under Public Health, Smith included "A study of the flora of normal udders and udder ducts, the methods of maintaining a relatively bacteria-free environment during milking . . . and the nature of bacteria which enter the milk during milking time." Also advocated were careful sanitary inspection and interrogation, and routine laboratory testing of all milk handlers. (All the laboratory tests were serological, except for a proposed "study of mouth and throat bacteria.")

Progress on all fronts might best be secured by sharing equally the responsibility for the salary of a well-trained resident veterinarian (who would keep all records), and by an agreement covering the costs of new buildings, apparatus and equipment incidental to the Cooperation. The company would pay for new buildings and all remedial agents; the Institute for research apparatus and supplies. Needed were a new building for the isolation of individual animals, as well as such miscellaneous items as a cheap automobile and surgical instruments. The arrangements would be terminable after due notice by either party.

Both Prudden and Flexner approved the proposals. The latter readily confirmed Smith's recommendation that his department should pay "up to one thousand dollars for one half of the salary of the veterinarian, who will carry out the plan of statistical study set forth in Dr. Smith's memorandum . . . I am very pleased to have work started."[61] Now and again, Theobald Smith and Jeffers discussed some troublesome aspect of their joint venture, e.g., "Confer with Mr. Jeffers about cooperation,"[62] but on the whole, both company and department benefitted from having the health and morbidity records in competent hands, and from the access to abundant research material by trained investigators. The herd was practically tuberculosis-free, and seldom caused anxiety on that account. Besides, as a research field, tuberculosis was no longer so promising. "I don't think there is any gold mine in the investigation of tuberculosis," Smith had advised G.W. McCoy of the U.S. Public Health Service recently, through

Flexner. "It means very hard work and probably very little outcome."[63] On the other hand, bovine contagious abortion was in a different category.

An outbreak of infectious abortion at the Walker-Gordon farm coincided with the entry of the United States into World War I. Smith's daily comments highlighted the story. The entry for April 7, 1917—"War officially declared by Congress"—preceded many references to autopsies of diseased calves, cultures of cows' uterine and fetal tissues, inoculations into guinea pigs, and "thinking about problems." Some of the specimens yielded pure cultures of a spirillum instead of the anticipated *Bacillus abortus* Bang. Between June 1917 and September 1918, the spirillum was isolated in fourteen cases and Bang's bacillus in twenty-seven.[64] By June 1919, an additional twelve strains of the spirillum (twenty-six in all) had been isolated by Smith in pure culture from the placenta, as well as various organs and tissues of aborted fetuses. In only one instance, near the end of the series, was there an apparent case of dual infection with the spirillum and *B. abortus.* He established an etiological relationship of *V. fetus* to bovine abortion by isolating this organism in pure culture from the abortion complex of several cows, and by inducing abortion in two of four pregnant cows injected with spirillary culture intravenously.[65] He later confirmed these results on a larger scale.[66]

Before Smith published these findings, he had noted a British report[67] on abortion in both cattle and sheep, which MacFadyean and Stockman (representing the Committee concerned) attributed to a spirillum whose properties resembled those of the Walker-Gordon isolates. Theobald Smith, who had first reported the microbiological and pathogenic properties of this spirillum in December 1918,[68] within a year, assisted by Marian S. Taylor, extended his observations. They designated this spirillum a new species, *Vibrio fetus,* and showed twenty-four strains to be (with a single exception) agglutinogenically homogeneous.[69] Meanwhile, Smith procured, for comparative purposes, cultures of the spirillum isolated from sheep in England. The results of any such comparative tests were apparently not published.

In the post-War period, December 1918 to March 1923, Theobald Smith published six technical articles (four as sole author) about *Vibrio fetus.* A relatively unimportant seventh paper appeared in 1927, by himself and Marion L. Orcutt. In 100 consecutive cases of abortion in the Walker-Gordon herd, twenty-six (about one-quarter) were due to *V. fetus* while sixty-two, or 57%, were associated with *B. abortus.* Vibrionic abortions affected the older cows. *V. fetus* was never isolated in an aborted first pregnancy, whereas *B. abortus* was involved generally with the first or early pregnancies. Smith attributed the mutual exclusiveness of these two abortion-inducing agents to the higher immunizing efficiency of *B. abortus,* and to the particular system locally adopted for separating or intermingling old and new stock.[70] His studies on vibrionic abortion ceased rather abruptly. The local outbreak was extinct by the end of 1920,[71] and he became preoccupied with other problems.

In contrast to his ephemeral concern with the vibrionic form of bovine abortion, Theobald Smith was frequently involved between 1894 and 1933—four-fifths of his working life—in some aspect of the commonest cause of bovine infectious abortion, *Bacillus abortus* Bang, or in modern terminology, *Brucella abortus*. In the period 1918–1924, four papers were published. The first of these recorded, in fine detail, the observation that the chorionic epithelium serves as a customary habitat for *B. abortus*. His compulsiveness about microscopic observations sometimes led to assertions of excessively dogmatic flavor, such as: "The bacilli do not lie on the cell or in the ectoplasm, but fill the cell body entirely. When the microscope is raised or lowered the cytoplasm appears filled in all optical sections."[72]

The chorion can be invaded by various microorganisms besides the two commonly associated with contagious abortion. In a series of 109 cases affecting the Walker-Gordon herd,[73] Smith noted two in which a pure culture of *Bacillus pyogenes* was isolated from fetal organs. He emphasized that an abortifacient role might be assigned fallaciously to such an organism normally associated with sepsis. However, early in 1920, he reported isolating a mould of the genus *Mucor* from the diseased chorion of a cow, and from the fetal lungs and digestive tract.[74] The general condition of the pregnant uterus, sent intact from a local abattoir, convinced Smith that abortion had been impending.

Many of Theobald Smith's publications of this era were superfluously detailed for most readers. Concern for minutiae in the planning and reporting of experiments typifies much of his work, but became very conspicuous during this post-war revival of laboratory activity. In the first of two papers by Smith on the cultural features and CO_2 requirements of *Br. abortus*, which appeared in August 1924,[75] the reader's patience is at times sorely taxed by the author's mixture of experimental thoroughness and interpretive caution. However, if an audience was known to prefer practicalities, Theobald Smith avoided laboratory details—although it was always difficult for him to unbend in style and manner.

He accepted an invitation from his former associate, Veranus A. Moore, to take part in the Thirteenth Annual Conference for Veterinarians, to be held on January 20, 1921, at Cornell University. Smith's scholarly well-rounded review of infectious abortion in cattle neither swamped the practitioner audience with technicalities nor over-simplified the situation. He prophesied that "The best result and the greatest progress in our knowledge of diseases are attainable only when the practitioner and the laboratory worker are cooperating." And characteristically, he exhorted both laboratory worker and practicing veterinarian to stretch their efforts far beyond their customary reach. Each party should "gather with minute and painstaking care all data accessible with current methods and work them over into a consistent whole to discover in it the residue of fact."[76]

Theobald Smith thoroughly enjoyed his three full days on the familiar campus. Dean Moore hosted a luncheon for him at the University Club on January 30 with several of his faculty and "J.R. Mohler of Wash" (Salmon's successor as Head of the Bureau of Animal Industry). The official lecture on infectious abortion of cattle followed that same afternoon. Next day, Smith addressed about 100 veterinarians banqueting at the Ithaca Hotel on "Research versus Practice." He repeated much of this informal talk on the final day: "All of the staff of the Vet. School at Univ. Club for lunch and I speak again on research teaching & practice."[77] Gage accompanied him almost everywhere. He met the arrival train at 7 A.M., took him to breakfast, and then drove Smith over rough roads to his home across Fall Creek. There he put up the guest for two nights.

In a few years, Theobald Smith's bitter sense of research deprivation had been replaced by a scramble for time and personnel to handle a research renewal. He adjusted well and promptly to the changed situation—he had never minded lab. work all day, including Sundays. Administrative problems often could be settled at departmental staff meetings, only the most prickly issues being referred to New York. Additional duties were delegated to Smillie, and many humdrum diversions avoided by Smith simply intensifying his natural air of Olympian detachment. As for research associates, Grayhill was encouraged to round out his turkey blackhead studies before moving on to greener pastures.[78] Little was trained to become a useful collaborator; and Smith mastered his fear of a "feminized" department to the extent of accepting as laboratory coworkers certain senior female technicians stationed at Princeton, such as Marian Taylor, Laura Florence, and Marion Orcutt. But he still preferred usually to work alone.

Prior to the Cornell visit, Theobald Smith submitted for publication the second of three papers on a pleomorphic microorganism from bronchopneumonia in calves.[79] In the spring of 1917, and again in the fall of 1919, small outbreaks of acute exudative bronchopneumonia (ten and eleven cases, respectively), occurred among the 100 or so calves raised annually in the Walker-Gordon herd. In each outbreak, there were a few fatalities. The other affected animals were killed and autopsied. From the lungs of several of the affected calves, Smith isolated pleomorphic bacillus, which he named *B. acteroides,* from its supposed resemblance to the *Actinomyces* genus. Cultures were harmless to small laboratory animals. However, subcutaneous injection of *B. acteroides* into healthy calves caused extensive local induration ending in necrosis. Intrathecal injections of this bacillus also produced localized indurations and necrosis.

Smith determined the cultural conditions for development of the various phases of this complex microorganism in the laboratory; he also prepared numerous sections, variously stained, for study of the affected tissues. Small clusters of slender, Gram-negative bacilli were noted in the exudate from the cut surface of acutely infected foci. Such areas might yield *Bacillus actinoides* in one of three forms, depending upon the cultural conditions. Grown on agar containing horse serum, *B. actinoides* might develop into bundles of slim, chaining bacilli within "sheathing filaments," which, after several days of incubation, appeared largely replaced by coccoid bodies, interpreted as spores by Smith. In the condensation water of a coagulated horse-serum slope, *Actinomyces*-like flakes developed, comprising chains of bacilli with terminal "clubs."

Any microbiologist, on first encountering a pleomorphic organism such as *B. actinoides,* or the more established *Streptobacillus moniliformis* and its "L" (pleuropneumonia-like) derivative[80] or even a representative of the currently-designated *Mycoplasma* genus, is liable to some degree of shock or incredulity. Despite having pioneered more than thirty years before in his observations of "bacterial variability," Theobald Smith found *Bacillus actinoides* an unavoidable challenge. His consummate technique, experimental ingenuity, and descriptive accuracy were unquestioned and widely acknowledged. According to his day card entries, *B. actinoides* distracted him for several years.

In February 1922, Theobald Smith was still preoccupied with *Vibrio fetus* and *Bacillus actinoides* when Little and Orcutt,[81] of his department, reported that colostrum played an important role in the transfer of antibodies from the dam to her suckling calf. Colostrum—the mammary gland's secretion during the first few hours after parturition—was the vehicle for transferring *Brucella abortus* agglutinins from the immune infected dam to the previously agglutinin-free blood of the new-born calf. Realizing the importance of this observation, Smith teamed up with that enterprising veterinarian, Ralph B. Little, and before the end of 1924, published with him four papers about colostrum; and in his last working years, Smith alone published four reports on this agent.

The first joint paper, which appeared in August 1922, reported a high mortality in calves during the first week of life, unless they received maternal colostrum. Of ten new-born calves allowed to suckle, all survived. Of twelve calves from the same herd who got no colostrum, eight died and two were killed, one being moribund and the other having multiple abscesses. The cause of death in all instances appeared to be a heavy invasion of vital organs by *Bacillus coli.*[82] These authors next sought to verify the inference that if colostrum protected the new-born calf through its mother's circulating antibody content, then the blood serum of a healthy cow should be capable of protecting calves unfortified by suckling.

To test this hypothesis, three groups of five new-born calves were kept isolated and variously treated with blood serum from one healthy cow. All calves were fed on mid-lactation milk from healthy cows. The serum was administered orally in 100 cc. amounts; or in 20 cc. amounts injected subcutaneously, and sometimes intravenously. The copious notes on individual calves only partially compensate for the small numbers of animals used; but it was concluded that the blood serum of a healthy cow, properly administered, can effectively substitute for colostrum. The best results were shown by the group which received serum both by mouth and by injection. All five of these calves survived.[83] Here likewise, the production afforded by the serum in these experiments was against the invasion and multiplication of *B. coli*.

A few months later, Smith and Little supplemented these findings, testing the specific agglutinin levels against *Br. abortus* reached in the blood of new-born calves fed on cow's serum and colostrum, respectively. The donor cow's serum had an artificially-induced high titer of *Br. abortus* agglutinins. The results indicated that colostrum is probably the most efficient transporting agent for such antibodies. However, 500 to 700 cc. of high-titer cow serum taken orally shortly after birth can serve protectively, especially if reinforced by subcutaneous and intravenous injections of the serum.[84]

The last in this series of dual-authorship reports on colostrum, sought an explanation for the proteinuria in new-born calves following the feeding of colostrum, or noted at autopsy during the first week of life. The extra permeability of the kidneys was a temporary aberration, associated with the ingestion of colostrum.[85] About half-way through the foregoing series of reports, Marion Orcutt joined the other two authors in a complex inquiry into the source of *Brucella abortus* agglutinins in cow's milk. Although the experimental data are too detailed, and the tentative explanations too wide-ranging for discussion here, the justifiable conclusion seems to be that the udder actively participates in the production of *Br. abortus* agglutinins when that gland is invaded by living, or flooded by dead, bacteria.[86]

These researches showed that colostrum effectively protected the new-born calf against a natural hazard—a generalized invasion by *B. coli*, commonly fatal during the first week of life. Colostrum, or alternatively, cow's serum with a high titer of *Br. abortus* agglutinins, proved an efficient vehicle for transferring this antibody to the calf. But a high titer of specific agglutinins alone did not ensure invulnerability of heifers to Bang's disease; so Smith and Little investigated the possibility of developing a vaccine to protect heifers against infectious abortion due to *Brucella abortus*. In the first of two papers, Smith and Little demonstrated that partial protection during the first pregnancy was afforded by four injections of a heat-killed vaccine. Superior results were obtained from a single injection of live vaccine prepared from a culture of relatively low virulence.[87] Their findings led elsewhere to the selection of a strain of *Br. abortus* of low virulence and high immunogenic properties, which now has international acceptance in the manufacture of the vaccine.

The generous reception of Theobald Smith's doctrines about infection and immunity, and the satisfaction brought by his recent outpouring of researches on cattle diseases, were not lost upon Simon Flexner. The two men had mutual respect, but each was jealous of his own prerogatives, and their egos were not soothed by the same balm. Neither was content with the *status quo*. Smith prepared a fifteen-page report (double-spaced typing) apparently for presentation at the April 1923 meeting of the Board of Scientific Directors. Entitled "Suggestions Concerning Directions of Growth of the Department of Animal Pathology in the Near Future," it told that "the work of the Department to date has been largely governed by environment and opportunity."[88]

The Directors were reminded that the Department had operated on the assumption that its "greatest field of usefulness . . . lay in research into the diseases of domestic animals." They were further informed that this policy had found favor, and formed "a bulwark behind which the less practical and more fundamental" aspects of pathology might be pursued. Animal pathology had been divided into specialties, the foremost being diseases of "domesticated animals useful to man as producers of food and raw material for clothing." Recently recognized hazards affecting marine and fresh water (aquatic) fauna included "the pouring of poisons from industrial plants into streams."

Another form of specialization among animal pathologists was now indicated; namely, that each host species had its own pattern of disease susceptibility. "Hitherto the rapid expansion of microbiology and parasitology has placed the emphasis too much on the parasite, whereas the determining factors towards disease rest largely with the host." Local circumstances had dictated that no attempt be made "to extend the researches beyond cattle." The concentration of effort upon known cattle problems had revealed unexpected complexities, e.g., *V. fetus* as a causal parasite in bovine abortion; the immunological significance of colostrum; and the udder as a locus for the production of agglutinins. Swine and poultry problems—the latter particularly suited to women—should be similarly approached.

The criticism that "such a heterogeneous mass as the different diseases of one species" should not be brought together in a single division was dismissed on the grounds that the "etiological grouping" had been in vogue for over forty years and it was time for a regrouping based on host species. The development of special fields in nutrition, genetics, morphology, cytology, immunology, protozoology, and, "in reproduction," should come "*after* the divisions of porcine, avian and ovine pathology have been organized and manned." To secure interdivisional cooperation would "be the most important duty of the director."

According to Smith, his main proposal promoted *comparative* pathology, which "assumes the underlying oneness of cell processes in different species." Study of the reaction to injury of the lower forms also facilitates "tracing the evolution of protective mechanisms in higher animals." Under the proposed plan, "the temporary exhaustion of local material for study" raises questions of cooperation with similar institutions, to ensure a continued, balanced research program. Smith outlined the resources of existing organizations concerned with animal diseases.

The National Research Council supplied figures for State Experiment Stations and Agricultural Colleges as well as for the National Bureau of Animal Industry. Total annual expenditures (exclusive of salaries and plant maintenance) were $277,166.00, of which the B.A.I. accounted for $122,000.00 or 44%. The comparable total for the Rockefeller Institute's Department of Animal Pathology was between $25,000 and $30,000. The chair of comparative pathology at Harvard Medical School had funds for "purchase of animals and material and assistance," largely from donations, amounting to "a few thousand dollars" each year. Apart from the excellent work carried out in research institutes in South Africa and East Prussia, there was nothing significant elsewhere to report.

Such meager fiscal allotments reflect the fact that "economic considerations dominate all transactions with animals. Again, animal pathology is of value in so far as it reduces pecuniary losses due to disease;" and the ultimate beneficiaries, the farmers and livestock owners, are "primarily interested in productivity." In human medicine, on the other hand, "the high value placed upon health and life . . . has built up between medical research and the community a highly trained class of medical practitioners and efficient health organizations . . . through which new ideas percolate with amazing rapidity." By contrast, "in the domain of animal pathology, the distributing apparatus is as yet poorly organized, and the receptive attitude only partially developed;" and there was not a single independent periodical in the field.

The Report was, in some respects, disappointing. Quotable phrases, often so candidly critical as almost to command reform, were weakened by verbiage and anticlimactic conclusions. According to Theobald Smith, "The work to be done is to take certain diseases, examine existing literature, study such diseases *de novo* and present the results monographically. The unexpected problems which invariably arise during such work can be dealt with at the same time." This plan had been followed exactly by Smith himself for the past few years. His suggestions regarding the crucial recruitment of suitable staff were no more novel or uplifting. "The only method for obtaining young men of the training indicated is for the Institute to find promising young men and direct the training into the desired channels."

Data bearing on the Report's submission and reception are scant and inconclusive. Smith's day card of April 9, 1923 records two hours set aside for "Rep. on Dept for Directors." The Report received attention for a further three hours on October 6, six months later. About then, meetings of the Board were liable to postponement because of illness or death among the membership. Some meetings were held with only four Directors present. Items might be withdrawn from the agenda if the attendance were less than anticipated. The Report's presentation was thus probably delayed for several weeks after its completion.

Suddenly and unexpectedly (but with Flexner's approval) Theobald Smith took off for the United Kingdom, taking his wife with him on what proved to be his last overseas mission. They left New York on November 3 and returned to Princeton on December 18. The main purposes of this trip will be outlined separately. Meanwhile, the Report on near-term growth for the Department of Animal pathology lay dormant.

An important clue to the date of presentation or release of the Report is revealed by an entry in Simon Flexner's own diary for Sunday, January 20, 1924, relating to events of the previous day. "Bd. of Sc. Directors v. much disorganized. Dr. S. negative. Neglected to mention discussion of reorganization plan of Dr. S's at Princeton." Flexner wrote to Welch that he had been perhaps "too harsh" with Smith at the meeting. He had accordingly telephone Princeton on Sunday morning to convey his apologies; but Smith had seemed "not offended." Smith's own day card for that day, January 19, was unruffled, "Leave early for N.Y. Quarterly meeting of Directors—only 4 present. Lunch with members of Institute. Meeting continues till 4.30." But only three days before, on January 16, Smith had gone to New York, to attend an all-morning meeting of Directors of the National Tuberculosis Association. An Executive Committee meeting of the Rockefeller Institute's Scientific Directors was held in the late afternoon at Prudden's home. Perhaps the Report was unveiled then, with discussion deferred until the next quarterly meeting.

25

LAST EUROPEAN JOURNEY
BACILLUS ABORTUS AND BACILLUS MELITENSIS
CONTINUING RESEARCHES AND
PUBLICATIONS

Theobald Smith seems to have been secretive about his fifth and last over-seas journey to Europe. When he and his wife boarded the S.S. *Rotterdam* on November 3, 1923, they had kept quiet about their plans for fifteen weeks. At Silver Lake, on July 18, he had received an invitation from J. Lorain Smith, Dean of the Faculty of Medicine at Edinburgh University, to deliver an address at the Centenary Celebration of the founding of the Edinburgh Veteri-nary College by William Dick. The University and College jointly wished to arouse public interest in the "important domain of Comparative Pathology." The latter's final sentence appealed irresistibly: "I trust you may see your way to ac-cede to the very cordial invitation of the University and the College to aid us in the advance of the Department of Science with which your name is so conspicu-ously and so indissolubly associated."[1]

Smith found Flexner summering a few miles away and secured his approval. In accepting the invitation, he requested advice about the address and about clothing.

> I shall be sixty four years this month. I have never been robust and my capacity to make myself understood to a large audience is somewhat limited . . . I expect to

be accompanied by Mrs. Smith. We will take this journey as a vacation in place of a European trip projected for next year . . . We are assuming that warm clothing will be needed, but it is easy to go to extremes . . . I am accustomed to protect myself here during the winter with a fur lined overcoat.[2]

By the time the voyagers embarked, the Centenary plans in Edinburgh had expanded. Everyone was plainly delighted at Theobald Smith's acceptance. The University wanted his address to be delivered under its official auspices, and in due course Principal Sir Alfred Ewing presided. "We shall arrange to have the Address in a room of the size you wish," wrote Lorain Smith. "As to clothing, you will realise that . . . in winter we wear warm underclothing even in the house. A fur lined overcoat would be suitable."[3] The visitors would stay at Dr. and Mrs. F.G. Nasmyth's comfortable home. Nasmyth was Vice-Chairman of the Board of Management of the Veterinary College. Finally, Sir Robert Philip (President of the Tuberculosis Society of Scotland, of the Medico-Chirurgical Society of Edinburgh, and also of the Royal College of Physicians of Edinburgh) invited him to address the two first-named Societies on tuberculosis, and to dine with himself and some Royal College and University colleagues in the Physicians' Hall, on dates to be arranged.

The Smiths thus knew they faced a heavy program for two or three days in Edinburgh. Since Theobald had not written a word of his Address, time must be found *en route* for that. The voyage started auspiciously. They passed the inbound *Leviathan,* and then the *Majestic* "with Lloyd George on board." But overnight the sea became choppy, the boat began to pitch, and Lilian took to bed (for two days). Theobald assumed daily shipboard habits—four hours of writing, and three to four miles of brisk walking. The wet and foggy weather cleared in time for a glimpse of the Scilly Isles early on the eighth day. That afternoon a tender landed them at Plymouth. They stayed overnight at the "cold and chilly" Grand Hotel, explored the Hoe and the Pilgrims' Landing, and entrained for Paddington.

Five days were spent in London in a succession of cold hotel rooms, shopping expeditions, work on the address, and a good luncheon at the University Club with Sir Walter Fletcher, who had directed the Medical Research Council since 1920. On November 17, they left for Cambridge, where some mutual scientific interests and friendships helped to warm things up. On Sunday, November 18, they lunched with Sir Hugh Anderson and family, and then went on to King's College Chapel, where they shivered on the hard, cold choir stalls through the service. To fulfil social obligations, they took tea with Sir Clifford and Lady Allbutt, and called on Lady Woodhead (widow of Sir G. Sims Woodhead) and Lady Anderson. Theobald, now freed to seek whom and what he wanted, saw plenty of Henry J. Dean, Professor of Pathology, and of G.H.F. Nuttall; met Griffith, still working on the tubercle bacillus; visited the "field laboratories"— numerous small, brick animal houses and adjacent small laboratories; and finally, talked shop with the Master of Gonville and Caius College, Sir Hugh Anderson, and with "Prof. Wood & Dr. Buxton, on the new Dept. of Compar. Pathol. Then luncheon in Caius Hall with them & Dr. Allbutt . . . then home & start a fire."[4] Whenever opportunity offered, Theobald worked on his Address, and had nearly straightened things out before leaving Cambridge for Edinburgh via York on November 24.

They caught a tantalizing view of Lincoln Cathedral's three towers from the train; whereas throughout the two-night stay at York's Royal Station Hotel it was so "hoary and foggy" that the Minster was almost invisible at any hour. Their room was just under the roof, so icy that the coal fire made no impression. During the first night, Theobald got quite panicky: "fail to warm up, rapid pulse, fear of pneumonia, all right towards morning."[5] They left for Edinburgh on the morning of November 26, arriving after lunch. Nasmyth drove them to the Morningside suburbs "to a beautiful new house in a large garden, enclosed with a stone wall. Central heating & electric stove in room. Tea & dinner at home."[6]

The Nasmyths thoughtfully left the travellers to themselves until the afternoon of Tuesday, November 27. Then, after a quick breakfast and a brisk walk, Theobald huddled for a long last look over his Address, by now entitled "Comparative Pathology: Its Biological and Economic Significance." He avoided the distraction of the first social gathering of the Centenary, an "At Home" held in the early afternoon at the Veterinary College by the Principal, Dr. Channock Bradley. Here Sir John MacFadyean, in the presence of a distinguished company of citizens and visitors, presented to the College a portrait of its founder, William Dick. This was a gift from Dr. Duncan McEachran, who had established in Montreal a famous Veterinary College, later affiliated with McGill University. Unfortunately, Dr. McEachran was too ill to travel.

The visitors from North America were fetched by limousine around 4:15 and brought to the Medical School, where they were met by Prof. J. Lorain Smith, and introduced to the Principal of the University, Sir James Ewing, and Dr. Channock Bradley. This welcoming committee had escaped from the "At Home." The address was delivered in the anatomic amphitheater to a responsive audience of 200 to 300. *The Scotsman* reported next day that "Professor Smith had a most enthusiastic reception." His own comment was less effusive: "Got through pretty well & talk well rec'd by the students."[7]

The Chairman introduced their guest as the leading authority in comparative pathology. In an eloquent and thought-provoking address, Theobald Smith expanded the scope and enhanced the prestige of that subject. His own forty years' contributions were so modestly cloaked that listeners were both charmed and edified. He reviewed historically the evolution of pathology into human and animal divisions, with comparative pathology an important though somewhat nebulous off-shoot of the latter. Smith's own role would be that of the research worker (discovery of new facts) rather than that of the better-known educator (acceptance and assimilation). The early pathologist, who used his unaided senses to examine the sick body, was "a naturalist of the world of disease." With development of the microscope and the emergence of the precision-minded bacteriologist and the other specialists, he became a laboratory worker; but the pathologist's main task has remained the study of the diseased body, with the primary object of discovering causal or contributory factors. A subsidiary function persists "to supply the raw material of important discoveries to the vigorous, younger specialties."

Animal pathology covers diseases of wild mammals and birds, insects and aquatic life, as well as of domesticated livestock. In the early days of domestication, diseases may have been latent because natural selection reduced virulence and raised resistance. This equilibrium generally persists in the wild, but is easily upset by various types of human intervention, such as herding and forced migrations. Interplay between wild and domesticated mammals and birds, on pastures and poultry yards, may also disturb the balance between host and parasite, causing an epizootic. Some of the disease-promoting mechanisms are very complex, e.g., more than one parasite, or a combination of improper diet and parasite, may be required to cause a virulent outbreak.

A major difficulty in animal pathology stems from the fact that the livestock owner is highly sensitive to profit and loss considerations. Economic factors that may influence the susceptibility of domesticated animals to disease cover a wide range—from deliberate breeding for better yields of milk and butterfat, or eggs, or meat protein, regardless of the consequences in terms of hardiness, to the increased risks of importing diseased cattle or poultry into the larger herds and flocks now being established further from city land. Despite great progress in pathology, many problems remain which may yield solutions to the animal pathologist through the advantage denied to the human pathologist, the ability to examine the *diseased* body at any chosen stage of the disease. The *dead* carcass often yields little and sometimes misleading information.

Among humanitarian contributions of animal pathology are the direct control of diseases transmissible from animals to man, notably rabies, anthrax, glanders, and tuberculosis. More valuable, in Smith's view, would be the knowledge gained from researches into the disease processes provoked in different animal species by the same parasite, e.g. the "natural" paratyphoid diseases of small mammals. If variable and unknown factors were reduced to a minimum, and assuming the underlying cell processes to be similar for all host species, animal and comparative pathology could merge with marked benefit to human pathology.

The animal pathologist's obligations should include applying conservative methods of controlling the parasitic agents which human exploitation has often encouraged to spread among the local fauna. Of the measures available, preventive mass vaccination is the one most favored, but has an inherent weakness: "the highly susceptible are not protected, and the highly resistant do not need vaccination." Two animal diseases were being eradicated in the United States by governmental decree—Texas fever and tuberculosis. In the former, all cattle are dipped to destroy ticks, the only vector. In tuberculosis, all cattle giving a positive tuberculin reaction are slaughtered. Whatever the remedy or preventive measure adopted, it must pay for itself with some form of aid from public funds, and must leave the animal with health and vigor unimpaired.

In human medicine by contrast, everything may be done to save a life, irrespective of its value and regardless of costs. The stock owner should be educated in the principles underlying disease, to the point of understanding at least that the health of his animals cannot be maintained or restored on a cost-free basis. Meanwhile, research in animal pathology goes on. Theobald Smith concluded his Address by proclaiming what he considered the proper job specifications for his favorite specialty: "To draw capable men into animal pathology presupposes adequate remuneration, permanency, and a standing not below that of the workers engaged in the investigation of human diseases."[8]

His main task accomplished, Theobald was ready to attend the social events for which they had official invitations. On the evening of the 27th, he and Lilian, with over 200 other guests, attended an 8 P.M. Reception at the City Chambers, where they were warmly welcomed by the Lord Provost, Magistrates and Council of the City of Edinburgh. The Lord Provost (The Right Hon. W.L. Sleigh) and the Councillors wore their civic robes. A high-class program of light music, instrumental and vocal, was provided; and the murals depicting episodes of Scottish history were interpreted.

The next morning, they were driven by Mrs. Nasmyth first to Holyrood, and then to the Veterinary College for the noon-time William Dick Oration by Sir John MacFadyean, under the chairmanship of the Duke of Atholl. The Chairman introduced Sir John as the most illustrious Dick College alumnus. The orator reviewed the history of veterinary science, emphasizing the contributions of William Dick. Among many unsolved problems was foot-and-mouth disease, which had been ravaging Great Britain. Theobald Smith had processed in academic robes to the stage, where he found himself seated beside the University Principal. That evening, a Reunion Dinner was held in the Hall of the Royal College of

Surgeons, where a large company of eminent men dined together, under the chairmanship of The Right Hon. Lord Forteviot. Many fine after-dinner speeches were made. Theobald Smith was seated next to the Lord Provost and spoke on the Rockefeller Institute.

The main events of the two-day Centenary Celebrations were followed by a fund-raising bazaar on each of the three succeeding afternoons. They were officially opened each day, the first on November 29 by Field Marshal Earl Haig; the second on November 30 by the Duchess of Atholl; and the third on December 1 by Lady Craig of Ulster. Earl Haig extolled the splendid contribution of the Veterinary Corps during the war. He launched the campaign to raise the sum of £10,000 to institute a post-graduate Fellowship as a permanent memorial of the College. The Smiths attended the opening of the first day's bazaar. Theobald had already spontaneously offered to relinquish the honorarium of £100 (which Lorain Smith had written "attaches to the Address") and had suggested the sum "should be applied to some purpose in connection with the subject of Comparative Pathology." But in a subsequent note, the offer had been courteously rejected: "This proposal is altogether too generous, and we would be glad if you would allow the arrangement to stand."[9] Nevertheless, family legend has the honorarium transferred to some worthy educational purpose.

After listening sympathetically to Earl Haig's speech, Theobald had one last obligation to fulfill: "4.15 go to College of Physicians & give an extempore address on tuberculosis chiefly historical & comparative. Then back to dress for dinner given by Sir Robt. Philip at the same place in my honor. Sit at right of Sir Robt. & on left of Prof. Ellinger, Copenhagen, Dir. of vet. school. Do a little speaking after dinner."[10] His remarks on tuberculosis were synopsized in the *Edinburgh Medical Journal.*[11]

Although Theobald Smith reported nothing new in his address, his audience might well have been impressed by the privilege of hearing perhaps the world's greatest expert on tuberculosis review the highlights of this widespread plague. Smith's reported reactions to some of Koch's work are noteworthy. First, he praised unstintedly Koch's 1882 report on the discovery of the tubercle bacillus. "No bacteriological research work since then has been carried out in a more thorough and systematic manner." Secondly, Koch took too long to acknowledge Smith's personal disclosure, twelve years before, that he had differentiated two types of tubercle bacilli, human and bovine. Smith's exasperation at this cavalier treatment, seldom revealed, here becomes apparent. "When the speaker visited Koch in 1896, he suggested to him that all tubercle bacilli were not the same, and Koch acknowledged at the Washington meeting in 1908 that he had got the idea from the speaker, but this never appeared in any of the publications subsequently."[12]

Leaders of the medical profession in Scotland were most favorably impressed by Theobald Smith: for at an Extraordinary Meeting of the Royal College of Physicians of Edinburgh held on February 5, 1924, "the motion previously blessed by the Council, was acclaimed unanimously by the Fellows," that he be offered the Honorary Fellowship of the College on account of "eminent services to medical science." Sir Robert Philip, in his handwritten letter, added that the list of Honorary Fellows, currently totaling nineteen, included the names of Edward Jenner, William Welch, Emile Roux, Shihasaburo Kitasato, and Jules Bordet.[13] Sir Robert also wrote a very warm, almost poetic, farewell note:

> In the stress of busy . . . days, it is pleasing when the breeze wafts some of the bouquet of the spiritual life . . . I am happy to think that it may perhaps be my good fortune to greet you on your side of the ferry in 1926, when . . . the International union against Tuberculosis will meet somewhere near your home and be presided over by yourself. The absolute unanimity of choice on the part of your colleagues when the question of Presidency presented itself, cannot but be a pleasing foretaste of the judgement of history.[14]

Other tokens of appreciation included conferment of the honorary degree of LL.D. by the University of Edinburgh. This was approved by the University Senate in 1924, but the laureation was postponed in the hope that a return visit might soon be made. Ten years later, when Smith reluctantly decided he could not revisit Edinburgh, the Secretary to the University notified him that the degree would be awarded *in absentia*.[15] Within six months of this interchange, Theobald Smith had died.

On November 30, Theobald and Lilian felt they had no further call on the kind hospitality of the Nasmyths during the remaining week of their stay in Edinburgh; so they took their leave and went to a private hotel. It was penetratingly cold, in spite of keeping the fire going all night. The citizens of Edinburgh have a very profound sense of history, and the Smiths found these days full of interest through visits to friends sandwiched between pilgrimages to monuments, relics and sites. On Sunday, December 2, they lunched at the home of Prof. J. Lorain Smith on Carlton Terrace, meeting his three daughters and one son. He took them through the private gardens of several terraces on Carlton Hill to get a fine view of Nelson's Monument. Then they proceeded to Sir David Wallace's house on Charlotte Square for tea.

On December 3, Smith visited the laboratories of the Royal College of Physicians, where he was shown some research projects; and on the 4th, Prof. Ashworth at the University produced memorabilia of Darwin and Lister, and manuscripts of Burns and Carlyle. Then they both had tea with the Nasmyths, to whom they said grateful goodbyes. On December 5, Lady Wallace took them by limousine to the Firth of Forth Bridge, and back by way of the Zoo to a Women's Club on Charlotte Square for lunch. Lilian was then taken to a Faculty Women's Tea while Theobald was guided around the Veterinary College. The last full day in Edinburgh was spent in shopping and resting, "chilled and tired out by the cold sharp air and the strolling."

On December 7, they took the east coast train for King's Cross, and arrived in the early evening, "the air full of fog & mist & landscape obscured." They taxied to a hotel in "Buckingham Palace Rd. just opp. the Royal Mews. Room with a small radiator, temp about 58°F." During the next brief days of shopping and loafing, the two republicans walked twice around the Royal Palace and Gardens. On December 11, Theobald set out early for the National Institute for Medical Research at Hampstead. Henry Dale, who was in charge, took him to see various workers. Next day they left after breakfast for Waterloo Station, whence a special train brought them to Southampton Wharf, where they boarded the *Berengaria,* a large German prize-of-war with many amenities. The liner sidestepped to pick up some passengers at Cherbourg, and an uneventful crossing ended on the afternoon of the sixth day. After fretting for two hours on the pier waiting for baggage & trunks inspection, they "see Phil & Dorothy who help us to get off to Pr. after a supper at Sta. Dr. Smillie waiting at Jc. House heated up & water turned on, etc. comfortable night on porch."[16]

As usual, Theobald slept soundly on his porch bed that first night back from Edinburgh. Philip sometimes wondered at his father's spiritual resilience and objectivity, his ability to appraise calmly, without bias, assorted problems that most businessmen would avoid or find unbearable. In view of his impatient yearnings to resume laboratory researches, this equanimity was paradoxical. Theobald Smith believed, according to his son Philip, that such inner conflicts might be resolved, or held in check, by efforts of the will—"the human will is the strongest force in the universe." Lilian Smith observed that sometimes his absorption in a problem seemed impenetrable.

When he returned to Princeton, after an absence of six or seven weeks, his outlook began to change. Edinburgh was noted for its rich sense of history and kind hospitality, but not for spurious enthusiasms. Those Scots had made him humbly aware of his world leadership in animal pathology, and especially in tuberculosis. Within the Rockefeller organization, the lines of communication grew blurred as old friends and colleagues died or retired; and the rate of recruitment seemed extravagant. Without feeling disloyal, Smith began to ponder his own retirement. After all, he was in his sixty-fifth year, his health was not robust, and he had served the Institute in a senior capacity for over twenty years. Some months later, he actually raised the question of his retirement at a meeting of the Board of Scientific Directors: "My retirement discussed and turned down temporarily," was his curt Day Book entry.[17]

Although Theobald Smith no longer pined for the laboratory, there were, nonetheless, still some left over problems he wanted to tackle, while others had arisen because shedding light on an obscure question often cast new shadows. He would get busy in his laboratory soon. Meanwhile, he would allow himself to brood a little. A famous fellow scientist had died (Samuel Meltzer, 1920) and another would soon pass on (Jacques Loeb, February, 1924). Death was also invading the ranks of the original Scientific Directors. At the end of June 1923, he had attended the funeral of Hermann Biggs—his organ-playing rival at Cornell—and in 1924, two more of them died—Mitchell Prudden in April and Emmett Holt in May. Prudden's special relationship with Smith warrants commemoration. They had known and admired each other for over thirty years.

Theophilus Mitchell Prudden (1849–1924), fourth son of a Congregational clergyman, was the oldest and most popular of the Institute's Board of Scientific Directors. William Welch, a close friend and fellow bachelor, was about one year younger, while Theobald Smith was his junior by ten years and Simon Flexner by seventeen. This remarkably kind, sensitive and talented man was a pioneer pathologist, an ardent apostle of public health, and a distinguished authority on the archaeology of the cliff-dwelling ancestors of the Navajos and kindred tribes of the North American Southwest. The Rockefeller Institute was indeed fortunate to have enjoyed Prudden's allegiance since its inception. His felicitous command of the English language is already apparent in the note of thanks he sent to Theobald Smith for some culture "bulbs," shortly after the Texas fever monograph appeared in 1893: "I should think you justified in being very proud of your work," Prudden wrote, "I am, anyhow, and admire the courage and cleverness which has already given us many good things."[18] Subsequently, as colleagues on the Board of Directors of the Rockefeller Institute for Medical Research, Prudden and Smith often worked together as an advisory subcommittee of the Board. They were usually in accord and dispensed sound advice. The older man sized up the other as taking his job and himself too somberly, jeopardizing his health by unremittent effort. Many a serious memorandum ended with a gentle chuckle or a whimsy of corrective advice.

For example, near the end of the War, he writes: "I don't a bit like your plan to go over into the winter without any sort of reasonable vacation break. I do not think anybody does well on that sort of plan. While your men are still there, why don't you pike off, if only for a week or ten days, and go back to the job with a fresh view. These are the golden days in this country;" and he added by way of encouragement, his observation that "No one man related to the Institute . . . has made a contribution comparable to your own."[19] The War being over, Alexis

Carrel returned. Smith was bedridden when he read Prudden's recent news: "We hear that Carrel's steamer is docking this morning, so I suppose we shall have some fresh problems in the way of experimental surgery. I hope Mrs. Smith has hidden your clothes, so that you will not be able to get up until the rest of them say so."[20]

The War Demonstration Hospital was to be demolished or otherwise disposed of. Prudden had been urging Smith to transfer parts of it to Princeton. "Wouldn't they make good shelters for many purposes on a farm? We might get them for nothing. One of the smaller ones when taken down in panels would pack in a big truck. Say what and say quick lest the cat jump and catch us unaware."[21] Four months later: "The fate of the poor old War Demolition Hospital is apparently not yet clear . . . I am grieved to hear that you are going back to the job too soon. You surely haven't had time for the vacation benefits to soak in properly as yet."[22] When the newspapers announced that Harvard University had awarded the Flattery Medal and $500 to Theobald Smith, Prudden wrote: "I see by the papers that you have lots of money these days. Perhaps you would lend a fellow a couple of bucks if he got hard up. At any rate, show us the Medal and receive our felicitations."[23]

Prudden had been unwell himself. "Now don't go working hard this summer; the country is too fine not to use it for its own said."[24] When Theobald was laid up again with sacro-iliac trouble, Prudden could not resist once more giving him a piece of advice:

> We have been watching your career as an invalid with great interest . . . But if you will let a hoary old sage like me give you a bit of counsel from experience, it is that for most folks it is a mighty good thing to round up a convalescence not by just plumb going to work but by a little change of scene, like Atlantic City, for three or four days. Why don't you do it? I'll bet you a new hat of the latest style that it would do you a lot of good.[25]

Soon after his return to Princeton in late December 1923, Theobald Smith sought out Prudden in his Institute office, and was relieved to find him at work, diminished in vigor, but with mental acuity unimpaired. Meetings of the Executive Committee were held in the New Year as usual, at Prudden's New York apartment. On March 14, 1924, the two old friends lunched together at the Institute. On April 12, Theobald noted in his Day Card: "Go to Prudden's funeral in the assembly room at the Institute. The heart has failed quietly during the night."[26] John D. Rockefeller, Jr. had assured Prudden, in a letter written during his last illness, that "No man related to the Institute . . . has made a contribution comparable to your own."[27]

"Scours," *B. Coli,* and Colostrum

Shortly before leaving for Scotland, Theobald Smith had submitted for publication two papers on the bacteriology of the intestinal tract of young calves and on the disease "Scours." Originating out of his studies on colostrum, both appeared in print at the beginning of January 1925 in the same issue of the *Journal of Experimental Medicine.* In the first, under his sole authorship, entitled, "Hydropic Changes in the Intestinal Epithelium of New-Born Calves,"[28] Smith described vacuolation of the epithelium of the lower intestine, originating in the late intrauterine life of the fetal calf. The vacuoles became more abundant during the first twenty-four hours after birth, and then began to disappear, until very few remained by the end of the third day. The dropsical epithelium contained coagulable protein. The process was apparently not connected with "scours," a diarrhea affecting calves during the first few days of life caused by a septicemia infection through the umbilical chord, which might occur with or without such changes. The second paper, coauthored with Marion Orcutt, attempted to correlate the bacteriology of the intestinal tract of young calves with the development of early diarrhea.[29] The intestinal flora was methodically investigated in a large number of young calves, all from the same herd, grouped according to the extent they showed evidence of "scours," in a range from healthy animals to calves recently dead from this disease. The authors concluded that "scours" was a local manifestation of *B. coli* septicemia; that this potential pathogen was probably present normally in small numbers at all intestinal levels; but that in the event of a disequilibrium between *B. coli* and such inhibitory factors as colostrum intake, the numbers of living bacilli might increase locally and "carpet" (his description) the intestine to the duodenum. The possible occurrence of especially toxigenic strains of *B. coli* remained to be investigated.

Two publications dealing directly with colostrum then followed. In mid-January 1925, Smith addressed the 17th Annual Conference of Veterinarians at the New York State Veterinary College, Cornell University. His review of colostrum[30] was of the same fine quality as was his address on bovine infectious abortion to the 13th Conference, four years earlier. He also spoke informally to a large gathering of professors and students on the nature and needs of research. Dean Veranus Moore arranged a lunch for him and staff members, and President L. Ferrand gave a very pleasant dinner in his honor. Professor George L. Burr served as genial go-between. Simon Gage was unavoidably away.

In 1922, Theobald Smith and associates had demonstrated the life-saving properties of specific antibodies in colostrum against microbic hazards, especially *B. coli.* In a solo paper completed in 1925, "Focal Interstitial Nephritis in the Calf following Interference with the Normal Intake of Colostrum,"[31] Smith now attributed "white spotted kidney" in young calves to a virulent strain of *B. coli* following and resulting from colostrum deprivation. The deficiency of colostrum could be induced by mere postponement of feedings for from twenty-four to thirty-six hours. When colostrum was withheld totally, very few calves survived their first week of life.

Counterattractions

Smith's researches were interrupted by the intrusion of new duties. Extra responsibilities occasionally arose because he was the foremost survivor among senior staff members qualified to administer, at least temporarily, the Rockefeller Institute's complex affairs. When Simon Flexner journeyed to the Middle East in 1925, Smith was appointed Acting Chairman of the Board of Scientific Directors. Again, when illness forced Welch's resignation from the Board in October 1933, Smith was nominated to succeed him as its President.

Another type of diversion arose because Theobald Smith felt he must uphold his reputation for preeminence in knowledge of tuberculosis and of bovine contagious abortion. Notwithstanding his outward modesty, self-esteem was abundant. His future duties as incumbent President of the International Union against Tuberculosis, and as President-Elect of the National Tuberculosis Association, presented no small challenge. Incidentally, he had been elected to the International Union's presidency at its Philadelphia meeting in 1921. The first inkling of the other honor came from a friendly emissary in July 1925: "Dr. Hatfield, Lilian and I lunch at Martha's Kitchen. Dr. H. . . . informs me of my election to Presidency of the American Tuberculosis Society."[32] He foresaw countless meetings to chair and train journeys to endure, as well as repeated attempts to reconcile the clinician's efforts with those of public health and the laboratory.

Smith's discomfiture and fatigue were hidden with composure and dignity. For example, in September 1925, the National Tuberculosis Association met for two days at Lansing, Michigan. After the Executive Committee had completed the business of the morning session, Theobald was the luncheon guest of three local clubs—with "Singing & rapid eating"—before returning to the afternoon executive session. Next day, after exploring the State Health Department Laboratories, and listening to some of the Mississippi Valley Tuberculosis Society's papers, he attended the evening reunion, when "all members driven to Country Club, where a banquet of 250 men & women is staged. Singing & eating . . . Introduced & audience rises. Speak a few desultory words."[33] He then left to catch a midnight train. One other example must suffice. Late in November 1925, Theobald left home early for New York to attend three days of conferences with the delegates of various Tuberculosis Associations and the Milbank Fund. He resented the time-wasting habits of these representatives, and was tempted to spurn their routine expressions of goodwill, their windy speeches and costly hospitality at the Biltmore Hotel. By contrast, near the end of his visit, a select committee settled in three hours all of the main issues of the coming year's International Union program and "foreign guest invitations."[34]

During the week beginning September 28, 1926, Smith was headquartered at the Mayflower Hotel in Washington. The two meetings—the International Union against Tuberculosis and the National Tuberculosis Association—were separated by Sunday, October 3, which he spent with Paul Howe and his wife. Howe, a friendly member of Smith's staff, drove his chief over to inspect the Beltsville plant of the U.S. Department of Agriculture. The International meeting had many absentees, including Sir Robert Philip. It opened on September 30, with an address of Welcome by U.S. Treasury Secretary Andrew W. Mellon, with Theobald's presidential address following. Secretary Mellon hosted a luncheon-reception on the opening day. The Union's program covered three themes: 1, Secondary infection in adults; 2, Tuberculosis from Beginning to Cavitation (one speaker held forth for two-and-a-half hours on this theme); and 3, Milk and Tuberculosis. In the afternoon of the final day the attendees were taken by bus to Mt. Vernon and Arlington. They returned for a farewell dinner, with toastmaster and numerous speeches.

Theobald's presidential address, entitled "Remarks on the Cooperation of Science and Practice in Tuberculosis," was a model of pertinence and literary elegance.[35] "We are here to devise new and strengthen old defenses against the tubercle bacillus," he reminded the audience. "We are assured by the history of science that our differences will be ironed out . . . and that the final results cannot be successfully disguised by propaganda, negatived by legal enactments, or exploited for personal gain. The truth will come to light. Whatever is accomplished is for the benefit of humanity in its broadest dimensions." Noteworthy also was a charitable reference to Robert Koch's part in the 1908 International Congress of Tuberculosis, likewise held in Washington. "Among the important problems still agitating the members at that time," Smith recalled, "was the relation between human and animal tuberculosis, and it was our good fortune to have as one of our distinguished guests Robert Koch, whom we could meet face to face and ply with questions *ad libitum* to bring out his point of view."

Theobald Smith's Day Card for Monday, October 4, indicates that his presidential duties at the second tuberculosis meeting followed without respite. "Nat'l[.] Tuberc. Association opens. I read Presidents Address. Business meeting. Sessions P.M. very hot. In evening I preside to hear Sir Henry Gauvain on Home for crippled children . . . I receive Trudeau Medal for Tuberc. work. First presentation."[36] The title of Theobald's presidential address on this occasion, "The Problem of Natural and Acquired Resistance to Tuberculosis,"[37] foretold a complex, lengthy and perhaps baffling message. He stressed the importance of validating hypotheses and organized research. "Without a second base-line of fact, ideas simply represent the ploy of the imagination . . . When, as in tuberculosis, the same problem is attacked from several directions, each field of work has within its horizon, data not accessible to other groups of workers. Only by coordination and cooperation can the subject be fully explored." After analyzing the interaction between the human host and the bacillary parasite, he asserted: "Nothing in biology is foreign or alien to the problem of tuberculosis, for parasitism is a universal phenomenon of life." Sanitation and preventive medicine were largely responsible for the epidemiological improvement (the declining death rate) in tuberculosis. Additional benefits might be expected from immunological sources, natural or acquired. The Association was praised for broadening "the anti-tuberculosis movement into a general health campaign," in which all types of immunity might flourish. Theobald closed by quoting the now well-known maxim of a colleague who had recently died, Hermann L. Briggs—"Health is purchasable."

Bacillus Abortus and *Bacillus Melitensis*

Theobald Smith's knowledge of tuberculosis covered practically every aspect of the disease, as his complete bibliography indicates. He was unquestionably the leading authority on the pathogenicity of *Mycobacterium tuberculosis bovis* for man. His authority on bovine contagious abortion was also unrivalled (between 1911 and 1929, for example, he published approximately a dozen articles on *Bacillus abortus* and related bacteria), except for his unwillingness to acknowledge that the strong resemblance of *Bacillus abortus* to *Bacillus melitensis,* the etiologic agent of Malta fever, later named, alternatively, Brucellosis after Sir David Bruce, the British army surgeon who first cultivated the organism from the goat in Malta in 1887, made plausible the existence of cow's milk-borne undulant fever.

Alice C. Evans, a 1909 graduate of Smith's alma mater, Cornell University, and a long-time bacteriologist of the U.S. Public Health Service, was assigned a project to study the bacteria that occur in milk freshly drawn from the cow when beginning work in the Dairy Division of the Bureau of Animal Industry in 1913. Among the bacterial flora she found commonly present was *Bacillus abortus,* which was suspected by some as being dangerous to human health. Although *B. abortus* at the time appeared to be an unlikely relative of *B. melitensis,* Evans was sufficiently impressed by the fact that both organisms shared the same habitat, the udders of apparently healthy animals, to undertake a bacteriological comparison of the two. To her amazement, she found that *B. abortus* of bovine origin and *B. melitensis* of human origin behaved essentially the same in all cultures.[38] In 1918, when drawing attention to the close morphological and biochemical relationship of the two microbes, she anticipated that *B. abortus* could likewise infect human beings. "Considering the close relationship between the two organisms, and the reported frequency of virulent strains of bac. abortus in cow's milk," she observed, "it would seem remarkable that we do not have a disease resembling Malta fever prevalent in this country."[39] Although these forecasts were later amplified and confirmed by herself and were supported by others, Smith felt that the evidence then available and the scarcity of known human infections did not justify such a conclusion—at least not yet.

As an early observer of the relatively mild pathogenicity of *B. abortus* toward small laboratory animal species, and from his continuing researches on infectious abortion in cattle,[40] Smith could not bring himself to agree with Evans and she resented with persistent bitterness his paternalistic attitude toward her findings. In 1919, he published a paper on the bacteriology of bovine abortion with special reference to acquired immunity.[41] In this study of a large herd in which a fair proportion of its members had been bred on the spot, he concluded that, while *Bacillus abortus* might be the sole agency of abortion in certain herds, this proved clearly not to be true of the herd under investigation, where 57% of the infected cases were associated with that organism, 23.8% with *spirilla* (*Vibrio fetus*), 1.8% with *Bacillus pyogenes,* and 17.4% had been invaded by miscellaneous bacteria.

Smith stated in a paper on "The Relation of Bacillus Abortus from Bovine Sources to Malta Fever," published in 1926,[42] that the existence of races indistinguishable fundamentally and differing only in minor physiological characters had presented a major problem to comparative pathologists since the methods of Koch had come into use. Citing the tubercle bacillus and the streptococci as well-known examples of this genre, he conceded that to this group must now be added the *Melitensis abortus* species; but while statements based on recent comparative studies of *B. abortus* and *B. melitensis* had been made to the effect that these two microorganisms were identical and that a clinical complex similar to Malta or undulant fever might be produced in man, he asserted, in opposition, that the well-defined geographical limitations of Malta fever and its relation to goat's milk, the high degree of infectiveness of *B. melitensis* toward laboratory workers handling the organism, and the wide diffusion of infectious abortion in cattle throughout Europe and the United States militated against this definition. There were three known widely diffused animal sources of the brucella group, he declared: the cow, the pig, and the goat (although in some European countries where sheep were hosts, he assumed that the goat and sheep races of *B. melitensis* were the same). And he claimed that "The bovine disease and its affiliated microbe, *Bacillus abortus,* may be regarded as highly specialized types." Except for another, minor study appearing immediately afterward,[43] Theobald published nothing more on this problem for several years.

In February 1928, when delivering a lecture before the New York Academy of Medicine on "Animal Reservoirs of Human Disease with Special Reference to Microbic Variability,"[44] Smith once more took notice of the subject of Malta or undulant fever, telling that since the great war attention had been called by clinicians to an affection appearing in our midst sporadically and usually in isolated cases which was characterized by prolonged fever without recognizable local manifestations, and its similarity to Malta fever had been emphasized. Furthermore, from a great number of recent cases a bacillus had been obtained from the blood which closely resembled *Bacillus melitensis* or Brucella. In 1918, he recounted, Alice Evans, while studying the bacteria of cow's milk, showed that *B. melitensis* was closely related to *B. abortus* from the cow. Although the former had been isolated in 1889 (actually, in 1887) and the latter, by Bang, in 1897, the close relationship of the two was not pointed out until twenty years later. "This condition may be ascribed to the fact that the two streams of information resulting from investigations in human and animal pathology rarely mingle."

"The appearance of an undulant type of fever in man in our midst associated with an organism up to the present not distinguishable by routine bacteriological and serological methods from either *B. melitensis* or *B. abortus* raises many important problems which cannot be reviewed at this time and which demand more detailed study." The situation at the present time, he believed, was that, of the three different hosts of Brucella, the bovine organism had been thoroughly studied; the pig organism much less thoroughly; and the goat organism, known to exist among goats in southern Europe and in several southern states in America as coming directly from goat's milk, was still to be comparatively studied. Only through an extensive comparative investigation of the three races of Brucella, he contended, would the problem of human undulant fever be solved. "The burden of proof still rests upon those who claim that the bovine type of *Brucella* produced undulant fever in man."

Theobald pointed out that bacteriologists working with cultures of Malta fever were frequently laid low with the disease in spite of the usual care observed in bacteriological laboratories, while, on the other hand, *B. abortus* from the cow had been under investigation for more than a quarter of a century the world over without being suspected of producing any febrile condition in laboratory workers. Nor had veterinarians coming directly into contact with the diseased tissues in their daily practices presented any grievances against the bovine bacillus.

In April 1929, Smith published an article on "A Strain of Bacillus Abortus from Swine"[45] in which he told that "The economic significance of abortion among swine and the evidence already presented that the particular race or races of *Bacillus abortus* causing this disease may be involved in undulant fever in man justify a better detailed study of this disease and the strains of *Bacillus abortus* associated with it." He noted that he had published a review of the early work with the porcine disease in 1926,[46] at which time the evidence, although quite incomplete, pointed to an identity with the bovine race in terms of specific agglutination but to differences in growth in sealed and unsealed cultures and in lesions produced in guinea pigs.

Late in May 1927, he reported, after his attention had been called to an outbreak of swine abortion in a herd belonging to a state institution, "we obtained a few fetuses and learned at the same time that the animals had not been fed cow's milk, nor was there any record of abortion in this herd prior to March 1928. In addition, there had been no fresh pigs introduced into the herd except a boar in 1926 which came from a herd free from the disease." Since the porcine disease had been subjected to but little detailed study, perhaps owing to its relatively infrequent occurrence, several cases were studied. It appeared from protocols that bacilli resembling *B. abortus* had been isolated from the fetuses of three out of four sows, while the fourth had had a normal litter and was evidently not a carrier.

From post-mortem examinations and serological tests, it was determined that this outbreak of infectious abortion in swine, probably the first reported from the eastern United States, was associated with a strain of *Bacillus abortus,* though presenting certain slight pathological deviations from the bovine form of the disease in guinea pigs. The specific bacilli were widely disseminated in the tissues of the fetuses. He concluded that the pathogenic action of this swine strain on guinea pigs was evidently much feebler than that of most swine strains as reported and it approached more closely that of the bovine strains. The culture fed to a pregnant sow failed to produce abortion, possibly because of the advanced state of pregnancy, and the organism was not recovered from the uterus but was found in the sow's milk.

In his October 1928 De Lamar Lecture, "Undulant Fever, Its Relation to New Problems in Bacteriology and Public Health,"[47] Smith told his Johns Hopkins School of Public Health audience that "As in nearly all somewhat unexpected developments in science, the new problem of undulant fever in populations not using goat's milk seemed at first simple," with the cow being regarded as the source of infection owing to the wide dissemination of the bovine disease. His intention, he declared was to learn from existing data whether or not the bovine type of *Bacillus abortus* produced undulant fever in man, primarily and not as a secondary invader.

After referring to the three known sources of the Brucella group, Theobald stated that the bovine disease and its affiliated microbe, *B. abortus,* may be regarded as a highly specialized disease, and he went on to review the progress of the research of the disease in guinea pigs since he and Fabyan had observed and reported it in 1911. Turning to the porcine variety of *B. abortus,* which had been under observation since J. Traum had first isolated it from swine in 1914, he told that it had since been encountered in various states of the Middle West and the Pacific Coast, and according to reports, had been more virulent. Of the three animal races of *B. abortus,* Smith assumed that the bovine and caprine races had been adapted to their respective hosts through a long series of passages, adding that the caprine race of *B. abortus* had been much less thoroughly studied than the bovine disease, although longer under observation, and nothing was known of its behavior in the guinea pig, nor its relation to disease or abortion in the goat.

Turning his attention to the subject of undulant fever in man, he reported that there was a considerable background of studies in the human disease as produced by ingestion of cow's milk, and that the most impressive physiological distinction among the animal races was the relation to CO_2 (in the investigation of which Theobald had published two studies);[48] and from inoculation in man and from the determination of CO_2 requirements of cultures, the following inferences could be drawn:

1. Bovine strains or strains not distinguishable from them had been cultured from patients in a small percent of cases.
2. The caprine strains isolated directly from goat's milk needed more detailed study before this type could be used in comparative studies.
3. Cultures isolated from man and presumably ingested in cow's milk but not fitting the bovine type may have been swine strains introduced into that receptive organ, the cow's udder.
4. The partly saprophytized cultures which had been used on a large scale in vaccinating cows against infectious abortion might be another possible source of bovine strains.
5. The swine type of *B. abortus* might have been developed in the midwestern states in recent years, where the enormous development of the swine industry, the feeding of by-products of the dairy, as well as association between the two species in feed lots, have given Nature opportunities to form new varieties.
6. The further internal differentiation of the non-bovine types found in man suggested other possible forms of aberrant parasitism of a more or less permanent character developed locally in rats, mice, wild rabbits, ground squirrels and other rodents.

7. The gradual development of the milch-goat industry in northern states required supervision as a possible source of human disease.

Smith concluded his De Lamar Lecture with the remark that, "As to active measures against undulant fever, if it should be made fairly clear that the bovine race
of *B. abortus* is the real source of the other races, then the time would be ripe for
an active campaign against it," and the same held true for goats if the parent race
was found to be harbored in that species.

In August 1929 was published an abstract, entitled "Undulant Fever,"[49] of an
address Theobald Smith had given before the annual State Health Conference at
Saratoga Springs, New York, the previous June 24. In this lecture, he pointed
out again that the discovery of Malta or undulant fever in southern Europe as a
distinct disease in the 1880s, appearing wherever milch goats from such countries had been introduced, had within the prior six years been recognized as occurring in the northern United States and central and northern Europe. This
discovery had raised several questions. Had the disease prevailed for several generations and had the medical profession failed to distinguish it from other febrile
diseases? Had the general and specific resistance of the population declined? Or
had the microbe of this disease undergone recent changes or a redistribution
owing to the vastly increased and world-wide commercial activities? In response, he stated that "These questions cannot be answered and they may seem
academic but they have fundamental significance in epidemiology."

He observed that bacteria closely related to the original Malta fever bacillus
and isolated from the human patient had been found in goats, cattle, swine,
sheep and horses, in cattle producing the so-called infectious abortion which
was now distributed worldwide and which, in this and perhaps other countries,
few large herds were free of five or ten years before. The problem confronting
health officers was the source of the bacilli from the different animal sources.
"While slight differences may be brought out by bacteriological technique and
animal inoculation they are neither sharp nor constant." In this country, the
problem had practically narrowed down to two sources, cattle or swine. In view
of the prevalence of infectious bovine abortion in this country for some thirty or
forty years, with a peak probably ten years before, the question arose as to why
there had not been more cases and even local epidemics.

The tentative explanation he proposed, based upon studies of human strains of
the bacilli, was that the genuine bovine type was relatively harmless to man and
that the swine type was largely responsible, either directly or in the handling of
swine or raw pork or indirectly when the swine bacillus was introduced into the
cow's udder in one of several ways. He concluded with the statement: "This pos-

sible explanation of the increase in undulant fever does not justify any relaxation in the movement for more pasteurization but it does indicate the need for more investigation into the swine disease and other non-bovine types of *Brucella abortus*."

In 1929 and 1930, reports began to come out of Europe and other world regions with increasing frequency of cases of Malta fever of bovine origin, supplying evidence beyond resasonable doubt that raw cow's milk was a likely causal agent in the transmission of the disease to humans, a matter that Smith referred to in his final pronouncement on the various strains of Brucella made at the third Annual Eastern States Conference on Bang's Disease held at Trenton, New Jersey, on November 9, 1934.[50] After noting that much had been written in the previous ten years about infectious abortion in cattle, the occurrence of related bacteria in other animal species, and the effects of agents of these diseases on the human subject, he asked, "Have we learned enough to suppress the bovine disease successfully and economically, or do we need more light?" He suggested that "we can add to our understanding of infectious abortion . . . from whatever source it comes," and that more knowledge of the disease itself was needed. In a recent study of thirty-nine cases of abortion, he had found seventeen associated with *B. abortus*, five with vibrios, and fifteen with these bacteria absent, and he wondered what those fifteen abortions were due to. He asserted that the abortion disease was not stationary, in fact, no active infectious disease remained the same, and changes undergone by the infectious agent and the race in the past made current tests misleading.

In his discussion of what relation the Brucella races from other species of animals bore to the bovine disease, he told that through careful tests the swine and the goat types could be distinguished from the bovine type, and that the outstanding fact of the prior ten years of investigation was the susceptibility of man to one or another of these Brucella races. The fact that undulant fever occurred in man had greatly stimulated the study of Brucella, and although studies of strains isolated from man in this country had put the swine type as the chief cause of undulant fever in man, there was evidence also that this type could occur in the cow's udder. While he still believed that in America the bovine type was of minor significance in human disease, he acknowledged that in Europe and South America the opposite was true; and he theorized that it was possible that geographic races existed which could be ascribed to the widely different methods of feeding livestock.

Theobald Smith's preserved correspondence contains many inquiries he received between 1928 and 1934 from clinicians who had inquired about suspected undulant fever in patients under their care, from state, local and private bacteriological institutions and laboratories, from industry, and from other sources; and, in addition to exchanging cultures with them, his answer to their inquiries about the disease was constantly the same: that there were several varieties of bacteria which might produce the malady in man, of which the swine type was the chief culprit in this country, and the bovine type the least dangerous; that "we have been unable to distinguish the various races satisfactorily in serological test," and that it was possible that individuals might have a relatively high agglutination content in their blood without being ill; that the danger from the strictly bovine bacillus in this country had been exaggerated, and although attention should be given to the prevalence of the swine type, it was a wise policy gradually to eliminate, or at least reduce the bovine disease to its lowest terms; that if milch goats are kept, they will require supervision; and that the pasteurizing temperature killed all types of bacteria responsible for the disease.[51] Since hard evidence had still not been produced to convince him to think otherwise, he almost invariably referred inquirers asking for more information to his 1928 De Lamar Lecture or to the address he had delivered at Saratoga Springs the year afterward.

As Alice Evans's biographer has observed,[52] Evans became ill with brucellosis in late 1922, and *B. melitensis* was shown as the etiologic agent by positive cultures obtained from the first attack and subsequent episodes in 1923, 1928 and 1931, with many years of ill health, and periods of complete incapacitation alternating with periods of recovery, following. Evans published the first paper in the United States on chronic brucellosis in 1934, the year of Theobald Smith's death, and by 1936, when she undertook a more detailed study of chronic brucellosis, acute cases were being reported from all over the United States and the problem of chronic disease was emerging. Evans set up and coordinated a project utilizing field investigations by young physicians in three separate cities where a large percentage of milk was still consumed raw, despite knowledge that the herds supplying the milk were infected with brucellae. Results of the survey exposed a total of twenty-two human cases and probable or proven brucellosis among the 325 cases of chronic illness studied. Since none had a history of exposure to brucellae by other means than the ingestion of milk and dairy products, this survey supplied the data upon which Evans based her early estimate that the actual number of cases of brucellosis occurring in the United States was at least ten times the number of reported cases, results which were supported by investigators in other parts of the country. The overall figures explained the reasons why Theobald Smith had observed so few human cases of brucellosis in proportion to the far larger number who had been exposed by consuming raw milk from infected cows.

Paul de Kruif and *Microbe Hunters*

In the last half of the 1920 decade, Theobald Smith had some contact with a former employee of the Rockefeller Institute, Paul de Kruif, a young and rather li-
bidinous American of Dutch stock who acquired a celebrity of a sort from writing about the lives and discoveries of various famous figures who had
contributed to the control of infectious diseases. De Kruif had received a Ph.D.
in bacteriology from the University of Michigan in 1912 and had served with the
U.S. Sanitary Corps in France during the last year of the war. Afterwards, as an
assistant professor at the University of Michigan, he, a married man with two
children, became intrigued with a woman working in the bacteriological laboratories there. Dissatisfied with the limitations of his work at Michigan, and desirous of escaping his unhappy marriage situation, in 1920 de Kruif went to work
as a research assistant at the Rockefeller Institute in New York. While there,
with the encouragement of Henry L. Mencken, he began to write popular articles about science and scientists, an avocation which eventually got him in trouble with the administration of the Institute and led to his second career as a popular science writer. And in 1922, he divorced his wife and married the lab
assistant.

In the early 1920s, de Kruif began publishing such articles in *The Century Magazine,* Hearst's *International Magazine,* and elsewhere. And in 1926, these and
other vignettes of "fighters against disease" were gathered together and published in the hardbound volume entitled *Microbe Hunters.* De Kruif had, in 1923
and 1924, also collaborated with Sinclair Lewis in preparing Lewis's novel
Arrowsmith, which appeared in 1925, and which was also, as one critic has
pointed out,[53] a fictionalized version of de Kruif's early career. De Kruif had
been employed as a research assistant at the Institute for a few years prior to his
dismissal in September 1922 for having, in Simon Flexner's opinion, mocked the
Institute, and for indirectly associating his name in doing so. Flexner felt that he
had taken unfair advantage of his employers under whom he had done good
work on rabbit septicemia (*Bacillus pneumosintes*), despite some warnings from
Flexner about his flirting with female technicians. However, while the matter
was never publicized and remains somewhat unclear, the reason for his firing reportedly stemmed from the fact that de Kruif wrote an anonymous attack on the
Institute in a popular magazine which he signed "K——, M.D.," and when
Flexner discovered that it was de Kruif who had written the article, he fired
him.

In the opinion of Tom Rivers,[54] de Kruif was fired—reportedly in Flexner's
words to Rivers as well as to de Kruif—for *not* signing his name to the article. It

was anathema to a scientist such as Flexner to publish an article, even a fictionalized or romanticized piece about science, without signing one's name to it, and Rivers later opined, "I don't think de Kruif would have been fired if he had signed the article." In his later memoir, *The Sweeping Wind,* de Kruif, in answer to his question, "Why did Dr. Flexner want to get rid of me?" answered himself, saying, "he was disturbed [because] it had been reported to him that I was fooling around with not one but two young women in the Institute," which, "was, to say the least, improper here."[55] But later on in the memoir, de Kruif talked about his anonymous articles that were appearing in *The Century Magazine* signed "K——, M.D.," and of Flexner's reaction to them. This led him to resign from the Institute on September 1, 1922, with the remark, "My microbe-hunting days were done."[56]

Nonetheless, according to Rivers, de Kruif soon after took great public revenge. As an advisor on *Arrowsmith,* the loquacious Dutchman saw to it that the McGirk Institute of Lewis's novel was a beautiful satirization of the Rockefeller Institute, and many of the members of the Institute found their way into the novel, Jacques Loeb, John Northrop, Rivers himself, Simon Flexner, and others. As Rivers put it, "Some of these portraits were etched in acid, and the book remained a topic of conversation at the Institute for a long time."[57]

When *Microbe Hunters* appeared in print in February 1926, only four of the leading characters of the book were still alive, among them Theobald Smith, who appeared under the chapter heading, "Theobald Smith: Ticks and Texas Fever."[58] The essay's opening sentences were characteristic of de Kruif's overly dramatic and romantic style: "It was Theobald Smith who made mankind turn a corner. He was the first, and remains the captain, of American microbe hunters." Emile Roux, David Bruce and Ronald Ross were the other remaining survivors when the book appeared. Ross attacked de Kruif's article on him on the basis of historical inaccuracy and invasion of privacy,[59] while Smith, on the other hand, took the matter good-humoredly at the time, although he expressed strong disfavor later on, as is evident from a letter written by him to Simon Flexner in 1931:[60] "I am told there was a radio talk recently on Texas Fever, dramatized from *Microbe Hunters.* I suppose with introduction of a plot and mythical love affair between two people created for the occasion. Next week, Walter Reed. Could not the nonsense be stopped and the chewing gum firm [the program's sponsor] be forced to give the facts." In his response, Flexner said, "Yes, I heard something of the radio talk based on de Kruif's book. It's an age of forced and painful publicity. I fear nothing can be done, and perhaps the least done will insure quickest forgetfulness."[61]

Earlier on, however, de Kruif's contacts with Smith seemed to have been marked by genuine appreciation for the outline on the Texas fever problem given him; but de Kruif made characteristic use of details which again he could have got only from Smith, a matter that was indiscreet of the writer to mention. For instance, he stirred up animosity by disparaging references to Alexander, "a darkie ex-slave who sat solemnly," and to "Bachelor Kilborne, who rejoiced in the Degree of Bachelor of Agriculture and was something of a horse doctor (he now runs a hardware business near New York)." These disparaging details of his co-workers were magnified by Smith's antagonists in the veterinary profession which later presented the gold medal to Kilborne at a ceremony to which Smith was not invited.

Continuing Labors in the Vineyard of Science: Enteric Disease, Immunology, and Public Health Concerns

In the last half of the 1920s, Theobald Smith interested himself in several other scientific problems in addition to colostrum, *Bacillus abortus* and its relationship to undulant fever, and the other researches that have been reviewed previously. His bibliography from the beginning of 1925 through the year 1929 numbered no less than thirty items, with ten of them appearing in 1927 alone; although a few of them were philosophical and not devoted to hard science, his output during these years matched or at least approximated the production of all but his peak years. Theobald had got himself back into the saddle following his sojourn to Edinburgh and was transgressing his familiar terrain at an invigorated pace.

During the year 1926 he submitted for publication three papers related to paratyphoid disease. The first was undertaken for the purpose of shedding more light on an unsolved problem of the past, while the second two capitalized on an unexpected opportunity occasioned by a spontaneous outbreak of a paratyphoid infection in a colony of guinea pigs maintained for breeding purposes at the Princeton laboratories, allowing Theobald and John B. Nelson to observe the cause and effects of the disease. (Smith modestly described these paratyphoid papers to Simon Flexner as being "of no striking importance and bring only some new sidelights perhaps.")[62] In the first paper, by Smith and Helena Tibbetts, "The Relation between Invasion of the Digestive Tract by Paratyphoid Bacilli and Disease,"[63] the authors reported that they had artificially induced a paratyphoid disease in mice to study its effects and resulting pathology. To bring the problem within the field of experiment, the hog cholera bacillus and the white mouse were chosen, the authors noting that the susceptibility of grey mice to this bacillus had been studied by one of them (Smith) in 1885, white mice being unavailable for laboratory research at the time.

Their investigations determined that the bacilli fed to mice disappeared from the stomach within twenty-four hours, but remained and perhaps multiplied in the ileum for at least several weeks, and that they also promptly penetrated the mucosa and could be found in the spleen. On the other hand, bacilli introduced subcutaneously quickly passed into the intestinal tract where they might be found for several weeks, and the infected mice might harbor bacilli in the spleen for several months. Smith and Tibbetts determined that mice harbor a relatively high degree of natural resistance towards the hog cholera bacillus, which gave way to large doses; and that the disease was probably the result of an invasion of the viscera from the digestive tract following feeding, but the relation between the dose fed and the numbers penetrating the mucosa was a variable one, although conditions favoring such an invasion had not been established.

During the summer of 1924 the spontaneous outbreak of paratyphoid disease occurring in one guinea pig colony was studied by Smith and Nelson. Their first report, of which Theobald was the secondary author,[64] was directed towards the gross pathology resulting from the infection and the bacteriology of the causal organism, with a single strain of *B. paratyphi* appearing to be the culprit. In the second paper, by Smith and Nelson,[65] the authors told that spontaneous epidemics in small animals had not been studied in the past with the care warranted by the importance of the phenomenon. In this investigation they observed factors bearing on the maintenance of the paratyphoid condition in an endemic state for approximately two years (from mid-1924 until June 1926), during which time there was no evidence of any increase nor any demonstrable proof of a decline in virulence of the causative agent. The transition of the outbreak from epidemic to endemic phase was believed to be due to a weeding out of the individuals of low natural resistance, with a gradual adjustment of the invading organism to the population on a lower lever of resistance.

The main thrust of Smith's publishing activity in 1927—a very prolific year— centered around three studies of pathogenic *B. coli* from bovine sources, with a fourth such report appearing in the following year. Theobald was following up a question he had posed in an earlier paper on scours,[66] which concluded that the disease was a local manifestation of *B. coli* septicemia and suggested that this matter was in need of further investigation. In the first such study,[67] Smith and Ralph Little, by inquiring into the pathogenic action of culture filtrates, determined that the relatively young bouillon filtrates, twenty-four and forty-eight hours old, of certain strains of *B. coli* obtained directly from the ileum of scouring calves were highly toxic for calves of about one month old, as well as for older calves and cows when given in the vein.

The second paper, by Smith and Gladys Bryant, investigated mutations and their immunological significance. On agar plates certain strains of *B. coli* from the ileums of calves suffering from diarrhea and scours were found to promptly mutate and give rise to forms which had lost capsular substance and whose virulence had been greatly reduced.[68] In the third publication, authored by Smith alone, entitled "Normal and Serologically Induced Resistance to B. Coli and Its Mutant,"[69] the interrelations between bacterial toxins, bacterial capsular substances, and certain normal protective factors in the guinea pig were studied with the aid of bacterial mutants and immune serum, with the results pointing to the capsular substance as the material carrying virulence, or, expressed somewhat differently, it being the factor which protected the organism in the host. The fourth *B. coli* study, reported by Smith alone and published in 1928, was concerned also with the relation of the capsular substance to antibody protection.[70]

Another paper published in 1927, reporting research conducted by Smith and Marion Orcutt on the life cycle of *Vibrio fetus,* the spiral organism found to cause abortion in animals,[71] has been referred to earlier as of little importance. The authors told that the occasional encounter of vibrios in the intestinal tract of young calves called attention to possible locus of *Vibrio fetus;* and that these vibrios might be survivors of a fetal infection with *Vibrio fetus,* or they might represent a different group, possibly associated with intestinal inflammation in calves after the first week of life.

On April 1, 1927, Smith delivered the Annual Samuel D. Gross Lecture before the Pathological Society of Philadelphia. His Day Card of that date contains the following interesting note: "9–12.30 prep. for lecture in Phila[.] leave 4.22—to Univ. Club—dinner given by Dr. Opie to about 15 men . . . to Coll. Phys. & Surgeons for lecture on passing of disease fr. one gen. to another etc. receive Gerhard medal & diploma of Hon. membership of Phil. Path. Society. Heavy thunder punctures my lecture. Stop with Opies over night & see son & 2 daughters."[72] Theobald's lecture, "The Passing of Disease from One Generation to Another and the Processes Tending to Counteract It," which appeared in print later that year,[73] was a review of the mechanisms functioning in the host during the earliest days of life to defend it against potential disease germs and the parasitic enemies of the young, on the one hand, and the perpetuation of parasitism by transfer from one generation to another after birth, on the other.

The possibility of dispensing with colostrum and feeding an alien milk instead led to an experiment involving the attempt to raise lambs free from parasites, and after three years of experimentation, a small flock was all but free of them, Theobald Smith and T.R. Ring reported in their 1927 paper, "The Segregation of Lambs at Birth and the Feeding of Cow's Milk in the Elimination of Parasites."[74] Their study originated out of the question of the significance of colostrum to the new-born lamb. Experiments to test the protective value of colostrum were begun in 1924 (and concluded in late 1926) by substituting cow's milk for ewe's milk; and the results showed clearly that the ewe's colostrum was not necessary to protect the lamb against miscellaneous infections and that normal growth took place even when no colostrum was fed. In a letter to Simon Flexner in mid-January 1927, Smith reported that he had finished the manuscript and was a little puzzled as to what he should do with it, although he presumed that the *Journal of Parasitology* (which published it) might be a suitable depository for it. He concluded his letter with the remark, "What do you think of sending it to Dr. Nuttall's journal, *Parasitology?* The English are very interested in sheep and, as you know, flocks of them are everywhere in the landscape."[75]

Theobald Smith delivered several philosophical speeches and addresses before the 1920 decade had run its course, and two of them, because of the subject matter, their length, or the importance of the audiences should be given attention here. As his Presidential Address to the Congress of American Physicians and Surgeons at Washington on May 1, 1928, he delivered a long and somewhat involved oration on "The Decline of Infectious Diseases and Its Relation to Modern Medicine."[76] In reviewing half a century's progress in scientific microbiology since Pasteur, Lister and Koch began their pioneer work, he recalled some of the guiding theories that had survived and crystallized into actual facts and principles—immunology, the variability of organisms, parasitism, and others that had evolved—and he described the impact of these new concepts on microorganisms. In the process, he observed, the medical man had turned from the idea of cure to that of prevention, referring, first, to the public health movement to eliminate them, and, secondly, to means to neutralize their effects, such as vaccination and chemotherapy. Afterwards, he discussed factors that had led to a decline in mortality, such as changes in economic conditions, the application of medical science, and the interplay of natural forces which tended to raise resistance in the host and reduce virulence in the parasite.

He assured his audience that medical practice in all its forms was so thoroughly a part of human civilization that no surgical operation could remove it and that medical science and practice must go on and continue their evolution parallel with human society and maintain the barriers against environmental enemies that will be continually thrust at mankind; for while many animal infections of the past had been eliminated, others had taken their place due to the extreme mobility of modern life in bringing together elements from all over the globe. As an example of this occurrence, he cited the sudden, sporadic appearance of undulant or Malta fever at great distances from its supposed center around the Mediterranean, and discussed the possible role that *Bacillus abortus* might play in the phenomenon.

In the other, somewhat analogous address, "The Influence of Research in Bringing into Closer Relationship the Practice of Medicine and Public Health Activities,"[77] presented at the meeting of the Boards of Council of the Milbank

Fund in New York on March 13, 1929, Smith observed that the concept of public health or preventive medicine was new. Public health had developed out of medical practice, he reasoned, its germ being the causal concept of disease; it was thus the embodiment that much of the routine treatment had been ineffective, and sometimes injurious, and that the growing knowledge of causation had forced preventive measures to the foreground.

Research, he opined, was fundamentally a state of mind, involving continual reexamination of the doctrines and axioms upon which current thought and action were based. Thus, research was a vital part of both medical practice and public health activities, and the technique of both preventive and curative medicine was created and remodeled from time to time by medical research. Medical practice and preventive medicine, apparently facing one another as competitors at the beginning of the bacteriological era and getting their impetus from quite different medical theories and medical operations, had gradually been drawn together willy-nilly by the forces of truth developed by the underlying activities of research. However, while science sought the simplest experimental conditions to determine truth, the physician inherited all of the complications of nature. The experiment assumed uniformity, whereas the physician accepted diversity in his material. Thus, diverging views conditioned by the field work, the method of approaching it, and the direction taken in it, led naturally to a certain lack of appreciation on the respective functions of the other group.

As long as disease prevailed, Smith maintained, the physician could not be spared. The physician was the outpost of public health. He was often the first to scent new diseases and give warning of impending danger when he correctly diagnosed a case unexpected or out of the ordinary. Public health could not dispense with the support of practical medicine until the last case of some disease had been detected and restrained. As long as disease existed, the operations of preventive medicine must be found in the knowledge of disease. Disease is the positive pole from which the current of research flows. Demonstration must become a connecting link between the two kinds of activities, the preventive and the curative, for it must apply to both the results of scientific research and the experience of the individual physician. It should be the force that brings together the student of public health and the local doctor.

26

FINAL YEARS AT
THE ROCKEFELLER INSTITUTE,
AND RETIREMENT

Death of Hideyo Noguchi

On May 21, 1928, word arrived from Accra on the Gold Coast (now Ghana) that Hideyo Noguchi, one of the Rockefeller Institute for Medical Research's best known scientists, had died that day from laboratory-acquired yellow fever; and on the following day a fulsome eulogy of the man by Simon Flexner appeared in the *New York Times.*[1] Flexner's tribute was both fitting and ironic, because Noguchi not only owed his career to the director of the Institute's laboratories, but because it was Flexner who sent him first to Ecuador and later to Peru and Columbia between 1918 and 1924 to investigate the causal agent of yellow fever; and, by suggesting the nature of the causal agent to Noguchi, who was still pursuing it in Africa in 1927 and 1928, was ultimately involved in determining his downfall and death.

Flexner's association with Noguchi dated back to 1899, when Flexner led a Johns Hopkins University commission to study the diseases of American soldiers in the Philippine Islands. On a stop-over in Tokyo, Flexner requested permission to visit Prof. Kitasato's Institute, and a courteous invitation was brought to the hotel by Noguchi, then an assistant at the Institute with scant prospect for advancement. Noguchi expressed a desire to study pathology and bacteriology in America. Although Flexner gave him no particular encouragement, soon after Flexner became professor of pathology at the University of Pennsylvania that autumn, Noguchi turned up in Philadelphia, dressed in his finest and bringing an armful of presents, but otherwise penniless.

Flexner found him a place to live, bought him clothes, taught him English, and, with the financial help of S. Weir Mitchell, put Noguchi to work helping him study snake venoms, with Noguchi subsequently working with him on antivenoms, cytolysins and later on the spirochaete identified by Schaudinn as causing syphilis. Flexner long afterwards acknowledged that Noguchi had helped him make his career in Philadelphia just as he had helped make Noguchi's. "He was much the better craftsman, although he did not (or could not) I believe plan and think better than I."[2] When the Rockefeller Institute was inaugurated in 1904 under Flexner's directorship, Noguchi accompanied him to New York as his assistant. Here he devised methods of cultivating microorganisms that had not previously been grown in the test tube, succeeded in growing the spirochaetes that cause syphilis, and studied poliomyelitis and trachoma.

Noguchi had been appointed to a team of microbiologists in 1918 to determine why Guayaquil remained the last focus for endemic yellow fever in South America. It so happened that the communities in South America that were subject to yellow fever also had an endemic and occasionally epidemic outburst of spirochetal jaundice, in whose etiology Noguchi had been interested from the beginning because the discovery of *Leptospira icterohemorrhagia* (Weil's disease) had been made by Japanese friends of his (Inada, Ido et al.) and confirmed by Noguchi himself. The main cause of Noguchi's dismal failure in mistaken ardor was Flexner's suggestion, which is commemorated in Flexner's own diary,[3] perhaps not seen by many and ignored by a proportion of those who did see it, in which Flexner argued that since yellow fever and leptospiral jaundice resembled one another superficially at least in clinical manifestations, the cause of yellow fever must resemble the cause of leptospiral jaundice and therefore be a leptospira, and secondly, that Noguchi's naive but tragic assumption that diseases that looked clinically so similar were nevertheless differentiated by ordinary practitioners who referred these cases and these specimens to him. In other words, Noguchi had a strong motive for suspecting that the leptospira was the cause of yellow fever, and when he found leptospira present in the blood and viscera of patients, did not give sufficient weight to the possibility that they were victims, not of yellow fever, but of leptospiral jaundice.

Noguchi soon claimed to have isolated a leptospira, similar to *L. icterohemorrhagia* but distinguishable from it, which he termed *L. icteroides,* from six to twenty-seven cases of yellow fever. From the outset, some attempted laboratory confirmation failed to differentiate between *L. icteroides* and *L. icterohemorrhagia;* and the diagnostic acumen of local physicians in selecting yellow fever cases was questioned. Again, guinea-pigs succumbed to Noguchi's *L. icteroides* and also to

L. icterohemorrhagia, whereas Walter Reed's Yellow Fever Commission had found the usual small laboratory animals unaffected by all relevant specimens. The skepticism grew, and Noguchi's claims were openly challenged at the International Health Conference held at Kingston, Jamaica, in 1924, where it was shown that the claim made by Noguchi for protection against yellow fever by antiserum from horses prepared in the Rockefeller Institute and the prevention of the disease in certain communities given vaccine likewise prepared by the Rockefeller Institute were entirely fallacious based on false argument and false acceptance of the supposition that they had been cases of yellow fever. At the 1924 conference, A. Agramonte, the only surviving member of Reed's Commission, took the lead in emphasizing the evidence that the causal agent in yellow fever was not bacterial, but a filter-passing virus.

The search for the virus was intensified in West Africa, where in many areas yellow fever was endemic. In 1925, the Rockefeller Foundation set up its second West African Yellow Fever commission under Dr. Henry Beeuwkes, with headquarters near Lagos, Nigeria, and a subsidiary station at Accra, under Dr. Alexander Mahaffy. Skilled bacteriologists and pathologists attached to the Commission, notably Adrian Stokes, N. Paul Hudson and Johannes Bauer, tried in vain for more than a year to verify Noguchi's findings. All sixty-seven undoubted cases of yellow fever were bacteriologically negative. No leptospira were isolated from many possible sources. In June 1929, mild cases of yellow fever were identified among natives, about 100 miles north of Accra, and a shipment of *Macacus rhesus* monkeys arrived from India. Blood from one of the yellow fever cases proved harmless to various laboratory animals, but lethal to the monkey. This turning-point in the elucidation of the viral etiology of yellow fever was climaxed by Adrian Stoke's death in September from the laboratory-acquired disease.[4]

Consternation induced Simon Flexner to consent to Noguchi travelling to West Africa to attempt reconciliation of the conflicting findings. In November 1927, Noguchi established his laboratory in the British Colonial Medical Research Institute, in friendly collaboration with William Young, its director. The Institute was close to the Mahaffy household, which hosted Noguchi for much of his stay. Lagos supplied two technicians. Noguchi worked long hours, often at night, alone and secretively, so that his technicians became baffled, and he himself confused. He ordered extravagant numbers of monkeys, and used mosquito cages that were not proof against escape. His carelessness was encouraged by an attack of Salmonella-like food poisoning, which he claimed was yellow fever, and upon recovery, he considered himself to have acquired immunity to the disease. In May 1928, he left Accra in a distraught state, became ill at Lagos, and returned by ship to Accra, where he died of typical acute yellow fever in a few days. A team arrived overland from Lagos to pay last respects. Young, who performed the autopsy and supervised the clean-up of Noguchi's laboratory, also died of yellow fever a week later.

Noguchi's remains, his working notes and laboratory specimens, which were shipped to New York, failed to provide any evidence supporting the various claims made in his letters to Simon Flexner; in particular, that a spore-bearing bacillus played some etiological role in yellow fever, perhaps in association with a virus. Theobald Smith was prevailed upon by Flexner to speak in tribute at Noguchi's memorial service. Smith had been consulted often by Noguchi, sometimes on Flexner's instructions, before impetuously seeking to commit his latest findings in print. He had managed to help prevent premature announcements in connection with, for example, rabies, poliomyelitis, and trachoma. But this obituary tribute, which might be regarded as partly a gesture of exaggerated homage to please Flexner, probably reflected (as Smith himself generously explained) the sympathy of one laboratory man for another, who had identified a bacterium in place of a virus, because of inadequate or faulty clinical data.

In his memorial address delivered at the New York Academy of Medicine on December 20, 1928—seven months, almost to the day, following Noguchi's demise[5]—Smith extolled Noguchi as an individual of originality and one who had the capacity to bring that originality to fruition. He found it easy to analyze the forces that led him to so many successes. In technique, Noguchi was master in many fields, but he especially excelled in creating his own methods. While these were relatively simple, his craftsmanship was such that he accomplished wonders with them. But the most impressive thing about him was his marvelous energy; his numerous papers presented the internal evidence of laborious, time-consuming processes, carefully controlled. Smith divided Noguchi's career into periods according to his major problems: 1900–1908, snake venom; 1909–1918, syphilis and many forms of spirochaetes; 1919–1928, yellow fever, oroyo fever and trachoma. But his work with syphilis would perhaps leave the most prominent record of his output, Theobald believed. Telling that Noguchi's work on trachoma was a striking demonstration of his capacity to dig into the debris of earlier failures and bring success to the surface, he closed by relating that Noguchi had a remarkable achievement for three decades of life work; that he would stand out more and more, with the passing of time, as one of the greatest, if not the greatest figure in microbiology since Pasteur and Koch.

Less than three months later, Theobald received an inquiry from Gustav Eckstein, a physiologist at the University of Cincinnati who had earlier lived in Japan and had corresponded with the now dead scientist about that experience. Eckstein was proposing to write Noguchi's biography and was seeking any information that Smith might have on him.[6] Despite the fact that Smith answered him negatively—"I think it is well to bear in mind that I had not been associated with him at any time," and that Flexner was the one he should see[7]—the two did get together at Princeton in late March during Eckstein's visit east. In a letter of thanks sent to Theobald shortly afterewards,[8] Eckstein wrote: "I will never forget the wonder—if you will allow so big a word—of that afternoon with you. It will touch, for good, the work I have in hand. And it will touch also, for good, my life." Eckstein's biography of Hideyo Noguchi came into print in 1931.[9]

In his oral history memoir, Tom Rivers did not award Noguchi the high marks that many others have done, saying that, "after I got to know Noguchi better, I did not consider him a great scientist."[10] Nor did he think much of Noguchi's knowledge of yellow fever: "He knew nothing about the pathology of yellow fever and wouldn't know a case of yellow fever if it hit him in the face." In a footnote elsewhere in Rivers's memoir appears a letter of the Rockefeller virologist Peter Olitsky,[11] who asserted that the culture medium attributed to Noguchi's discovery was, in fact, first devised by Theobald Smith in 1899, its chief ingredients being a fragment of kidney, plus fresh, unheated ascitic fluid collected under sterile conditions from human beings. "Dr. Fred Gates and I renamed it the Smith-Noguchi, for Noguchi only added some modification." In summing up Noguchi's overall career and impact, a recent evaluation of his life and work perhaps best expresses the matter: "Noguchi's quick perceptivity and remarkable energy often permitted him to correct or amplify the original discoveries of others. Unfortunately, he applied bacteriologic techniques to many viral diseases."[12]

The Predicament of Paul Lewis

On July 1, 1929, Theobald Smith and Simon Flexner received cable messages informing them of the death by yellow fever in Brazil of another Rockefeller Institute colleague, Paul A. Lewis; and although in his association with Smith and Flexner Lewis did not enjoy the paternal relationship that had existed between Flexner and Noguchi, the news nevertheless came as something of a shock to both men. Paul Lewis went as far back in Smith's experience as his Boston days, and in Flexner's to his early years at the Institute. The son of a local physician, Lewis studied medicine at the College of Physicians and Surgeons in Milwaukee and completed his training at the University of Pennsylvania, which awarded him the M.D. degree in 1904. While still a medical student at Pennsylvania, Lewis decided upon a laboratory career rather than the practice of medicine and gave special attention to the study of bacteriology and pathology. He subsequently obtained a residency in pathology at the Boston City Hospital, where he came under the tutorage of one of the outstanding pathologists of the day, Frank B. Mallory. The following year was spent as assistant in the Antitoxin Laboratory of the Massachusetts State Department of Health under Theobald Smith, with Lewis serving also from 1906 to 1908 as the Austin Teaching Fellow in comparative pathology at the Harvard Medical School. In 1908, he entered the Rockefeller Institute as an assistant in pathology.

Lewis's connection with the Rockefeller Institute covered two periods, from 1908 to 1910 at the laboratories in New York City, and from 1923 until his death in the laboratories at Princeton. Between 1910 and 1923, he was Director of Laboratories at the Henry Phipps Institute in Philadelphia as well as Professor of Experimental Pathology at the University of Pennsylvania. While at the Phipps Institute, he studied the influence of heredity in tuberculosis. Lewis's earlier work with Flexner in New York on poliomyelitis had brought him into contact with the widening subject of the filter-passing viruses as excitants of disease in man and the lower animals; this experience dominated his investigative interests during his Princeton connection with the Rockefeller Institute and was a motivating impulse that led him to volunteer for yellow fever work in Brazil in the 1928–1929 period.

It is obvious from correspondence between Lewis and Smith in mid-1921, and between Lewis, Smith and Flexner in early 1923, that Lewis was desirous of closing up his research in Philadelphia and returning to work at the Rockefeller Institute, preferably at Princeton with Smith. In a May 1921 letter to Smith he proposed, as his program there, to start with the best of the tuberculosis work —"to develop the heredity matter a little more broadly perhaps if it proved feasible"[13]—and to devote a considerable amount of effort to the problems being investigated in Smith's department. The matter came up again in January 1923, and after an exchange of letters between the three,[14] Lewis rejoined the Institute on a three-year trial period and by July had moved his animals and files to Princeton, with Dr. Opie succeeding to his place at the Phipps.

From letters exchanged between Lewis and Smith from mid-1923 on, it is clear that he was back at work on his heredity in tuberculosis study and on the transmissibility of the disease.[15] It is also evident from succeeding correspondence that he was also assisting in some of Theobald's work or cooperating on problems being studied by the senior scientists. For example, in a letter to Smith on August 20, 1925 he informed Smith that he was once more "unreasonably absorbed over the hog cholera virus, again in an unproductive way I fear."[16] Lewis also mentioned in that letter that "the Iowa people" had called on Flexner in London to obtain his assistance in filling a pathology chair there, and Flexner could recommend no one but Lewis, with Flexner later telling Lewis that his departure would be a serious loss to the Institute.

In a long letter written by Flexner to Lewis on December 4, 1925, in which the director expressed his concern about Lewis's pension situation—when leaving the Phipps, Lewis had forfeited his pension privileges, and no provision had yet been made for his trail period at the Institute—Flexner discussed at length another problem which had in the meantime become apparent, Lewis's interest in succeeding Smith to the directorship of the Department of Animal Pathology.[17] Lewis had earlier written to Flexner acknowledging this ambition, and Flexner now replied that he was a good deal upset by the letter, "and I have not yet and I fear I shall not ever, feel wholly comfortable about it." It indicated to him that Lewis's coming to the Institute had a different significance than he had gathered from their earlier talks together. "I was further disturbed by our conference in the autumn of 1924, based on your letter to me, in which you intimated an 'ambition' to become the future director of the Department of Animal Pathology;" furthermore, Flexner commented that Lewis's letter so closely coincided with Smith's sixty-fifth birthday that he could not help connecting the two events.

These circumstances had led Flexner to present the case of Lewis's future relationship to the Institute to its Board of Scientific Directors at its October meeting and to discuss it with Smith. "As the Iowa chair is still open and you very much wanted to fill it," Flexner informed Lewis, "and the University of Iowa would make a supreme effort to secure you, I believe it due you to be minutely informed just what the position is which the Board of Scientific Directors has taken with reference to you." He advised Lewis that the Board was unequivocally opposed to the appointment of one primarily a human pathologist to the directorship of the Department of Animal Pathology at any future time. In addition, as it was hoped that Smith would continue to serve as director for a number of years more, the question of successor did not have to be decided immediately. He also told Lewis that doubt had been expressed by the Board concerning his future, and "it is probable that in the event of reappointment at the end of the present year no change in your status would be made." Flexner also acknowledged that it seemed certain that the next director would be a person with a wide interest in the problem of animal pathology and one whose work showed a comprehensive interest in biological problems in general, and if such a person were appointed, he would unavoidably be Lewis's superior. "You can only judge of the effect of such a contingency on your happiness, and on your work, assuming that you were still at the Institute at that time."

In a communication to Smith some two weeks later, Flexner, who, in the meantime had had a personal interview with Lewis, told him that "if Lewis stays I think his relationship to and value for the Institute improved and increased by experience."[18] Coming, as he did, from a semi-administrative post, Flexner supposed that it was inevitable that Lewis should plan ahead as he did. "From now on his future in science is in his own hands . . . There is no doubt in my mind that

Lewis can make himself very valuable to your Department, and I believe he means to do so."

Writing to Lewis on August 1, 1927 from Chocorua, where he had had several talks with Smith who was summering at nearby Silver Lake, Flexner informed Lewis that he and Smith had discussed the upcoming report that Flexner normally made to the Board of Scientific Directors in October, summing up the past year's work.[19] Flexner explained that the report that year would be different; instead of surveying all of the work of the year, it would be devoted to selected topics, drawn from the year's work. In reviewing problems pursued at the Institute in the recent period, he naturally thought of Lewis's studies on the hereditary influence of tuberculosis on guinea pigs. Believing that Lewis must have records extending over his four years at the Department of Animal Pathology, from which he could doubtless have indications of the way the result was shaping itself, he asked Lewis to prepare a statement for him so that he could determine whether or not to include that topic in the October report. On September 8 following, Lewis sent on the desired material, which ran over four and a half typewritten pages.

In September, Flexner forwarded Lewis's report to Smith and told him that he would like his analysis of the statement before seeing Lewis personally.[20] "It is obvious that he has very little to go on," Flexner commented, although he believed that one point had been established, the factor of nutrition in tuberculosis infection; and he asked Smith to provide him with some idea of what the cost per year of the experiment amounted to. He concluded his letter, saying, "With the closing of the tuberculosis work, Lewis will be left without a major problem or sense of problem to be attacked. This is quite serious at the end of five years. If, therefore, he is to be encouraged to accept a teaching position, this should be the proper time to discuss the subject with him."

Flexner wrote to Lewis on September 22, telling him that he had had time to go over his report and to think about it, and also to discuss it with Dr. Smith.[21] While Lewis had arrived at one definite point, namely that nutrition made a difference in susceptibility, in a major problem that had been underway for four years, this was minimal; and furthermore, the outcome, even if continued many years longer, was uncertain, and the yield of side issues, often the most fruitful of all the problems, had been small. Since he did not believe in sticking to a rather barren subject, he asked Lewis to wind up the tuberculosis problem as quickly as possible, but certainly within a year. He told Lewis that because his status and future were bound up with the remaining two years of his appointment at Princeton, he desired to have a "pretty full talk" with him. And in a letter to Smith early in the New Year, Flexner mentioned that he would talk with Lewis and with Smith very soon.[22] "I think it not impossible that he may be asked again about teaching. He would be well advised to accept a good school appointment."

In a communication to Flexner about a month later,[23] Smith stated that he was at a loss to make suggestions concerning some new problems for Dr. Lewis. He thought that Lewis might well study other diseases of swine and let hog cholera alone until he could muster new lines of investigation. Theobald believed that Dr. Lewis had two ideas in mind when he came to the Institute: 1, that under the cover of animal pathology he could work on anything he pleased; and 2, that he would be Smith's successor. "Whether he can be influenced to dig into an. path. wherever it presents an opening or not remains to be seen."

Flexner wrote to Lewis again on April 27, informing him about the discussion of his tuberculosis work at the meeting of the Board of Scientific Directors six days earlier.[24] Reminding him that his tuberculosis problem was in its fifth year, and that when he had brought it over from Philadelphia the notion was that it would be completed in a year or so, he told Lewis that it was the opinion of the Board that his search for the food factor or factors responsible for the change was too indefinite to be continued at the Institute. The Board had therefore decided that he should be requested to discontinue the experiment during the present academic year.

Flexner notified Smith on June 18 that Dr. Henry Houghton, formerly director of the Peking Union Medical College and now medical dean at the University of Iowa, had spoken to him about recruiting a head of the department of pathology.[25] "He may come to Princeton to see you. If the opportunity should come to Lewis again, he would make a great mistake not to seize it." Two days later, Flexner informed Smith that Lewis had come to New York to talk with Houghton about the Iowa position, and while he appreciated the offer of the position that might come, "his 'compelling' interest lies in Princeton."[26] Lewis's attitude puzzled Flexner, especially since he had no great security at Princeton and his years were increasing (he was then forty-nine years old). Flexner considered this a pity, because at Iowa "His quite unusual gifts of exposition would be used, and he might really come to exercise a real influence on medical teaching and research." Two days afterward, Flexner informed Smith that he had had a talk with Lewis and "Lewis's mind is, I think, absolutely made up not to go to Iowa if the position is offered to him."[27] Flexner spoke of sensing that Lewis now felt the uncertainty of his future at Princeton. "If the next year does not develop something quite certain in him for the future, he expects not to be reappointed."

Flexner wrote to Smith again on June 30, telling him that "he would write a little more about Lewis especially as Houghton spoke to me before I left N.Y." He reported that Lewis was entirely unaffected by Flexner's frank talk with him and the possibility that his appointment at the Institute might not be renewed a year hence, even after Flexner told Lewis that, as far as he could see, "he was not essentially of the investigative type." Flexner clearly encouraged Lewis to take the Iowa job, assuring him that things would go well at Iowa under him. Houghton had offered him $10,000 a year (a great deal more than his Institute salary) and a very good budget, as well as a free hand in organizing a department. Flexner recommended to Lewis that he go to Vienna, under leave from the Institute, and see a lot of human pathological material, then go to Iowa and make himself indispensable, believing that "He could become a great figure there," that he would be far happier than he was now. He said that Lewis had become a disappointment to him and that his obstinacy was something that they were not responsible for and "for which he will have to pay, I fear."[28]

In October, Dr. Frederick F. Russell, Director of the Institute's International Health Board, wrote to Flexner, telling him that he had talked with Theobald Smith about a bacteriologist for yellow fever work then going on in South America.[29] Theobald had suggested Dr. Richard E. Shope, a young member of the Princeton department, who had expressed his interest in the possibility; but in a response to Russell three days later, Flexner told him that Shope was not available that year, because work he was carrying on required that he remain in Princeton through the following June.[30] Smith had also sent a letter to Russell three days afterwards, reinforcing Flexner's decision, and asking Russell if he would like him to discuss the matter with Dr. Nelson, a member of Smith's staff; but in a letter to Smith on the following day,[31] Russell told Smith that he should let the follow-up with Nelson rest, because that morning he had received a call from Paul lewis, who said that he would like to talk with Russell about the yellow fever position.

After both Smith and Flexner agreed to release Lewis on leave from his Institute commitment, he was hired by Russell and sailed for Brazil on December 29. In a long letter written to Smith on February 1,[32] Lewis related that he had arrived in Brazil a few weeks earlier and had gone right to work with the idea of sending virus material to New York. He reported that the laboratory arrangements were as good as possible, from the view of both safety and efficiency, and that he had no reason to be apprehensive of any difficulty concerning health. He spoke also of having read most of the yellow fever literature since Noguchi's first paper, which "certainly is confusing enough." He believed the whole business should be gone through again thoroughly and little taken for granted, and he was starting fresh with guinea-pigs, which seemed to have been neglected recently.

When replying to Lewis on February 19, Smith told of noting what Lewis had said about the confused state of yellow fever etiology, expressing his feeling that the study should take into account the West African work, as well s the Brazilian virus work done thus far.[33] "I agree that it is desirable to work again with the guinea pig, but that animal will not suffice for the study from the virus point of view;" and he added, "I write about it merely because you did not mention the use of the monkey in our letter." On April 12, Lewis sent a lengthy communication to Flexner from Bahia, reporting on his "work with the virus proper."[34] Telling that Davis, who was in charge, had made full use of his available space and supply of monkeys, he said that he did not feel it necessary to order a great increase in either until he had really seen a little of the disease in operation. He reported that the monkeys arrived there in monthly shipments, and from work he had seen thus far with about 100 animals, "There seems to be no doubt that the disease represents yellow fever very well, and I think their work is ample to show that the South American virus is fundamentally the same as the African." Suggesting that there may be a difference in virulence, due, perhaps to differences in manipulation, he told that what he could do in this direction was to try by passage to get a fully virulent South American virus to bring back to New York.

"Using the material presented by the experiments going on here," he next reported to Flexner, "I have now had a good 'look' for the virus," but "I have not been able to locate anything," despite the fact that bacteria were extremely abundant. He revealed that in two instances thus far, "both monkeys well treated with mosquito virus," he had recovered a very interesting spirillum that had presented under the dark field every morphological feature of changing conditions of growth—"vibriospirillum, spirochete and Vincent bacilliform." This material had failed to produce disease in the one monkey he had tested it on, and "I have failed to find it so often that I do not think it is 'yellow fever' either." He mentioned that he had promised Dr. Russell to stay in Brazil for at least six months, and he still had in mind the idea of returning to the swine influenza work that he had been helping Smith carry on at Princeton. The preceding was the last communication that Lewis would make to Simon Flexner.

On June 30, Flexner wrote to Smith that when he had arrived at the Plaza Hotel that night, he had received the disturbing message that Lewis had been diagnosed with yellow fever.[35] "I am taking hope that the South American fever is less fatal than the African," and he raised the possibility that the case might prove to be one of laboratory infection with the African virus, which had been sent to South America for comparative purposes. Then, on July 1, came the dire cable message of Lewis's death. When writing to Smith that same day, Flexner related that the fatalities from the disease had been entirely among laboratory workers. "The clinicians in the field seem to escape. I suppose it is the handling of the infectious organs of animals which leads to inoculation." He closed by saying that "Lewis's death changes so many things."[36] Flexner then set to work preparing an obituary of Lewis, which appeared in *Science* magazine soon afterwards.[37]

In a letter sent to Smith in late July,[38] Flexner reflected that Lewis had spent twenty-five years after taking his M.D. degree in the laboratory with the two of them. When looking over Lewis's publications in light of Theobald's comments on the obituary notice he had sent on, Flexner opined that it was evident that he was not originally gifted or "lucky" in his work; that he had remained pretty closely chained to the subjects he worked with under direction and never secured a field or rewarding set of problems of his own. Letters sent to Flexner by Dr. Russell indicated that he had worked hard in Bahia, looking for a lead, and he thought he had secured one or two, but they proved to be false. "Perhaps the Lewis type of man should always have a routine and try to do research on the side," Flexner reflected. "It would make for his happiness as satisfying a natural feeling of something accomplished. Pure research positions should, I think, be reserved for more ingenious if not more original minds, so that as age comes on they have individual accomplishments to look back on." He then told Theobald, "I always admired the way in which you kept intellectual, scientific interests uppermost in your mind."

While Flexner's remarks honestly expressed his philosophical view of the matter, he might have been harsh with poor Lewis, who did accomplish something in his career in that his name appears on two classic contributions to the literature of medicine, in both instances growing out of research he participated in in 1910 during his first stint at the Rockefeller Institute: with John Auer on an important study of anaphylaxis in the guinea-pig,[39] and with Flexner himself, for developing experimental poliomyelitis in monkeys.[40] In the reports of both accomplishments, however, appropriately, his name appeared in the secondary role.

Director Designate TenBroeck

Carl TenBroeck's return to the Princeton laboratories and his later career there was not, like Lewis's, ill-fated—indeed, quite the opposite. TenBroeck had remained at the Peking Union Medical College and by 1925 was head of its Department of Pathology; and Flexner, who was always on the lookout for good laboratory experimenters, and Smith had discussed him a number of times in their frequent correspondence with one another. In fact, some of their letters relating to Lewis's return to the Institute and his eventual downward spiral there contain references to their desire to bring TenBroeck back into the fold should events prove favorable to the accomplishment of such a goal. For example, in his letter to Smith of October 26, 1925, after mentioning that he wanted to have a talk with Lewis about the pension matter, Flexner remarked, "What you said at the meeting about Ten Broeck interested me very much." He felt confident that his experience as head of the department of pathology in Peking would help in his development, and in another two years his term there would expire and he would be free to choose whether he wished to remain in China or return to the United States. "I do not think that the Rockefeller Foundation considers any of its men in Peking bound beyond their terms of appointment."

TenBroeck was not discussed again in the Smith-Flexner correspondence until the end of July 1926, when Theobald mentioned to Flexner[41] that Lilian had received a letter from Janet TenBroeck telling that they expected to spend the following year, from the beginning of the summer of 1927, in Europe, he to study there. She thought that she would like to stay in China indefinitely, but it might not be best for her husband and children, since the political outlook seemed to be worrying them some. "If he is to follow me," Theobald remarked, "we should be doing something about it. I am 67 today and you know, we are likely to be extinguished any moment. Besides, the dept. needs a strong man with its increased size and activities who will take an interest in its various details and ramifications. I think Ten Broeck will. He has a conscience about his work and is no bluff. It would be unfortunate if a sudden gap should occur with no one in sight to fill it."

In a note to Edric Smith on August 4, Flexner told him to mark TenBroeck for discussion at the upcoming October Board meeting in executive session. And in replying to Theobald Smith two days later,[42] he said, "I agree with what you write of taking Ten Broeck under serious consideration for Princeton. He has solid qualities and from all accounts has acquitted himself well in Peking." Mentioning his intention to discuss the matter at the October meeting, he indicated that if TenBroeck wanted to return to Princeton, he would make him a member of the Institute with a suitable salary. Hoping that Smith would remain in the directorship, health permitting, for another period, within that time TenBroeck could "be gathering up threads and getting himself to work on some problem or problems in animal pathology," under Smith's direction, of course. Then, when the time came for Smith to lay aside the directorship, the transition would occur naturally with no break with the past. "The essential point is, I think, to secure a working, productive director and not merely an intelligent executive. We cannot hope to succeed your admirable administration by one who is essentially an investigator, but we should approximate this as nearly as possible." He viewed as the most unfortunate thing that could happen, either at Princeton or New York, would be to develop a bureaucratic type of director. "I do not fear this from Ten Broeck, but if he could first go to work on a problem or two, I should feel more confident about the future."

Theobald Smith afterwards wrote to TenBroeck hinting at what he and Flexner had in mind. And in a letter that Flexner sent to Smith in late November,[43] he said that once TenBroeck was presented with a choice of spending years in China or coming back to the remarkable opportunities with Smith at Princeton, he and his wife would probably view the future in a somewhat different light. Then, on the last day of the year 1926, Theobald wrote to Flexner, telling him that his surmise was correct: "I have just received a letter from Ten Broeck in which he accepts the position for member[ship] if appointed."[44] Owing to his earlier plans for spending some time in Europe, Theobald suggested that they should take some action at the coming meeting, saying, "I am greatly pleased for the department needs pathologists to balance the present structure."

When communicating with Smith a few weeks later,[45] TenBroeck reported to his future chief that work he had completed that day led him to the conclusion that most of the reports he and his colleagues had published on tetanus had been secured by a cunning, deliberate modification of the various substances used for animal inoculation; and he admitted to having been too cunning, perhaps even dishonest, because they had since had trouble carrying out the work—in other words, work he had believed to be good had since turned out to be false—and he now felt contrite. "As the tentative offer of an appointment as a member of the Institute staff was no doubt based largely on my research work, I should like to have it reviewed by the Board of Scientific Directors with this letter before them with the understanding that they are in no way committed by any previous action they have taken." In a cablegram to TenBroeck on February 7, or thereabout, Smith wired: "Advise against science statement Appointment unaffected Writing."[46]

The next time TenBroeck was mentioned in the Smith-Flexner correspondence was on July 29, 1927, when, writing from Silver Lake, Smith reported that he was expecting Dr. TenBroeck that afternoon to stay for a few days before sailing.[47] He also related that Lilian had fallen on the camp floor the previous Sunday with an impacted fracture of the right radius resulting. TenBroeck and his family subsequently embarked for that planned year abroad; and on September 21 following, Simon Flexner wrote to his brother Abraham of the Rockefeller's General Education Board,[48] telling him that he and Smith were willing to cooperate with him in a survey of European and American veterinary schools, with the possibility of TenBroeck undertaking the survey during his year in Europe. Flexner explained that Smith did not favor TenBroeck making a survey of the United States, and for this he advised him to procure the services of Veranus Moore, who had recently retired from Cornell and was available, he handling the American survey and TenBroeck the European. And in a follow-up letter to TenBroeck then in Paris, Abraham Flexner outlined the financial support that would be provided him in the completion of that work.[49]

When in communication with Smith on January 25, 1928,[50] Flexner referred to having read TenBroeck's letters and memoranda, commenting: "There is no doubt, I think, that he is learning a very great deal abroad, is having his vision widened, and will be all the more valuable to us for his experience." Flexner hoped that when TenBroeck returned to them he could start at once on some animal disease that occurred naturally and follow it as closely as possible; he would be sorry, however, to see him start with the disease in mice, unless it had wider implications, or return to the tetanus toxoid problem, except at second hand. In reply,[51] Smith expressed the view that TenBroeck was perhaps unnecessarily anxious about problems, since he had been absorbed in human pathology. "I wrote to him recently that there was no dearth of problems here." Theobald thought it best for the present not to suggest any, but "to keep his mind open to his environment," and he referred to several problems that TenBroeck might attack.

The TenBroecks returned to America in August and were in Princeton about the 25th; on September 22 Smith informed Flexner that he was starting in with his work as well as possible without an outfit.[52] In another letter to his chief about two months later,[53] Smith regretted to report that "there is afloat a story that TenBroeck is to be made the next director." Someone had heard it in Princeton and had reported it to Shaw, the former superintendent, who had telephoned Smith's son in New York to find out. Smith related that Philip knew nothing and was not interested in speculation, having his hands full getting on. He concluded the matter, saying, "To be sure, there is always much gossip by putting 2 and 2 together."

In early December, TenBroeck asked or was asked to visit Flexner in New York, and on December 12 Smith communicated to Flexner TenBroeck's trepidation about the impending interview.[54] "We have been talking housing with him as he is nervous about next year." After Theobald suggested "various quiet possibilities," TenBroeck causally told him that he might not wish to remain under some other administration à propos of the housing problem. Smith quieted him down and told him he might wish to get something more definite on the matter from Flexner. He also told Flexner that TenBroeck might have found his job more difficult than he had anticipated, as there was much to learn about animal diseases before knowledge could be advanced. The Peking appointment had been attractive because TenBroeck liked teaching, which was lacking here. "He may need a little encouragement," Theobald believed,

> and perhaps some statement that the Directors do not expect anything unusual for the present from him unless accident throws something in his way. The situation here is not ideal and the difficulties with large animals trying. He is broken down nervously and every obstacle might look mountainous to him. Your assurances

would do much to help as he knows my time is up and I cannot hope to do much for him beyond suggestions now and then.

When contacting Smith late in January,[55] Flexner expressed his pleasure with the report "on the Shope-Ten Broeck matter," saying that he appreciated the great complications of working with pigs. "Hence the importance of a man of Ten Broeck's knowledge and reliability being really in charge." Then, near the end of April,[56] Flexner informed Smith that it would be well for the two of them to talk before the next Executive Committee meeting at which the question of "Acting Director" would come up for definite discussion, as the final decision would doubtless be made at the June meeting in Princeton. From his reflections on this very important matter, Flexner believed that there was real merit in Welch's suggestion of Dr. Stockard, for Stockard's work on dogs on a small farm near Peekskill, conducted under a General Education Board grant, showed his interest in animal physiology and pathology, and he had a wide knowledge of animal biology, including parasitology, in general, although he was not an animal pathologist in the usual sense. Flexner thought him remarkably equipped in breadth.[57]

In his response written the following day,[58] Smith told Flexner that "The essential fact in the future development of the department here is whether we shall keep in view the study of disease as the major function and whether other specialties are to be grouped around this central idea or whether we shall then have what businessmen called 'Kampff der Theile' and the more aggressive . . . or persistent . . . will beat out pathology." While he had no doubt that Stockard would make an excellent director, "no matter how widely read we are or how generally informed we cannot direct other lines in the most forward & intelligent way without depending on the men in other lines for key advice." He felt that if Stockard was asked and accepted, someone should be authorized to direct the pathology work and its contacts with other fields there.

On May 27, Smith advised Flexner that it might be desirable for him to confer with TenBroeck before the Executive Committee meeting the following Saturday.[59] "He might decline or wish to consider it. In either case we would have something definite by Saturday." Then, on the following day,[60] he told Flexner that while he and Edric Smith had been inspecting Princeton sites, he had referred to Flexner's hesitation about TenBroeck and the following had suggested itself: "After definitely retiring on June 30, I might be appointed 'acting director' until successor is appointed. The announcement of this step might bring to the surface other candidates not now within our horizon and by the autumn we might be in better shape to commit ourselves." Flexner's letter to Smith a day later[61] was concerned with the directorship job and the complications of

TenBroeck's salary. He felt that there was scarcely an argument to be made for increasing his salary before he had produced any work except that of increasing his responsibilities by an executive position, because his salary then equalled or exceeded that of all Princeton professors except the recently endowed "research professorships." Telling that "his value to the Department has yet to be shown unless he can fill an executive position," he indicated that he would prefer to negotiate both things together.

On June 6, Flexner informed Smith about an extremely interesting and pleasant talk he had had with TenBroeck.[62] "He will act as Director in the Department of Animal Pathology for a year and leave the future to be determined. He impressed me as having an understanding of the grasp of the Princeton Department situation which should make it not difficult for him to take over the administration, relieving you quite completely, when your term of office comes to an end." Flexner said that TenBroeck felt, as he did, that he could not replace Smith; "he merely follows you." He continued: "Ten Broeck's administration must invariably be his own; and indeed I feel that it is only by making it his own that he can possibly succeed with it." TenBroeck would, of course, continue to consult with Smith, Flexner went on, but he hoped that in a short time very little of this would be required, so that Smith need not carry executive matters in his mind as he had done so continually for the past fifteen years. While Flexner was content to give TenBroeck a free hand, he believed that for the most part things would go on as before. He closed his letter, saying, "I hope that you will find the release from executive occupations a happy circumstance in the very full life of scientific work which you have had. Fortunately you are at the height of your powers so that the next years may well prove the most fruitful in a career of extraordinary productivity and significance."

On June 27, three days before Theobald's term of office ended, he wrote to Flexner, telling that he thought it best to move out of his office to relieve the space tensions there;[63] but in his reply on July 1—the same day he wrote another letter to Smith about Paul Lewis's death—Flexner stated that he was not disposed to make any changes in TenBroeck's status except to have him act as director during the year.[64] Therefore, the small office space that TenBroeck would need could be found near his present laboratory. He also confessed that he was hoping for the best for TenBroeck. "I have as you know explained to you that there is no great confidence in his being able to administer the Department executively and scientifically. There should be no misconception about this being a trial year and to move into your permanent quarters would establish him much more definitely and permanently than I am willing should happen."

Flexner believed that the trial year would prove most whether or not

TenBroeck could deal with him directly about everything that required attention. "It will hasten decision on his power to carry on executive duties while conducting scientific work for him to stand on his own feet immediately; and it will help my relations with him to work directly with him rather than through you." By adhering closely to this plan, Flexner explained, "I shall come to learn the quality of Ten Broeck's mind in a way I cannot do unless I deal with him directly. I am sure that you also prefer this plan." And with that, Theobald Smith's fifteen year tenure as Director of the Department of Animal Pathology of the Rockefeller Institute for Medical Research came to a close. The torch had been passed.

On Monday, July 1, 1929, his first day of release from the administrative chain of the Director's position, Theobald Smith recorded in his diary, "Lab. all day."[65] However, the days following were spent running errands, for at week's end, the diary also discloses, he was off to Boston and ultimately Silver Lake, where, as in many summers past, he rested and relaxed and worked on his camp, with scientific studies and researches and writing intermittently sandwiched in. On July 8, while passing through Boston, he paid visits to his bank and to the investment firm of Lee, Higginson & Company to attend to financial matters before proceeding on to the New Hampshire camp, where he arrived at a few minutes before 5 P.M.[66] After spending a day or two repairing an engine and the plumbing, and unpacking his microscope and numerous notes made at the Institute, he settled in for the summer, which was largely passed making further repairs, putting in another camp house for visitors and children, cutting up fallen trees in the woods, receiving visits from family and friends (Flexner, TenBroeck, etc.), relaxing and engaging in water play and rowing some with children and grandchildren and pursuing other restful activities, with scientific work taking place in-between.

On July 27, Simon Flexner again wrote to Smith; after discussing Lewis and TenBroeck, he commented that "About the time this letter reaches you you will be celebrating your 70th birthday. How nice it is that you should be having it with your family and at your house beside the lake! In Germany there would be a great Fest. It would be well deserved but I am not certain you would enjoy the occasion as much as you will enjoy your family circle." Reminding him that "We are to have an 'occasion' in the autumn as you know," he ended with the thought, "I hope you will let your mind rest momentarily on the great fact that you have made contributions to knowledge of pathology which place you in the very first rank among investigators of all times."[67] And a few days later Flexner sent on a congratulatory editorial, "A Scientist's Birthday," which had appeared in the *New York Times* on July 29.[68] Thus passed the summer of 1929. After breaking camp at the end of September, and arriving home on October 3, Theobald entered into his diary on the 5th, "Autopsy cow this A.M.;" and on the 7th, "Lilian 72 years old. Lab. and work on report."[69]

Smith interrupted his daily routine early in November and took the train to Albany—"weather clear, cold. Take fur coat"[70]—where, on November 8, he listened to papers delivered at a meeting at the State Laboratories, saw old friends, and gave a talk on "varieties among bacteria—good effect." That same day, he also drove eight miles to the new animal quarters of the State Labs and then back to Albany to call on his old medical school teacher, Dr. Albert Van Derveer, then nearly ninety years old.[71] On the day following, he toured the new buildings of the Albany Medical College and afterwards was driven by Dr. Wadsworth to Williamstown via Rensselaar, Sandlake, Stephentown and Hancock, arriving at the Prentice farm around noon ("wonderful estate, wonderful house"). Following lunch with Mr. and Mrs. Prentice, he inspected cattle and cattle barns, and after dinner heard organ music. After staying overnight in a "Beautifully furnished bedchamber about 30 ft. sq.," he was driven to Albany in the morning by one of the Prentices' chauffeurs and entrained for Princeton.[72]

Further interruptions in his schedule followed. On November 19, at the meeting of the National Academy of Sciences at Princeton, he listened to Simon Flexner lecture on filterable viruses and on the following day he read a paper on streptococcal diseases in guinea-pigs, afterwards lunching at the Institute's director's house with about 105 guests present; and at the Academy's dinner that evening, he sat at the high table.[73] On November 23, Smith attended a dinner with fifteen members of the Holland Society; and on November 26, he was back in New York, where, at another meeting of the Holland Society with about 200 members in attendance, he spoke on Texas fever, blackhead, colostrum and toxin and antitoxins, afterwards receiving the Society's gold medal and diploma.[74] On December 19, while in New York for a meeting of the Tuberculosis Committee of Cattarangus County, he saw Veranus Moore and other friends.[75]

When in communication with Smith in late September, Flexner mentioned that "You may recall our little talk about your portrait." Thus far, Flexner explained, the Scientific Directors had merely made the recommendation to the Trustees, who would at the upcoming meeting be requested to vote on the needed funds. "As Mr. Rockefeller, Jr. and possibly some other of the Trustees are interested in portrait painting, it may so happen that they will have suggestions as to particular artists. Portrait painting is always a gamble and it would be well to reduce the stake as much as possible."[76] In his response two days later, Smith was noncommittal. "Would it not be as wise to pass the portrait by," he suggested. "There is a Harvard plaque in the Harvard Med. School which may serve to keep my memory green! Why not let it go."[77]

In mid December 1929, Flexner made another proposal to Theobald Smith, although he claimed that the idea had originally come from Smith himself.[78] "It is your suggestion, made on several occasions, of a high type of Journal of Animal Pathology, running say, about six numbers a year (bi-monthly) as the J. G. P. [*Journal of General Pathology*] does, and subsidized by the Institute." He reminded Theobald that he had spoken of being willing to assume editorial control, and that either Williams and Wilkins or the Science Press could be interested. He suggested that Smith consider the matter before the January meeting of the Board, at which time it could be discussed. Again Smith made a discouraging reply—commenting that it was a big problem to assume editorial control of a journal especially during the first two years, with much depending upon the work that was being done at the time.[79] And after Flexner brought up the matter once more,[80] it was dropped for the moment.

On February 3, 1930, Flexner sent Smith a letter of transmittal[81] and an enclosed typescript transcription of a brief note that had appeared initially in *Science*[82] and had afterwards been printed in reduced form in the *Journal of the American Medical Association*.[83] He questioned the correctness of the *Science* note, and, when sending it to Theobald, said, "I am inclined to set both journals right on your Texas fever work, unless you disapprove." The article or note in question, written by the London correspondent of *JAMA,* reported that Sir Patrick Manson, who died in 1922, had established the principle of the insect transmission of disease, and at the international Medical Congress held in London in 1913 was acclaimed the father of tropical medicine.

In 1907, Manson had helped found the Society of Tropical Medicine and Hygiene and had served as its first president. Since the work of the Society was now hindered by the lack of suitable quarters, its members had decided to establish a home and name it after Manson. Although $30,000 had been subscribed, another $100,000 was being sought. The article told that Manson began his great work at Amoy, China in 1877 with the demonstration that the filaria of elephantiasis was transmitted by certain mosquitos and that this was not a chance discovery but a labor done in isolation. Thus, Manson's conviction that malaria was transmitted by mosquitos was no inspired guess, but was founded on his long critical observation of the malarial parasite in human blood and led Ronald Ross to final victory. Flexner had underlined the phrase, "*established the principle of the insect transmission of disease,*" which he knew conflicted with Smith's priority in the discovery of Texas fever, and he now wanted clarification and permission before contesting it.

Smith replied two days later. He told Flexner that when determining that the larvae of *Filaria sanguinis hominis* entered the bodies of mosquitos and developed there, Manson supposed at the time that the mosquito containing the larva or larvae died in water and that the larva was set free and entered the human body in the drinking water. "He did not, therefore, establish the cycle." Smith said that it was as late as 1900 that Lowe (i.e., Low) finally demonstrated the presence of the larvae in the proboscis of mosquitos and their injection into the next patient.[84] "This work is sometimes parallel to demonstrations of the intermediation of ectoparasites such as lice and fleas, in the transmission of tapeworms. It could take some time to determine whether the establishment of the cycle of the tapeworm in these ectoparasites preceded the preliminary work of Manson."

In general, he believed, it was difficult to give anyone credit for any so-called principle. "I think the English might well be allowed to give Sir Patrick Manson the title of 'Father of Tropical Medicine' or 'pioneer.' He did a great deal of good work which stimulated later on the intensive work in tropical diseases." Smith doubted whether it was worthwhile to enter into any controversy concerning these various facts. The judgment would, on the whole, be subjective in any case and likely to be called in question by some other person. "The Europeans have been very careful to give the nationals credit for work done. I have recently been reading in Lubarsch and Ostertag's Ergebnisse the work on influenza as written up by Walter Levinthaal in 1922. He gives fulsome credit to Pfeiffer on almost every page. In this country we have rather downed our own people and given credit to foreigners."

When writing to Flexner again on February 7, Smith revealed that he was debating whether or not to accept an invitation to speak on undulant fever in Little Rock, Arkansas, in May before the Southwestern Tuberculosis Association in connection with the National Association's meeting.[85] "The invitation refers to the benefits derived from the Texas fever work by the SW states. It occurred to me that if I accept I will ask them to hunt up copies of the original report as compensation for my trouble." In his reply a few days later,[86] Flexner said that the judgment about going to the meeting was Theobald's. "If the meeting is one you think important and the journey is not too strenuous, I am sure the board would wish to defray expenses." And, regarding the *Science* article he had sent on earlier, he commented: "I see the complexities of the historical problem." Agreeing that Smith was quite right about the American attitude regarding precedence, he reflected: "At first there is skepticism, and afterwards an effort to find a European precursor. I think we are improving. Perhaps being less chauvinistic has its good, as well as its less good side. The Germans are rather inclined to claim too much; we claim too little. What is the wise and modest and honest thing to do?" When in contact with Flexner again, Smith indicated that he had decided not to make the Little Rock expedition: "It is merely a side show, Little Rock being about four hour's railroad journey from Memphis, where the National Tuberculosis Association would do something about the matter." Nonetheless, he thanked Flexner for the offer.[87]

In a letter of February 10 Flexner once more referred to the oil portrait of Smith that had been suggested. Mentioning that an important National Academy exhibition was then taking place in Philadelphia, and offering to pay Smith's expenses to go and view it, he told that a Philadelphia painter, Mr. Adolphe Borie, had been recommended. "If you go to Philadelphia, I think it would be nice for you and Mrs. Smith to visit his studio. This can be conveniently arranged." Subsequently, Flexner sent on photographs of some of Borie's work, and on April 1 told Smith that he had suggested to Borie that he come to New York and view the place where the portrait was to be hung before Theobald sat for it, adding, "Perhaps at some later day when there is a 'common room' at the Princeton Department it should go there."[88] Borie afterwards did visit the Institute[89] and Smith finally did agree to sit for the portrait, telling Flexner that the artist had come to Princeton and that they had made a satisfactory arrangement with him.[90] "I shall go to Philadelphia on May 1st and 2nd to start work and then at intervals of a week, since he prefers it that way."[91]

In March and April three more of Smith's studies on colostrum appeared in the *Journal of Experimental Medicine,* although they had been completed the year before. (He informed Flexner in September 1929 that they were being typed up,[92] and Flexner afterwards told of having read them and that "They are of course intrinsically very important, and the presentation is most excellent."[93]) Under the series title, "The Immunological Significance of Colostrum," the first and third were undertaken and reported by Smith alone, while the second was the work of Smith and Ralph Little.[94] Telling, in the first paper, subtitled "The Relation between Colostrum, Serum and Milk Cows Normal and Immunized toward *B. coli,*" that the passing on from one generation to another of parasites took place most frequently after birth and that the mortality of the young generation was governed largely by the variety, concentration and virulence of the infectious agents and parasites, Smith also noted that in certain species the uterine transmission of antibodies toward certain enzootic diseases occurred in the blood of the female parent, while in others, such as the bovine species, temporary protection of the young was accomplished by storage of antibodies in the udder, quiescent before parturition. He pointed out that the importance of colostrum in controlling the mortality due to *B. coli,* which tended to parasitize the udder, had been brought forward in another publication,[95] at which time the possibility of substituting normal cow serum for colostrum had been indicated in certain experiments with calves. In this first study involving the substitution of cow serum for colostrum, it had been determined that the antibody content of normal cow serum was below that of colostrum in the same animal.

In the second study, "The Initial Feeding of Serum from Normal Cows and Cows Immunized towards B. Coli in Place of Colostrum," calves from the same dairy had been raised by feeding normal and immune cow serum (serum containing a high concentration of *B. coli* antibodies) in place of colostrum, with the result that losses were one in ten. The third study, "Internuclear Bodies in Renal Disease in Calves," investigated the so-called "white spotted kidney," a peculiar focal interstitial nephritis, a common lesion found in calves in which colostrum feeding had been withheld (which Smith had discussed earlier).[96] The evidence in the condition pointed to a sublethal infection with *B. coli,* but it produced no conclusive results, and the investigation was discontinued and its protocols were now being published because of the interest in similar structures associated with certain infectious diseases.

On April 4, the Rockefeller Institute for Medical Research sponsored a dinner in honor of William Henry Welch on his eightieth birthday, and Theobald Smith was among the four main speakers commemorating the occasion (the others being C.M. Camac of Columbia University's College of Physicians and Surgeons, Rufus Cole, Director of the Hospital of the Rockefeller Institute, and James Ewing, Professor of Pathology at Cornell University). In his address, which appeared in print later that year,[97] Theobald related that, unfortunately, his early contacts with Welch were not those of student and cooperating research worker, but were limited to occasional visits to him in Baltimore while he was working in Washington. Whenever Smith felt troubled in his work, he found consolation talking to Welch, who was nine years his senior. Baltimore had already become the Mecca for research workers, who appealed to Dr. Welch for ideas. Smith's own acquaintance with Welch began with the biological era when young men were drawn into the maelstrom that had been created by the significant discoveries of Koch and his school. "I read every word that he published during this time," which Theobald described as unsurpassed in lucid style, accuracy of expression, thoroughness of work, and great judiciousness. He also recalled Welch from early meetings of the Association of American Physicians as the one who carried the burden of discussion. "It is said of Buddha that after he had learned all there was to be learned he went into retirement and considered whether to give the world his knowledge or keep it to himself . . . I know from my own contact with Dr. Welch that he made up his mind to give his wisdom to the world."

On April 27, Smith informed Flexner that he and Mrs. Smith greatly appreciated the gracious action of the Board of Scientific Directors in conferring on him the honor of representing the Institute at the forthcoming meetings of the Bacteriological, Veterinary and Tuberculosis Congresses that would be held in Europe that summer.[98] Because he felt that the Institute's representative should take some active part in the proceedings, and, secondly, because they were confronted with a change of residence and the problems associated with it, he and Lilian did not feel equal to the undertaking.

Theobald Smith's diary for April contains many notations of working in the laboratory, and in May of sitting for his portrait. On May 5, he entrained, with Kendal Emerson on board, for Memphis to attend the meeting of the National Tuberculosis Association; and his diary entry on the 6th discloses that he did change his mind about that Southwestern Veterinary Association talk, for it records him going to Little Rock (149 miles away) and talking on undulant fever to an interested audience of 100, and returning to Memphis in mid-evening—"walk to hotel through negro quarters. Bad conditions." After spending May 7 and 8 in Memphis hearing papers, he boarded the train home.[99] In a later letter to Simon Flexner, in which he reported that the Department was going on as usual and that TenBroeck dropped by occasionally, he admitted that "The trip to the Southwest may or may not have been worthwhile," and in a blind allusion to his Texas fever work, remarked, "The dept. was put on the map in Little Rock, or rather seeds were scattered or bread cast on the waters," which was his way of explaining his change of plans.[100] On May 16, he recorded his forty-second wedding anniversary and on June 2 his purchase from Robert Hetherington for $5,700 a lot on Battle Road in Princeton, which was to be the site of their future home. And on June 29, he boarded the train for Boston for another summer's stay at his Silver Lake camp.[101]

When Theobald Smith retired from the directorship of the Princeton Institute, he and Lilian were allowed to stay in the Director's House for another year, but now, upon their return to Princeton in late September, they were busy packing their belongings for another move. Pending completion of their jointly-designed home on Battle Road, they once more arranged to board at the Peacock Inn, to which they moved on October 1, taking some of their furniture with them but storing most of it in daughter Lilian's garage or at a warehouse in Trenton. On September 19, Theobald heard from his old Harvard comrade, Marshal Fabyan, who wrote from his summer home at Beverly Farms, north of Boston. Fabyan informed his mentor that his health had not been behaving well for the past two years. "They have finally come down to the diagnosis of Meniere's Disease as I have severe attacks of dizziness associated with deafness in the left ear and with terrible nausea and vomiting." He related that he had done little at the School, "and I think I will resign this year."[102] In a letter written the following January, Smith enclosed a photograph of his oil portrait, and Fabyan afterwards critiqued it:[103] "I think the forehead & eyes very good but somehow I can never get used to your pointed beard. The gown would not aid in doing a horse autopsy and I suppose you borrowed the microscope from Ernst. I wonder how Mrs. Smith likes it. I think she is the best judge."

Back in February, Smith had received a letter from Flexner relative to a letter Flexner had received from B.S. Oppenheimer of the Mt. Sinai Hospital. The hospital had established a named lecture in honor of Dr. Welch, and Theobald had been invited to be a Welch Lecturer. Apparently he had failed to respond to the invitation, and Flexner now seemed determined to prod him into committing himself. He wrote: "The Welch lecturers at Mt. Sinai have in the past, I think, been selected with very great care; and I take it that in your case, as in mine, there is something of an obligation to give these lectures established in honor of Dr. Welch, if it is possible to do so." He therefore hoped that Smith would be able to comply with Dr. Oppenheimer's request, "although of course I am not in a position of urging you to do anything that will put too much pressure on you."[104] Smith replied two days later, informing Flexner that he had declined the Mt. Sinai lecture twice because each time he had a presidential address to write. He did not recall that it was a Welch lecture, but now knowing the full situation, he authorized Flexner to advise Dr. Oppenheimer that he would be delighted to give the lecture, provided that he was allowed sufficient time to prepare one that would dignify the Foundation and satisfy the lecturer.[105]

As it turned out, Theobald gave not one, but two Welch Lectures, on October 17 and 18, 1930. The initial lecture, entitled "The General Problem of Respiratory Diseases as Illuminated by Comparative Data," was delivered to a full house.[106] Theobald began by pointing out that in the early days of bacteriology, the first successes were achieved in the study of septic or blood diseases, where conditions were simple. However, with certain diseases in which the mucous membranes were the scene of multiplication and injury, the problem became more difficult. While the lower digestive tract was more or less guarded by the destructive action of the stomach secretions from incoming bacteria, with regard to the respiratory tract, which was open to all floating matter in the air, the situation became more complicated; and his lecture became a long, involved review of the pneumonias, endemic plagues (bubonic, pneumonic), endemic influenza, and the mounting number of respiratory infections associated with filterable viruses.

At his second Welch Lecture, on "Spontaneous and Induced Streptococcal Diseases in Guinea-Pigs,"[107] the hall was only two thirds full.[108] Smith reviewed the history of a colony of guinea-pigs suffering from naturally acquired streptococcal infection through many generations, comparing it with the conditions in another colony in which the disease had been purposely transmitted or induced. The talk was quite convoluted and technical. It is obvious from his records that much of the material presented here had been derived from the talk on "Streptococcal Disease in Guinea-Pigs" that he had delivered to the National Academy of Sciences nearly a year before but had been left unpublished. Having had the lectures cast upon him, Theobald turned back to material he had utilized before and expanded it to meet the exigency of the situation.

Two single honors were bestowed on Theobald Smith during the year 1930. In late April, a message from Howard T. Krasner, Secretary of the American Association of Pathologists and Bacteriologists, informed him that he had been presented with the gold-headed cane that Harold Ernst had donated to the Society a few years before his death, hoping that it might have a career somewhat comparable to the gold-headed cane deposited in the Royal College of Physicians of London.[109] The first holder of the Ernst cane, Dr. Welch, had been advised that he was being relieved of its custody and was requested to transfer it to Theobald Smith, and in due time it reached him. And in September, Homer N.C. Iver, Executive Secretary of the American Public Health Association, informed him[110] that Milton Rosenau, head of the Association's Sedgwick Memorial Medal Committee, had told him that Smith had been voted the Sedgwick Medal that year. Because Theobald was unable to attend the Association's convention in Fort Worth, Texas in late October, formal presentation would have to be made *in absentia* and Rosenau subsequently offered to come to Princeton and present it to him in person, or, alternatively, to pass it on to him at some future meeting which both might happen to attend.[111]

A letter written by Smith to Flexner at the beginning of the year 1931 indicates that the issue of publishing a journal on animal pathology by the Rockefeller Institute was still very much alive. Smith mentioned in that letter[112] that since the proposed journal would be discussed at a staff meeting the following week, from which Flexner would be absent, he would gather information about various aspects of the subject for the April Board meeting, and he recommended that they get together before he undertook the report. Flexner, who had been away in Baltimore attending a dinner given in Dr. Welch's honor, proposed, upon his return to New York on January 31, that they discuss the journal in early April.[113] Smith, however, wrote to Flexner on February 1, saying that in a talk with TenBroeck about the necessity of such a journal to give animal pathology impetus and perhaps to draw qualified people into the field, TenBroeck mentioned causally that, if they had such a journal, he would probably have something to do with it, or words to that effect, with Theobald then adding, "this rather meant to the editorship."[114]

Stating that it was highly desirable that nothing come between him and TenBroeck, Smith recommended that everything pertaining to the new journal, if any was launched, should come from the Board directly and nothing from

Smith himself—he did not even want to talk to TenBroeck about the matter. If the Board thought that Smith should act as editor, at least for a time, he would not shirk the responsibility. However, it would be a great relief to see someone else begin that undertaking and continue it. Responding soon thereafter,[115] Flexner thanked Theobald for TenBroeck's "reaction." He felt that Smith was indeed correct that the invitation to undertake editorial supervision of any such journal should come from the Board of Scientific Directors; he also believed that TenBroeck should be spared obligations of that sort for a few years. "There are far more important things for him to do—he is a slow worker and to cover the literature is a heavy burden. I don't anticipate difficulties and of course your relations with him must not be disturbed in any way." There is nothing further in the Smith-Flexner correspondence on the publication of such a journal, and it seems a likely conclusion that at the April meeting of the Board the matter was shelved or dropped altogether.

Puerto Rican Interlude

Theobald Smith had been contacted in early January 1930 by Frederick P. Gay of the Department of Bacteriology of Columbia University's College of Physicians and Surgeons, inviting him, at the request of Earl B. McKinley, a member of Gay's department, to serve during the academic year 1930–1931 as visiting professor at the School of Tropical Medicine and Hygiene of the University of Puerto Rico, of which McKinley was director. Since the Puerto Rican facility operated under the auspices of Columbia University, McKinley had sent news of Theobald's selection to Gay with the request that he extend the invitation in the hope that Gay might exert some personal influence to induce Smith to accept the offer.[116] When transmitting McKinley's letter to Smith, Gay stated that Columbia University was proud of the excellent laboratories and hospital that had been established in San Juan and was anxious that a number of eminent American scientists might realize the great opportunities available there for the study of tropical disease. Several were invited to visit each year, and they now desired him to be a participant. Smith could choose his own time for the trip and stay on the island for ten days or longer.

Smith's reply to Gay was noncommittal.[117] He expressed his concern about the kind of service he might render. "You know that I have not given any course of lectures since leaving Boston in 1915. I need therefore rather precise instructions as more or less thought would go into the preparation," stating also that "I should need to go during the *lowest* temperature period since I have grown sensitive to conditions of heat and moisture which render my stay in Princeton during the summer unsafe." Gay's answer[118] informed him that the audience would be entirely medical graduates, the staff of the Institute, and some of the more advanced local physicians interested in tropical disease. As to the content of the lectures, he suggested anything in the field of parasitology would suffice, "although McKinley's own work, as you may know, emphasizes the filterable viruses."

Earl McKinley wrote a follow-up letter on January 27,[119] expressing his hope that Smith would come to the school sometime next year, and he extolled the climate. In responding,[120] Smith accepted the invitation and suggested March 1931 as the time of his and Lilian's visit, telling that the lectures would probably be on the general subject of immunology and perhaps more generally the host-parasite relationship of bacteria to the higher animals. From a more detailed list of possible subjects that Smith later sent on, from which he might select those most appropriate for the Puerto Rican environment, McKinley chose four, the etiology of respiratory diseases, immunity towards *B. coli,* cell parasitism, and animal sources of *Brucella abortus.*[121]

Theobald's diary entries from January into early February 1931 show him at work on the Puerto Rico lectures, and on February 19, while in New York for a Milbank Fund conference, he traveled to the foot of Wall Street to purchase a pair of tickets from The New York and Puerto Rico Steamship Company. After completing a trip to Jacksonville, Florida from February 27 to March 3 to inspect Robert Yerkes's Anthropoid Ape Colony, which was being supported by the Rockefeller Institute,[122] he and Lilian set out on their tropical adventure, sailing on the S.S. *Borinquin* that day and arriving at San Juan early on March 16. They were picked up by Dr. McKinley at 8:30 A.M. and taken for a ride around the town and delivered to the Condado Hotel. The next ten days were filled with rounds of lunches and dinners, inspection trips to hospitals and the School of Tropical Medicine, enjoying the climate and amenities of San Juan, and, of course, the lectures. On March 26 the Smiths boarded the steamer *Cuomo* for their return voyage to New York, passing out of the harbor past the Spanish fortifications into the open ocean. After experiencing heavy seas and rain and thunder on March 29, they arrived in New York harbor early the next morning and were met at the gate by Philip and Dorothea, reaching Princeton at 2:00 P.M.[123] McKinley, in a letter of April 8, expressed his regrets that Theobald had found the weather very cold upon his return to New York, attributing his discomfort to the change from the tropics.[124]

27

AND SO TO ALL MUST END

On April 16, 1931, a fine spring day, Smith's diary informs us, he prepared to set out on a trip to Boston to deliver an address to the Harvard Medical Alumni Association. After packing for the journey and working on his address in the morning, daughter Lilian drove him to the station to catch the train for New York and Boston, where he arrived at 10:00 P.M. and put up at the Statler Hotel. On the following morning, he visited with E.E. Tyzzer at the Harvard Medical School before attending a luncheon at Vanderbilt Hall, the school's new dormitory that had opened in 1929. At the Association's meeting in the gymnasium in the afternoon, he listened to papers by Otto Folin, Wilson G. Smilie, Hugh Cabot and Francis G. Blake until it came time for his own. Owing to the lateness of the hour, he declined to give his speech, but after a vote of the audience was taken, he began to read his address on "Disease as a Biological Problem."[1]

Smith defined diseases as disturbances of equilibrium between the human race and nature, with overpopulation exerting the greatest strain on that equilibrium. It caused the pollution of soil, water and air, the loss of soil fertility, and the impending loss of water through deforestation to pose constant threats of biological upheaval. Thus, disease was a biological entity conjured up by the herding and domesticating factors of civilization. It involved not mere states of degeneration, but a mass of biological reactions. "We are indebted to bacteriology for this changed conception," he reassured his audience, "for it gave us immunology," which he defined as a general term for reactions against disease agents. "These reactions taught us to respect and study symptoms rather than to drown them in drugs." Theobald believed that the continuing largest problem before the human race was still the infectious and parasitic diseases, and the most interesting of present-day activities the attempt to eradicate them completely or annihilate certain infectious diseases, with the problem before the race being what methods should be used to preserve its dominance. While at the present an eclectic combination of suppression and vaccination was perhaps the most easily carried out toward a few diseases, for the bulk a rigid delimitation, suppression and exclusion were the only applicable safeguards. "We are forever mortgaged to nature by civilization, and it remains for medical science to see that the mortgage is not unexpectedly foreclosed." It would appear that Theobald Smith's thinking had advanced markedly since his Anaconda smelter days.

During his address, his diary reveals, Smith's heart accelerated to a rapid beat and he had to stop. He was driven to his hotel where he rested; at 10:00, when Dr. Broughton called on him, he had recovered his balance and his heart was beating regularly. On April 18, Dr. Broughton took him to Dr. Cleaves, who X-rayed his heart and left leg, then to Dr. Hamilton's office, were Miss May worked the electrocardiograph and Dr. Hamilton once more examined his heart. Afterwards he journeyed by trolley to have four savings bank books verified and interest added. Then, following a brief nap, he proceeded to Charles H. Tyler's residence at 83 Bay State Road to confer about the "Distemper Fund" and, after taking tea with the Fabyans and their daughter Frances at their home nearby on Commonwealth Avenue, he was driven in Fabyan's car to call on Dr. Walcott, who was nearly blind. On the morning following, he began an uneventful journey home.[2]

On May 18, Simon Gage drove down to Princeton and stayed overnight with the Smiths before going on to Philadelphia the next day. And on May 20, Theobald caught a train to Philadelphia and walked from the 30th Street Station to the Wistar Institute, where friends of Dr. Gage were gathering to celebrate his eightieth birthday. At noon on the 20th, they were driven in a bus to the Institute's Morris Biological Farm where they lunched and inspected the new buildings for the Director and houses for rats and opposums. About twenty-five guests were present at the dinner for Professor Gage that evening. If Theobald Smith gave a speech on this occasion, it was, unlike the one he delivered at his mentor's sixty-fifth birthday tribute in May 1916, informal and unrecorded. After breakfasting the following morning at the Bellevue Stratford, where most of the guests stayed, he and Gage parted, he returning by train to Princeton and Gage motoring on to New York.[3]

After spending many intervening days in the laboratory, Smith, on June 8, departed for Silver Lake where he passed a mostly uneventful summer, intermingling resting and leisure activities with some scientific work as well as repairing and painting and cleaning up and making improvements around the place. The children came and went intermittently, and not many visitors arrived that summer. On July 24, a sultry day, after painting and attending to chores and busying himself with "some vibrio study," his diary records that he found his "Heart very irregular. Arry[th]mitic feels like 'palpitation'." Nonetheless, he took a short row on the lake in the evening.

On the following day he entered in his diary, "Keeping rather quiet. Heart irregular indicating injury. Do regular chores only." And again on August 18 he encountered some problems: "Trying to keep quiet to see if premature heart beat could be relieved." But afterwards, things seemed to clear up, and he was busy at work trimming trees and cutting down dead ones, painting, raking, rowing across the lake and undertaking other somewhat strenuous activities. He broke camp on September 22 and proceeded to Boston where, on the following day, he spent an hour at Lee, Higginson & Company "Talking finances with Mr. M.J. Cooney—Nothing encouraging concerning possible losses." He then caught the 3:00 P.M. train to Williamstown, arriving after dinner, and meeting Lilian. The two spent the next few days visiting old friends before returning to Princeton.[4]

The "Theobald Smith House"

When Theobald Smith retired as Director of the Division of Animal Pathology of the Rockefeller Institute, his successor, TenBroeck, had no interest in occupying the Director's House, having previously purchased a farm in the vicinity, to which he became devoted. As a result, the Smiths were allowed to remain at Larkfields for another year, a term that was later lengthened by several months.[5] What use to make of the house was afterwards the subject of many discussions among the Institute's Board of Scientific Directors. Flexner thought that the Director's House could be converted to multiple uses as a staff club. After this had been agreed upon, it was decided to discard the name "Larkfields" and name it after Theobald Smith, so that the house would also commemorate its distinguished eponym. (On November 1, 1930, after attending the quarterly meeting of the Board, Smith entered into his diary: "By vote of directors a class members emeritus created [that is, he was granted the status of Director Emeritus]. Also the Dir. house, Larkfields to be called Theobald Smith House.")

On November 20, 1931, the opportunity came to ceremonialize Theobald Smith's retirement and to open the renovated house simultaneously; Smith himself became interested in this proposal, and was asked to prepare some notes on his early years for Mr. Rockefeller, Jr.'s use on the occasion.[6] But how to plan for opening of the house remained a big problem, for Smith himself shrank from any large formal gathering. Moreover, he was a man of few pupils, even among the working group of his department, who always seemed distant from him. It must not be an occasion for jollification or weeping sentimentality. Yet, as Simon

Flexner wrote, "he was a great force in American medical science . . . [and] his individuality made him to be thoughtful and gifted beyond the ordinary. He always thought around a subject, never just at one or another narrow edge, and yet his work was always on specific problems—fertile, highly original and meticulously accurate."[7] The Director's House was really too large and too remote for servants, and there were plenty of critics who considered it unsuitable for conversion into the sort of clubhouse Flexner envisioned. However, as the scientific directors and even the trustees were favorable to the idea, the Coolidge architectural firm was instructed to go ahead with the alterations.

Living quarters for young, unmarried assistants and a guest room for visiting scientists were provided. A billiard table was installed in the reconstructed attic. Yet another development was the use of the house as a place to serve lunch for the scientific staff on working days. This measure was popular, and sometimes Smith could be seen at the table. (Peyton Rous remembered with pleasure walking with him to the Theobald Smith House occasionally for lunch.)[8] The main credit for the transformation should go to Simon Flexner. He thought that "something was needed to stir the staff into a community interest. The house can be used as an entertaining centre for the staff and wives etc. With plant physiology going on, it will make a real centre of contact, bringing it together in a wholesome way."[9]

On November 20, 1931, the Director's House was the setting for a formal dinner commemorating Theobald Smith's sixteen years of directorship of the Princeton Division. The whole scientific and administrative staff of the Division, with spouses, was invited, and absentees were very few. Mr. and Mrs. John D. Rockefeller, Jr. headed a gracious, friendly gathering. Every department of the Institute was represented by a senior scientist, while the Board of Scientific Directors and Trustees attended in full force. "Outsiders" included groups from Princeton and Harvard Universities, and a few special friends of the Smiths, with, of course, Simon Henry Gage, jovial and hearty at eighty, among them. The entire Smith family was present, looking very well pleased with this genuine tribute to Theobald. The former Director's House stood open for inspection, spruced up and welcoming. The new billiard room was a popular show-piece, evidently already well patronized. An informal reception lasting for about forty-five minutes preceded the nicely served dinner. And there, for all to see and critique, was the Borie portrait, commissioned by Flexner, hanging in the Smith's old living room; previewers had thought it a good likeness of the Director Emeritus, capturing his frequent expression of aloneness.

Flexner presided, with Mrs. Rockefeller seated on his right and Mrs. Smith on his left; Theobald was seated between William Welch and Simon Gage. Speeches began at nine o'clock. Mr. Rockefeller started with the eulogies, outlining Smith's early educational history, gleaned from notes supplied by Theobald himself (annotated with handwritten addenda, frequently inaccurate and hard to read, by Simon Flexner). Rockefeller acquitted himself quite well in this tricky undertaking, and ended by offering appropriate toasts to the guests of honor and his wife. Although Flexner's speech contained much conventional praise, which he thought lacked sparkle and fell a little flat, the general opinion was that he spoke well, with sincerely-voiced homage. William Welch, as was often the case, made some brilliant observations, allegedly jotted down in the train at the last moment (as was also often the case when he was expected to make a speech). He spoke perceptively, without manuscript, of Smith's scientific achievements. Fortunately, arrangements had been made for a stenographic transcription.[10] Theobald Smith, looking dignified but rather frail in full evening dress, replied with some interesting and enlightening reflections, and thanked the assembly for honoring him by attending this gratifying occasion.[11]

The Smith-Flexner Relationship and Correspondence

When reading the correspondence between Theobald Smith and Simon Flexner, one is impressed with how much enjoyment two outstanding scientists seemed to derive from the interplay of their minds; each man certainly understood and appreciated the high quality of the other's thoughts, and found much pleasure in the contact. Their thinking seemed to synchronize perfectly, as occurred rarely in other of their relationships; they conversed freely in a common language that few others knew or understood as well. Smith frequently was the senior partner and received greater homage in the interchange. Flexner deferred to his wide knowledge and experience and to his keen powers of observation and perception, as well as to his originality of thought. He often bounced ideas off of Smith and gauged his reactions in order to form his own line of thought and action. In almost every instance, he was respectful or deferent or patronizing, particularly now that public relations or administrative duties were no longer a deterrent. Flexner considered Theobald Smith one of the most brilliant jewels in the Rockefeller Institute's crown, looking upon him as an original thinker and innovator in American medical science. After all, he had spent liberally to build a large, separate department at the Institute in order to entice him there, and to retain his services.

While still at Silver Lake, Theobald had, on August 7, received a letter from Flexner expressing his disappointment in having to delay for so long a visit to Smith's lodge. He had been called to New York City three times that summer for several days on each occasion because of a poliomyelitis epidemic that was raging there.[12] In his reply a few days later,[13] Smith sympathized with his chief for having his vacation broken into by the outbreak of polio, saying, "There is certainly something mysterious about the disease and I am inclined to think that when the whole plot is laid bare it will be a surprise to everybody even to the 'discoverer'." He added an afterthought: "Dr. M.W. Richardson[14] writes me again about rats and rat fleas as a possibility. He lost two boys, as you will recall, many years ago."

In his next communication,[15] Flexner reported that while the epidemic in New York was severe, it was less so than in 1916, he being in daily contact with the situation. "There is a general increase in cases of poliomyelitis east of the Mississippi River . . . There's still a great deal to find out about the epidemiology." And in another letter to Smith on the day following,[16] Flexner related that in a conference the week before Rosenau had brought up again the subject of the rat carrier; but the tissue of rats caught in a highly affected district had been inoculated into monkeys and rats had been injected with virus to determine its survival in the brain with no determinable results. "Perhaps if we get a culture method for the virus (& filterables in general) we shall learn something very new."

When informing Flexner in early September that they were about to close up camp, Theobald commented on the unusual abundance and activity among mammals up there that season.[17] Believing that "There is evidently a peak of cycles going on," he asked if someone could compare these with polio epidemics. And in a subsequent letter to Flexner from Silver Lake, Smith remarked, when referring once more to poliomyelitis, that "this year has been exceedingly rich in floral exhibits." He told of trees being covered with blossoms in the spring, and pines unusually rich in cones, with blossoms very abundant also, although insects were not unusually abundant; and he mentioned seeing several new (to him) plant diseases. "The entire faunal and floral situation was greatly exaggerated."[18]

In his response to Smith's initial letter,[19] Flexner remarked that Theobald's allusion to the unusual abundance of mammals appeared to be very timely. His own house had been invaded by field mice, and there seemed to be more than the usual number of squirrels and chipmunks about. "I would like to know what you have observed as you are much more out of doors & so much more observant." Flexner told that his interest had been aroused by Ellsworth Huntington's article on "Biological Cycles" in the September 4 issue of *Science*.[20] Noting that the epidemic curves of the 1916 and 1931 polio outbreaks, when superimposed, were very much alike, he wondered if this was a mass immunization problem or whether it had to do with the mode of infection?

On November 16 following, Smith sent to Leslie T. Webster, a young Rockefeller scientist, a long letter containing his comments on Webster's forthcoming paper on the factors that govern epidemics as well as the intervals between epidemics, being sure to send Flexner copies of both.[21] He told Webster that, as he understood it, Webster's observations had led him to conclude that the variable factors were much more prominent and distinct in the host than in the infecting agent, which Theobald believed to be quite true. He pointed out, however, that there were certain modifying conditions (a matter that Webster had not discussed in his manuscript): that bacteria can vary within certain limits that were relatively narrow, one being a quantitative increase in capsular formation that would increase the virulence; and, on the other hand, that the limits of variation within much larger hosts were probably much greater, having not only heredity, but also environmental factors to govern such variation.

In the study of animal disease, he continued, "we come upon another group of conditions which do not obtain in your experiments, namely, what happens to bacteria when they pass from one host species to another." As a result of this passage, either from ancestral forms or from present living forms, definite variations resulted. "For example, we have three quite distinct varieties of the tubercle bacillus and we have marked varieties of the *Pasteurella* group," with the *Brucella* races being perhaps the most striking of all. And because there were distinctions between the lability of bacteria in the same host species and in passing from one host species to another, the question arose, "what happens when such modified races of bacteria go back to their original host?" Although, admittedly, this was a phenomenon that would be exceedingly difficult to control by observation, it was the only way he thought possible to account for the varieties of types of bacteria even in the same host that were found, for example, among the tubercle bacilli affecting cattle.

Another factor that should be borne in mind, he believed, was the size and physical capacity of the host. "Mice are small animals, and whether they are capable of multiplying bacteria is a question. When we come to larger animals I think that the host must then have a much more pronounced influence on the organism and in them we must look for the formation of races that I mention above." Flexner thanked Smith for the copy of the letter he had sent on, commenting that "It is just what he needs."[22] He thought that there was a good deal of substance in Webster; he was thoughtful and was a good experimenter, and he was learning something by earlier work "although like so many young men he lives entirely in the present."

When thanking Smith on November 22 for sending his criticisms of Leslie Webster's paper to him for review, Flexner interjected a bit of self-criticism: "Our trouble in New York is that we 'laboratize' our subjects too much. It is a constant struggle to have men 'take' their problems and not 'invent' them. I do not think it so much a misfortune that in your extraordinary career you were led or compelled to accept problems set by nature." It was at about this time also that Flexner called Smith's attention[23] to the recent paper Fred Neufeld had published in the *Centralblatt für Bakteriologie* "in which correctly of course he credits you with being the first to distinguish 'types' among bacteria. This refers to the tubercle bacilli. I suppose that Neufeld had to add Koch's name to yours. He points out that the word 'type' was first used at this time."[24] Theobald's response to Flexner's allusion has previously been noted in Chapter 10.[25]

Theobald's publications during the year 1931 included the two Welch lectures he had delivered at Mt. Sinai Hospital in October 1930 and a more recent article on "The Agglutinating Action of Agar on Bacteria."[26] In the latter, Smith related that a recent statement by C.P. Fitch and associates in Technical Bulletin 73 of the Minnesota Agricultural Experimental Station (1930) that small amounts of agar had some influence on thermoagglutination of the *Brucella abortus* group led him to state some facts in reference to the same or similar phenomenon not associated with heat that he had observed a dozen years before in the study of *Brucella abortus,* and he then described the process.

A report appearing in the *New York Herald Tribune* on February 23, 1932 told that Theobald Smith, "of Princeton University," had that day been elected a Corresponding Member of the French Academy of Sciences; and Flexner sent on his congratulations on the following day,[27] saying, "It gives us all the greatest pleasure to have your remarkable scientific achievements recognized by scientific men and organizations," although he noted that Smith had been credited to Princeton University, an error he thought unimportant. ("I am sure you will not mind and of course they will not mind.") Smith's reply disclosed that he had been rather surprised by the notice "because my scientific affiliations have been chiefly on the other side of the Rhone."[28] He also indicated his willingness to take part in a Koch celebration at the Rockefeller Institute of the fiftieth anniversary of the discovery of the tubercle bacillus, which Flexner had proposed in a separate letter sent to him the previous day.[29] He confessed, however, that the prior fall he had accepted an invitation of the Philadelphia Medical Society to participate in a similar program on March 14, choosing as his subject Koch's views on the stability of species among bacteria. As he intended to write this out, might it not serve a second time with perhaps a slightly modified title, he asked, adding, "I never like to use material over again but the subject is quite important historically." Flexner's reaction was, "If you could turn the Philadelphia lecture a little in the direction of the tubercle bacillus, I think it would be splendid."[30]

While in New York City on March 8 for the meeting of the National Tuberculosis Association, Smith was finally presented the American Public Health Association's Sedgwick memorial gold medal that had been eluding him since mid-1930;[31] and on March 14, he journeyed to Philadelphia to fulfill his commitment on the Koch celebration. After registering at the University Club as the guest of

Dr. Hatfield, he accompanied him to the Art Club for dinner with about twenty guests, among them Francis Packard, Dr. Opie and Edward B. Krumbhaar; after a "Dinner of terrapin chiefly," they went on to the College of Physicians, where, before a "Large audience, many standing," Smith delivered the talk on the stability of bacterial species.[32] Appearing in print later that year, it was his only publication in 1932.[33] Then, ten days later, he was in New York fulfilling his commitment to Simon Flexner and the Institute, speaking—"Myself, Landsteiner, Welch, Flexner"—on Koch's discovery of the tubercle bacillus.[34]

In a letter dated April 1, 1932, C.M. Wenyon, Honorary Secretary of the Royal Society of Tropical Medicine and Hygiene, informed Smith that he had been designated the recipient of its Manson Medal. Commemorating Sir Patrick Manson, this was awarded triennially to the "living author of such original work in any branch of Tropical Hygiene as the Council may consider to be deserving of the honour."[35] The Council had voted unanimously on March 22 to award the medal to Smith, its second paragraph told, "for your fundamental observations and experiments—the first of their kind—on the transmission of a blood inhibiting protozoon by a blood sucking arthropod and for your many contributions to knowledge which are of world-wide importance." The medal was to be awarded at the general meeting of the Society on June 16, and Wenyon expressed the hope that Smith could attend in person to receive it. After a formal announcement appeared in the journal *Nature*, Simon Flexner wrote to Theobald on May 29 conveying his delight and congratulations on the honor. "The award is most appropriate and the citation is most proper," he believed; and he offered to send Theobald and Lilian to London to receive it in person.[36] But when replying on June 1, Smith told Flexner, regarding Flexner's kind "proposition to our going abroad," that the matter "Of course, is out of the question. Even if conditions were favorable I should hesitate to accept the invitation as hardly having been earned."[37] It was eventually arranged by F.F. Russell that the medal would be accepted for Theobald by Dr. George K. Stroude, a member of the Foundation's International Health Division, who was then working in Paris.

On May 11, Theobald departed at 10:00 P.M. on the Lehigh Valley Railroad to deliver a Schiff Foundation lecture at Cornell University on the following evening. Carl TenBroeck accompanied him, desirous of seeing the Cornell Veterinary School. They were met on arriving in the morning by Drs. Gage and Kerr who drove them about the campus, and they visited Cascadilla Gorge to see it lined with forsythias in bloom. After stopping at Willard Straight Hall, where they were being put up, Smith worked on his lecture until noon; ate dinner with Gage at 4:00 P.M.; and afterwards went to the Veterinary School where he listened to TenBroeck talk on filterable viruses. After taking supper with Gage, he dressed in a dinner coat for his 8:15 lecture on "Cell Parasitism and

Phagocytosis" before a crowded hall, with many standees, coming through without fatigue. After breakfast the next morning, he took a familiar walk up Cascadilla Gorge with Gage and TenBroeck on the new Sackett walk. The falls looked beautiful, with large columns of water pouring over them. At noon, Gage and the Veterinary School combined to give the guests dinner at the W. Straight, with about thirty present. Theobald sat next to Dean Mann and Norman Moore, Veranus Moore's son, who was in medical practice in Ithaca (Veranus Moore had died on February 11, 1931). In the afternoon, Kerr drove them about the country, to the entrance of Enfield Falls, then north to Taughannock Park—"Falls beautiful"—and in the evening Professor Gage demonstrated to them ultraviolet light effects, using a mercury vapor lamp quartz condenser on his microscope. After passing the time with Gage on the following morning, he and TenBroeck boarded a train home—he departing for the last time after a visit to a favorite haunt of his youth.[38]

Following a director's meeting at Larkfields (Smith continued to use the original name of the Director's House) on June 4, about which his diary records "Dr. Welch absent," he left on the 9th for Silver Lake, to pass another restful summer at his New Hampshire retreat, occupying himself with chores and scientific work alternately and sporadically. The summer was uneventful, except for the arrival of a letter in late June from Lord Rayleigh in London, informing him that he had been elected a Foreign Member of England's Royal Society.[39] During the summer, his diary discloses, he read Walter B. Cannon's *The Wisdom of the Body,* Pearl Buck's *The Good Earth,* and bits of Otto Lubarsch's autobiography; in-between, he recorded "Lilian 2d 40 years old today" (August 21) and "Dorothea 42 years old today" (August 28).

Smith left Silver Lake on September 19 and proceeded to Boston, where, as usual, he stayed at the Statler. On the next day, he paid a visit to the defunct Lee, Higginson company to check over and take into a safety deposit box all of his securities that had been held by it for many years. Lee, Higginson & Company, which traditionally had been the pet investment firm of the Boston social and academic communities, had in the 1920s invested heavily in stock issued by Ivar Krueger, the Swedish "match king," and in the spring of 1932 a scandal broke out after Krueger shot himself in Paris. It was soon determined that Krueger's multi-faceted dealings had been so strained by the world-wide Depression that the assets and profits recorded for his business were largely fictitious. Walter Cannon, Harvey Cushing and other of Smith's Boston friends were hit hard by the failure, and were either financially embarrassed or wiped out, and the Lee, Higginson firm was eventually put out of business.[40] It is impossible to know how adversely the Smiths were affected in this matter; Theobald made a return trip to the firm on September 21, his diary discloses, and was persuaded to reverse the procedure of his prior visit and hand over to the new Lee, Higginson Corporation some of his securities and stock certificates, taking others to Princeton. While in Boston, he visited J. Mahler, the son of his cousin, and learned from him that cousins Rosy, Katie and Louise were still alive and in Albany. He also called on his nephew, Edward Theobald Murphy, and lunched with him at the Statler. Following another visit to Lee, Higginson, he walked in the public gardens with Lilian, who had joined him, and they dined together before starting home on the 22nd. Theobald's diary locates him back at work in his laboratory on September 30, where he began an autopsy on a tubercular cow, spending most of the day examining tissues and cultures. And on October 6 he recorded that he was planning work on new subjects.[41]

Upon the Smiths return to Princeton from their summer vacation they stayed for a few days with the TenBroecks, for the new house was not quite ready for occupation. Following the purchase of the lot on Battle Road in mid-May 1930, the Smiths in July of 1931 engaged the firm of Coolidge, Shepley, Bulfinch and Abbot to design their projected home. After a great deal of time and effort had gone into drafting and altering and revising plans, Theobald began negotiations with the Matthews Construction Company of Princeton to erect a brick house on the property. He signed a contract with the Matthews firm on February 16, 1932, and by the 25th excavation was underway. Theobald recorded in his diary throughout that winter and spring the progress that was being made—"cinder blocks going up; first floor timbers laid; second floor framing in; electricians running wires; brick work being put up; chimneys in;" and the like—with stone laid on the front porch and slate on the roof in late May. When they left for Silver Lake in June there still remained work to be done. Finally, on September 8, he informed his diary, "Set up bed and slept alone in new home." Moving in followed, with the retrieval of their stored belongings, and afterwards, unpacking and arranging furniture and papers. On October 14, Smith recorded, "First breakfast in our house pre. by Lilian."[42] And in late October, he informed Flexner, "We are now in our home with our belongings and quite happy with the outcome."[43]

The year 1933 was an uneventful one in the life of Theobald Smith—his time and his energy were beginning to run out. It commenced, as in the past, with many diary entries telling of work at the laboratory: January 3, "Lab. till 2 P.M.;" January 4, "Lab. all day;" January 6, "Lab. A.M. writing chiefly and ex. placenta & inoc. g. pig with strept. A 8;" January 7, "Saturday half lab-day;" January 9, "Lab. all day;" January 10, "lab."[44] And so passed the winter and spring, with many other diary references to reading, listening to music on the radio, attending to chores at home, entertaining friends, attending informal lectures at the nearby university, and being visited occasionally by Flexner and other scientists. But the year was not totally devoid of the unusual; there occurred a number of "out of ordinary" events which are worthy of mention. On January 13 and 14, Smith was in Washington at the invitation of Earl McKinley, now Dean of the George Washington University School of Medicine, attending the first meeting of the newly-formed "Smith Reed Russell Society." And on January 18, he and Lilian traveled to New York to view a movie at the Rockefeller Institute of Dr. Welch reminiscing, which Simon Flexner had promoted.[45]

Theobald had been invited by Princeton University to deliver a series of lectures sponsored by the Louis Clark Vanuxem Foundation. His diary shows him hard at work on them in early March, and delivering them on March 7, 9, 14, 16 and 21.[46] They were devoted to the topic of "parasitism and disease," and in order to complete them, he drew upon material he had used, but had not published, when giving the Herter lectures in early May of 1916, supplementing it with a great deal of information he had since learned. And afterwards, he began to edit and prepare them with the view of issuing them as a book.

In early April, he was busy lecturing again, this time in Baltimore at Johns Hopkins University, where he gave three on April 5, 6 and 7 in a series commemorating the memory of William Sidney Thayer and his wife Susan Read Thayer. On April 6, he was honored with a dinner at the Chesapeake Club, and on April 7, after finishing preparations on the third lecture that would be delivered late that afternoon, he taxied to the Brady Institute to "see Dr. Welch for 5 min. Seems much changed after operation."[47]

Smith's Thayer lectures were divided into two parts under the general title, "Focal Cell Reactions in Tuberculosis and Allied Diseases," with the first part subtitled "Epithelioid Cell Reactions," and the second, "The Succession of Cell Relations."[48] In a long technical discussion that was intended to emphasize the stimulating activities of the tubercle bacillus, Smith told that, while all studies of focal cell reactions revolved around tuberculosis, an immense amount of patient research concerning the tubercle had not brought unanimity in the interpretation of its various phases. However, his long-time comparative study of the lesions of bovine tuberculosis and paratuberculosis had led him to make certain conclusions regarding cell reactions. Due to Metchnikoff's concept of phagocytosis, for half a century pathologists had been inclined to view all local cell gatherings as an active resistance on the part of the host. "All that we can really postulate, however, is that certain bacteria and cell types have an affinity for each other, with either death of the host or suppression of the parasite resulting.

He pointed out that certain bacteria associated themselves with connective and adenoid tissue of the epithelioid type, others had an affinity for vascular endothelium, while still others manifested a chemotactic affinity for endothelial leucocytes. The epithelioid type of cell reaction appeared in tuberculosis and bovine paratuberculosis. Each group of cells was the product of a specific action of the corresponding infectious agent and the expanding cytoplasm modified specifically, since there was no cross immunization among these diseases. They were the result either of direct contact of the bacteria with the progenitor cell or of diffusible metabolic products, or of products resulting from disintegration or dismantling of the bacteria, dependent upon genetic and acquired host factors of the epithelioid cell as well as the virulence of the bacteria.

The earliest phases of spontaneous bovine tuberculosis were assumed to consist in the multiplication of the deposited bacilli, followed by a prompt swelling of the cytoplasm of the local cells subsequent necrosis. The outward spread and diminishing activity of the metabolic products of the tubercle bacilli led to the epithelioid-cell mantle and finally the connective-tissue capsule. In paratuberculosis, the association of bacilli with the normal reticulo-endothelial system was observable and the presence of various swollen cells could be seen in the progressive disease. The increasing resistance of the tissues was due to the discharge of diffusible products of the living cell bacilli and their impact on the forerunners of the epithelioid cells throughout the system. When bacilli escaped from a primary focus, the secondary foci were built under the influence of this increased resistance.

From the evolutionary standpoint the gradual loss of diffusible aggressive metabolic products by the invading parasite reduced the systemic effect and tended to localize and make chronic the disease process, provided the parasite at the same time gained in protective capacity. Host specialization rose and the host-parasite conflict became a purely cellular one. In general, the focal lesions in any infectious disease represented the conditions under which the bacterium could multiply and survive and eventually leave the host. Paradoxically, however, these foci, owing to active cell immigrations and proliferations, had been considered the sites where the organism was suppressed, despite the fact that the same organisms were unable to survive elsewhere in the host, should they break away from the primary focus, unless similar foci had been established.

In mid-April, Smith was in Washington for the National Academy of Sciences meeting, and in early May he attended the advisory council meeting of the Phipps Institute in Philadelphia, acting as chairman.[49] His diary entry for May 31 shows him at work writing up the Thayer lectures, and in early July he headed for Silver Lake for the summer (of course, during his stop in Boston, having his bank books verified and interest added). His usual routines around the camp that summer were interrupted on August 14 by the need to proofread the Thayer lectures; and on August 30, his diary reveals, "Dr. Yerkes and Cannon unexpectedly appear as I was staining" the front porch floor. (When writing to Flexner in late August and telling that he had recently read galley proof on the Thayer lectures, Smith informed him that "The material is in a sense original."[50] There is no reply from Flexner to Smith's letter extant, which is regrettable, for it would be most interesting to know his reaction to Smith's novel and interesting theory of cell reactions.) By September 19, Theobald was back in Princeton and the next day at work in his laboratory. On October 5, while autopsying a calf exposed to paratuberculosis, his diary reveals, he cut his finger badly; and on October 9, Simon Flexner paid him a visit to discuss the future membership of the Board of Scientific Advisors.[51]

On October 28, while in New York for a meeting of the Board, Smith afterwards confided to his diary: "Dr. Welch resigns o/a of illness. I elected president." On November 20–22, while attending meetings of the National Academy of Sciences at M.I.T., he again met his old friends Cannon and Folin, paid a visit to the Lee, Higginson firm, saw Mr. Ames about the remnant of the dog distemper fund, and met with the Fabyans. When returning home, he stopped in New York for a meeting of the Rockefeller Institute directors and talked with Charles Stockard, now a Board member, about current dog distemper work. (Before his departure for the Boston meetings, news reached him from Sir Henry Dale in London that he had been awarded the Copley Medal of the Royal Society, then thought by many to be the most distinguished scientific award in the world.)[52] On December 5, he discussed with the editor of the Princeton University Press the publication of his Vanuxem lectures. On December 21, Charles Stockard arrived for lunch and the two once more discussed current work on dog distemper. And on the last day of the year, Theobald recorded that he was at work on the final draft of the Vanuxem lectures, typewriting some of its pages, "The first typewriting since June 1932."[53]

On January 3, 1934, Theobald began the new year the same way he had commenced new years for many decades now, entering into his diary, "Lab. all day. Working over notes & animals & cult.," but adding now, "Mss ready to send to Univ. Press." The manuscript was, of course, for his book, *Parasitism and Disease,* and it appeared in print about six months later. Meanwhile, he was in New York on January 20 for a meeting of the Rockefeller Institute's Board of Scientific Directors, which on that occasion included himself, Flexner, Francis Blake, and Stockard. They had a lengthy discussion concerning its future make-up and the Institute's next Director, for Simon Flexner had indicated his desire to retire in 1935. On January 30, due to a cold snap and storm, Smith remained at home, "reading on Texas fever and anaplasmosis." Following another bout of unusually cold weather and much snow, Smith was in New York once more on February 15 for another Rockefeller Executive Committee meeting and another discussion as to the choice of Flexner's successor. March brought more trips to New York—on the 12th for a Leonard Wood Memorial Fund council meeting and on the 14th and 15th for the Milbank Fund's council meeting, at which, after lunch on the 15th, he heard Mayor La Guardia speak.

While at dinner at the Veblen's on March 16, he encountered Frau Landau, the daughter of Paul Ehrlich, who was now resident in the United States. On the 19th, Lilian had her to tea, and on March 22 she and Lilian visited Smith in his laboratory. On April 12, he received the proofs of his forthcoming book and set about reading them. On April 14, Smith recorded in his diary, "Daffodils out in force," and on April 18, "Forsythias coming out. Buds on trees swelling. Maples in bloom." It was a fine spring, which was fortunate, for it was to be the last one he would see. Theobald and Lilian were in New York again on April 20 for a dinner party given by the Flexners, at which Rufus Cole, Charles Stockard, Francis Blake and Warfield Longcope and spouses also were present, and on the next day he attended another meeting of the Board of Scientific Directors. May 1 brought news that Dr. Welch had died the previous night, and on the 2nd Smith and TenBroeck proceeded to Baltimore to attend the funeral service at St. Paul's Church, accompanying Flexner and other Rockefeller men on the return trip as far as Princeton. On May 4 he attended a meeting of the New York Society of Tropical Medicine at the Cornell Medical College, giving an address on Texas fever, which he had been preparing for several months, to about twenty-five guests. Lab work and chores at home consumed most of his time thereafter until he headed north on June 29, lunching with Dorothy and Phil in New York, and stopping overnight in Boston before going on to New Hampshire.[54]

Although he did not record the event in his diary, his book, *Parasitism and Disease,* came out in late June, for on July 3, Simon Flexner wrote to him, just before leaving for Connecticut two days previously, and thanked him for the author's complimentary copy he had received.[55] Flexner described the book as a "really masterly piece of work;" he believed that no one else could have developed even remotely the main theme of the book as he had done so admirably and successfully. He only wished that Dr. Welch had lived to see it. "He would have appreciated it wholly." With regard to Welch, Flexner told that he had been asked by the Johns Hopkins authorities to prepare a biography, and he asked Theobald if he would jot down his experiences and episodes for his use in that work.[56] "For example, you can tell me, as no one else can, about the period around 1890 when Dr. Welch was studying hog cholera and associated diseases in swine. It was that period which I recall so well because of your visits to the laboratory at the Johns Hopkins Hospital . . . and there were doubtless many other occasions on which you conferred about problems in which you were jointly interested." And he asked for specific information about both Smith's and Welch's work on mutation or variation in colony formation and about the pneunococcus work on which Welch had for so long been engaged.

In *Parasitism and Disease*,[57] a book of nearly 200 pages, Theobald Smith summarized everything of importance that he had learned over his long and distinguished career about the role of parasites in animal pathology and their relationship to human disease—fields that he had helped bring to maturity and over which he was an acknowledged master. He classified the potential living agents of parasitism into six categories: (1), the higher animal parasites, of which worms were the largest group; (2), certain molds causing skin or lung affections; (3), minute, single-cell animal forms, barely visible to the higher powers of the microscope, known as protozoa (including coccidia); (4), bacteria, justifiably regarded as forms of vegetable origin and just visible with the highest power of the microscope, producing some of the most formidable diseases and plagues of man and animals; (5), a group of organisms smaller than bacteria, but still visible under the microscope and cultured with greater difficulty, which produced diseases such as typhus and Rocky Mountain spotted fever, and known as Rickettsia (after their discoverer, Howard Taylor Ricketts); and (6), a large group of organisms below the resolving power of the microscope termed viruses, which passed through the pores of filters restraining the bacteria and vied with them in their capacity for destroying human, animal and plant life, and which, when inhaled, might start certain processes in the body cells which, in turn, reproduced the invading agent for further dissemination.

In nine chapters, he attempted to explain what parasitism was; detailed the life cycles of parasites; described aberrant parasitism, or incomplete cycles; sketched out the nature of the conflict between host and invading parasites; took account of cell parasitism and phagocytosis, that is, the destruction of the invaders by host cells dedicated to that purpose; surveyed the variation and mutation among parasites as protective devices and their survival and movement from host to host; outlined the epidemiology or destructive spreading of microorganisms and other parasites; and discussed the utilization of discoveries about parasitism as a means of annihilating or checking them, such as modifying or attenuating their destructiveness by heat, alcohol, carbolic acid and formalin, or extinguishing their virulence by passing the original virus through a series of small animals and modifying it into a vaccine.

The following may be cited as an index of Smith's exactness in and command of his subject. While busy at work transforming his Vanuxem lectures into book form in late December 1933, he asked Flexner about the correctness of his views on poliomyelitis, telling him that what he had said in his lectures might have to be modified to accord with Flexner's most recent investigations.[58] Flexner's response[59] was that the paragraph on infantile paralysis taken from the Herter Lectures of 1917 was a very interesting statement and a significant one also, "and might well hold even today." He mentioned that "Such modification as is called for might relate merely to the varying degrees or grades of immunity in poliomyelitis." And after summarizing everything that then was known about the disease, Flexner suggested only a few changes.

And when writing to Smith in late July of 1934,[60] and congratulating him on news of his final receipt of the honorary LL.D. degree from the University of Edinburgh, Flexner told him that he was reading the Vanuxem lectures, lecture by lecture, with pleasure, profit and admiration. In this way, he believed, he could better appreciate the vast experience, knowledge and thought that went into their preparation. "The volume will be prized most by those whose judgment you will value best; and it will be a permanent addition to the literature of parasitology in disease." William Bulloch, a British bacteriologist of world repute and author of a classic history of that science,[61] described *Parasitism and Disease* as "a wide survey of the whole field written with undimmed mental faculties, a remarkable effort for a man of seventy-five."[62]

Most of Theobald's summer vacation at Silver Lake in 1934 was spent cleaning up and making repairs around the place; little time was devoted to reading and scientific work. On August 7, he interrupted his relaxed life-style to make a trip to Boston where, after a hurried trip to Lee, Higginson, he attended a meeting with Stockard and others on the dog distemper fund: "Stockard to write a report for Sept. to reach full committee." The Smiths' vacation ended on September 13 when Lilian and he took the train to Boston, afterwards catching the Boston-to-Washington "Senator," which stopped at Princeton Junction. On the 17th, he was back in his laboratory as usual, working until after lunch, and continuing an almost daily work routine during the weeks following.[63]

On October 6, while Lilian attended a departmental tea, Theobald stayed home, "slight temp. palpitation etc." Two days later he was back in his lab. On October 16, his diary entry reads, , "lab. till bus time[.] errands[,] then walk home. Very tired. Too much exercise." But he was back in the laboratory the following day. On October 19, he recorded, "Cardiac difficulties," and on the following day, "Personal condition poor. Lost 3–4 lbs. Cardiac irritability, Weariness." On October 21, a Sunday, he was "moping around because not well." Nonetheless, on October 27, he was in New York for a meeting of the Institute's Directors: "Annual meeting election of officers. I elected President again nominations for director." At a special meeting of the Board of Scientific Directors on June 1, Theobald, Charles Stockard and Flexner himself were appointed a committee to nominate a new director, and after long and thorough consideration they recommended the distinguished physiologist Herbert S. Gasser, with Flexner's resignation becoming effective October 1, 1935. On October 30, Robert Yerkes called "to talk over the Florida chimpanzee plant." And on the day following he noted "L1 in bed with symptoms of renal calculi," he himself

"Moving about aimlessly, accomplish nothing." And so it went for the next two weeks, "stomach painful," "no appetite," "lying down most of the day. Swallowing painful."[64]

On November 18, Simon Flexner stopped in Princeton on his way back from Washington to see Theobald Smith. "Looks badly," he jotted in his diary.[65] "Obviously apprehensive about himself." After consultations with TenBroeck and others, Flexner conveyed the wish that he should come into the Institute hospital. They would send a Packard car with pillows for comfort. Theobald asked for a few days delay as his temperature was normal for the first time that day. Moreover, Mrs. Smith was ill with cystitis and pyelitis. But on November 18 also, Smith recorded in his diary—the last entry in it—"Packing for R.I. Hospital tomorrow.[66] He entered the Rockefeller Hospital on November 19, and on that same day his wife went into the Princeton Hospital for treatment. Flexner saw him in the hospital at noon, observing that "his face was a little flushed from fever and excitement. I think he's glad to be there."[67]

Smith had been out of sorts for weeks but it was impossible to persuade him to see a doctor. He was convinced that he had a mortal disease, but he dodged verification. A few days after admission, he seemed better and it was difficult to keep him in the hospital. Although he had always tended to be apprehensive about his health, he now tried the deception that a slight respiratory infection caused the fever, the irregular heart, the gastrointestinal disturbance and the prostration. At home, he had preferred staying up and moving around to maintain his strength, although it was apparent that he was growing weaker. Flexner recorded in his diary that "Yesterday Cohn called me up at nine to report that Dr. S. had bleeding from the intestine during the night. A mass had been felt low in the right abdominal region. [Dr.] Heuer of the New York Hospital was called in and diagnosed a possibly malignant tumor of the ileocolic region. I saw Smith today. He looks pretty white but is in better condition than yesterday."[68]

Mrs. Flexner was ill and had been ordered to take a holiday. Flexner was reluctant to depart for Egypt since he knew Smith's days were numbered. So they left word to be posted on details. "It was a hard getaway in which my duty to Helen and my wish to be near Dr. Smith conflicted," he confided to his diary.[69] "It was of course no telling how long he might linger . . . [though] I did not believe the illness would be a long one, since he was already weakened by intensive dietary treatment." It was decided that if he gained strength an exploratory operation would be necessary, for which he would be transferred to the New York Hospital. Simon Flexner saw Theobald Smith for the last time on November 30, when he was having a "solid" meal with mashed potatoes. "But I had been apprehensive right along and every day expected a radio message. It never came. Yesterday a telephone call from Cook's [travel agency] announced that after several hemorrhages and blood transfusions, Smith was transported to the New York Hospital. Before any anesthetic was given, he suddenly developed pulmonary edema and succumbed." The funeral was to take place on the following day at the Theobald Smith House with the Dean of Divinity at Princeton officiating, and Stockard speaking on behalf of the Scientific Directors.[70]

Ten days later, Flexner recorded in his diary that "Fortunately Mrs. S. could come to New York and spent the 9th there and saw Dr. S. before he was taken to the operating room" on December 10th. A letter from Alfred Cohn on the 11th revealed the nature and details of his illness.

> He became much agitated; his heart failed and he suddenly died of pulmonary edema before an anesthetic could be administered. The autopsy revealed hopeless conditions; a carcinoma of the ileocecum with mesenteric gland metastases and metastasis in the ventricle, a rare condition. In view of this, it was better that there was no operation, and that death, which was inevitable and imminent, came swiftly. Apparently up to the end Dr. Smith conducted himself in the "grand manner" but he could not wholly conceal his suppressed emotional reactions.[71]

In a later note to Mr. and Mrs. Edric Smith, who had sent roses to her at the hospital, Lilian wrote: "I took some to his room when they came to me and we admired them together and again when I went in to say good morning—just before he slipped away he noticed the fragrance. Thank you for giving me this little memory."[72]

A January 28, 1935 letter from Edric Smith to Lilian[73] informed her that by action of the Board of Scientific Directors, Theobald's entire salary would be continued through June of that year, after which she would be eligible for a retirement allowance of half of his retiring salary for life, which left her in comfortable circumstances. Theobald had made a handwritten will with everything left to his widow. He had transferred all ready cash on hand to her a few days before his death. Everything pointed to the belief that he knew his end had come.

In January 1935, Flexner visited Lilian in Princeton. It was a very pleasant and satisfactory visit. He had written ahead and had asked her to lunch with him and TenBroeck at the staff house. Lilian talked very quietly about her husband, emotion being apparent only by two red spots on her checks. Otherwise she appeared composed. She talked about the autopsy findings and was glad that "Theo" was spared a long hopeless illness. He had thought out his future entirely and every detail of his affairs was in order. The house had been paid for as built, and Mrs. Smith confidentially told Dr. Flexner that she thought the estate would reach $150,000, a tidy sum in those days. Son Philip proved very helpful as executor. Daughter Dorothy was working at Princeton University. Although

Theobald had thought that she should give this up and be with her mother, Flexner, however, believed otherwise.

> I agreed with Mrs. S. that this was not best. Mrs. S. is not well and only a little younger than Dr. S. [she was actually two years older]. TenBroeck is like another son and spoke of Dr. Smith's papers and thought they should be kept. A biography should be written, and we talked about putting the papers at the RI in New York. Mrs. Smith raised the question of a memorial meeting. She seemed to dread it and I did not press the subject. On the contrary I said that the exercise at the Theobald Smith House might well stand instead.[74]

Burial

Theobald Smith asked Philip to see that he should wear a pair of trousers made by his father of fine greenish colored cloth. Philip went to some trouble to find these and eventually did, and his father's wishes were carried out. Theobald was, however, cremated and his ashes placed in a bronze casket, to be buried on his Silver Lake property among the roots of a white pine tree, of which he was very fond and whose growth he had watched since it had been a young sapling. Upon her death in June 1940, Lilian's ashes were buried in another bronze casket adjacent to her husband's.

In 1967, when both daughters were still alive, they conceived the notion that their parents' ashes deserved a more accessible and conventional burial place. Philip agreed to this proposal and between them they bought a headstone of Vermont marble with appropriate curbing, which would be set up in Chocorua Cemetery, three miles or so from Silver Lake, which they had both enjoyed so much. First the ashes had to be retrieved, and the author (Dolman) had the privilege of helping Philip do so while Jeanne, his wife, looked on. Both caskets containing their ashes were extricated without much difficulty and were driven northward along the lake to the Chocorua Churchyard. During the drive, we discussed whether the caskets should be buried at the same level, side by side, or one above the other. It was resolved that they should be buried side by side. The proceeding was very informal, with no one present for the ceremony other than Philip, Jeanne and the author. It was a windy day, and blown leaves abounded, but we dug away with our trowels. The ashes were buried a good two feet down, and covered with turf and fern roots. The author's camera misbehaved, so that memorable photos of the pine root and burial are lacking, but Lilian Foerster went to Chocorua later and took photos that showed that the ferns had grown well. Everything looked neat and proper. Their names and dates were easy to read. Their nearest neighbor was William James, the famous professor of philosophy at Harvard, a friendly contemporary of Theobald Smith and uncle to Henry James, Jr.

While on the subject of the cessation of vital functions, it would be appropriate to follow briefly the fortunes of Theobald Smith's Department of Animal Pathology. In 1935, in the wake of Smith's death, Carl TenBroeck was appointed Director and served for the next fifteen years of so. But in 1948, beset with changes in philosophy and constriction of funds, the Board of Trustees of the Rockefeller Institute began to question the necessity or wisdom of maintaining extensive laboratories in Princeton as well as in New York where some duplication of work went on; and after much discussion and soul-searching as to whether the Princeton laboratories should be closed down and their functions moved to New York, of whether the Institute itself should move to Princeton, they chose in favor of the former and in 1950 the Princeton facilities were closed. Afterwards, all employees were moved to New York or located elsewhere; but Carl TenBroeck, desiring not to move away from Princeton, chose retirement in 1951. And the Institute itself underwent further changes as well. In 1954, the Rockefeller Institute began to alter its role, becoming part of the University of the State of New York, and in 1965, changed its name to Rockefeller University, devoted to graduate education as well as research.

Theobald Smith and the Nobel Prize

Theobald Smith was several times nominated by friends, colleagues and admirers for consideration for a Nobel Prize. The earliest proposal came from his worthy successor at Harvard, E.E. Tyzzer,[75] who in January 1921, having been invited to propose candidates for a Nobel award, wrote to the Caroline Medico-Chirurgical Institute in Stockholm recommending Smith for that honor.[76] His primary reason for this action was that Smith, with Kilborne, had in 1893 demonstrated that Texas fever or piroplasmosis of cattle was transmitted in mammals through the agency of an invertebrate host, and that this finding paved the way for a similar discovery with respect to the transmission of malaria, for which Ronald Ross had been granted a Nobel Prize nine years later. Tyzzer thought Smith deserving of a prize also because he had shown that the bacilli of human and bovine tuberculosis were culturally and biologically distinct, a matter that was later corroborated by Koch. And he referred to a number of other fundamental contributions by Smith: his invention of a fermentation tube for the determination of the gas production of bacteria; for having discovered the causal agent of blackhead; and for his important work on the aetiology of hog cholera, abortion in cattle, and other animal diseases.

In the following year, Howard Krasner of the Department of Pathology of

Western Reserve University wrote to Theobald, informing him that he and several others had been consulted by the Nobel Committee and had recommended him. "We feel that you are the one living individual who by his original work has led to a distinct epoch of medical discovery," growing out of his discovery of the insect transmission of disease. Furthermore, "No other American and probably no one else in the world, has so continually offered original and highly valued contributions."[77] Smith replied that such a matter "rests with time and the mature opinion of peers, usually formulated only after his death." He understood also, from colleagues who had consulted the Foundation, that "my work of 1899–1893 [sic] was outlawed by time," and he also mentioned that he had taken no interest in the matter.[78]

In January 1925, Peyton Rous sent another letter to the Nobel Committee suggesting that Smith was worthy of a prize. He contended that the influence of his discoveries, some of which dated back fifty years, was a vital force at the present time, and one affecting knowledge widely.[79] He also pointed out that Smith's demonstration that a disease, Texas fever, caused by a protozoon and transmitted by an insect host, had led to an understanding of analogous conditions which obtain in malaria, nagana, yellow fever, sleeping sickness, and other diseases. "Can anyone doubt that this discovery will continue to be fruitful in the future?" And furthermore, he observed, his work on swine plague led him to recognize the existence of sub-types within the bacterial species. "How many sub-types are now known to be of import!" he asked. "One thinks immediately of the paratyphoid and pneumococcus organisms." And he declared that Smith's demonstrations of the differences among mammalian tubercle bacilli (bovine and human) had been fundamental in its effect upon the investigation of tuberculosis. "His observations of the so-called Theobald Smith phenomenon opened the door to present knowledge of anaphylaxis," and "his demonstration of the possibilities of immunization with balanced toxin-antitoxin mixtures has been responsible for a great advance in serum treatment of disease." In all these ways, Rous argued, "Dr. Smith's past work is of the present in its implications and of the future in its possibilities." Rous also noted that within the prior three or four years Smith's study of the disease of turkeys called "blackhead" had shown that for the production of this infection an association of a protozoan parasite with an intestinal worm was necessary, a finding that might have an applicability as wide as that of his demonstration of the role of insects as intermediate hosts.

In October 1931, Rous wrote to Carl TenBroeck transmitting a draft of another letter he was sending to the Nobel Committee once more proposing Smith for an award. He asked TenBroeck what points he should stress, and informed him that numerous other people were proposing Smith as well. He said that the Nobel Committee had given no prize in 1925, claiming that no one who had been proposed was worthy.[80] (As pointed out in Chapter 6, Smith may have been denied the 1925 prize for his Texas fever work because the Nobel Committee objected to the fact that Kilborne had not been included in the nomination.) TenBroeck subsequently sent to Rous a bibliography of Smith's scientific publications and suggested that he bring up Smith's recent work on the transmission of immunity by colostrum,[81] to which Rous replied that Smith's colostrum work was too specialized; and with respect to TenBroeck's comment that the Texas fever work and work on the differential of tubercle bacilli were too old for Nobel consideration, he suggested, "why not point out five or six discoveries of larger importance by Dr. Smith and let them make their own choice. If they can go all the way back to Landsteiner's blood group discovery, they can certainly do so in the case of Dr. Smith, should they so wish."

Writing to Simon Gage in late 1935, the Stanford University anatomist A.W. Meyer said that it might interest Gage to know that when he was first asked regarding a candidate for the Nobel Prize he suggested Theobald Smith, "and even today I am at a loss to account for the fact that this honor was never shown him." Meyer felt that the oversight would not redound to the credit of the Foundation. "I do not feel that Professor Smith needed that honor but it always seemed to me that he deserved it more than several others who were granted it."[82]

Finally, Frederick B. Bang, Professor of Pathology at the Johns Hopkins School of Hygiene, wrote to the Nobel Foundation in 1958. Reporting that he was proposing a biography of Theobald Smith, he asked for information on proposals made in 1922 and 1923 on his behalf.[83] Nils K. Ståhle replied for the Foundation in typical bureaucratic style that the prize was distributed annually to those "who, *during the preceding year* [italics his] shall have conferred the greatest benefit on mankind," or "for older works only when their significance has not become apparent until recently. Thus, it seems quite clear that the Prize must have failed on the above reasons, or, perhaps, there were still more deserving candidates in the year in question."[84]

It is relevant to point out here that Peyton Rous was himself awarded a Nobel Prize for Physiology of Medicine in 1955 for work on cancer-inducing viruses—work that he had actually completed and published in 1910, over fifty years before! His award was apparently justified under Ståhle's alternative explanation—that its significance or importance had not become clear until long afterwards. And indeed, his fellow Rockefeller Institute virologist Tom Rivers later discussed this very matter.[85] He told that in 1911 Rous had demonstrated the existence of the virus of chicken sarcoma and helped prove that it was transmissible, which he referred to as "an important watershed in cancer as well as virus research." Rivers commented that Rous did not know how to stress the importance of this work, and its relevance was not widely recognized or appreciated until much later, in the 1960s, "when virologists, particularly those at the National Institute of Health, were hell bent on proving that a virus is the cause of cancer in man," and thus were in a position to at last appreciate and promote Rous's early work connecting viruses with the induction of cancer.

Rivers also talked about Charles Richet, the French physiologist who had been awarded a Nobel Prize in 1913 for his 1907 work on anaphylaxis. Rivers told about giving a speech at a medical meeting in Montana in 1931 in which he referred to Richet's book, titled in English *The Natural History of a Savant,* and being roundly criticized for doing so by Ajax Carlson, who was in the audience. Carlson didn't think much of River's quoting from a book that had been written by a man who, in later life, espoused spiritualism, and whose book had been translated by another scientist who did the same. It made no difference to Carlson, Rivers pointed out, that Richet had won a Nobel Prize for his work on anaphylaxis; and he went on to add, "I don't care what they believed in their old age. Hell, if Carlson had argued that the Nobel Prize committee made a mistake in giving the prize to Richet for his work on anaphylasix, why then I might have gone along with him. I have always believed that the prize for that work should have gone to Theobald Smith."[86]

Reflections

Theobald Smith's death was much on Simon Flexner's mind in late 1934. Flexner's diary recordings in Naples, Italy on December 13 and 14 contained many reminiscences and appreciations of his work and of the man himself. "So ended the life of perhaps the most original and technically skilled pathologist in the modern sense that the U.S. had ever produced," he reflected in his initial thoughts on the man recently deceased.

> Indeed Dr. Smith was far more than a pathologist. He was a comprehensively minded biologist [to whom] all problems in pathology resolved themselves into biological processes. I think no one has ever comprehended pathology with all its side or main issues (bacteriology, immunology, parasitism), in the broad way in which he always viewed biological problems.
>
> A remarkable pathfinder, he had the merit of seeing problems so cleanly and clearly that relatively few experiments served his ends. He was the antithesis of those experimenters who get lost in the maze of excessive experiment and observation. He tapped some phenomena, the full implications of which he did not perceive, a notable instance being serum sensitization in the guinea-pig. But his path-breaking proof of the insect-transmission of Texas fever of cattle—a particularly baffling form of such transmission of disease; his distinction of different types of

tubercle bacilli; his determination of the importance of colostrum as a carrier of possible immunizing substances—are master observations.

Smith was undoubtedly the discoverer of the immunizing effect of killed bacteria. It is questionable whether this is a purely original new observation or an acute interpretation of Pasteur's experiments with "attenuated chick cholera organisms." Smith once told me the old culture which Pasteur used were doubtlesss dead. I do not know whether this idea came to him before he tried killed cultures, or having found killed cultures to be effective, he inferred Pasteur's experiments were comparable.[87]

Flexner's diary entry on the following day contained additional reflections and reminiscences.

There was a great reserve about Theobald Smith, so that I wonder if anyone besides his wife ever reached into his inner thoughts. I never did, I am sure. There were admirable sides to his reticence for he did not speak of the scientific work of others, and spoke little of his own. He could be drawn out, but he did not talk about work. He was free of obvious striving, or speciousness.

I do not regard him as a successful trainer of men. No pupil of his ever reached real distinction. Tyzzer was not I believe a real pupil, although influenced by him. TenBroeck is useful in consolidating and improving the staff, but he is not unusual in any way. He is not, as Dr. Smith was, a natural investigator. Smith's interest was in his own mind and work, not in an organization. No one excelled him in making crucial experiments. His animal experiments were never so numerous as to be confusing. This is a real Virtue. He never lost the sense of economy enforced at Washington and Boston.[88]

Following Theobald Smith's death there occurred an outpouring of eulogies. All of the leading bacteriological, pathological and medical journals in the United States and Great Britain, as well as some in France, Canada and elsewhere, published accounts and appreciations of his life and work. (Germany, which was feeling the tightening of the Nazi grip, seems to have taken almost no public notice of his passing.) Two stand out as catching Smith's uniqueness in an economy of words. Charles Stockard, who succeeded Smith as President of the Board of Scientific Directors of the Rockefeller Institute, in his December 14 memorial tribute at the Theobald Smith House, identified him as one of the originators and builders of opportunities and fields in which he worked.

Theobald Smith was one of nature's high priests. He believed with Pasteur that science in obeying the law of humanity, will always labor to enlarge the frontiers of life; and with Goethe, that the first and last thing required of genius is the love of truth. He built temples to nature and communed in them by whispering questions to her. And nature answered back to this favorite son—and he understood.[89]

William Bulloch characterized Smith appropriately as the greatest bacteriologist the United States had produced and the contemporary of many founders of that science, observing, "He may be regarded as the Last of the Mohicans."[90] But Theobald Smith needed no eulogy, for he was well aware of what he had achieved and for him this was eulogy enough. He accomplished the prodigious feats that made him stand out as extraordinary among his peers as well as those who followed him by also constructing a temple to truth, which he dedicated on September 24, 1878, when but nineteen years old. This is proved by an entry in his diary under that date of a self-rule of conduct he continued to follow diligently throughout the remainder of his life:

> "Seek the truth earnestly, humbly and for the truth's sake."

BIBLIOGRAPHY OF

THEOBALD SMITH

1880–1934

1880

1. Letter to the Editors [on the alternatives of economy and useless extravagance in college life]. *Cornell Era,* 13 (Oct. 29), pp. 69–71.

1881

2. The ideals destroyed by science and their substitutes. *Cornell Review,* 8 (March), pp. 202–206.

1883

3. GAGE, S.H. and SMITH, T. Serial microscopic sections. *The Medical Student,* 1 (November), pp. 14–16.

1884

4. GAGE, S.H. and SMITH, T. Section flattener for dry section cutting. (Note 1 & 2). *The Microscope,* 4 (February), pp. 25–26.

5. The diagnostic and prognostic value of the bacillus tuberculosis in the sputum of pulmonary diseases. *Albany Medical Annals,* 5 (July), pp. 193–198.

6. Method of demonstrating the presence of the tubercle bacillus in sputum. *Albany Medical Annals,* 5 (August), pp. 233-236.

7. SALMON, D.E. [and SMITH, T.]. Investigations of swine plague. In U.S. Department of Agriculture. *Contagious Diseases of Domesticated Animals. Investigations by Department of Agriculture, 1883–1884.* Washington, pp. 78–88. Reproduced in U.S. Department of Agriculture. *Report of the Commissioner of Agriculture for the year 1884.* Washington, pp. 258–267; and U.S. Department of Agriculture. *First Annual Report of the Bureau of Animal Industry for the Year 1884.* Washington (1885), pp. 221–232 (3 Pl.). Includes: A new form of culture tube used in the preceding investigation, pp. 229–232 (1 Pl.).

8. The gape disease of fowls, and the parasite by which it is caused. Translation of M.P. Mégnin's Memoir on a verminous epizootic disease of the pheasantries and on the parasite which causes it, the Syngamus Trachealis (Sieb.), Sclerostoma Syngamus (Dies.). In U.S. Department of Agriculture. *Contagious Diseases of Domesticated Animals. Investigations by Department of Agriculture, 1883–1884.* Washington, pp. 103–121. Reproduced in U.S. Department of Agriculture. *Report of the Commissioner of Agriculture for the Year 1884.*

Washington, pp. 268–284 (2 Pl.); and U.S. Department of Agriculture. *First Annual Report of the Bureau of Animal Industry for the Year 1884.* Washington (1885), pp. 280–296 (2 Pl.).

1885

9. Remarks on fluid and gelatinous media for cultivating micro-organisms, with description of Salmon's new culture-tube, and demonstrations of the process of using it. *Proceedings of the American Association for the Advancement of Science,* 33, pp. 556–559. Abstract of paper (read by Romyn Hitchcock) before the Section of Histology and Microscopy, American Association for the Advancement of Science, thirty-third Annual Meeting, Philadelphia, beginning September 3, 1884.

10. Pathogenic bacteria and wandering cells. *Albany Medical Annals,* 6, pp. 50–56.

11. SALMON, D.E. and SMITH, T. Koch's method of isolating and cultivating bacteria as used in the Laboratory of the Bureau of Animal Industry, Deptartment of Agriculture. *American Monthly Microscopical Journal,* 6 (May), pp. 81–84. Also abstracted in *The National Republican,* April 23, 1885. Abstract of communication to the seventy-eighth Meeting of the Biological Society of Washington, April 18, 1885. Cited in *Proceedings of the Biological Society of Washington,* 3 (1884–1886), p. XXXVII, with T.S. as sole author.

12. Woodhead & Hare's "Pathological mycology." Letter to Editor. *Science,* 6 (October), p. 316.

1886

13. SALMON, D.E. and SMITH, T. A new chromogenous bacillus. *Proceedings of the American Association for the Advancement of Science,* 34, pp. 303–309. Read before the Section of Biology, American Association for the Advancement of Science, thirty-fourth Annual Meeting, Ann Arbor, Michigan, beginning August 26, 1885.

14. Investigations in swine plague. In U.S. Department of Agriculture. *Report of the Commissioner of Agriculture, 1885.* Washington, pp. 476–522 (2 Pl.). Reproduced, with new section headed "Other microbes found in swine-plague," and 5 additional plates, in U.S. Department of Agriculture. *Second Annual Report of the Bureau of Animal Industry for the Year 1885.* Washington (1886), pp. 184–246 (7 Pl.).

15. SALMON, D.E. and SMITH, T. On a new method of producing immunity from contagious diseases. *Proceedings of the Biological Society of Washington,* 3, pp. 29–33. Reproduced in full in *American Veterinary Review,* 10 (1886–1887), pp. 63–67. Read before the ninetieth Meeting of the Biological Society of Washington, February 20, 1886. Cited in *Proceedings of the Biological Society of Washington,* 4 (1886–1888), p. VII.

16. Notes on the biological examination of water, with a few statistics of Potomac drinking water. *American Monthly Microscopical Journal,* 7 (April), pp. 61–64; *Washington Post,* March 23, 1886. (Abstract). Abstracts of communication presented to the Biological Society of Washington, March 20, 1886. Cited in *Proceedings of the Biological Society of Washington,* 4 (1886–1888), p. VIII, as: Notes on some biological analyses of Potomac drinking water, by D.E. Salmon and Theobald Smith. In the published abstracts Salmon's name was dropped.

17. A few simple methods of obtaining pure cultures of bacteria for microscopical examination. *American Monthly Microscopical Journal,* 7 (July), pp. 124–125. (Discussion, p. 139). Abstract of a communication to the Washington Microscopical Society, May 25, 1886.

18. Some recent investigations concerning bacteria in drinking water. *Medical News,* 49 (October), pp. 399–401.

19. The relative value of cultures in liquid and solid media in the diagnoses of bacteria. *Botanical Gazette,* 11 (November), pp. 294–297; *Medical News,* 49 (November), pp. 571–573.

20. On the variability of pathogenic organisms, as illustrated by the bacterium of swine-plague. *American Monthly Microscopical Journal,* 7 (November), pp. 201–203; *Proceedings of the American Association for the Advancement of Science,* 35 (1887), pp. 267–268. Abstract. "On" omitted from title. Read before the thirty-fifth Meeting of the American Association for the Advancement of Science, Buffalo, beginning August 18, 1886.

21. SALMON, D.E. and SMITH, T. The bacterium of swine-plauge. *American Monthly Microscopical Journal,* 7 (November), pp. 204–205; *Proceedings of the American Association for the Advancement of Science,* 35 (1887), p. 268. (Abstract). Read before the thirty-fifth Meeting of the American Association for the Advancement of Science, Buffalo, beginning August 18, 1886.

1887

22. Parasitic bacteria and their relation to saprophytes. *American Naturalist,* 21 (January), pp. 1–9. Read before the Biological Society of Washington, December 11, 1886. Cited in *Proceedings of the Biological Society of Washington,* 4 (1886–1888), p. XII.

23. A contribution to the study of the microbe of rabbit septicaemia. *Journal of Comparative Medicine and Surgery,* 8, pp. 24–37.

24. Investigations of swine diseases. In U.S. Department of Agriculture. *Report of the Commissioner of Agriculture. 1886.* Washington, pp. 603–686 (9 Pl.). Reproduced in U.S. Department of Agriculture. *Third Annual Report of the Bureau of Animal Industry for the Year 1886.* Washington (1887), pp. 20–100, 103–104 (9 Pl.).

25. The preparation of blood serum. Letter to Editor. *Medical News,* 50 (March 3), p. 307.

26. Quantitative variations in the germ life of Potomac water during the year 1886. *Medical News* (April), pp. 404–405; *American Monthly Microscopical Journal,* 8 (July), pp. 129–130. Read before the Biological Society of Washington, April 2, 1887. Cited in *Proceedings of the Biological Society of Washington,* 4 (1886–1888), p. XVI.

27. Spirillum, Finkler and Prior, in hepatized lung-tissue. *Medical News,* 51 (November 5), pp. 536–538.

28. SALMON, D.E. and SMITH, T. Experiments on the production of immunity by the hypodermic injection of sterilized cultures. *Transactions of the IX International Medical Congress,* 3, pp. 403–407. Read by T.S. before the IX International Medical Congress, Washington, D.C., September 6, 1887.

1888

29. Bacteriology as a study in schools. Letter to Editor. (January 23). *Science,* 11 (February), pp. 61–62.

30. Further investigations on the nature and prevention of hog cholera. In U.S. Department of Agriculture. *Report of the Commissioner of Agriculture. 1887.* Washington, pp. 481–491. Amplified as Nature and prevention of hog cholera. Investigations of 1887. In U.S. Department of Agriculture. *Fourth and Fifth Annual Reports of the Bureau of Animal Industry for the Years 1887 and 1888.* Washington (1889), pp. 63–86.

31. Further investigations on the etiology of infectious pneumonia in swine plague. In U.S.

Department of Agriculture. *Report of the Commissioner of Agriculture, 1887.* Washington, pp. 491–520, 522 (4 Pl.). Reproduced with additional plates as Investigations on the etiology of infectious pneumonia in swine (swine plague). In U.S. Department of Agriculture. *Fourth and Fifth Annual Reports of the Bureau of Animal Industry for the Years 1887 and 1888.* Washington (1889), pp. 86–116 (9 Pl.).

32. Recent advances in the disinfection of dwellings as illustrated by the Berlin rules. *New York Medical Journal,* 48 (August), pp. 117–120.

33. The relation of drinking water to some infectious diseases. *Albany Medical Annals,* 9 (November), pp. 297–302.

1889

34. Prevention of hog cholera. In U.S. Department of Agriculture. *Report of the Commissioner of Agriculture, 1888.* Washington, pp. 156–175. Reproduced in U.S. Department of Agriculture. *Fourth and Fifth Annual Reports of the Bureau of Animal Industry for the Years 1887 and 1888.* Washington, pp. 148–166.

35. Experiments on the attenuation of hog cholera by heat. In U.S. Department of Agriculture. *Report of the Commissioner of Agriculture, 1888.* Washington, pp. 175–205. Reproduced in U.S. Department of Agriculture. *Fourth and Fifth Annual Reports of the Bureau of Animal Industry for the Years 1887 and 1888.* Washington, pp. 117–147.

36. The etiology and diagnosis of glanders. In U.S. Department of Agriculture. *Report of the Commissioner of Agriculture, 1888.* Washington, pp. 206–219. Reproduced in U.S. Department of Agriculture. *Fourth and Fifth Annual Reports of the Bureau of Animal Industry for the Years 1887 and 1888.* Washington, pp. 49–62.

37. Some observations on the origin and sources of pathogenic bacteria. *The Sanitarian,* 22, pp. 110–119. Read before the American Public Health Association, Milwaukee, Wisconsin, November 22, 1888.

38. SMITH, T., SALMON, D.E. and KILBORNE, F.L. *Hog cholera: its history, nature, and treatment, as determined by the inquiries and investigations of the Bureau of Animal Industry.* Washington, U.S. Department of Agriculture, Bureau of Industry, 193 pp. (16 Pl.).

39. Some observations on coccidia in the renal epithelium of the mouse. *Journal of Comparative Medicine and Surgery,* 10 (July), pp. 211–217. Read before the Biological Society of Washington, May 4, 1889. Cited in *Proceedings of the Biological Society of Washington,* 5 (1888–1890), p. XIX, as: Parasitic protozoa (Coccidia) in the renal epithelium of the mouse.

40. Preliminary observations on the microorganism of Texas fever. *Medical News,* 55 (December), pp. 689–693; *American Public Health Association Reports,* 15, pp. 178–185; *Veterinary Journal and Annals of Comparative Pathology,* 30, pp. 153–161. Read before the American Public Health Association, Brooklyn, N.Y., October 23, 1889.

41. Investigations of infectious animal diseases. In U.S. Department of Agriculture. *First Report of the Secretary of Agriculture, 1889.* Washington, pp. 75–110. Reproduced in U.S. Department of Agriculture. *Sixth and Seventh Annual Reports of the Bureau of Animal Industry for the Years 1889 and 1890.* Washington (1891), pp. 28–62.

1890

42. On the influence of slight modifications of culture media on the growth of bacteria as illustrated by the glanders bacillus. *Journal of Comparative Medicine and Veterinary Archives,* 11 (March), pp. 158–161.

43. Das Gährungskölbchen in der Bakteriologie. *Centralblatt für Bakteriologie,* 7 (April), pp. 502–506.

44. Einige Bemerkungen über Säure- und Alkalibildung bei Bakterien. *Centralblatt für Bakteriologie,* 8 (September), pp. 389–391.

45. Observations of the variability of disease germs. *New York Medical Journal,* 52 (November), pp. 485–487. See also: Observations on the variability of disease-germs. (Title only). *Proceedings of the American Association for the Advancement of Science,* 39 (1891), p. 348. Read by title before the Biology Section, American Association for the Advancement of Science, thirty-ninth Annual Meeting, Indianapolis, Indiana, beginning August 19, 1890.

46. Investigations of the infectious diseases of animals. In U.S. Department of Agriculture. *Report of the Secretary of Agriculture, 1890.* Washington, pp. 105–122. Reproduced in U.S. Department of Agriculture. *Sixth and Seventh Annual Reports of the Bureau of Animal Industry for the Years 1889 and 1890.* Washington (1891), pp. 93–110.

1891

47. Einige Bemerkungen zu dem Aufsatze "Eine Methode der Blutentnahme beim Menschen." *Centralblatt für Bakteriologie,* 9 (January 8), pp. 48–49.

48. Bacteriology and Koch's lymph. *Kate Field's Washington,* 3 (January 14), pp. 20–21. Subtitled "A leading young scientist on the topic of the hour." Based on a telephone interview edited by T.S.

49. Zur Kenntnis des Hogcholerabacillus. *Centralblatt für Bakteriologie,* 9 (March), pp. 253–257, 307–311, 339–343.

50. Kleine bakteriologische Mittheilungen. *Centralblatt für Bakteriologie,* 10 (August), pp. 177–186.

51. On changes in the red blood-corpuscles in the pernicious anaemia of Texas cattle fever. *Transactions of the Association of American Physicians,* 6, pp. 263–277. (Discussion, pp. 277–278). Read by invitation at the sixth Annual Meeting, Association of American Physicians, Washington, D.C., September 25, 1891. This paper was rearranged and presented at the one hundred and eighty-seventh meeting of the Biological Society of Washington, under the title "Peculiar forms of red corpuscles in mammalia in anaemic conditions." Cited in *Proceedings of the Biological Society of Washington,* 7 (1892–1893), p. xviii.

52. U.S. Department of Agriculture. *Special Report on the Cause and Prevention of Swine Plague. Results of Experiments Conducted under the Direction of Dr. D.E. Salmon, Chief of the Bureau of Animal Industry.* Washington. 166 pp. (12 Pl.). Includes appendix by V.A. Moore on "The presence of septic bacteria, probably identical with those of swine plague, in the upper air passages of domesticated animals other than swine," pp. 151–159.

53. Zur Kenntniss der amerikanischen Schweineseuche. *Zeitschrift für Hygiene,* 10, pp. 480–508.

54. Washington drinking-water. Letter to Editor (October 31). *Medical News,* 59, pp. 525–526.

1892

55. Investigation of infectious diseases of domesticated animals. In U.S. Department of Agriculture. *Report of the Secretary of Agriculture, 1891.* Washington, pp. 117–138. Reproduced in U.S. Department of Agriculture. *Eighth and Ninth Annual Reports of the Bureau of Animal Industry for the Years 1891 and 1892.* Washington (1893), pp. 45–66.

56. Uses of the fermentation tube in bacteriology with demonstrations. *Proceedings of the American Association for the Advancement of Science,* 40, p. 319. (Abstract). Read before the Biology Section, American Association for the Advancement of Science, fortieth Annual Meeting, Washington, D.C., August 21, 1891.

57. BROWN, C.C. and SMITH, T. Third report on Hudson River. In New York. State Board of Health. *Twelfth Annual Report for 1891.* Albany, N.Y., pp. 533–540.

58. Zur Unterscheidung zwischen Typhus- und Kolonbacillen. *Centralblatt für Bakteriologie* (Originale), 11 (March), pp. 367–370.

59. On pathogenic bacteria in drinking water and the means employed for their removal. *Albany Medical Annals,* 13 (May), pp. 129–150. Lecture delivered before the Albany Medical College Alumni Association, at Albany, N.Y., April 27, 1892.

60. U.S. Department of Agriculture. Bureau of Animal Industry. *Special Report on Diseases of Cattle and on Cattle Feeding.* Washington. 496 pp. (44 Pl.). By Murray, A.J., Atkinson, V.T., and 8 other authors, including T.S. Reprinted 1896.

61. SALMON, D.E. and SMITH, T. Infectious diseases of cattle. In U.S. Department of Agriculture. Bureau of Animal Industry. *Special Report on Diseases of Cattle and on Cattle Feeding.* Washington, pp. 371–438 (16 Pl.). Revised in 1904, 1908 and 1912 by D.E. Salmon and J.R. Mohler. Section headed "Texas Fever, or Southern Cattle Fever" by Salmon and Smith, reissued as B.A.I. Circular No. 69. (Revised in 1904 by Salmon and Mohler).

62. SMITH, T. and MOORE, V.A. Zur Prüfung der Pasteur-Chamberland-Filter. *Centralblatt für Bakteriologie* (Originale), 12 (November), pp. 628–629. Cited as "The growth of bacteria through the Pasteur-Chamberland filter" in *Proceedings of the Biological Society of Washington,* 8 (1893), p. V. Read at the two hundred and fourth meeting of the Biological Society of Washington, January 14, 1893.

1893

63. Investigation of infectious diseases of domesticated animals. In U.S. Department of Agriculture. *Report of the Secretary of Agriculture, 1892.* Washington, pp. 110–118. Reproduced in U.S. Department of Agriculture. *Eighth and Ninth Annual Reports of the Bureau of Animal Industry for the Years 1891 and 1892.* Washington, pp. 96–104.

64. SMITH, T. and KILBORNE, F.L. *Investigations into the Nature, Causation, and Prevention of Texas or Southern Cattle Fever.* U.S. Department of Agriculture. Bureau of Animal Industry. Bulletin No. 1. Washington. 301 pp. (10 Pl.). Reproduced, but with Appendix (showing details of field experiments) omitted, and with a differently worded Letter of Transmittal from D.E. Salmon to the Secretary of Agriculture, in U.S. Department of Agriculture. *Eighth and Ninth Annual Reports of the Bureau of Animal Industry for the Years 1891 and 1892.* Washington, pp. 177–304. The latter version was reprinted in *Medical Classics,* 1 (January), 1937), pp. 327–597.

65. Die Aetiologie der Texasfieberseuche des Rindes. *Centralblatt für Bakteriologie* (Originale), 13 (April), pp. 511–527.

66. Some problems in the etiology and pathology of Texas cattle fever, and their bearing on the comparative study of protozoan diseases. *Transactions of the Association of American Physicians,* 8, pp. 117–134. Read at the eighth Annual Meeting, Association of American Physicians, Washington, D.C., May 31, 1893.

67. Potomac river water. *Popular Health Magazine,* 1 (September), p. 104.

68. The fermentation tube with special reference to anaërobiosis and gas production among bacteria. In *The Wilder Quarter-Century Book, 1868–1893.* Ithaca, N.Y., Comstock Pub-

lishing Co., pp. 187–233; *Centralblatt für Bakteriologie* (Referate), 14 (December), pp. 864–867. (Abstract).

69. Presentation Address. In *The Wilder Quarter-Century Book, 1868–1893*. Ithaca, N.Y., Comstock Publishing Co., pp. 69–74. Proceedings and Addresses at the Twenty-fifth Anniversary [of the Opening of] Cornell University, Ithaca, N.Y. Published by the University, 1893. Reprinted, with revisions, in *Cornell Era,* October 9, 1893, 8 pp.; *Ithaca Daily Journal,* October 9, 1893, pp. 18–20. Delivered at the twenty-fifth Anniversary of Cornell University Exercises, Ithaca, N.Y., October 7, 1893.

70. KILBORNE, F.L., MOORE, V.A., SCHROEDER, E.C., SMITH, T. and STILES, C.W. *Miscellaneous Investigations Concerning Infectious and Parasitic Diseases of Domesticated Animals.* U.S. Department of Agriculture. Bureau of Animal Industry. Bulletin No. 3. Washington. 88 pp. (3 Pl.).

71. On a pathogenic bacillus from the vagina of a mare after abortion. In U.S. Department of Agriculture. Bureau of Animal Industry. Bulletin, No. 3, pp. 53–59.

72. SMITH, T. and SCHROEDER, E.C. Some experimental observations on the presence of tubercle bacilli in the milk of tuberculous cows when the udder is not visibly diseased. In U.S. Department of Agriculture. Bureau of Animal Industry. Bulletin No. 3, pp. 60–66.

73. SMITH, T., KILBORNE, F.L., and SCHROEDER, E.C. Additional observations on Texas Cattle fever. In U.S. Department of Agriculture. Bureau of Animal Industry. Bulletin No. 3, pp. 67–72.

74. Preliminary notes on a sporozoön in the intestinal villi of cattle. In U.S. Department of Agriculture. Bureau of Animal Industry. Bulletin No. 3, pp. 73–78. Read before the Biology Section, American Association for the Advancement of Science, forty-second Annual Meeting, Madison, Wisconsin, August 18, 1893, under the title "A new sporozoon in the intestinal villi of cattle." See *Proceedings of the American Association for the Advancement of Science,* 42 (1894), p. 232.

75. A new method for determining quantitatively the pollution of water by fecal bacteria. In New York State Board of Health. *Thirteenth Annual Report for 1892.* Albany, N.Y., pp. 712–722.

1894

76. The production of races and varieties of bacteria in mixed cultures. *Proceedings of the American Association for the Advancement of Science,* 42, p. 232. (Abstract). Read before the Biology Section, American Association for the Advancement of Science, forty-second Annual Meeting, Madison, Wisconsin, August 18, 1893.

77. Further observations on the fermentation tube with special reference to anaërobiosis reduction, and gas production. *Proceedings of the American Association for the Advancement of Science,* 42, p. 261. Abstract read before the American Association for the Advancement of Science, forty-second Annual Meeting, Madison, Wisconsin, August 17, 1893.

78. Investigation of infectious diseases of domesticated animals. In U.S. Department of Agriculture. *Report of the Secretary of Agriculture. 1893.* Washington. pp. 140–160.

79. Channels of infection, with special reference to water and milk. *Popular Health Magazine,* 1 (April), pp. 279–287. (Excerpts in Washington *Evening Star,* February 22, 1894, headed Water and Milk.) A popular lecture delivered under the auspices of the Sanitary League of Washington, in Washington, D.C., February 21, 1894.

80. The restriction and prevention of tuberculosis. *Food. A Journal of Hygiene & Nutrition,* 4,

pp. 564–565. Smith's contribution appears in the discussion, following presentation of report (pp. 535–538) of the Committee appointed by the Medical Society, District of Columbia, on May 9, 1894.

81. SMITH, T. and MOORE, V.A. *Additional Investigations Concerning Infectious Swine Diseases.* U.S. Department of Agriculture. Bureau of Animal Industry. Bulletin No. 6. Washington. 117 pp.

82. The hog-cholera group of bacteria. In U.S. Department of Agriculture. Bureau of Animal Industry. Bulletin No. 6, pp. 9–40.

83. SMITH, T. and MOORE, V.A. Experiments in the production of immunity in rabbits and guinea-pigs with reference to hog-cholera and swine-plague bacteria. In U.S. Department of Agriculture. Bureau of Animal Industry. Bulletin No. 6, pp. 41–80.

84. SMITH, T. and MOORE, V.A. On the variability of infectious diseases as illustrated by hog cholera and swine plague. In U.S. Department of Agriculture. Bureau of Animal Industry. Bulletin No. 6, pp. 81–95.

85. Practical bearing of the preceding investigations. In U.S. Department of Agriculture. Bureau of Animal Industry. Bulletin No. 6, pp. 109–114.

86. Arbeiten aus dem pathologischen Laboratorium des Bureau of Animal Industry in Washington, U.S.A. [Bulletin No. 6 (1894)]. *Centralblatt für Bakteriologie* (Original-Referate), 16 (August), pp. 231–241. [Reviews of items 82, 83, 84, 85, and of two papers by Moore alone in Bulletin No. 6.]

87. Modification, temporary and permanent, of the physiological characters of bacteria in mixed cultures. *Transactions of the Association of American Physicians,* 9, pp. 85–106. (Discussion, pp. 106–109). Read at the ninth Annual Meeting, Association of American Physicians, Washington, D.C., May 30, 1894.

88. Grobe und feine Spirillen im Darme eines Schweines. *Centralblatt für Bakteriologie* (Originale), 16 (September), p. 324.

89. SMITH, T., KILBORNE, F.L., and SCHROEDER, E.C. *Investigations Concerning Bovine Tuberculosis, with Special Reference to Diagnosis and Prevention.* U.S. Department of Agriculture. Bureau of Animal Industry. Bulletin No. 7. Washington. 178 pp. (6 Pl.).

90. Clinical and pathological notes on a herd of 60 cattle tested with tuberculin (Soldiers' Home herd). Pathological part. In U.S. Department of Agriculture. Bureau of Animal Industry. Bulletin No. 7, pp. 25–59.

91. Studies in bovine tuberculosis with special reference to prevention. In U.S. Department of Agriculture. Bureau of Animal Industry. Bulletin No. 7, pp. 88–128 (6 Pl.).

92. Some practical suggestions for the suppression and prevention of tuberculosis. In U.S. Department of Agriculture. Bureau of Animal Industry. Bulletin No. 7, pp. 129–144. Reproduced in *Yearbook of the U.S. Department of Agriculture for 1894.* Washington (1895), pp. 317–330.

93. Notes on the peptonizing or digestive action of sterile tissues of animals. *New York Medical Journal,* 60 (November), pp. 590–592; *Centralblatt für Bakteriologie,* I. Abteilung (Referate), 18 (December, 1895), p. 696. (Abstract).

1895

94. On a local vascular disturbance of the foetus, probably due to the injection of tuberculin in the pregnant cow. *New York Medical Journal,* 61 (February), pp. 233–234; *Centralblatt für Bakteriologie,* I. Abteilung (Referate), 18 (November), p. 570. (Abstract).

95. Ueber die Bedeutung des Zuckers in Kulturmedien für Bakterien. *Centralblatt für Bakteriologie,* I. Abteilung (Originale), 18 (July), pp. 1–9.

96. Notes on Bacillus coli communis and related forms, together with some suggestions concerning the bacteriological examination of drinking-water. *American Journal of the Medical Sciences,* 110 (September), pp. 283–302.

97. Antitoxic and microbicide powers of the blood serum after immunization, with special reference to diphtheria. *Albany Medical Annals,* 16, pp. 175–189. Address delivered to the Albany Medical College Alumni Association at its twenty-second Annual Meeting, Albany, N.Y., April 16, 1895.

98. Ueber den Nachweis des Bacillus coli communis im Wasser. *Centralblatt für Bakteriologie,* I. Abteilung (Originale), 18 (October), pp. 494–495.

99. SMITH, T. and MOORE, V.A. *Investigations Concerning Infectious Diseases among Poultry.* U.S. Department of Agriculture. Bureau of Animal Industry. Bulletin No. 8. Washington. 90 pp. (6 Pl.).

100. An infectious disease among turkeys caused by protozoa (infectious entero-hepatitis). In U.S. Department of Agriculture. Bureau of Animal Industry. Bulletin No. 8, pp. 7–38 (6 Pl.); *Centralblatt für Bakteriologie,* I. Abteilung (Referate), 18 (December), pp. 785–787. (Abstract). Read by title, "On infectious entero-hepatitis of fowls due to protozoa," at the two hundred and forty-third meeting of the Biological Society of Washington, April 20, 1895. Cited in *Proceedings of the Biological Society of Washington,* 9 (1894–1895), p. xiii.

1896

101. Reduktionserscheinungen bei Bakterien und ihre Beziehungen zur Bakterienzelle, nebst Bemerkungen über Reduktionserscheinungen in steriler Bouillon. *Centralblatt für Bakteriologie,* I. Abteilung (Originale), 19 (February), pp. 181–187.

102. SMITH, T. and DAWSON, C.F. Injuries to cattle from swallowing pointed objects. In U.S. Department of Agriculture. *Tenth and Eleventh Annual Reports of the Bureau of Animal Industry for the Years 1893 and 1894.* Washington, pp. 78–81. Reissued as Bureau of Animal Industry Circular No. 8. 4 pp.

103. Preliminary Investigations of unknown diseases in turkeys. In U.S. Department of Agriculture. *Tenth and Eleventh Annual Reports of the Bureau of Animal Industry for the Years 1893 and 1894.* Washington, pp. 82–83.

104. The production of diphtheria antitoxin. *Journal of the Association of Engineering Societies,* 16 (March), pp. 83–92. Read before the Boston Society of Civil Engineers, Boston, Mass., February 19, 1896.

105. Comparative pathology in its relation to human medicine. *Bulletin of the Harvard Medical Alumni Association,* 9 (June 23), pp. 50–69; *Boston Medical and Surgical Journal,* 135 (September), pp. 318–322. Speech delivered at the Harvard Medical Alumni Association's sixth Annual Dinner, Boston, Mass., June 23, 1896.

106. Water-borne diseases. *Journal of the New England Water Works Association,* 10, pp. 203–225. Address before the New England Water Works Association, Boston, Mass., January 8, 1896.

107. Presidential address. *Albany Medical Annals,* 17, pp. 132–138. Presidential Address (mainly on preventive medicine and water supplies), to the Albany Medical College Alumni Association at its twenty-third Annual Meeting, Albany, N.Y., April 14, 1896.

108. The conditions which influence the appearance of toxin in cultures of the diphtheria bacillus. *Transactions of the Association of American Physicians,* 11, pp. 37–61. Read at the eleventh Annual Meeting, Association of American Physicians, Washington, D.C., April 30, 1896.

109. Two varieties of the tubercle bacillus from mammals. *Transactions of the Association of American Physicians,* 11, pp. 75–93. (Discussion pp. 93–95.) Reproduced in U.S. Department of Agriculture. *Twelfth and Thirteenth Annual Reports of the Bureau of Animal Industry for the Fiscal Years 1895 and 1896.* Washington (1897), pp. 149–161.

110. *Sewage disposal on the farm, and the protection of drinking water. Farmers' Bulletin* (U.S. Department of Agriculture), No. 43. Washington. 19 pp.

1897

111. Sanitation on the farm. *New Bedford Evening Standard,* January 12, 1897.
     Abstract of lecture delivered to the South Bristol Farmers' Club on January 10, 1897.

112. The destruction of diphthereia toxin by other products of the diphtheria bacillus. *Journal of the Boston Society of Medical Sciences,* 1, No. 12 (April), pp. 5–8. Presented at meeting of the Boston Society of Medical Sciences, April 20, 1897.

113. Letter-Report to Tuberculosis Committee, Massachusetts Legislature. May 10, 1897. In Massachusetts Legislative Documents. House. No. 1341. Boston, Mass., Wright & Potter, pp. 9–10.

114. SMITH, T. and STEWART, J.R. spontaneous pseudo-tuberculosis in a guinea-pig, and the bacillus causing it. *Journal of the Boston Society of Medical Sciences,* 1, No. 16 (June), pp. 12–17. Presented at meeting of the Boston Society of Medical Sciences, June 15, 1897.

115. Investigations of diseases of domesticated animals. In U.S. Department of Agriculture. *Twelfth and Thirteenth Annual Reports of the Bureau of Animal Industry for the Fiscal Years 1895 and 1896.* Washington, pp. 119–183 (5 Pl.). Includes: Notes on sporadic pneumonia in cattle; its causation and differentiation from contagious pleuropneumonia, pp. 119–149; Two varieties of the tubercle bacillus from mammals, pp. 149–161; Notes on the evolution of hog-cholera outbreaks, pp. 161–166; Swine erysipelas or mouse-septicaemia bacilli from an outbreak of swine disease, pp. 166–174; Notes on peculiar parasitic affections of the liver in domesticated animals, pp. 174–179; Two cases of cirrhosis of the liver, pp. 179–183.

116. A modification of the method for determining the production of indol by bacteria. *Journal of Experimental Medicine,* 2 (September), pp. 543–547; *Journal of the Boston Society of Medical Sciences,* 2, No. 3 (November), pp. 23–24. (Abstract). Presented by title at meeting of the Boston Society of Medical Sciences, November 16, 1897.

117. SMITH, T. and WALKER, E.L. A comparative study of the toxin production of diphtheria bacilli. In Massachusetts. State Board of Health. *28th Annual Report for 1896–97.* Public Document No. 34, pp. 649–672. T.S. alone, Introduction, pp. 649–658. T.S. with E.L.W., Comparative study of forty-two cultures of diphtheria bacilli and of four cultures of pseudo-diphtheria bacilli from different localities in Massachusetts, pp. 659–672; *Centralblatt für Bakteriologie,* I. Abteilung (Referate), 23 (March, 1898), 554–556. (Abstract); *Journal of the Boston Society of Medical Sciences,* 2, No. 2 (November), pp. 12–15. The last being a summary presented at meeting of the Boston Society of Medical Sciences, November 2, 1897.

118. Ueber Fehlerquellen bei Prüfung der Gas- und Säurebildung bei Bakterien und deren Vermeidung. *Centralblatt für Bakteriologie.* I. Abteilung (Originale), 22 (August), pp. 45–59. See also: On sources of error in determining the production of gases and acids by bacteria and the means of avoiding them. *Journal of the Boston Society of Medical Sciences,* 2, No. 3 (November), p. 24. (Abstract). Given by title at meeting of the Boston Society of Medical Sciences, November 16, 1897.

1898

119. Preliminary report upon a comparative study of tubercle bacilli from man (sputum) and from cattle. In Massachusetts. Board of Cattle Commissioners of the Commonwealth of Massachusetts, *Annual Report.* Public Document No. 51 (January), Appendix B. (Boston, Mass., Wright & Potter), pp. 126–143.

120. One of the conditions under which discontinuous sterilization may be ineffective. *Journal of Experimental Medicine,* 3 (November), pp. 647–650; *Journal of the Boston Society of Medical Sciences,* 2, No. 8 (March), pp. 133–134. (Abstract).

121. The waste and destruction of wholesome meat. (Editorial). *Boston Medical and Surgical Journal,* 138 (March), pp. 282–283.

122. The toxin and antitoxin of tetanus. *Boston Medical and Surgical Journal,* 138 (December), pp. 292–295. (Discussion, pp. 303–305). Read before the Clinical Section of the Suffolk District Medical Society, December 15, 1897.

123. A comparative study of bovine tubercle bacilli and of human bacilli from sputum. *Journal of the Boston Society of Medical Sciences,* 2, No. 11 (May), pp. 187–189. (Summary): *Transactions of the Association of American Physicians,* 13, pp. 417–470; *Journal of Experimental Medicine,* 3 (September), pp. 451–511. Reprinted in *Medical Classics,* 1 (January, 1937), pp. 599–669. Read at the thirteenth Annual Meeting, Association of American Physicians, Washington, D.C., on May 4, 1898 and communicated in summary at a meeting of the Boston Society of Medical Sciences, Boston, Mass., May 24, 1898.

124. The action of typhoid bacilli on milk and its probable relation to a second carbohydrate in that fluid. *Journal of the Boston Society of Medical Sciences,* 2, No. 12 (June), pp. 236–244. Read before the Boston Society of Medical Sciences, Boston, Mass., June 21, 1898.

125. The toxin of diphtheria and its antitoxin. *Boston Medical and Surgical Journal,* 139 (August), pp. 157–160, 192–194; Massachusetts Medical Society. *Medical Communications,* 17 (August), pp. 709–728. (Discussion, p. 729). Read by invitation at the Annual Meeting, Massachusetts Medical Society, Boston, Mass., June 7, 1898.

126. ADAMI, J.G., ABBOTT, A.C., CHEESMAN, T.M., FULLER, G.W., SEDGWICK, W.T., SMART, C., SMITH, T. and WELCH, W. *Procedures Recommended for the Study of Bacteria, with especial reference to greater uniformity in the description and differentiation of species. Being the report of a Committee of American Bacteriologists to the Committee on the Pollution of Water Supplies of the American Public Health Association.* Concord, New Hampshire. 47 pp. (5 Charts).

127. Notes on a tubercle bacillus having a low degree of virulence. *Journal of the Boston Society of Medical Sciences,* 3, No. 2 (November), pp. 33–38. Presented at meeting of the Boston Society of Medical Sciences, Boston, Mass., November 15, 1898.

128. The sanitary aspects of dairying. *Maine Farmer,* December 15, 1898. No. 7 (pp. 1 & 4). Lecture before the Maine Dairy Association, Portland, Maine, December 8, 1898.

1899

129. Variations in pathogenic activity among tubercle bacilli. *Boston Medical and Surgical Journal,* 140 (January), pp. 31–33; *Climate,* 2, pp. 5–10. Presented by invitation at the fifteenth Annual Meeting of the American Climatological Association, Maplewood, New Hampshire, September 1, 1898.

130. Ueber einen unbeweglichen Hogcholera-(Schweinepest-) Bacillus. *Centralblatt für Bakteriologie,* I. Abteilung (Originale), 25 (February), pp. 241–244.

131. The thermal death-point of tubercle bacilli in milk and some other fluids. *Journal of Experimental Medicine,* 4 (March), pp. 217–233.

132. Harvard University. *Suggestions for a reorganization of the Harvard Veterinary School.* Cambridge, Mass. 4 pp. Statement prepared at the request of President Eliot.

133. The relation of dextrose to toxin production in bouillon cultures of the diphtheria bacillus. Preliminary note. *Journal of the Boston Society of Medical Sciences,* 3, No. 11 (June), pp. 315–318. Presented at meeting of the Boston Society of Medical Sciences, Boston, Mass., June 6, 1899.

134. Some devices for the cultivation of anaërobic bacteria in fluid media without the use of inert gases. *Journal of the Boston Society of Medical Sciences,* 3, No. 12 (June), pp. 340–343. Presented at meeting of the Boston Society of Medical Sciences, Boston, Mass., June 20, 1899.

135. The relation of dextrose to the production of toxin in bouillon cultures of the diphtheria bacillus. *Journal of Experimental Medicine,* 4 (July), pp. 373–397.

136. The aetiology of Texas cattle fever, with special reference to recent hypotheses concerning the transmission of malaria. *New York Medical Journal,* 70 (July), pp. 47–51. Read before the New York Academy of Medicine, New York, N.Y., April 6, 1899.

1900

137. Variation among pathogenic bacteria. *Journal of the Boston Society of Medical Sciences,* 4, No. 5 (January), pp. 95–109. Read before the Boston Society of Medical Sciences, January 16, 1900; and previously under the title "The significance of varieties among pathogenic bacteria" at the first meeting, Society of American Bacteriologists, New Haven, Connecticut, December 27, 1899.

138. Adaptation of pathogenic bacteria to different species of animals. *Transactions of the Congress of American Physicians and Surgeons,* 5, pp. 1–11; *Boston Medical and Surgical Journal,* 142 (May), pp. 473–476; *Philadelphia Medical Journal,* 5 (May), pp. 1018–1022. Read before the fifth Congress of American Physicians and Surgeons, Washington, D.C., May 1, 1900.

139. Comparative pathology: its relation to biology and medicine. *Transactions of the Congress of American Physicians and Surgeons,* 6 (September), pp. 409–414. Address delivered by invitation at the Annual Conversational Meeting of the Philadelphia Pathological Society, Philadelphia, Pennsylvania, April 26, 1900.

140. The antitoxin unit in diphtheria. *Journal of the Boston Society of Medical Sciences,* 5, No. 1 (October), pp. 1–11. Presented at a meeting of the Boston Society of Medical Sciences, Boston, Mass., October 16, 1900.

141. Public health laboratorires. *Boston Medical and Surgical Journal,* 143 (November), pp. 491–493. Chairman's introductory address at the opening of the second Annual Meeting, Section in Bacteriology and Chemistry, American Public Health Association, Indianapolis, Indiana, October 22, 1900.

1901

142. Harvard Medical School. *Animal Parasites and Their Relation to Pathological Processes. Syllabus.* Boston, Mass. 18 pp. Outline of a course in medical protozoology and parasitology that Smith had initiated at the Harvard Medical School the preceding year.

143. Notes on the occurrence of Anopheles punctipennis and a quadri- maculatus in the Boston suburbs. *Journal of the Boston Society of Medical Sciences,* 5, No. 6 (January), pp. 321–324. Presented at meeting of the Boston Society of Medical Sciences, January 15, 1901.

144. The etiology of malaria with special reference to the mosquito as an intermediate host. *Journal of the Massachusetts Association of Boards of Health,* 11 (October), pp. 99–113. Read before the Massachusetts Association of Boards of Health, Boston, Mass., May 14, 1900.

145. The production of sarcosporidiosis in the mouse by feeding infected muscular tissue. *Journal of Experimental Medicine,* 6, pp. 1–21; *Transactions of the Association of American Physicians,* 16 (November), pp. 576–594. Read by title at the sixteenth Annual Meeting, Association of American Physicians, Washington, D.C., May 2, 1901.

1902

146. The relation between bovine and human tuberculosis. *Medical News,* 80 (February), pp. 343–346. Read at meeting of the New York Academy of Medicine, New York, N.Y., December 19, 1901.

147. *Animal Experimentation. A Series of Statements Indicating its Value to Biological and Medical Science.* (30 authors). Edited by H.C. Ernst. Boston, Mass. Little, Brown, and Company. Smith's statement appears on pp. 113–120.

148. SMITH, T. and JOHNSON. H.P. On a coccidium (*Klossiella muris,* gen. et spec. nov.) parasitic in the renal epithelium of the mouse. *Journal of Experimental Medicine,* 6 (March), pp. 303–316 (3 Pl.).

149. The preparation of animal vaccine. *Boston Medical and Surgical Journal,* 147 (August), pp. 197–201; Massachusetts Medical Society. *Medical Communications,* 19, pp. 103–116. Read at the Annual Meeting, Massachustets Medical Society, Boston, Mass., June 10, 1902.

150. Foot-and-mouth disease. (Editorial). *Boston Medical and Surgical Journal,* 147 (December), pp. 626–627.

1903

151. The preparation and distribution of antitoxin by the Massachusetts Board of Health. Letter to Editor (April 13). *Boston Medical and Surgical Journal,* 148 pp. 431–433.

152. SMITH, T. and REAGH, A.L. The agglutination affinities of related bacteria parasitic in different hosts. *Journal of Medical Research,* 9 (n.s. 4) (May), pp. 270–300. Reproduced in *Studies from the Rockefeller Institute for Medical Research,* 1, No. 12 (1904), pp. 250–280. Read before the Boston Society of Medicial Sciences, April 7, 1903.

153. Studies in mammalian tubercle bacilli. III. Description of a bovine bacillus from the human body. A culture test for distinguishing the human from the bovine type of bacilli. *Transactions of the Association of American Physicians,* 18, pp. 109–151. Reprinted in *Journal of Medical Research,* 13 (n.s. 8) (February, 1905), pp. 253–300. Summarized in U.S. Department of Agriculture. *Twentieth Annual Report of the Bureau of Animal Industry for the Year 1903.* Washington (1904), pp. 73–74; and in *Centralblatt für Bakteriologie,* I. Abteilung

(Referate), 35 (July, 1904), pp. 170–174. Presented at the sixth Congress of Physicians and Surgeons, Washington, D.C., May 12, 1903.

154. The sources, favoring conditions and prophylaxis of malaria in temperate climates, with special reference to Massachusetts. *Boston Medical and Surgical Journal,* 149 (July), pp. 57–64, 87–92, 115–118, 139–144; Massachusetts Medical Society. *Medical Communications,* 19, pp. 337–410. The Shattuck Lecture. Delivered at the Annual Meeting, Massachusetts Medical Society, Boston, Mass., June 9, 1903.

155. SMITH, T. and REAGH, A.L. The non-identity of agglutinins acting upon the flagella and upon the body of bacteria. *Journal of Medical Research,* 10 (n.s.5) (August), pp. 89–100. Reproduced in *Studies from the Rockefeller Institute for Medical Research,* 1, No. 18 (1904), pp. 349–360. Read at the third Annual Meeting, American Association of Pathologists and Bacteriologists, Washington, D.C., May 14, 1903.

156. Malaria. Concerning the probable effect of the proposed fresh-water basin upon the occurrence of malaria in the territory adjoining the basin. Massachusetts. Committee on Charles River Dam. *Report,* Appendix No. 1, pp. 111–129.

1904

157. Some of the ways in which infection is disseminated. *Journal of the Massachusetts Association of Boards of Health,* 14, pp. 19–31. Read before the Massachusetts Association of Boards of Health, Boston, Mass., January 25, 1904.

158. The new laboratory of the Massachusetts State Board of Health for the preparation of diphtheria antitoxin and vaccine. *Journal of the Massachusetts Association of Boards of Health,* 14, pp. 231–236.

159. U.S. Department of Agriculture. Bureau of Animal Industry. *Special Report on Diseases of Cattle.* Prepared by L. Pearson, A.J. Murray, and 10 other authors, including T. Smith. Washington. 533 pp. (52 Pl.).

160. A study of the tubercle bacilli isolated from three cases of tuberculosis of the mesenteric lymph nodes. *American Journal of the Medical Sciences,* n.s. 128 (August), pp. 216–225; *Transactions of the Association of American Physicians,* 19, pp. 373–382. Read by title before the Boston Society of Medical Sciences, February 16, 1904; and at the nineteenth Annual Meeting, Association of American Physicians, Washington, D.C., May 11, 1904.

161. The pathological effects of periodic losses of blood. - An experimental study. *Journal of Medical Research,* 12 (n.s. 7) (October), pp. 385–406. Reproduced in *Studies from the Rockefeller Institute for Medical Research,* 3, No. 12 (1905), pp. 217–238.

162. Some problems in the life history of pathogenic microorganisms. *American Medicine,* 8 (October), pp. 711–718; *Science,* n.s. 20 (December), pp. 817–832. Also appeared in German, translated by H.B., as Über einige Probleme aus der Lebensgeschichte der pathogenen Mikroorganismen. *Die Umschau,* 9 (June, 1905), pp. 466–471. Address before the Section of Bacteriology, International Congress of Arts and Sciences, St. Louis, Mo., September 24, 1904.

163. Leprosy. *Boston Medical and Surgical Journal,* 151 (December), pp. 675–676. Based on paper read at the Annual Meeting, Massachusetts Association of Boards of Health, Boston, Mass., July 28, 1904.

1905

164. Degrees of susceptibility to diphtheria toxin among guinea-pigs. Transmission from parents to offspring. *Journal of Medical Research,* 13 (n.s. 8) (February), pp. 341–348.

165. Medical research: its place in the university medical school. *Popular Science Monthly,* 66 (April), pp. 515–530; *Boston Medical and Surgical Journal,* 152, pp. 466–471. Reproduced in Cattell, J.M., ed., *Medical Research and Education,* by R.M. Pearce, W.H. Welch, and many others, including T.S. (pp. 319–366). New York, Science Press, 1913. Address before the Harvard Medical Alumni Association of New York City, N.Y., November 26, 1904.

166. The reaction curve of tubercle bacilli from different sources in bouillon containing different amounts of glycerine. *Journal of Medical Research,* 13 (n.s. 8) (May), pp. 405–408.

167. Further observations on the transmission of Sarcocystis muris by feeding. *Journal of Medical Research,* 13 (n.s. 8) (May), pp. 429–430.

168. Note on the stability of the cultural characters of tubercle bacilli, with special reference to the production of capsules. *Transactions of the National Association for the Study and Prevention of Tuberculosis,* 1, pp. 211–220 (2 Pl.). Presented at the first Annual Meeting, National Association for the Study and Prevention of Tuberculosis, Washington, D.C., May 18–19, 1905.

169. SALMON, D.E. and SMITH, T. *Texas Fever, or Southern Cattle Fever.* U.S. Department of Agriculture. Bureau of Animal Industry. Circular No. 69. Washington. 13 pp. Reprinted from the Bureau's Special Report on Diseases of Cattle, 1904, with revision by D.E. Salmon and J.R. Mohler.

170. SALMON, D.E. and SMITH, T. *Tuberculosis of cattle.* U.S. Department of Agriculture. Bureau of Animal Industry. Circular No. 70. Washington. 28 pp. Reprinted from the Bureau's Special Report on Diseases of Cattle, 1904, with revision by D.E. Salmon and J.R. Mohler.

171. SALMON, D.E. and SMITH, T. *Anthrax in cattle, horses and men.* U.S. Department of Agriculture. Bureau of Animal Industry. Circular No. 71. Washington. 10 pp. Reprinted from the Bureau's Special Report on Diseases of Cattle, 1904, with revision by D.E. Salmon and J.R. Mohler.

172. Research into the causes and antecedents of disease, its importance to society. *Boston Medical and Surgical Journal,* 153 (July), pp. 6–11. Read by invitation before the Section on Hygiene of the American Social Science Association, Boston, Mass., May 12, 1905.

173. Über einige Kulturmerkmale des Rauschbrandbazillus. *Zeitschrift für Infektionskrankheiten, parasitäre Krankheiten und Hygiene der Haustiere,* 1 (September), pp. 26–31.

174. SMITH, T., BROWN, H.R. and WALKER, E.L. The fermentation tube in the study of anaërobic bacteria with special reference to gas production and the use of milk as a culture medium. *Journal of Medical Research,* 14 (n.s. 9) (November), pp. 193–206; *American Public Health Association Reports,* 31, pp. 229–240. Read before the Laboratory Section, American Public Health Association, Boston, Mass., September 25, 1905, and before the Boston Society of Medical Sciences, November 21, 1905.

175. The relation of animal life to human diseases. *Boston Medical Surgical Journal,* 153 (November), pp. 485–489; *American Public Health Associa- tion Reports,* 31, pp. 328–338. Read at the thirty-third Annual Meeting, American Public Health Association, Boston, Mass., September 29, 1905.

1906

176. What is the relation between human and bovine tuberculosis, and how does it affect inmates of public institutions? *Boston Medical and Surgical Journal,* 154 (January), pp. 60–62;

American Journal of Public Hygiene, 16 (n.s. 2), pp. 516–521. (Discussion, pp. 522–528). Read at the Boston Tuberculosis Exhibition, January 5, 1906.

177. The parasitism of the tubercle bacillus and its bearing on infection and immunity. *Journal of the American Medical Association,* 46 (April), pp. 1247–1254, 1345–1348; *Harvey Lectures,* 1, pp. 272–304. Lecture delivered under the auspices of the Harvey Society of New York, March 10, 1906.

178. A description of the new antitoxin and vaccine laboratory, together with a ten years' retrospect of the production and distribution of diphtheria antitoxin. In Massachusetts. State Board of Health. *Annual Report, 1905.* Public Document No. 34, pp. 527–546.

179. SALMON, D.E. and SMITH, T. *Actinomycosis, or lumpy jaw.* U.S. Department of Agriculture. Bureau of Animal Industry. Circular No. 96. Washington. 10 pp. Reprinted from the Bureau's Special Report on Diseases of Cattle, 1904, with revision by D.E. Salmon and J.R. Mohler.

180. The Department of Comparative Pathology. 1896. In Harvard University. *The Harvard Medical School. 1782–1906,* Boston, pp. 157–161.

181. SMITH, T. and BROWN, H.R. The resistance of the red blood corpuscles of the horse to salt solutions of different tonicities before and after repeated withdrawals of blood. *Journal of Medical Research,* 15 (n.s. 10) (December), pp. 425–447. Reproduced in *Studies from the Rockefeller Institute for Medical Research,* 7, No. 8 (1907), pp. 85–107.

1907

182. The degree and duration of passive immunity to diphtheria toxin transmitted by immunized female guinea-pigs to their immediate offspring. *Journal of Medical Research,* 16 (n.s. 11) (May), pp. 359–379.

183. SMITH, T. and BROWN, H.R. Studies in mammalian tubercle bacilli. IV. Bacilli resembling the bovine type from four cases in man. *Journal of Medical Research,* 16 (n.s. 11) (July), pp. 435–450.

184. The channels of infection in tuberculosis, together with some remarks on the outlook concerning a specific therapy. *Boston Medical and Surgical Journal,* 157 (September), pp. 420–427; Massachusetts Medical Society. *Medical Communications,* 20, pp. 447–472. Read before the Massachusetts Medical Society, Boston, Mass., June 11, 1907.

1908

185. Some neglected facts in the biology of the tetanus bacillus. Their bearing on the safety of the so-called biologic products. *Journal of the American Medical Association,* 50 (March), pp. 929–934; *Chicago Pathological Society. Transactions,* 7, No. 41 (1906–1909), pp. 1–14. Read at the joint meeting, Chicago Pathological Society and Chicago Medical Society, Chicago, December 18, 1907.

186. SALMON, D.E. and SMITH, T. *Foot-and-mouth disease.* U.S. Department of Agriculture. Bureau of Animal Industry. Circular No. 141. Washington. 8 pp. Reprinted from the Department's Special Report on Diseases of Cattle, 1904.

187. The vaccination of cattle against tuberculosis. Experiments conducted under the auspices of the Massachusetts Society for Promoting Agriculture. *Journal of Medical Research,* 18 (n.s. 13) (June), pp. 451–485.

188. The house-fly as an agent in the dissemination of infectious diseases. *American Journal of Public Hygiene,* 18 (n.s. 4), pp. 312–317. (Discussion, pp. 317–324). Reproduced in Mas-

sachusetts. State Board of Health. *Monthly Bulletin,* 4 (April, 1909), pp. 68–71. Read before Massachusetts Association of Boards of Health, Boston, July 23, 1908.

189. Experimental researches in tuberculosis, with special reference to etiology, pathology and immunity. In Locke, E.A., ed. *Tuberculosis in Massachusetts.* Boston, Wright and Potter, Chapter XII, pp. 158–174. Reprinted in Massachusetts. State Board of Health. *Monthly Bulletin,* 3 (September), pp. 191–203.

190. The relation between human and animal tuberculosis, with special reference to the question of the transformation of human and other types of the tubercle bacillus. *Boston Medical and Surgical Journal,* 159 (November), pp. 707–711. Read before International Congress on Tuberculosis, Washington, D.C., September 10, 1908.

1909

191. Active immunity produced by so-called balanced or neutral mixtures of diphtheria toxin and antitoxin. *Journal of Experimental Medicine,* 11 (March), pp. 241–256.

192. COUNCILMAN, W.T., SMITH, T. and ERNST, H.C. Letter to Editor (April 24): An appeal in behalf of a suffering benefactor of humanity. *Boston Medical and Surgical Journal,* 160, p. 561. An appeal for funds to aid John R. Kissinger and family. He was the first volunteer in the Walter Reed Yellow Fever Commission.

193. What is diseased meat, and what is its relation to meat inspection? *American Journal of Public Hygiene,* 19 (n.s. 5), pp. 397–411; Massachusetts. State Board of Health. *Monthly Bulletin,* 4 (October), pp. 220–229. Read at the quarterly meeting of the Massachusetts Association of Boards of Health, April 29, 1909.

194. Animal diseases transmissible to man. Massachusetts. State Board of Health. *Monthly Bulletin,* 4 (December), pp. 264–276. A public lecture in the Columbia University series on *Sanitary Science and Public Health.* Read at the Columbia College of Physicians and Surgeons, New York, April 12, 1909.

1910

195. Insects as carriers of disease. Massachusetts. State Board of Health. *Monthly Bulletin,* 5 (April), pp. 112–119.

196. What is the experimental basis for vaccine therapy? *Boston Medical and Surgical Journal,* 163 (August), pp. 275–278. (Discussion, pp. 278–279); Massachusetts Medical Society. *Medical Communications,* 21, pp. 761–773. (Discussion, pp. 774–776). Read at the Annual Meeting, Massachusetts Medical Society, Boston, Mass., June 8, 1910.

197. Amoeba meleagridis. Letter to Editor (Sept. 20). *Science,* n.s. 32 (October), pp. 509–512.

198. The reaction curve of the human and the bovine type of the tubercle bacillus in glycerine bouillon. *Journal of Medical Research,* 23 (n.s. 18) (October), pp. 185–204. Read at the sixth Annual Meeting, National Association for the Study and Prevention of Tuberculosis, Washington, D.C., May 3, 1910.

199. A protective reaction of the host in intestinal coccidiosis of the rabbit. *Journal of Medical Research,* 23 (n.s. 18) (November), pp. 407–415 (4 Pl.).

200. Note on the influence of infectious diseases upon a preexisting parasitism. *Journal of Medical Research,* 23 (n.s. 18) (November), pp. 417–422 (1 Pl.).

201. Intestinal amebiasis in the domestic pig. *Journal of Medical Research,* 23 (n.s. 18) (November), pp. 423–432 (2 Pl.).

202. SMITH, T. and BROWN, H.R. Further studies on the immunizing effect of mixtures of diphtheria toxin and antitoxin. *Journal of Medical Research,* 23 (n.s. 18) (November), pp. 433–449; *Transactions of the Association of American Physicians,* 25, pp. 212–222. Based on a paper read at the twenty-fifth Annual Meeting, Association of American Physicians, Washington, D.C., May 4, 1910.

1911

203. The vaccination of cattle against tuberculosis. II. The pathogenic effect of certain cultures of the human type on calves. *Journal of Medical Research,* 25 (n.s. 20) (September), pp. 1–33. (Investigations conducted under the auspices of the Massachusetts Society for Promoting Agriculture). Address before the Massachusetts Society for Promoting Agriculture, Boston, Mass., February 19, 1911.

1912

204. SMITH, T. and FABYAN, M. Ueber die pathogene Wirkung des Bacillus abortus Bang. *Centralblatt für Bakteriologie,* I. Abteilung (Originale), 61 (January 6), pp. 549–555.

205. Parasitismus und Krankheit. *Deutsche Medizinische Wochenschrift,* 38 (February), pp. 276–279. Formal Address as Visiting Professor, University of Berlin, January 13, 1912.

206. Demonstration mikroskopischer Präparate von mit dem Bacillus des Abortus geimpften Meerschweincher. *Berliner Klinische Wochenschrift,* 49 (April), p. 715. (Discussion, pp. 715–716). Also (with Oberstadt), Demonstration verschiedener Anwendungen des Gärungskölbchens in der Bakteriologie. *Berliner Klinische Wochenschrift,* 49 (April), p. 716. Demonstrations before the Berliner mikrobiologische Gesellschaft, Berlin, Germany, March 7, 1912.

1913

207. The etiology of hay fever. *Boston Medical and Surgical Journal,* 168 (April), pp. 504–506. Substance of a discussion on hay fever before the New England Otological and Laryngological Society, Boston, Mass., November 19, 1912.

208. An attempt to interpret present-day uses of vaccine. *Journal of the American Medical Association,* 60 (May), pp. 1591–1599. Address at the Annual Conversational Meeting of the Philadelphia Pathological Society, Philadelphia, Penn., April 24, 1913.

209. Notes on the biology of the tubercle bacillus. *Journal of Medical Research,* 28 (n.s. 23) (May), pp. 91–110.

210. REMSEN, I., CHITTENDEN, R.H., LONG, J.H., TAYLOR, A.E. AND SMITH, T. *Influence of Vegetables Greened with Copper Salts on the Nutrition and Health of Man.* (Report of the Referee board of Consulting Scientific Experts). U.S. Department of Agriculture, *Report No. 97.* Washington. 461 pp.

211. Histological examination of the tissues of dogs and monkeys. In U.S. Department of Agriculture, *Report No. 97.* Washington. pp. 449–461.

212. Some bacteriological and environmental factors in the pneumonias of lower animals with special reference to the guinea-pig. *Journal of Medical Research,* 29 (n.s. 24) (December), pp. 291–323 (3 Pl.). Read before the Boston Society of Medical Sciences, December 16, 1913.

1914

213. Foreword to Carl TenBroeck's "Experiments to determine if paralyzed domestic animals and those associated with cases of infantile paralysis may transmit this disease." Massachusetts. State Board of Health. *Forty-fifth Annual Report.* pp. 1–6.

214. BROWN, H.R. and SMITH, T. Notes on two "atoxic" strains of diphtheria bacilli. *Journal of Medical Research,* 30 (n.s. 25) (July), pp. 443–454.

215. The danger of transmitting disease by the feeding of offal to animals. New York State. Department of Health. *Monthly Bulletin,* 30 (October), p. 337.

1915

216. SMITH, T. and BROWN, J.H. A study of streptococci isolated from certain presumably milk-borne epidemics of tonsillitis occurring in Massachusetts in 1913 and 1914. *Journal of Medical Research,* 31 (n.s. 26) (January), pp. 455–502. Based on a paper presented to the Boston Society of Medical Sciences, Boston, Mass., November 17, 1914.

217. SMITH, T. and TENBROECK, C. Agglutination affinities of a pathogenic bacillus from fowls (fowl typhoid) (*Bacterium sanguinarium,* Moore) with the typhoid bacillus of man. *Journal of Medical Research,* 31 (n.s. 26) (January), pp. 503–521. Based on papers presented at the ninth Triennial Session, Congress of American Physicians and Surgeons, and the twenty-eighth Annual Meeting, Association of American Physicians, Washington, D.C., May 6, 1914, and also to the Boston Society of Medical Sciences, Boston, Mass., November 17, 1914.

218. SMITH, T. and TENBROECK, C. The pathogenic action of the fowl typhoid bacillus with special reference to certain toxins. *Journal of Medical Research,* 31 (n.s. 26) (January), pp. 523–546.

219. SMITH, T. and TENBROECK, C. A note on the relation between *B. pullorum* (Rettger) and the fowl typhoid bacillus (Moore). *Journal of Medical Research,* 31 (n.s. 26) (January), pp. 547–555.

220. Scholarship in medicine. *Boston Medical and Surgical Journal,* 172 (January), pp. 121–124. Address to the students of the Harvard Medical School on the occasion of the presentation of the John Harvard Fellowships, December 2, 1914.

221. SMITH, T. (Chairman), and 19 others. New York State. Commission for the Investigation of Bovine Tuberculosis. *Report.* (Albany, N.Y., March, 1915). 46 pp.

222. The anatomical and histological expression of increased resistance towards tuberculosis in cattle following the intravenous injection of human and attenuated bovine tubercle bacilli. *Journal of Medical Research,* 32 (n.s. 27) (July), pp. 455–469 (4 Pl.). Reproduced without plates, and with "to" in title replacing "towards," in *Transactions of the Association of American Physicians,* 30, pp. 7–19. Read by title at the thirtieth Annual Meeting, Association of American Physicians, Washington, D.C., May 11, 1915.

223. SMITH, T. and FABYAN, M. The vaccination of cattle against tuberculosis. III. The occasional persistence of the human type of tubercle bacillus in cattle. *Transactions of the Association of American Physicians,* 30, pp. 523–537. Investigations conducted under the auspices of the Massachusetts Society for Promoting Agriculture.

224. Further investigations into the etiology of the protozoan disease of turkeys known as blackhead, entero-hepatitis, typhlitis, etc. *Transactions of the Association of American Physicians,* 33 (n.s. 28) (November), pp. 243–270 (5 Pl.). Field work of this investigation made possible through a grant from the Massachusetts Society for Promoting Agriculture.

1916

225. Aberrant intestinal protozoan parasites in the turkey. *Journal of Experimental Medicine,* 23 (March), pp. 293–300 (1 Pl.).

226. Professor Gage: The Friend. In *The Gage Memorial*. Ithaca, N.Y., Cornell University, pp. 13–14. Tribute published in commemoration of S.H. Gage's sixty-fifth birthday, May 20, 1916. This was volume 7, number F of Cornell University's Official Publications.

227. The underlying problems of immunization. *Transactions of the Congress of American Physicians and Surgeons*, 10, pp. 99–109. Reproduced in *Studies from the Rockefeller Institute for Medical Research*, 27, pp. 489–500. Read at the tenth Triennial Session, Congress of American Physicians and Surgeons, Washington, D.C., May 10, 1916.

1917

228. Some field experiments bearing on the transmission of blackhead in turkeys. *Journal of Experimental Medicine*, 25 (March), pp. 405–414. Reproduced in *Studies from the Rockefeller Institute for Medical Research*, 27, pp. 501–510.

229. SMITH, T. and SMILLIE, E.W. A note on coccidia in sparrows and their assumed relation to blackhead in turkeys. *Journal of Experimental Medicine*, 25 (March), pp. 415–420. Reproduced in *Studies from the Rockefeller Institute for Medical Research*, 27, pp. 511–516.

230. Certain aspects of natural and acquired resistance to tuberculosis and their bearing on preventive measure. *Journal of the American Medical Association*, 68 (March), pp. 669–674, 764–769. Reproduced in *Studies from the Rockefeller Institute for Medical Research*, 27, pp. 517–552. Also published as a separate pamphlet by University of Pittsburgh (1916), 39 pp. The second Mellon Lecture, delivered before the Society for Biological Research, University of Pittsburgh, Penn., May 17, 1916.

231. The significance of laboratory research in medical education. *Albany Medical Annals*, 38 (August), pp. 351–360. Address at the eighty-sixth commencement of Albany Medical College, June 8, 1917.

1918

232. SMITH, T. and GRAYBILL, H.W. Coccidiosis in young calves. *Journal of Experimental Medicine*, 28 (July), pp. 89–108 (3 Pl.). Reproduced in *Studies from the Rockefeller Institute for Medical Research*, 31 (1919), pp. 555–574 (3 Pl.).

233. A pleomorphic bacillus from pneumonic lungs of calves simulating actinomyces. *Journal of Experimental Medicine*, 28 (September), pp. 333–344 (4 Pl.). Reproduced in *Studies from the Rockefeller Institute for Medical Research*, 32 (1920), pp. 475–486 (4 Pl.).

234. Spirilla associated with disease of the fetal membranes in cattle (infectious abortion). *Journal of Experimental Medicine*, 28 (December), pp. 701–719 (2 Pl.). Reproduced in *Studies from the Rockefeller Institute for Medical Research*, 32 (1920), pp. 519–537 (2 Pl.).

1919

235. A characteristic localization of Bacillus abortus in the bovine fetal membranes. *Journal of Experimental Medicine*, 29 (May), pp. 451–456 (3 Pl.). Reproduced in *Studies from the Rockefeller Institute for Medical Research*, 33 (1920), pp. 589–594 (3 Pl.).

236. SMITH, T. and TAYLOR, M.S. Some morphological and biological characters of the spirilla (Vibrio fetus, N.Sp.) associated with disease of the fetal membranes in cattle. *Journal of Experimental Medicine*, 30 (October), pp. 299–311 (1 Pl.). Reproduced in *Studies from the Rockefeller Institute for Medical Research*, 35 (1920), pp. 545–557 (1 Pl.).

237. The etiological relation of spirilla (Vibrio fetus) to bovine abortion. *Journal of Experimental Medicine*, 30 (October), pp. 313–323. Reproduced in *Studies from the Rockefeller Institute for Medical Research*, 35 (1920), pp. 559–569.

238. The bacteriology of bovine abortion, with special reference to acquired immunity. *Journal of Experimental Medicine,* 30 (October), pp. 325–339. Reproduced in *Studies from the Rockefeller Institute for Medical Research,* 35 (1920), pp. 571–585.

1920

239. Mycosis of the bovine fetal membranes due to a mould of the genus Mucor. *Journal of Experimental Medicine,* 31 (February), pp. 115–122. Reproduced in *Studies from the Rockefeller Institute for Medical Research,* 36 (1921), pp. 539–546.

240. SMITH, T. and GRAYBILL, H.W. Epidemiology of blackhead in turkeys under approximately natural conditions. *Journal of Experimental Medicine,* 31 (May), pp. 633–645. Reproduced in *Studies from the Rockefeller Institute for Medical Research,* 36 (1921), pp. 563–575.

241. GRAYBILL, H.W. and SMITH, T. Production of fatal blackhead in turkeys by feeding embryonated eggs of Heterakis papillosa. *Journal of Experimental Medicine,* 31 (May), pp. 647–655. Reproduced in *Studies from the Rockefeller Institute for Medical Research,* 36 (1921), pp. 577–585.

242. SMITH, T. and GRAYBILL, H.W. Blackhead in chickens and its experimental production by feeding embryonated eggs of Heterakis papillosa. *Journal of Experimental Medicine,* 32 (August), pp. 143–152. Reproduced in *Studies from the Rockefeller Institute for Medical Research,* 37 (1921), pp. 519–528.

243. SMITH, T. and SMITH, D.E. Inhibitory action of paratyphoid bacilli on the fermentation of lactose by Bacillus coli. I. *Journal of General Physiology,* 3 (September), pp. 21–33. Reproduced in *Studies from the Rockefeller Institute for Medical Research,* 37 (1921), pp. 589–601.

244. University of Nebraska College of Education. *The Importance of Research in Animal Pathology to Agriculture.* Lincoln, Ne. 23 pp. Address delivered at the dedication of the Animal Pathology and Hygiene Laboratories, University of Nebraska, College of Agriculture, Lincoln, Nebraska, September 24, 1920.

245. SMITH, T., LITTLE, R.B. and TAYLOR, M.S. Further studies on the etiological role of Vibrio fetus. *Journal of Experimental Medicine,* 32 (December), pp. 683–689. Reproduced in *Studies from the Rockefeller Institute for Medical Research,* 38 (1921), pp. 565–571.

246. The relation of animal to human diseases. In *Nelson's Loose-Leaf Medicine,* 7, pp. 399–413. Reproduced unchanged in *Nelson's Loose-Leaf Living Medicine* (1928), Chap. V, pp. 185–200.

1921

247. Remarks on the etiology of infectious abortion in cattle. *Cornell Veterinarian,* 11 (April), pp. 85–91. Presented at the thirteenth Annual Conference for Veterinarians, New York State Veterinary College, Cornell University, Ithaca, N.Y., January 20, 1921.

248. The etiological relation of Bacillus actinoides to bronchopneumonia in calves. *Journal of Experimental Medicine,* 33 (April), pp. 441–469 (9 Pl.). Reproduced in *Studies from the Rockefeller Institute for Medical Research,* 40 (1922), pp. 557–585 (9 Pl.).

249. Parasitism as a factor in disease. *Science,* 54 (August), pp. 99–108; *Transactions of the Association of American Physicians,* 36, pp. 172–187. Contributed to a symposium under the general title, "Discussion on the Causation or Etiology of Infectious and Parasitic Diseases," at the thirty-sixth Annual Meeting, Association of American Physicians, Washington, D.C., May 10, 1921.

250. Theories of susceptibility and resistance in relation to methods of artificial immuniza-tion. *Proceedings of the Institute of Medicine of Chicago,* 3, pp. 243–265. The second Pasteur Lecture, delivered at Chicago, October 21, 1921.

251. The capsules or sheaths of Bacillus actinoides. *Journal of Experimental Medicine,* 34 (De-cember), pp. 593–598 (1 Pl.). Reproduced in *Studies from the Rockefeller Institute for Medi-cal Research,* 42 (1922), pp. 559–564 (1 Pl.).

1922

252. Bovine tuberculosis as a contributory source of human tuberculosis. *Proceedings of the 47th Annual Meeting of the New Jersey Sanitary Association.* pp. 21–24. Address given under the auspices of the New Jersey Tuberculosis League, at Lakewood, N.J., December 9, 1921.

253. SMITH, T. and LITTLE, R.B. The significance of colostrum to the new-born calf. *Journal of Experimental Medicine,* 36 (August), pp. 181–198. Reproduced in *Studies from the Rockefeller Institute for Medical Research,* 44 (1923), pp. 523–540.

254. SMITH, T. and LITTLE, R.B. Cow serum as a substitute for colostrum in new-born calves. *Journal of Experimental Medicine,* 36 (October), pp. 453–468. Reproduced in *Studies from the Rockefeller Institute for Medical Research,* 45 (1923), pp. 531–546.

1923

255. SMITH, T., ORCUTT, M.L. and LITTLE, R.B. The source of agglutinins in the milk of cows. *Journal of Experimental Medicine,* 37 (February), pp. 153–174. Reproduced in *Studies from the Rockefeller Institute for Medical Research,* 46, pp. 621–642.

256. Further studies on the etiological significance of Vibrio fetus. *Journal of Experimental Med-icine,* 37 (March), pp. 341–356 (2 Pl.). Reproduced in *Studies from the Rockefeller Institute for Medical Research,* 46, pp. 643–658 (2 Pl.).

257. SMITH, T. and LITTLE, R.B. The absorption of specific agglutinins in homologous se-rum fed to calves during the early hours of life. *Journal of Experimental Medicine,* 37 (May), pp. 671–683. Reproduced in *Studies from the Rockefeller Institute for Medical Research,* 46, pp. 659–671.

258. SMITH, T. and LITTLE, R.B. *Studies in Vaccinal Immunity Towards Diasease of the Bovine Pla-centa due to Bacillus Abortus (Infectious Abortion).* Rockefeller Institute for Medical Re-search, Monograph No. 19, 124 pp.

1924

259. SMITH, T. and LITTLE, R.B. Proteinuria in new-born calves following the feeding of colostrum. *Journal of Experimental Medicine,* 39 (February), pp. 303–312. Reproduced in *Studies from the Rockefeller Institute for Medical Research,* 49, pp. 551–560.

260. Some aspects of the tuberculosis problem from the experimental and comparative stand-point. *Edinburgh Medical Journal,* 31 (Ser. 3, 74) (March), pp. 176–181. Synopsis of ad-dress to Joint Meeting of the Edinburgh Medico-Chirurgical Society and the Tuberculo-sis Society of Scotland, Edinburgh, November 29, 1923.

261. Some biological and economic aspects of comparative pathology. *Edinburgh Medical Jour-nal,* 31 (Ser. 3, 74) (April), pp. 221–240. Address delivered at the Centenary Celebra-tions, Royal (Dick) Veterinary College, Edinburgh, Scotland, November 27, 1923.

262. Some cultural characters of Bacillus abortus (Bang) with special reference to CO_2 re-

quirements. *Journal of Experimental Medicine,* 40 (August), pp. 219–232. Reproduced in *Studies from the Rockefeller Institute for Medical Research,* 52 (1925), pp. 501–514.

1925

263. SMITH, T. and FLORENCE, L. Encephalitozoon cuniculi as a kidney parasite in the rabbit. *Journal of Experimental Medicine,* 41 (January), pp. 25–35 (3 Pl.). Reproduced in *Studies from the Rockefeller Institute for Medical Research,* 53, pp. 543–553 (3 Pl.).

264. Hydropic stages in the intestinal epithelium of new-born calves. *Journal of Experimental Medicine,* 41 (January), pp. 81–88 (3 Pl.). Reproduced in *Studies from the Rockefeller Institute for Medical Research,* 53, pp. 555–562 (3 Pl.).

265. SMITH, T. and ORCUTT, M.L. The bacteriology of the intestinal tract of young calves with special reference to the early diarrhea ("scours"). *Journal of Experimental Medicine,* 41 (January), pp. 89–106 (1 Pl.). Reproduced in *Studies from the Rockefeller Institute for Medical Research,* 53, pp. 563–580 (1 Pl.).

266. Focal interstitial nephritis in the calf following interference with the normal intake of colostrum. *Journal of Experimental Medicine,* 41 (March), pp. 413–425 (3 Pl.). Reproduced in *Studies from the Rockefeller Institute for Medical Research,* 54, pp. 567–579 (3 Pl.).

267. The significance of colostrum in the prevention of the diseases of young calves. *Cornell Veterinarian,* 15 (April), pp. 173–180. Presented at the seventeenth Annual Conference for Veterinarians, New York State Veterinary College, Cornell University, Ithaca, N.Y., January 15, 1925.

268. Pneumonia associated with Bacillus abortus (Bang) in fetuses and new-born calves. *Journal of Experimental Medicine,* 41 (May), pp. 639–647 (2 Pl.). Reproduced in *Studies from the Rockefeller Institute for Medical Research,* 54, pp. 581–589 (2 Pl.).

1926

269. The relation of Bacillus abortus from bovine sources to Malta fever. *Journal of Experimental Medicine,* 43 (February), pp. 207–223. Reproduced in *Studies from the Rockefeller Institute for Medical Research,* 57, pp. 501–517.

270. Variations in CO_2 requirements among bovine strains of Bacillus abortus. *Journal of Experimental Medicine,* 43 (March), pp. 317–325. Reproduced in *Studies from the Rockefeller Institute for Medical Research,* 57, pp. 539–547.

271. SMITH, T. and LITTLE, R.B. Further data on the effect of vaccination against bovine infectious abortion. *Journal of Experimental Medicine,* 43 (March), pp. 327–330. Reproduced in *Studies from the Rockefeller Institute for Medical Research,* 57, pp. 549–552.

272. The problem of natural and acquired resistance to tuberculosis. *American Review of Tuberculosis,* 14 (November), pp. 485–495. President's address at the twenty-second Annual Meeting, National Tuberculosis Association, Washington, D.C., October 4, 1926.

273. Remarks on the cooperation of science and practice in tuberculosis. *American Review of Tuberculosis,* 14 (December), pp. 597–599. President's address at the opening of the fifth Conference, International Union Against Tuberculosis, Washington, D.C., September 30, 1926.

1927

274. SMITH, T. and TIBBETTS, H.A.M. The relation between invasion of the digestive tract by paratyphoid bacilli and disease. *Journal of Experimental Medicine,* 45 (February), pp. 337–352. Reproduced in *Studies from the Rockefeller Institute for Medical Research,* 61, pp. 535–550.

275. NELSON, J.B. and SMITH, T. Studies on a paratyphoid infection in guinea pigs. I. Report of a natural outbreak of paratyphoid in a guinea pig population. *Journal of Experimental Medicine*, 45 (February), pp. 353–363. Reproduced in *Studies from the Rockefeller Institute for Medical Research*, 61, pp. 551–561.

276. SMITH, T. and NELSON, J.B. Studies on a paratyphoid infection in guinea pigs. II. Factors involved in the transition from epidemic to endemic phase. *Journal of Experimental Medicine*, 45 (February), pp. 365–377. Reproduced in *Studies from the Rockefeller Institute for Medical Research*, 61, pp. 563–575.

277. SMITH, T. and ORCUTT, M.L. Vibrios from calves and their serological relation to Vibrio fetus. *Journal of Experimental Medicine*, 45 (February), pp. 391–397. Reproduced in *Studies from the Rockefeller Institute for Medical Research*, 61, pp. 589–595.

278. The passing of disease from one generation to another and the processes tending to counteract it. *International Clinics*, 3, Ser. 37, pp. 1–15. Reproduced in *Studies from the Rockefeller Institute for Medical Research*, 65 (1928), pp. 537–551. The Annual Samuel D. Gross Lecture, delivered before the Pathological Society of Philadelphia, April 21, 1927.

279. SMITH, T. and RING, E.R. The segregation of lambs at birth and the feeding of cow's milk in the elimination of parasites. *Journal of Parasitology*, 13 (June), pp. 260–269. Reproduced in *Studies from the Rockefeller Institute for Medical Research*, 64 (1928), pp. 579–590.

280. SMITH, T. and LITTLE, R.B. Studies on pathogenic B. coli from bovine sources. I. The pathogenic action of culture filtrates. *Journal of Experimental Medicine*, 46 (July), pp. 123–131. Reproduced in *Studies from the Rockefeller Institute for Medical Research*, 63 (1928), pp. 527–535.

281. SMITH, T. and BRYANT, G. Studies on pathogenic B. coli from bovine sources. II. Mutations and their immunological significance. *Journal of Experimental Medicine*, 46 (July), pp. 133–140 (2 Pl.). Reproduced in *Studies from* the Rockefeller Institute for Medical Research, 63 (1928), pp. 537–544 (2 Pl.).

282. Studies on pathogenic B. coli from bovine sources. III. Normal and serologically induced resistance to B. coli and its mutant. *Journal of Experimental Medicine*, 46 (July), pp. 141–154. Reproduced in *Studies from the Rockefeller Institute for Medical Research*, 63 (1928), pp. 545–558.

283. Public health progress and race progress—are they incompatible? *Transactions of the Twenty-third Annual Meeting of the National Tuberculosis Association*, pp. 135–139. Discussion, following paper on this topic by H.S. Jennings (pp. 125–135), Indianapolis, Ind., May 24, 1927.

1928

284. Animal reservoirs of human disease with special reference to microbic variability. *Bulletin of the New York Academy of Medicine*, 2nd ser., 4, pp. 476–496. Delivered before the New York Academy of Medicine, New York, N.Y., February 16, 1928.

285. The relation of the capsular substance of B. coli to anitbody production. *Journal of Experimental Medicine*, 48 (September), pp. 351–361. Reproduced in *Studies from the Rockefeller Institute for Medical Research*, 67 (1929), pp. 621–631.

286. The decline of infectious diseases in its relation to modern medicine. *Journal of Preventive Medicine*, 2 (September), pp. 345–363; *Transactions of the Congress of American Physicians and Surgeons*, 14 (1929), pp. 1–18. Reproduced in *Studies from the Rockefeller Institute for Medical Research*, 68 (1929), pp. 593–611; and also, somewhat abridged, in *Canadian Med-*

ical *Association Journal,* 19 (September), pp. 283–287. Presidential Address, fourteenth Triennial Session, Congress of American Physicians and Surgeons, Washington, D.C., May 1, 1928.

1929

287. Hideyo Noguchi. 1876–1928. *Bulletin of the New York Academy of Medicine,* 2nd ser., 5, pp. 877–886.

288. A strain of Bacillus abortus from swine. *Journal of Experimental Medicine,* 49 (April), pp. 671–679. Reproduced in *Studies from the Rockefeller Institute for Medical Research,* 70 (1930), pp. 615–623.

289. Undulant fever. Its relation to new problems in bacteriology and public health. *Medicine,* 8 (May), pp. 193–209. Reproduced in *Studies from the Rockefeller Institute for Medical Research,* 71 (1930), pp. 579–595. De Lamar lecture delivered before the Johns Hopkins University School of Hygiene, Baltimore, Maryland, October 30, 1928.

290. Undulant fever. *Health News,* 6 (August), pp. 121–122. (Abstract); *Bulletin of the Dairy Research Division of Mathews Industries Inc.,* 8 (September), pp. 113–114. (Abstract). Abstracts of address given before the Annual State Health Conference, Saratoga Springs, N.Y., June 24, 1929. Date confirmed by T.S. Diary; erroneously published as given on June 25.

291. The influence of research in bringing into closer relationship the practice of medicine and public health activities. *American Journal of the Medical Sciences,* 178 (December), pp. 741–747. Reproduced in booklet of three lectures by J.A. Miller, L.R. Williams, and T. Smith, respectively, under the general heading *Public Health and the Practising Physician.* New York, N.Y., Milbank Memorial Fund, pp. 17–27. Presented at the seventh Annual Meeting, Boards of Counsel of the Milbank Memorial Fund, New York, N.Y., March 13, 1929.

292. The clinical and pathological significance of races and varieties among pathogenic bacteria. New York State Association of Public Health Laboratories. *Proceedings,* 9 (No. 2), pp. 15–18. Abstract of paper presented at mid-year meeting, New York State Association of Public Health Laboratories, Albany, N.Y., November 8, 1929.

1930

293. The immunological significance of colostrum. I. The relation between colostrum, serum, and the milk of cows normal and immunized towards B. coli. *Journal of Experimental Medicine,* 51 (March), pp. 473–481. Reproduced in *Studies from the Rockefeller Institute for Medical Research,* 74 (1931), pp. 495–503.

294. SMITH, T. and LITTLE, R.B. The immunological significance of colostrum. II. The initial feeding of serum from normal cows and cows immunized towards B. coli in place of colostrum. *Journal of Experimental Medicine,* 51 (March), pp. 483–492. Reproduced in *Studies from the Rockefeller Institute for Medical Research,* 74 (1931), pp. 505–514.

295. The immunological significance of colostrum. III. Intranuclear bodies in renal disease of calves. *Journal of Experimental Medicine,* 51 (April), pp. 519–529 (2 Pl.). Reproduced in *Studies from the Rockefeller Institute for Medical Research,* 74 (1931), pp. 515–525 (2 Pl.).

296. Foreword to Wade W. Oliver's *Stalkers of Pestilence. The Story of Man's Ideas of Infection.* New York, N.Y., Paul B. Hoeber, pp. xi-xv.

297. Remarks made by Dr. Thoebald Smith. At a dinner in honor of Dr. William H. Welch, commemorating his eightieth birthday. *Bulletin of the New York Academy of Medicine,* 6, pp. 474–477. (Based on an inaccurate stenographic record of the speech, uncorrected by

T.S.). Revised version published in *William Welch at Eighty.* New York, N.Y., Milbank Memorial Fund, pp. 46–48. Speech at New York Academy of Medicine Dinner, New York, N.Y., April 4, 1930.

298. The Department of Animal Pathology of the Rockefeller Institute, Princeton, N.J. In L. Brauer, A. Mendelssohn Bartholdy and A. Meyer, *Forschungsinstitute, ihre Geschichte, Organisation und Ziele.* Hamburg. pp. 45–48.

299. Disease a biological problem. *Bulletin of the Harvard Medical Alumni Association,* 5 (June), pp. 2–6. Address to Harvard Medical Alumni Association, Boston, Mass., April 17, 1931.

300. The agglutinating action of agar on bacteria. *Science,* 74 (July 3, 1931), p. 21.

301. The general problem of respiratory diseases as illumined by comparative data. *International Clinics,* 3 Ser., 41, pp. 254–275. Reproduced in *Studies from the Rockefeller Institute for Medical Research,* 81 (1932), pp. 513–534 (1 Pl.). Smith's first William Henry Welch Lecture, delivered at Mount Sinai Hospital, New York, N.Y., October 17, 1930.

302. Spontaneous and induced streptococcus disease in guinea-pig: an epidemiologic study. *International Clinics,* 3, Ser., 41, pp. 276–297. Reproduced in *Studies from the Rockefeller Institute for Medical Research,* 81 (1932), pp. 535–556 (2 Pl.). Smith's second William Henry Welch Lecture, delivered at Mount Sinai Hospital, New York, N.Y., October 18, 1930.

1932

303. Koch's views on the stability of species among bacteria. *Annals of Medical History,* (n.s.) 4 (November), pp. 524–530. Read before the Historical Section, College of Physicians of Philadelphia, March 14, 1932, to commemorate the fiftieth anniversary of the discovery of the tubercle bacillus.

304. The inter-relation of strains of Brucella. *Veterinary Medicine,* 28 (March), pp. 98–99; *Proceedings of the Third Annual Eastern States Conference on Bang's Disease,* 1932, pp. 38–40. Presented at the third Annual Eastern States Conference on Bang's Disease, Trenton, N.J., November 9, 1931.

305. Focal cell reactions in tuberculosis and allied diseases. Part I. The epithelioid cell reactions. Part II. The succession of cell reactions. *Bulletin of the Johns Hopkins Hospital,* 53 (October), pp. 197–213, 213–225. Reproduced in *Studies from the Rockefeller Institute for Medical Research,* 88 (1934), pp. 461–477, 477–489. The William Sidney Thayer and Susan Read Thayer Lectures for 1933, Baltimore, Maryland, April 5 and 6, 1933.

1934

306. Letter to Dr. E.B. Krumbhaar. (October 11, 1933). *Journal of Bacteriology,* 27 (January), pp. 19–20. (In response to a request from Dr. Krumbhaar to elaborate on "certain attitudes which had guided his research . . . for the inspiration and guidance of the students of the University of Pennsylvania.") A fascimile copy was distributed to everyone who attended the thirty-fifth Annual Meeting, Society of American Bacteriologists, Philadelphia, Pennsylvania, December 27–29, 1933.

307. *Parasitism and Disease.* Princeton, N.J., Princeton University Press, 196 pp. Reprinted, New York, Hafner Publishing Co., 1963. Based on five Vanuxem Lectures, delivered at Princeton, N.J., March 7, 9, 14, 16 and 21, 1933.

308. Presidential address to the Society of American Bacteriologists, 1903. *ASM News,* 47 (June), pp. 233–235.

NOTES

Although Dr. Dolman did an outstanding job of researching and compiling the foregoing work, the co-author discovered, after agreeing to complete his manuscript and bring it to publishable form, that it contained two impediments that could not be corrected or eliminated. The first was Dr. Dolman's failure to identify many of the sources listed in the Notes with the specific institution, library or archival collection in which they were found; the second related to a handful of cases in which he left references undated or incomplete (Notes 21 and 32 of Chapter 12, and Notes 38, 39, and 40 of Chapter 24.) Because many of the original source materials still remained in the hands of Theobald Smith's descendants in scattered locations, while the documentation that Dr. Dolman had collected in original or photocopy form had been stored away in a great many cartons in an inaccessible location following his death, it was impossible to remedy most of these problems—a situation that would frustrate interested readers and researchers when attempting to find the original sources for checking or for carrying on further research.

In order to remedy these impediments and go on with publication, it was decided by all parties concerned to gather together all of the sources employed in the making of this work and to deposit them permanently in a single location where they could readily be found and utilized by future researchers and medical historians. Because the Boston Medical Library authorities had agreed to sponsor this work, and because that institution holds one of the country's outstanding collections of medically-related manuscripts and has a deep commitment to medical history as well, it was chosen to be the repository of the Theobald Smith Papers. Arrangements are now being worked out to collect all of the manuscript records cited in the Notes and other pertinent materials and deposit them in that institution, where they can be sought out and referred to in the future in the pursuance of the aims and objectives of scholarship and medical historical resarch.

Richard J. Wolfe

Chapter 1:
1. From the opening paragraph of an autobiographical sketch prepared by Theobald Smith for John D. Rockefeller, Jr., in anticipation of the dinner in his honor at the opening of the Theobald Smith House at the Princeton Department of Animal Pathology, Rockefeller Institute for Medical Research, on November 20, 1931.
2. The marriage certificate of Philipp Schmitt and Theresia Kexel has been preserved in the Smith Papers.

3. Theobald Smith, Autobiographical letter written June 17–21, 1886 to Lilian Egleston, his future wife, in response to her question, "Who are you?"

4. In May 1968, the author inspected the baptismal certificates in the Parish Records of the Church of the Holy Cross, at 12 Rosemont Street, Albany, by courtesy of the Rev. Edward W. Durkin.

5. Theobald Smith, Diary, 1875.

6. Theobald Smith, Autobiographical letter to Lilian Egleston, June 17–21, 1886.

7. Ibid.

8. Ibid.

9. The Teutoburger Wald, a densely wooded mountain range in northwest Germany, was the setting for fierce warfare between early German tribes and their Roman overlords. In A.D. 9, the heavily-laden troops of Varus, the Governor, were decoyed into the Teutoburger Wald, and three legions virtually annihilated, thus preventing the Romanization of Germany between the Rhine and Elbe.

10. Theobald Smith, Autobiographical letter to Lilian Egleston, June 17–21, 1886.

11. When inspected by the author in 1968, the dilapidated property was in a deteriorating rooming-house neighborhood. The sights and sounds of demolition were creeping up the street from the direction of the Hudson waterfront.

12. Theobald Smith, Diary, July 11, 1876.

13. Theobald Smith, Diary, November 13, 1876.

14. Theobald Smith, Autobiographical letter to Lilian Egleston, June 17–21, 1886.

15. Theobald's diary is sprinkled with monetary references. "Income $0.05 (apparently a monthly allowance) is an early entry. Bonuses for special effort included 5 cents for taking a vest to a customer, or 6 cents for carrying off ashes. Private enterprise brought in sporadic earnings—2 cents won from his cousins at dominos; tips for clothes delivery ranged to 35 cents; six quarts of home-grown "wall-nuts" sold for 30 cents. When he mislaid 50 cents, consternation followed. His investment in a 60-cent shovel was ultimately recouped by coaling contracts with neighbors, despite its failure to yield a five percent return in the absence of snow: "No snow. My shovel alas! stands dormant on the backstairs not making interest, for $.60 x .005 ? $.03, which is not yet earned." (Diary, January 3, 1876). Even Christmas presents from his parents were priced meticulously: "Received toothbrush. 25, cuffs, $.40" was the entry for December 25, 1875.

16. Theobald Smith, Diary, September 18, 1876.

17. This medallion has been preserved. It is inscribed: "Annual Exhibit 1872. Albany Public Schools. Best in penmanship. Theobald J. Smith."

18. Theobald Smith, Autobiographical letter to Lilian Egleston, June 17–21, 1886.

19. In 1833, the Mohawk and Hudson Railroad Company erected a hotel and stable on State Street, whence passengers were conveyed by horse-drawn stage coaches over the State Street Branch to Madison Avenue, to board the steam train for Schenectady. Steam-powered vehicles could not surmount the grade between Eagle and Swan Streets. When Albany's railroad station was built near the waterfront in 1841, the first terminus was abandoned, becoming known as Van Vechten Hall. The Old State Street trackage appears on a map (ca. 1836) in the New York Public Library. See also Horace Porter, *Railway Passenger Travel* (New York, Scribner's, 1888).

20. Theobald Smith, Diary, September 18, 1876.

21. *Report on the Free Academy and Public Schools of the City of Albany* (Albany, 1872). Another

pamphlet, headed *Rejoinder of the Mayor* (Albany, 1873), which contains Thacher's "Protest Against the Last City Tax Budget," and a review of the Mayor's message by the three-man Committee on Academics and Schools, summarizes the opposing contentions.

22. J.E. Bradley, "Response" to "Address of Welcome" by Principal O.D. Robinson, in *General Catalog of Albany High School, and Account of the Celebration of the Twenty-Fifth Anniversary* (Albany, 1894).

23. Theobald Smith, Diary, April 18, 1876.

24. Theobald Smith, Diary, June 25, 1875.

25. Theobald Smith, Diary, May 17, 1875.

26. Theobald Smith, Diary, November 10, 1874.

27. Probably the 1870 reprinted edition of *Deutsche Grammatik* (1819), by Jacob Grimm (1785–1863), the great German philologist and mythologist. He and his younger brother Wilhelm together wrote *Kinder- und Hausmarchen* (1812–1815), which became widely known in the English-speaking world as *Grimm's Fairy Tales*.

28. T.J. Smith, "Visit to a Castle." This account occupied six small pages of lined notepaper. He later inscribed on its title-page, "Visited in 1869 near Limburg a/d Lahn." Theobald Smith, Scrapbook No. 1.

29. T.J. Smith, "A Journey to Mars." Theobald Smith, Scrapbook No. 1.

30. Theobald Smith, Diary, January 3, 1876.

31. Theobald Smith, Diary, January 17, 1877.
    The famed microbiologist Élie Metchnikoff is reputed to have been influenced greatly by Buckle's *History of Civilization in England*.

32. Theobald Smith, Autobiographical letter to Lilian Egleston, June 17–21, 1886.

33. Theobald Smith, Diary, December 2, 1875.

34. Theobald Smith, Diary, December 5, 1876.

35. Theobald Smith, Diary, September 22, 1876.

36. Theobald Smith, Diary, December 21, 1875. One such tribute, to John van Gassbeckgis, is in Smith's Scrapbook No. 1.

37. Theobald Smith, Diary, June 29, 1876.

38. A major event of the Albany High School year was the joint debate held annually in the chapel on the first Friday in February, in the presence of the Philodoxian and Philologian Societies, the assembled school, alumni, and friends. (See J.H. Strenge, "The 'Logian-Doxia' Joint Debates," in *Philologiensis*, 1901, pp. 34–36.) Prior to "Logian-Doxia" 1896, according to Strenge, "various other forms of literary work were provided for the entertainment of the audience." The debate reported by Theobald Smith in 1877 apparently initiated the custom.

39. Theobald Smith to John L. Sturtevant, February 22, 1915.

40. Theobald Smith, Diary, May 13, 1875.

41. The third edition of Tyndall's *Sound* (1875) refers to the fog-signalling investigations of Smith's fellow-Albanian, Joseph Henry, America's most famous early physicist, who discovered the principle of electrical induction. Henry died in 1878. He is commemorated by a bronze statue in the Park before the historic building of the Albany Academy (for boys), where he became professor of mathematics and physics in 1826. The Academy, designed by Philip Hooker in 1817, now houses the Administrative Office of the Albany Department of Education.

42. Theobald Smith, Diary, June 20, 1876.

43. Theobald Smith, Diary, June 25, 1876.
44. Fitzhugh, "Flag of Our Heroes."
45. T.S. Smith, "Valedictory Address, Albany High School," June 30, 1876, Theobald Smith, Scrapbook No. 1.
46. Theobald Smith, Diary, June 30, 1876. Bradley's engraved invitation to the evening reception is in Scrapbook No. 1. He left the High School in 1886, becoming superintendent of schools in Minneapolis. From 1896 to 1900 he was president of Illinois College. He died in 1912. Oscar Robinson, who succeeded him as principal of Albany High School in 1896, died in 1911. See C.W. Blessing, *Albany Schools and Colleges Yesterday and Today* (Albany, 1936).
47. Theobald Smith, Autobiographical letter to Lilian Egleston, June 17–21, 1886.
48. Ibid.
49. Theobald Smith, Diary, May 22, 1875.
50. Theobald Smith, Diary, May 29, 1875.
51. Theobald Smith, Diary, October 11, 1876.
52. Theobald Smith, Diary, August 25, 1876.
53. Ibid.
54. Theobald Smith, Diary, August 10, 1876.
55. Theobald Smith, Autobiographical letter to Lilian Egleston, June 17–21, 1886.
56. Theobald Smith, Diary, January 17, 1875.
57. Theobald Smith, Diary, July 29, 1875.
58. Theobald Smith, Diary, February 7, 1877.
59. Theobald Smith, Diary, April 18, 1877.
60. Theobald Smith, Diary, December 20, 1876.
61. Theobald Smith, Diary, March 31, 1878.
62. Theobald Smith, Diary, November 7, 1876.
63. Theobald Smith, Diary, September 10, 1876.
64. Theobald Smith, Diary, November 26, 1876 (in French).
65. Theobald Smith, Diary, March 17, 1876.
66. Theobald Smith, Diary, May 17, 1877.
67. Theobald Smith, Diary, June 4, 1877.
68. Theobald Smith, Autobiographical letter to Lilian Egleston, June 17–21, 1886.
69. Theobald Smith, Diary, January 19, 1877.
70. Theobald Smith, Diary, March 18, 1877.
71. Theobald Smith, Diary, May 21, 1877.
72. Theobald Smith, Diary, June 16, 1877.
73. Theobald Smith, Diary, June 20, 1877.
74. Theobald Smith, Diary, August 16, 1877.
75. John O. Cole to "Mr. Theobald Smith," September 6, 1877. "Squire Cole" was the father of Charles W. Cole, Professor of English Literature and History at Albany High School.
76. Theobald Smith, Diary, September 16 and 17, 1877 (in German).

Chapter 2:
1. Morris Bishop's sprightly *A History of Cornell* (Ithaca, Cornell University Press, 1962) has furnished much data and many quoted phrases on the early days of Cornell University. A.H. Wright's *Pre-Cornell and Early Cornell V* (Ithaca, 1954, Studies in History No. 19),

and C.V.P. Young's *Cornell in Pictures: 1868–1954* (Ithaca, Cornell University Press, 1954) have also been helpful. The quote from President White's "Plan of Organization for Cornell University," presented to the Board of Trustees, October 21, 1866, is from Bishop's *A History of Cornell,* p. 76.

2. Jennie McGraw, heir to her father's estate, approaching forty and afflicted with advanced tuberculosis, in 1877 married Daniel Willard Fiske, the University Librarian, and died four years later. She willed $300,000 to her husband, half a million to her relatives, and the bulk of the residual estate to Cornell University. Fiske challenged the will and was awarded half a million dollars, collateral relatives receiving one million. At his death, he left his fortune and library to Cornell University.

3. Theobald Smith, Diary, June 20, 1877.

4. Morris Bishop, *A History of Cornell,* p. 75.

5. Cornell University, *Course Book, 1877–78,* of which a copy is in Theobald Smith's Scrapbook No. 1.

6. This brilliantly versatile teacher, a graduate of Harvard Medical School, served professionally in the Civil War, and developed a great interest in hygiene. His broader interests in various aspects of biology did not displace the physician's compassion. When John Henry Comstock, his assistant and protégé, contracted typhoid fever, Wilder devotedly nursed him in his own study (Morris Bishop, *A History of Cornell,* p. 176).

7. Actually, diseases due to faulty sanitation were prevalent on the campus and also in Ithaca. According to Bishop (p. 202), six undergraduates died in 1875–77, and five in 1877–78, of a student body totalling about 500. In 1903, a water-borne typhoid epidemic in Ithaca affected 681 persons, with fifty-one deaths. Of this total, 131 were students, of whom thirteen died (Bishop, pp. 421–422).

8. Theobald Smith, "Presentation Address," *Wilder Quarter-Century Book, 1868–1893* (Ithaca, Comstock Publishing Co., 1893); *Cornell Era,* and *Ithaca Daily Journal,* October 9, 1893.

9. Theobald Smith, Diary, October 3, 1877.

10. Theobald Smith, Autobiographical letter to Lilian Egleston, June 17–21, 1886.

11. Theobald Smith, Diary, February 26, 1878.

12. Theobald Smith, Diary, May 21, 1878.

13. Theobald Smith, Diary, December 21, 1877.

14. Theobald Smith, Diary, February 22, 1878.

15. Simon H. Gage to Marion E. Black, October 26, 1932, Simon Henry Gage Papers, Cornell University Archives.

16. Theobald Smith, Diary, October 30, 1878. James Abram Garfield (1831–1881) was born in poverty on a farm in Ohio. In early years an evangelist and teacher, his political appeal as Republican senator was enhanced by a distinguished record in the Civil War. After a long and uncertain campaign, he won the 1880 presidential election by a narrow margin over the Democratic candidate, General Winfield S. Hancock. Within a few months of his inauguration as twenty-first President of the United States, Garfield was shot by a disaffected Republican, and died in September 1881, after two months of medical bungling.

17. Taughannock Falls are now part of an 825-acre State Park in a mile-long glen.

18. Theobald Smith, Diary, May 13, 1878. The quaint scene was similar "in thousands of small towns across the U.S. The day opened typically with a parade led by a brass band

and the volunteer firemen hand- pulling their pumping engine. Following them were the Mexican war veterans . . . and finally, splendid in their visored caps and coats, the Civil War veterans. At midday came the patriotic speeches" (From "America, 1870–1900," in *This Fabulous Century, Prelude, 1870–1900* (New York, Time-Life books, 1970), vol. 1, p. 56).

19. Theobald Smith, Diary, March 8, 1878.

20. Theobald Smith, Diary, March 13, 1878. Molière's *Le Misanthrope* depicts the conflict between the high-minded Alceste, exasperated by society's corruption, and his beloved coquette, Celimène.

21. In 1871, Ezra Cornell linked Cortland with Ithaca by a railroad that terminated in the present Engineering Quadrangle. The locomotive, named "Cornell University," had a view of the campus painted on her tender. The line was extended southward to Elmira, and acquired a right of way north of Cortland on the Delaware, Lackawanna and Western Railroad (Morris Bishop *A History of Cornell,* pp. 94, 185).

22. Theobald Smith, Diary, April 12, 1878.

23. Theobald Smith, Diary, June 27, 1878.

24. Theobald Smith, Diary, July 29, 1878.

25. Theobald Smith, Diary, September 11, 1878.

26. Theobald Smith, Diary, July 18, 1878. The Cornell Yell apparently originated in exultant imitation of Yale's famous song "Eli-Eli-Eli-U," when Cornell won both varsity and freshman rowing races in the 1875 Saratoga regatta. After a similar victory by Cornell in 1876, according to Bishop (pp. 135–136, 207), "Yale withdrew from the Rowing Association of American Colleges . . . The next year Harvard withdrew, and the Association collapsed." Nevertheless, the freshman eight-oared race with Harvard occurred in 1878.

27. Theobald Smith, Diary, July 13, 1878.

28. Theobald Smith, Diary, August 13, 1878.

29. Cornell University, *Course Book, 1878–79,* of which a copy is in Theobald Smith's Scrapbook No. 1.

30. Theobald Smith, Diary, October 2, 1878.

31. Theobald Smith, Diary, November 13, 1878.

32. Theobald Smith, "List of Plants Studied at Cornell University, Spring Term, 1878," Theobald Smith, Scrapbook No. 1.

33. Theobald Smith, Diary, January 10, 1879.

34. Theobald Smith, Bibliography No. 226.

35. Theobald Smith, Diary, November 13, 1878.

36. Theobald Smith, Diary, January 8, 1879.

37. Theobald Smith, Diary, February 9, 1879 (in German).

38. Theobald Smith, Diary, April 10, 1879.

39. Theobald Smith, Diary, April 5, 1878.

40. Cornell University, "Statistics of the Class of 1881," Theobald Smith, Scrapbook No. 1.

41. Theobald Smith, Diary, June 9, 1879.

42. Theobald Smith, Diary, February 23, 1879.

43. Anna Basford Comstock, *The Comstocks of Cornell* (Ithaca, 1953).

44. Theobald Smith, Diary, February 8, 1879. Alfreda Bosworth Withington graduated A.B., then studied at the Women's Medical College of the New York Infirmary, from which she obtained her M.D. in 1887. A pioneer woman doctor in many fields, she es-

poused general practice, rejecting offered Chairs of Physiology at Vassar and Smith Colleges. Dr. Withington worked for several years at Pittsfield, Mass. and later in the Kentucky hills, and spent a summer at Labrador with Wilfred Grenfell's Mission. She visited Theobald Smith more than once in Washington and Boston. Dr. Withington died in 1951, after a brief illness, aged ninety-one. In her eightieth year, she wrote an autobiography, *Mine Eyes Have Seen. A Woman Doctor's Saga* (New York, E.P. Dutton & Co., Inc., 1941). The first chapter, describing her undergraduate days at Cornell, refers to afternoons when "a few of us would be asked to hear our classmates, Theobald Smith . . . or Hermann Biggs . . . play Bach on the organ then pumped by hand from below" (p. 24). In her Acknowledgments (p. 11), Dr. Withington thanks Isabel Howland "for an interchange of memories of college life." Miss Howland graduated B.S. in Science. This charming-looking girl became involved in education and the current reform movements (See *Cornell University, Quarter Century Book,* Class of '81).

45. The competition for a $100 prize established in 1870 by Stewart L. Woodford, a former Trustee and Lieutenant-Governor of the State, was one of the best-attended public events of the University year. Theobald was a candidate for the Prize two years later. Chosen from numerous nightly speakers, six finalists competed for the Prize in the Library Hall.

46. Theobald Smith, Diary, March 5, 1879.

47. Llena di Murska was noted for her high F in the Queen of the Night's Aria in Mozart's *The Magic Flute*. See Herman Klein, *Great Women Singers of My Time* (London, 1931).

48. Theobald Smith, Diary, June 3, 1879.

49. Theobald Smith, Diary, December 28, 1878.

50. Theobald Smith, Diary, June 21, 1879.

51. Theobald Smith, Diary, April 5 and 22, 1880. Retrospective notes since late summer 1879.

52. The Helderbergs formed a striking topographic feature of central-eastern New York State. These scenic "mountains" (average elevation about 1,000 feet) rise abruptly from the plain about fourteen miles to the southwest of Albany, showing massive limestone cliffs—hence the name (Dutch *helder,* bright or light; *berg,* mountain). Just beyond them lie the Catskills. See Winifred Goldring, "Geology of the Berne Quadrangle," *New York State Museum Bulletin,* No. 303 (Albany, 1935). Although the Helderbergs were often referred to in his diary, Theobald had not visited them previously.

53. Theobald Smith, Diary, July 31, 1879.

54. Theobald Smith, Diary, April 5 and 22, 1880.

55. Theobald Smith, Autobiographical letter to Lilian Egleston, June 17–21, 1886.

56. Theobald Smith, Diary, May 17, 1880.

57. Theobald Smith, Diary, April 5 and 22, 1880.

58. Several years later in his 1886 autobiographical letter to his future bride, Theobald wrote: "It required a great force to overcome my constitutional dislike for everything connected with medicine. I remember well my first dissection of a cat. My cheeks burned with excitement. I disliked to touch the animal. And now I can . . . make an autopsy of a pig . . . easily and cheerfully . . . yet such changes do not dull our sensibilities . . . I feel just as outraged now at the sight of any cruel act to animals as I did, when a boy of eight, I wept over the death of a pet kitten."

59. Wilder's certificate of attestation is preserved in Smith's Scrapbook No. 1.

60. In 1873, Prof. Wilder got wind of an abandoned circus camel, with injured legs, on show at a nearby picnic ground. He dispatched a dray with driver, as well as Gage and another student, to capture the beast for the museum. After the owner surrendered all rights to the camel for about $20, it was captured by Gage and his associates. The camel was lassoed and its head tied to a tree; a hat soaked in chloroform was held ruthlessly over its muzzle; and eventually the corpse was loaded upon the dray for a slow march to Ithaca. See S.H. Gage, "The University Camel," *Cornell Era,* 40 (1907): 88–90.

61. Theobald Smith, Diary, April 5 and 22, 1880.

62. Hailes performed more than 1,600 intubations for laryngeal diphtheria. In 1880, he became Professor of Histology and Pathological Anatomy at his alma mater. Skilled in microscopy and microphotography, he devised a freezing microtome. After building a fine country home on the banks of the Hudson at Van Wie's Point, he suffered a severe stroke which abruptly ended his professional career in 1901, though he survived until 1912. His brother, C.J. Hailes, wrote a tribute: "In Memoriam. Dr. William Hailes," *Albany Medical Annals* 33 (1912): 505–513.

63. Theobald Smith, Diary, July 11, 1880.

64. Theobald Smith, Diary, August 29, 1880.

65. Theobald Smith, Diary, September 11, 1878.

66. Theobald Smith, Diary, August 3, 1880, and March 1, 1878.

67. Theobald Smith, Diary, August 14, 1880. The diary recorded the visit. Gage's widow (his second wife) related to the author her late husband's recollection of this occasion.

68. Theobald Smith, Diary, September 12, 1880 (mainly in German).

69. Cornell University, *Course Book, 1880–81,* in Theobald Smith, Scrapbook No. 1.

70. Theobald Smith, Diary, February 17, 1882. Retrospective notes, September 1880 to May 1881 (original entries partly in German).

71. Theobald Smith, Scrapbook No. 1.

72. Theobald Smith, Diary, February 17, 1882.

73. Theobald Smith, Autobiographical letter to Lilian Egleston, June 17–21, 1886.

74. Simon H. Gage to Marion E. Black, October 26, 1932.

75. R.H. Bainton, *George Lincoln Burr, His Life* (Ithaca, Cornell University Press, 1943), pp. 22–23.

76. Theobald Smith, Bibliography No. 1.

77. Burr became secretary to President White, and was the unofficial co-author of White's *The Warfare of Science with Theology* (1896), dedicated to Ezra Cornell. Later, as professor of ancient and medieval history, his "enormous erudition humbled his colleagues and terrified his students" (Morris Bishop, *A History of Cornell,* p. 288). Burr held Theobald Smith in high respect.

78. Theobald Smith, Diary, February 17, 1882.

79. Theobald Smith, Bibliography No. 2.

80. Theobald Smith, Diary, November 8, 1880.

81. Theobald Smith, Diary, January 16, 1881.

82. Theobald Smith, Diary, March 5, 1881.

83. Theobald Smith, Diary, February 17, 1882.

84. Ibid.

85. Theobald Smith, Scrapbook No. 1.

86. Ibid.

87. Morris Bishop, *A History of Cornell,* p. 206.

88. Theobald Smith, Diary, February 17, 1882.

89. Ibid.

90. Theobald Smith, Autobiographical letter to Lilian Egleston, June 17–21, 1886.

Chapter 3:

1. Theobald Smith, Diary, April 23, 1882. Retrospective notes, June and July 1881.

2. Abraham Flexner, *Medical Education in the United States and Canada. A Report to the Carnegie Foundation for the Advancement of Teaching* (New York, 1910, Bulletin No. 4), p. 6; reprint edition, New York, Arno Press, 1972.

3. In his autobiography, *I Remember* (New York, Simon & Schuster, 1940), pp. 120–121, Abraham Flexner outlined his system for rapidly appraising "the quality and value of a medical school:"

    In half an hour or less I could sample the credentials of students filed in the dean's office, ascertain the matriculation requirements . . . and determine whether or not the standards, low or high, set forth in the school catalogue were being eroded or enforced. A few inquiries made clear whether the faculty was composed of local doctors . . . A single question elicited the amount of income of a medical school . . . A stroll through the laboratories disclosed the presence or absence of apparatus, museum specimens, library, and students; and a "*whiff*" told the inside story regarding the manner in which anatomy was cultivated. Finally, the situation as respects clinical facilities was readily clarified by a few questions, directed in succession— and separately—to the dean of the school, the professors of medicine, surgery, and obstetrics, and the hospital superintendent.

4. J.J. Walsh, *History of Medicine in New York. Three Centuries of Medical Progress* (New York, National Americana Society, 1919), v. 2, pp. 643–649.

5. M.J. Lewi, "Presidential Address to Albany Medical Alumni," *Albany Medical Annals* 37 (1916): 396–402.

6. E.S. Van Olinda, "Tattle Tales of Old Albany," *The Times-Union,* Albany, September 16, 1945.

7. Theobald Smith, Autobiographical sketch prepared for John D. Rockefeller, Jr., in anticipation of dinner . . . November 20, 1931.

8. Theobald Smith, Diary, May 26, 1882. Retrospective notes, August 1881 to March 1882.

9. Theobald Smith, Diary, July 5, 1882. Retrospective notes, March 28 to July 5, 1882.

10. Ibid.

11. Ibid.

12. Gilman was selected by a three-man committee, which included Andrew D. White and Charles W. Eliot, presidents of Cornell and Harvard Universities, respectively. Some newspapers decried his inviting the atheistic Huxley to deliver the inaugural address at the official opening of Johns Hopkins University. The "well-known Donaldson" was Henry Herbert Donaldson (1857–1936), whose name may have been familiar to Smith through Prof. Wilder. Donaldson became distinguished as a neurologist and later visited Theobald Smith in Boston.

13. E.O. Jordan, G.C. Whipple, and E.E.A. Winslow, *A Pioneer of Public Health: William Thompson Sedgwick* (New Haven, Yale University Press, 1974), p. 13.

14. Theobald Smith, Diary, July 5, 1882.

15. Frederic Schiller Lee (1859–1939) obtained his Ph.D. at Johns Hopkins University after studying there from 1881 to 1885 as assistant, graduate scholar, and fellow in biology. Later, he was Professor of Physiology at Columbia University. He upheld physiology as a biological science and deplored restricting its main development to medical schools.

16. Theobald Smith, Diary, December 21, 1883. Retrospective notes, July 1882 to winter 1883.

17. Theobald Smith, Diary, July 5, 1882.

18. H.J. Conn, "Professor Herbert William Conn and the Founding of the Society," *Bacteriological Reviews* 12 (1948): 275–296. This was Conn's presidential address to the Society of American Bacteriologists.

19. Theobald Smith, Autobiographical sketch prepared for John D. Rockefeller, Jr. in anticipation of dinner . . . November 20, 1931.

20. Theobald Smith, Diary, December 21, 1883.

21. Ibid.

22. A copy of Theobald Smith's Graduating Thesis is in the Library of the Albany Medical College.

23. Theobald Smith, Diary, April 20, 1884. Retrospective notes, March to August 1883.

24. Theobald Smith, Autobiographical sketch prepared for Secretary A.A. Milne of the Liverpool School of Tropical Medicine, August 7, 1907.

25. Theobald Smith, Diary, April 20, 1884.

26. Theobald Smith, Autobiographical sketch prepared for Secretary A.A. Milne of the Liverpool School of Tropical Medicine, August 7, 1907.

27. Theobald Smith, Diary, April 20, 1884.

28. Ibid.

29. Theobald Smith, Diary, June 10, 1884. Retrospective note on August 1883.

30. Ibid.

31. Theobald Smith, Diary, June 29, 1884. Retrospective notes, September to November 1883. This entry and the preceeding ones dated April 20 and June 10, 1884, and a later one made on June 29, were made after his arrival in Washington and terminated his early diaries.

32. Morris Bishop, *A History of Cornell,* p. 84.

33. Simon H. Gage to Daniel E. Salmon, October 12, 1883. The paper referred to was presumably the one on "Several Microscopical Sections" (Theobald Smith, Bibliography No. 3).

34. E.A. Cameron to Theobald Smith, October 25, 1883.

35. *Cornell Daily Sun,* October 31, 1883. Quoted in A.H. Wright's *Pre-Cornell and Early Cornell V,* pp. 51–52.

36. Theobald Smith, Diary, June 29, 1884.

37. W.R. Rasmussen and Gladys L. Baker, *The Department of Agriculture* (New York, Praeger Publishing Company, 1972), pp. 3–13; U.G. Houck, *The Bureau of Animal Industry of the U. S. Department of Agriculture* (Washington, 1924), pp. 19–23; L.A. Merillat and D.M. Campbell, *Veterinary Military History of the United States* (Chicago, Veterinary Magazine Corp., 1935), pp. 229–230; and A.H. Dupree, *Science in the Federal Government* (Cambridge, Mass., Harvard University Press, 1957), p. 165.

38. Theobald Smith to Simon H. Gage, August 31, 1884.

39. Theobald Smith to Simon H. Gage, October 19, 1884.

40. Theobald Smith to Simon H. Gage, July 11, 1885.

41. Theobald Smith to Simon H. Gage, June 20, 1885.

42. Ernst Abbe (1840–1905) inherited the Zeiss optical plant at Jena in 1888, and bequeathed his estate to the Carl Zeiss Foundation. Volume 1 (pp. 15–24, 119–164) of his *Gesammelte Abhandlungen* (Jena, 1904) contains papers on his illuminator, or condenser (1871), and on the optical limits of microscopy, including the principle of immersion lenses (1876). James Law's microscope, a Jackson model, was presented by his Edinburgh students before he left for Cornell University. The instrument was donated to the New York State Veterinary College by Law's daughter. See S.H. Gage, "Microscopy in America (1830–1945)," *Transactions of the American Microscopical Society* 83, No. 4 (October 1964): Supplement.

43. Theobald Smith, Bibliography Nos. 3 and 4.

44. Theobald to Simon H. Gage, October 19, 1884.

45. Theobald Smith, Bibliography No. 5.

46. Theobald Smith, Bibliography No. 6.

47. Thobald Smith to Simon H. Gage, February 1, 1885.

48. Theobald Smith, Bibliography No. 10.

49. Theobald Smith, Bibliography No. 8.

50. F.A.T. Hueppe, *Die Methode der Bakterien-Forschung* (Wiesbaden, 1885).

51. Hermann Biggs's translation was published by Appleton in New York in 1886 under the title *The Methods of Bacteriological Investigation.*

52. Theobald Smith to Simon H. Gage, April 19, 1885.

53. Theobald Smith to Simon H. Gage, August 31, 1884.

54. Daniel E. Salmon, "A New Form of Culture Tube Used in the Preceding Investigation [of swine plague]," in U.S. Department of Agriculture, *First Annual Report of the Bureau of Animal Industry for the Year 1884* (Washington, 1885), pp. 229–232.

55. Theobald Smith, Bibliography No. 9.

56. Oscar Brefeld, author of the 15-volume treatise on mycology, *Botanische Untersuchungen über Schimmelpilze* (Leipzig, Munster, 1874), described in 1874 many of the pure culture techniques which Koch later improved. Brefeld stressed the heat sterilization of culture media, glassware and all utensils; precautions to exclude air-borne contaminants; and the addition of gelatine to stabilize fluid media. See C.E. Dolman, "Brefeld, Julius Oscar," in *Dictionary of Scientific Biography* (New York, Charles Scribner's Sons [1974], v. 2, pp. 436–438.

57. Theobald Smith, Bibliography No. 11.

58. Theobald Smith to Simon H. Gage, April 19, 1885.

59. Theobald Smith to Simon H. Gage, October 19, 1884.

60. Theobald Smith to Simon H. Gage, November 30, 1884.

61. Theobald Smith to Simon H. Gage, February 1, 1885.

62. A.F. King to Theobald Smith, February 2, 1886, in Theobald Smith, Scrapbook No. 1.

63. Simon H. Gage, *Notes on Histological Methods, Including a Brief Consideration of the Methods of Pathological and Vegetable Histology, and the Application of The Microscope to Jurisprudence. For the Use of Laboratory Students in the Anatomical Department of Cornell University* (Ithaca, Andrus & Church, 1885–6).

64. Theobald Smith to Simon H. Gage, March 16, 1886.

65. D.C. Peattie, "Burrill, Thomas Jonathan," *Dictionary of American Biography* (New York, Scribner's, 1928–1937), v. 3, pp. 326–327.

66. J. Ewan, "Trelease, William," *Dictionary of American Biography,* Supplement 3, 1941–1945, pp. 775–776.

67. Martha L. Sternberg, *George Miller Sternberg. A Biography* (Chicago, American Medical Association, 1920), pp. 74–87.

68. Lillian E. Pruden, ed., *Biographical Sketches and Letters of T. Mitchell Prudden, M.D.* (New Haven, Yale University Press, 1927), pp. 55–61, 79–93.

69. T. Mitchell Prudden, "Occurrences of the Bacillus Tuberculosis in Tuberculous Lesions," *Medical Record* 23 (1883): 397–400.

70. C.E.A. Winslow, *The Life of Hermann M. Biggs, M.D., D.Sc., LL.D., Physician and Statesman of the Public Health* (Philadelphia, Lea & Febiger, 1919), p. 65.

71. D.H. Bergey, "Early Instructors in Bacteriology in the United States," *Journal of Bacteriology* 11 (1917): 595–601.

72. Simon Flexner and James T. Flexner, *William Henry Welch and the Heroic Age of American Medicine* (New York, Viking Press, 1941), pp. 100–117, 138–153. For an amusing anecdote involving Koch, Welch, Prudden and *V. cholerae,* see pp. 148–149.

73. Theobald Smith to Simon H. Gage, August 31, 1884.

74. Theobald Smith to Simon H. Gage, July 11, 1885.

75. F. Cooper Curtice, undated, handwritten autobiographical letter, ca. 1921, probably intended for U.G. Houck, Bureau of Animal Industry, Washington, D.C., Cooper Curtice Papers, Library of Congress.

76. Theobald Smith to Simon H. Gage, April 19, 1885.

77. A copy of this can be found in Smith's Scrapbook No. 1.

78. Theobald Smith to Fred L. Kilbourne, July 9, 1885, in the Cornell University Archives, Collection on Regional History.

79. Theobald Smith to Simon H. Gage, January 10, 1886.

80. Theobald Smith to Simon H. Gage, February 5, 1886.

81. Theobald Smith to Simon H. Gage, January 10, 1886.

82. Theobald Smith to Simon H. Gage, February 5, 1886.

83. Ibid.

Chapter 4:

1. Theobald Smith to Simon H. Gage, August 31, 1884.

2. Theobald Smith to Simon H. Gage, February 1, 1885.

3. Theobald Smith to Simon H. Gage, November 30, 1884.

4. Theobald Smith to Simon H. Gage, November 4, 1885.

5. *Baird's Manual of American College Fraternities,* 17th ed., edited by John Robson (Menasha, Wis., George Banta Co., [1963]), pp. 618–623. Phi Beta Kappa was founded at the College of William and Mary in 1776.

6. Theobald Smith to Simon H. Gage, August 31, 1884.

7. Theobald Smith to Simon H. Gage, April 19, 1885.

8. Theobald Smith to Simon H. Gage, November 4, 1885.

9. Nathaniel H. Egleston, *Village and Village Life. With Hints for Their Improvement* (New York, Harper & Bros., 1878).

10. Arbor Day, one of several national holidays started in the decade following the Civil War,

was launched in 1875 by J. Sterling Morton of Nebraska, who became Secretary of Agriculture during President Cleveland's second term, 1893–1897. Well before then, most of the States had proclaimed it an official holiday, and "school children, church and temperance groups had adorned the plains with the awesome total of 600 million newly planted trees." From "America, 1870–1900," in *This Fabulous Century*, (New York, Time-Life Books, 1970), v. 1, p. 56.

11. Lilian Egleston to Theobald Smith, written on calling card, undated, but probably on April 23, 1886.
12. Lilian Egleston to Theobald Smith, undated, but written probably on May 6, 1886.
13. Lilian Egleston to Theobald Smith, May 13, 1886.
14. Theobald Smith to Lilian Egleston, May 31 (with additions dated June 1), 1886.
15. Lilian Egleston to Theobald Smith, June 3, 1886 (written at 6 A.M.).
16. Theobald Smith to Lilian Egleston, June 3, 1886 (written at 1 P.M.)
17. Theobald Smith to Lilian Egleston, June 17, 1886.
18. Lilian Egleston to Theobald Smith, June 18, 1886.
19. Theobald Smith, Autobiographical letter to Lilian Egleston, June 17–21, 1886.
20. Theobald Smith to Lilian Egleston, June 21, 1886.
21. Lilian Egleston to Theobald Smith, June 26, 1886.
22. Theobald Smith to Lilian Egleston, July 8, 1886.
23. Theobald Smith, Bibliography Nos. 20 and 21.
24. Theobald Smith to Lilian Egleston, August 11, 1886.
25. Lilian Egleston to Theobald Smith, September 10, 1886.
26. Theobald Smith to Lilian Egleston, September 12, 1886.
27. Lilian Egleston to Theobald Smith, September 26, 1886.
28. Theobald Smith to Lilian Egleston, October 12, 1886.
29. Lilian Egleston to Theobald Smith, October 13, 1886.
30. Theobald Smith to Lilian Egleston, October 16, 1886.
31. Lilian Egleston to Theobald Smith, October 22, 1886.
32. Theobald Smith to Lilian Egleston, November 2 (with additions dated November 6), 1886.
33. Lilian Egleston to Theobald Smith, November 8, 1886.
34. Theobald Smith to Lilian Egleston, November 15, 1886.
35. Theobald Smith, Bibliography No. 24.
36. Theobald Smith to Lilian Egleston, October 23, 1886.
37. Theobald Smith to Lilian Egleston, December 2, 1886.
38. Theobald Smith to Lilian Egleston, March 17, 1887.
39. Theobald Smith to Lilian Egleston, December 21, 1886.
40. *Cornell Sun,* May 11, 1887.
41. Theobald Smith to Lilian Egleston, May 13, May 16–17, May 19, 1887.
42. Lilian Egleston to Theobald Smith, May 19, 1887.
43. Theobald Smith to Lilian Egleston, May 25, 1887.
44. Theobald Smith to Lilian Egleston, August 31, 1887.
45. Lilian Egleston to Theobald Smith, September 3, 1887.
46. Theobald Smith to Lilian Egleston, March 1, 1888.
47. Theobald Smith to Lilian Egleston, April 29, 1888.
48. Theresia Schmitt to Lilian Egleston, May 2, 1888.

49. Theobald Smith to Lilian Egleston, May 2, 1888.
50. *Cornell Sun,* May 3, 1888.
51. Theobald Smith to Lilian Egleston, May 5, 1888.
52. Theobald Smith to Lilian Egleston, May 8, 1888.
53. The clipping is preserved in Theobald Smith's Scrapbook No. 1.
54. Theobald Smith, Bibliography No. 28.
55. Theobald Smith to Lilian Egleston Smith, August 12, 1891.
56. Theobald Smith, Diary, June 22, 1889.
57. Theobald Smith, Diary and Account Book, January 1902.
58. Theobald Smith to Lilian Egleston Smith, May 8, 1890.
59. Theobald Smith, Diary, May 31, June 2 and June 5, 1890.
60. Theobald Smith to Simon H. Gage, July 13, 1890.
61. Theobald Smith, Diary, June 24, 1891.
62. Theobald Smith to Lilian Egleston Smith, August 12, 1891.
63. Theobald Smith to Lilian Egleston Smith, June 24, 1891.
64. Theobald Smith, Diary, May 29 and June 6, 1889.
65. Theobald Smith to Lilian Egleston Smith, July 15, 1891.
66. Theobald Smith to Lilian Egleston Smith, July 19, 1891.
67. Lilian Egleston Smith to Theobald Smith, July , 1891.
68. Lilian Egleston Smith to Mrs. Simon H. Gage, August 9, 1891.
69. Theobald Smith, Diary, February 1, 1891.
70. Lilian Egleston Smith to Theobald Smith, August 14, 1891.
71. Ibid.
72. Lilian Egleston Smith to Mrs. Simon H. Gage, August 27, 1893.
73. Theobald Smith to Simon H. Gage, March , 1891
74. Theobald Smith, Diary, November 25, 1890.
75. Theobald Smith, Diary, July 5, 1890.
76. Theobald Smith, Diary, March 30 and April 18, 1889.
77. Theobald Smith to Lilian Egleston Smith, July 3, 1891, and Theobald Smith, Diary, July 2, 1891.
78. Lilian Egleston Smith to Mrs. Simon H. Gage, August 27, 1893.

Chapter 5:

1. U.S. Bureau of Animal Industry, *Hog Cholera: Its History, Nature, and Treatment, as Determined by the Inquiries and Investigations of the Bureau of Animal Industry. Special Report of the Bureau of Animal Industry, United States Department of Agriculture* (Washington, 1889).
2. E.E. Saulmon, "Hog Cholera Eradication—Dream or Reality," *Journal of the American Veterinary Association* 163 (November 1973): 1103–1105.
3. A.H. Quin, "The Past and Future of Hog Cholera Control," *Journal of the American Veterinary Association* 116 (1950): 411–415.
4. U.G. Houck, *The Bureau of Animal Industry of the United States Department of Agriculture, Its Establishment, Achievements and Current Activities* (Washington, 1924), p. 32.
5. Peter R. Ellis, *An Economic Evaluation of the Swine Fever Eradication Programme in Great Britain, Using Cost Benefit Analysis Techniques* (Reading, England, 1972).
6. *Animal Health, A Centenary (1865–1965)* (London, H. M. Stationary Office, 1965).

7. H.W. Dunne, "Hog Cholera," Chapter 8 in H.W. Dunne and A.D. Leman, eds., *Diseases of Swine,* 4th ed. (Ames, Iowa, Iowa State University Press, 1975), p. 190.

8. William Budd, "Typhoid Fever in Pigs," *Journal of the Royal Agricultural Society of England,* 2d ser. 1 (1865): 472–488. Budd is best known for his classic monograph on *Typhoid Fever* (London, Longman, 1873; reprint ed., New York, American Public Health Association, 1931).

9. William Osler, "On the Pathology of So-called Pig-typhoid," *Veterinary Journal and Annals of Comparative Pathology* 6 (June 1878): 385–402.

10. Edward Emanuel Klein, "Report on the So-called Enteric or Typhoid Fever of the Pig," in Great Britain. Privy Council. Medical Department, *Reports of the Medical Officer of the Privy Council and Local Government Board,* n.s. 8, *Report to the Lords of the Council on Scientific Investigations* (London, 1876), pp. 91–101.

11. Edward Emanuel Klein, "Experimental Contribution to the Etiology of Infectious Diseases with Special Reference to the Doctrine of Contagium Vivum," *Quarterly Journal of Microscopical Science,* n.s. 18 (1878): 170–177 (read before the Royal Society on February 17, 1878); and Edward Emanuel Klein, "Report on Infectious Pneumo-enteritis of the Pig (So-called Pig Typhoid)," in Great Britain. Privy Council. Medical Department, *Report of the Medical Officer of the Local Government Board* (London, 1877–1878), v. 7, pp. 169–290.

12. "Report of the Examiner. Investigation of Swine Plague," in U.S. Department of Agriculture, *Report of the Commissioner of Agriculture for the Year 1878* (Washington, 1879), pp. 321–331.

13. Ibid, pp. 331–365.

14. Ibid, pp. 365–383.

15. Ibid, pp. 432–443.

16. Louis Pasteur, "Sur le Rouget, ou Mal Rouge des Porcs," (extract from a letter to M. Dumas), *Comptes Rendus de l'Académie des Sciences* 94 (December 4, 1882): 1120–1121; "Sur le Mal Rouge, ou Rouget des Porcs," *Bulletin de la Société National d'Agriculture de France* 42 (December 13, 1882): 639–643 (Resumé). Also in *Oeuvres de Pasteur* 6 (1933): 524–527.

17. H.J. Detmers, "A Pathogenic Schizophyte of the Hog," *American Naturalist* 16 (March, April 1882): 195–203, 293–305.

18. Louis Pasteur and Louis Thuillier, "La Variation du Rouget des Porcs à l'Aide du Virus Mortel Atténué de Cette Maladies," *Comptes Rendus de l'Académie des Sciences* 97 (November 26, 1884): 1163–1169. Also in *Oeuvres de Pasteur,* 6 (1933): 527–543.

19. Edward Emanuel Klein, "The Bacteria of Swine Plague," *Journal of Physiology* 5 (January 19, 1884): 1–13; "Die Bakterien der Schweinesuche," *Virchows Archiv für Pathologische Anatomie und Physiologie und für Klinische Medizin* 95 (1884): 468–484.

20. Daniel E. Salmon, "Investigation of Swine Plague, Fowl-Cholera, and Southern Cattle Fever," [Part II., "Investigations of Swine Plague," pp. 267–272], in U.S. Department of Agriculture, *Report of the Commissioner of Agriculture for the Years 1881 and 1882* (Washington, 1882), pp. 258–316.

21. Theobald Smith to Simon H. Gage, October 19, 1884.

22. Theobald Smith to Simon H. Gage, November 2, 1884.

23. U.S. Department of Agriculture, *Contagious Diseases of Domesticated Animals, Investigations by Department of Agriculture, 1883–84* (Washington, 1885).

24. Theobald Smith to Simon H. Gage, November 30, 1884.

25. Daniel E. Salmon, "Investigations of Swine-Plague," in U.S. Bureau of Animal Industry, *First Annual Report of the Bureau of Animal Industry for the Year 1884* (Washington, 1885), pp. 221–229.

26. Theobald Smith to Simon H. Gage, April 19, 1885.

27. Daniel E. Salmon and Theobald Smith, "Remarks of Fluid and Gelatinous Media for Cultivating Micro-organisms, with Description of Salmon's New Culture-Tube and Demonstrations of the Process of Using It," Abstract in *Proceedings of the American Association for the Advancement of Science* 33 (1884): 556–559.

28. Theobald Smith to Simon H. Gage, July 11, 1885.

29. Theobald Smith to Simon H. Gage, November 4, 1885.

30. Theobald Smith, Bibliography No. 13.

31. Ibid.

32. Daniel E. Salmon, "Two Different Germs Found in Hog Cholera," *Breeder's Gazette,* November 11, 1886.

33. F. Loeffler, "Experimentelle Untersuchungen über Schweine-Rothlauf," *Arbeiten aus dem Kaiserlichen Gesundheitsamte* 1 (1885): 46–55; and W. Schütz, "Über den Rothlauf der Schweine und die Impfung Desselben," *Arbeiten aus dem Kaiserlichen Gesundheitsamte* 1 (1885): 56–75.

34. A. Lydtin and M. Schottelius, *Der Rothlauf der Schweine: Seine Entstehen und Verhütung (Schutzimpfung nach Pasteur)* (Wiesbaden, 1885).

35. Daniel E. Salmon, "Why Pasteur's Vaccine Fails to Prevent Hog Cholera," *Breeder's Gazette,* May 20 and 27, June 3 and 10, 1886; also in *American Veterinary Review* 10 (1886–1887): 175–183, 232–240.

36. Theobald Smith to Simon Flexner, December 1, 1931, Flexner Papers, American Philosophical Society.

37. Theobald Smith to Simon H. Gage, January 10, 1886.

38. See Daniel E. Salmon, "The Virus of Hog Cholera," *American Public Health Reports* 11 (1886): 73–77.

39. Theobald Smith to Lilian Egleston, September 9, 1886.

40. Theobald Smith, Bibliography No. 15.

41. James Law, Third Report, "Investigation of Swine Plague, in U.S. Department of Agriculture, *Report of the Commissioner of Agriculture for the Year 1880* (Washington, Government Printing Office, 1881), pp. 455–526.

42. Theobald Smith to Simon H. Gage, March 16, 1886.

43. Ibid.

44. Daniel E. Salmon, "The Theory of Immunity from Contagious Diseases," *Proceedings of the American Association for the Advancement of Science* 35 (1887): 262–266.

45. Theobald Smith, Bibliography No. 21.

46. Theobald Smith, Bibiliography No. 20.

47. U.S. Department of Agriculture, *Third Annual Report of the Bureau of Animal Industry for 1881* (Washington, 1887); Daniel E. Salmon, "Letter of Transmittal," pp. 6–7, "Investigations of Swine Diseases," pp. 20–100.

48. Theobald Smith to Lilian Egleston, September 6, 1887.

49. Daniel E. Salmon, "Investigations of Swine Diseases," in U.S. Department of Agricul-

ture, *Third Annual Report of the Bureau of Animal Industry for 1886*. The article (Theobald Smith, Bibliography No. 28) was, of course, written by Theobald Smith and not Salmon.

50. Ibid.

51. Theobald Smith, Bibliography No. 23.

52. Theobald Smith to Simon H. Gage, March 16, 1886.

53. Simon Flexner and James T. Flexner, *William Henry Welch and the Golden Age of American Medicine*, p. 78.

54. The Illinois Industrial University, located at Champaign and Urbana, was one of Senator Justin S. Morell's Land Grant colleges. Founded in 1867, it became officially designated the University of Illinois in 1885, but two years later had not assumed its new name. Theobald Smith revisited the University of Illinois repeatedly from 1907 onward, chiefly in connection with the work of its Nutrition Commission. He became friendly with President Edmund J. James, whom he met again in Berlin in 1912. H.W. Conn's fine work in dairy bacteriology was done at Wesleyan University, Bloomington, Illinois, about forty miles to the northwest.

55. W. Schütz, Über die Schweinseuche," *Arbeiten aus dem Kaiserlichen Gesundheitsamte* 1 (1886): 376–413.

56. Daniel E. Salmon, "Hog cholera," *American Veterinary Review* 12 (1888–1889): 6–20; also in *Journal of Comparative Medicine and Surgery* 9 (1888): 136–151. Salmon read the article before the United States Veterinary Medical Association at Baltimore on March 19, 1888.

57. Theobald Smith to Lilian Egleston, October 9, 1886.

58. Theobald Smith, Bibliography Nos. 16–20.

59. Theobald Smith, Bibliography No. 27.

60. Simon H. Gage, "Account of Retirement of Professor Veranus A. Moore, and Other Items on Prof. Moore," Gage Papers, Olin Library, Cornell University.

61. Theobald Smith, Bibliography No. 36.

62. Theobald Smith to Lilian Egleston Smith, September 28, 1888.

63. Theobald Smith to Lilian Egleston Smith, November 14, 1888.

64. Theobald Smith to Simon H. Gage, November 28, 1888.

65. William H. Welch to Theobald Smith, December 10, 1888.

66. L. Brieger, "Ueber Spaltungsprodukte der Bacterien," *Zeitschrift für Physiologische Chemie* 8 (1883–1884): 306–311; 9 (1885): 1–7.

67. F. Hueppe, "Historisch-kritisches über den Imfschutz, Welchen Stoff-wechselproducte gegen die Virulenten Parasiten Verleihen," *Fortschritte der Medizin* 6 (April 15, 1888): 289–295.

68. A. Chantemesse and F. Widal, "De l'Immunité contre le Virus de la Fièvre Typhoide Conférée par des Substances Solubles," *Annales de l'Institut Pasteur* 2 (1888): 54–59.

69. E. Roux and C. Chamberland, "Immunité contre la Septicémie Conférée par des Substances Solubles," *Annales de l'Institut Pasteur* 1 (December 1887): 561–580.

70. Daniel E. Salmon, "Discovery of the Production of Immunity from Contagious Diseases by Chemical Substances Formed during Bacterial Multiplication," *Proceedings of the American Association for the Advancement of Science, Section F (Biology)* 37 (May 1889): 275–280.

71. Selander, "Ueber die Bacterien der Schweinpest," *Centralblatt für Bacteriologie* 3 (1888): 361–365.

72. Elie Metchnikoff, "Etudes sur l'Immunité (5e Memoire). Immunité des Lapins Vaccines contre le Microbe du Hog-Cholera," *Annales de l'Institut Pasteur* 6 (May 1892): 289–320.

73. William H. Welch and A.W. Clement, *Remarks on Hog-Cholera and Swine Plague* (Philadelphia, 1934). This talk was originally delivered before the First International Veterinary Congress of America at Chicago on October 20, 1893. It was reprinted in *Papers and Addresses by William Henry Welch* (Baltimore, Johns Hopkins Press, 1920), v. 2, pp. 86–119.

74. Theobald Smith, "Investigation of Infectious Diseases of Domesticated Animals," in U.S. Bureau of Animal Industry, *Eighth and Ninth Annual Reports of the Bureau of Animal Industry from 1891–1892* (Washington, 1893), pp. 45–58, 104 (Bibliography No. 55).

75. Frank S. Billings, *Swine Plague, with Especial Reference to the Porcine Pests of the World. An Etiological, Patho-Anatomic, Prophylactic, and Critical Contribution to General Pathology and State Medicine* (Lincoln, Nebraska, State Printers, 1888).

76. Frank S. Billings, "The Germ of the Southern Cattle Plague," *American Naturalist* 22 (1888): 113–128.

77. "Report of the United States Board of Inquiry Concerning Epidemic Diseases among Swine," in U.S. Department of Animal Industry, *Sixth and Seventh Annual Reports of the Bureau of Animal Industry for 1889–1890* (Washington, 1891), pp. 129–143.

78. William H. Welch, "Preliminary Report of Investigations concerning the Hog Cholera," *Bulletin of the Johns Hopkins Hospital* 1 (1889): 9–10.

79. Simon Flexner and James T. Flexner, *William Henry Welch and the Golden Age of American Medicine*.

80. U.S. Department of Animal Industry, *Hog Cholera: Its History, Nature, and Treatment, as Determined by the Inquiries and Investigations of the Bureau of Animal Industry*.

81. Theobald Smith to Simon H. Gage, September 18, 1889.

82. U.S. Department of Animal Industry, *Fourth and Fifth Annual Reports of the Bureau of Animal Industry for 1887–1888* (Washington, 1889); Daniel E. Salmon, "Letter of Transmittal," pp. 5–7; "Investigations of 1887," pp. 63–115; "Investigations of 1888," pp. 117–159.

83. Theobald Smith to Simon H. Gage, November 4, 1885.

84. I. Saphra and M. Wassermann, "Salmonella Cholerae Suis. A Clinical and Epidemical Evaluation of 329 Infections Identified between 1940 and 1954 in the New York Salmonella Center," *American Journal of Medical Sciences* 228 (1954): 525–531.

85. Theobald Smith to Simon H. Gage, August 17, 1890.

86. Jeremiah M. Rusk to the President of the United States, Benjamin Harrison, October 26, 1889. Published in U.S. Department of Agriculture, *Report of the Secretary of Agriculture* (Washington, 1890), pp. 7–45.

87. Theobald Smith to Lilian Egleston Smith, May 13, 1890.

88. Theobald Smith, Bibliography No. 41.

89. E.A. von Schweinitz, "Results of Chemical Investigations for the Prevention of Disease," in U.S. Bureau of Animal Industry, *Sixth and Seventh Annual Reports of the Bureau of Animal Industry for 1889–1890* (Washington, 1891), pp. 110–128.

90. U.S. Department of Agriculture, *Report of the Secretary of Agriculture* (Washington, 1891). Quoted from Jeremiah M. Rusk's letter to President Benjamin Harrison, dated October 25, 1890, and appearing on p. 20.

91. Ibid.

92. E.A. von Schweinitz, "The Production of Immunity with the Chemical Substances Formed during the Growth of the Bacillus of Hog-Cholera," *Medical News* 57 (October 4, 1890): 332–335.

93. Theobald Smith, Bibliography No. 45.

94. Theobald Smith, Bibliography Nos. 43 and 44.

95. P. Frosch, "Ein Beitrag zur Kenntnis der Ursache der Amerikanischen Schweine-Seuche und Ihrer Beziehung zu den Bakteriologisch Verwandten Processen," *Zeitschrift für Hygiene* 9 (1890): 235–281.

96. Theobald Smith, Bibliography Nos. 49 and 53.

97. P. Frosch, "Entgegnung auf die Vorstehende Arbeit des Hrn. Dr. Th. Smith: Zur Kenntnis der Amerikanischen Schweineseuche," *Zeitschrift für Hygiene* 10 (1891): 509–512.

98. Jeremiah M. Rusk to Theobald Smith, March 27, 1891, preserved in Smith's Scrapbook No. 1.

99. Daniel E. Salmon to Theobald Smith, March 31, 1891, also found in Scrapbook No. 1.

100. Theobald Smith to Simon H. Gage, March 27, 1891.

101. Jeremiah M. Rusk to Benjamin Harrison, President of the United States, October 27, 1891, in U.S. Department of Agriculture, *Report of the Secretary of Agriculture* (Washington, 1892), pp. 28–29.

102. Theobald Smith, Diary, June 13, 1891.

103. Theobald Smith, Bibliography No. 52.

104. Theobald Smith, Bibliography No. 63.

105. Austin Peters, "Report of the Chairman of the Committee on Intelligence and Education of the U.S.V.M.A. for the Year Ending September, 1891," *Journal of Comparative Medicine and Veterinary Archives* 12 (1891): 514–527.

106. P. Frosch, "Ein Beitrag zur Kenntnis der Ursache der Amerikanischen Schweine-Seuche und Ihrer Beziehung zu den Bakteriologisch Verwandten Processen."

107. P. Frosch, "Entgegnung auf die Vorstenehde Arbeit des Hrn. Dr. Th. Smith: Zur Kenntnis der Amerikanischen Schweineseuche."

108. Daniel E. Salmon, "Reply to Dr. Austin Peters' Criticism of the Bureau of Animal Industry," *Journal of Comparative Medicine and Veterinary Archives* 13 (1892): 28–37; *American Veterinary Review* 15 (1892): 524–565.

109. Daniel E. Salmon, "The Scientific Investigations at the Bureau of Animal Industry," *Journal of Comparative Medicine and Veterinary Archives* 13 (1892): 692–719.

110. E.A. de Schweinitz, "Investigations of the Effects of Bacterial Products on the Prevention of Diseases," in U.S. Bureau of Animal Industry, *Eighth and Ninth Annual Reports of the Bureau of Animal Industry for 1891–1892* (Washington, 1893), pp. 66–70.

111. E.A. de Schweinitz, "The Enzymes of [i.e. or] Soluble Ferments of the Hog-Cholera Germ," *Medical News* 61 (October 1892): 376–377.

112. William H. Welch to Theobald Smith, October 2, 1892.

113. Theobald Smith, Bibliography No. 70.

114. Theobald Smith, Diary, May 8, 1893.

115. Theobald Smith, Bibliography No. 81.

116. William H. Welch and A.W. Clement, *Remarks on Hog Cholera and Swine Plague*.

117. William H. Welch to Theobald Smith, September 5, 1894.

118. Theobald Smith, Bibliography No. 71.

119. J. Lignières, "Etude et Classification des Septicémies Hemorrhagiques. Maladies du Porc," *Bulletin de la Société Centrale de Medécine Vetérinaire* 18 (1900): 389–431.

120. Organisms of the *Pasteurella* genus are now defined as small, non-motile, gram-negative ovoid rods, bipolar when appropriately stained, non-hemolytic, producing indol, and not liquefying gelatin or coagulating milk. They parasitize mammals (including man) and birds, causing hemorrhagic septicemia as Hueppe (1886) first pointed out. Since 1939, the comprehensive designation *Pasteurella multocida* has been favored for organisms having those characteristics, regardless of the host sources, whether fowl, rabbit, deer, swine, or man. *P. multocida* thus supersedes earlier designations for what were considered to be the related but distinctive bacterial agents of e.g., fowl cholera, rabbit septicemia, and *Wildseuche*.

121. J. Lignières, "Contribution à l'Etude et à la Classification des Septicémie Hemorrhagique. Les 'Pastuerelloses'," *Annales de l'Institut Pasteur* 15 (1901): 734–736.

122. J.C. Weedin, "The Colon-Typhoid Group of Bacteria and Related Forms. Relationships and Classification," *Iowa State College Journal of Science* 1 (1927): 121–197.

123. Theobald Smith to Simon H. Gage, December 21, 1933.

124. Theobald Smith, Bibliography No. 130.

125. Walter Reed and J. Carroll, "A Comparative Study of the Biological Characters and Pathogenesis of *Bacillus X* (Sternberg), *Bacillus Icteroides* (Sanarelli), and the Hog Cholera Bacillus (Salmon and Smith)," *Journal of Experimental Medicine* 5 (December 1900): 215–270.

126. J. [G.] Sanarelli, "Etiologie et Pathogénie de la Fièvre Jaune," *Annales de l'Institut Pasteur* 11 (1897): 433–522, 673–698.

127. E.A. de Schweinitz and M. Dorset, "A Form of Hog Cholera Not Caused by the Hog-Cholera Bacillus," in U.S. Department of Agriculture, Department of Animal Industry, *Circular No. 41* (Washington, 1903).

128. F. Loeffler and P. Frosch, "Berichte der Kommission zur Erforschung der Maul- und Klauenseuche bei dem Institut für Infektionskrankheiten in Berlin," *Centralblatt für Bakteriologie,* Abt. I. 23 (March 1898): 371–391.

129. M. Dorset, B.N. Bolton, and C.N. McBryde, "The Etiology of Hog Cholera" (condensed from U.S. Bureau of Animal Industry, *Bulletin No. 72* (Washington, 1905).

Chapter 6:

1. James Mease, "An Account of a Contagious Disease Propagated by a Drove of Southern Cattle in Perfect Health," *Memoirs of the Philadelphia Society for Promoting Agriculture* 5 (1826): 280–283. This was incorrectly cited by J.R. Dodge in Note 4 of this chapter to the year 1814. See J.F. Smithcors, "James Mease, M.D., on the Diseases of Domestric Animals," *Bulletin of the History of Medicine* 31 (March-April 1957): 122–131, particularly pp. 128–130. Interestingly, from a communicable disease standpoint, Mease published at Philadelphia in 1792 the first monograph in America on rabies—*An Inaugural dissertation on the Disease Produced by the Bite of a Mad Dog, or Other Rabid Animal.*

2. John Shaw Billings and Edward Curtis, "Examination of Blood and Secretions from Cattle Affected with the Texas or Splenic Fever," U. S. Commissioners of Agriculture, *Report on the Diseases of Cattle in the United States,* series II (Washington, 1871), v. 1, pp. 162–170.

3. J. Gamgee, "Report on the Splenic and Periodic Fever of Cattle," U. S. Commissioners of Agriculture, *Report on the Diseases of Cattle in the United States* (Washington, 1871), 82–132.

4. J.R. Dodge, "Report of Statistical and Historical Investigations of the Progress and Results of the Texas Cattle Disease," U. S. Commissioners of Agriculture, *Report on the Diseases of Cattle in the United States* (Washington, 1871), pp. 175–202.

5. Daniel E. Salmon, "Investigation of Southern Cattle Fever," U.S. Department of Agriculture, *Special Report for 1879 and 1880* (Washington, 1881), pp. 98–141.

6. Daniel E. Salmon, "Texas Cattle Fever," U.S. Department of Agriculture, *Report of the U. S. Commissioner of Agriculture for 1882* (Washington, 1883), pp. 19–44.

7. H.J. Detmers, "Investigations of Texas Cattle Fever," U.S. Department of Agriculture, *Report of the U. S. Commissioner of Agriculture for 1880* (Washington, 1881), pp. 595–601; *Special Report No. 34*, 1881, pp. 291–297.

8. H.J. Detmers, "Investigation of Southern Cattle Fever," U.S. Department of Agriculture, *First Annual Report of the Bureau of Animal Industry for 1884* (Washington, 1885), pp. 426–436.

9. Frank S. Billings, "The Germ of the Southern Cattle Plague," *American Naturalist* 22 (February 1888): 113–128; "Southern Cattle Plague and Yellow Fever from the Etiological and Prophylactic Viewpoints," *Bulletin of the Agricultural Station of Nebraska* 2, no. 3 (Lincoln, 1888); "The Causes and Nature of the Southern Cattle Plague of the United States," *Medical Register* 3 (1888): 252–254, 276–278, 300–302, 321–324, 343–346.

10. Frank S. Billings, "The Etiology of Southern Cattle Plague—Texas Fever," *Journal of Comparative Medicine and Veterinary Archives* 13 (July-November, 1892): 397–425, 467–486, 526–557, 613–629, 676–692.

11. Theobald Smith, Bibliography No. 64.

12. Paul Paquin, *Texas Fever (Southern Cattle Fever, etc.)*, Missouri Agricultural College Experiment Station, Bulletin No. 11 (Columbia, Missouri, May 1890); reprinted in *Journal of Comparative Medicine and Veterinary Archives* 11 (July and August, 1890): 367–383, 436–455.

13. Frank S. Billings, "The Recent Work on Texas Fever," Letter to the Editor, *The Breeder's Gazette* 31 (June 9, 1897): 413.

14. R.C. Stiles, "V. Report on the Pathology of Texas Cattle Disease," in "Report of the N.Y. State Commissioners, in Connection with the Special Report of the Metropolitan Board of Health, on the Texas Cattle Disease," *Transactions of the New York State Agricultural Society*. Part II, 27 (1869): 1134–1150.

15. E. Harris, ed., "Report upon the Investigations Concerning the Texas Cattle Disease," *Transactions of the New York State Agricultural Society*, 27 (1869): 985–1133, 1151–1170. Hallier's main commendable achievement in microbiology was to stress the germ theory of disease. W. Bulloch, in *The History of Bacteriology* (London, 1938, 1960, p. 188) mentions Hallier's claims to have "definitely settled the problem of the aetiology of many infective diseases of man, animals, and vegetables. He founded a phytopathological institute in Jena and issued therefrom a special journal, *Zeitschrift für Parasitenkunde*. Hallier's active reign was brief—the edifice which he had erected with so much diligence and by such defective methods was shaken to its foundations by the drastic criticisms of Anton de Bary (1868), and F. Cohn (1872) also pointed out that Hallier's cultural experiments possessed not the slightest value. Further, Bulloch quoted (p. 192) the mycologist Oscar

Brefeld: "If one does not work the pure cultures, 'da kommt nur Unsinn und Penicillium glaucum heraus'."

16. John Shaw Billings and Edward Curtis, "Examination of Blood and Secretions from Cattle Affected with the Texas Splenic Fever."

17. Theobald Smith to Simon H. Gage, November 30, 1884.

18. Theobald Smith, Bibliography No. 40.

19. Cooper Curtice, "Outbreaks of Southern Cattle Fever in Maryland," U.S. Bureau of Animal Industry, *Fourth and Fifth Annual Reports of the Bureau of Animal Industry for 1887 and 1888* (Washington, 1889), pp. 429–442.

20. Theobald Smith, Bibliography No. 40.

21. Theobald Smith, Diary, August 31, 1890.

22. Theobald Smith, Diary, September 7, 1889.

23. Theobald Smith, Diary, September 23, 1889.

24. Theobald Smith, Bibliography No. 40.

25. Victor Babes, "Sur l'Hémoglobinurie Bacterienne du Boeuf," *Comptes Rendus de l'Académie des Sciences* 107 (October 1888): 692–694.

26. Victor Babes, Die Aetiologie der Seuchenhaften Haemoglobinurie des Rindes," *Virchow's Archiv* 115 (January 1889): 81–108.

27. Theobald Smith, Bibliography No. 40.

28. Theobald Smith, Bibliography No. 41.

29. Theobald Smith to Simon H. Gage, July 13, 1890.

30. Theobald Smith, Bibliography No. 41.

31. Theobald Smith, Bibliography No. 51.

32. William H. Welch to Theobald Smith, October 2, 1892.

33. Theobald Smith, Bibliography No. 64.

34. T.M. Haygood has claimed that "from the mid-eighteenth century through the 1930's," most southern cattle were "permanently infected with babesiosis and anaplasmosis." See "Cows, Ticks and Disease: A Medical Interpretation of the Southern Cattle Industry," *Journal of Southern History* 52 (November 1986): 551–564.

35. W.H. Patton, "The Name of the Southern or Splenic Cattle-Fever Parasite," *American Naturalist* 28 (May 1895): 498.

36. Victor Babes, "Sur les Microbes de l'Hémiglobinurie de Boeuf," *Comptes Rendus de l'Académie des Sciences* 110 (April 1890): 800–802.

37. Victor Babes, "Note Asupra Cauzelor Unor Enzootii de Vite in Rromânie," *Analele Academiei Romône*, ser. II 16 (1894): 57–62.

38. C. Starcovici, "Bemerkungen über den durch Babes Entdeckten Blutparasiten und die durch Denselben Hervorgebrachten Krankheiten, die Seuchenhafte Hemoglobinurie des Rindes (Babes), das Texasfieber (Th. Smith) und der Carceaq der Schare (Babes)," *Centralblatt für Bakteriologie* 14 (July 1893): 1–8.

39. Shortly after Babes died in 1926, Wenyon's classification of the phylum Protozoa was widely adopted (C.M. Wenyon, "Subdivisions of the Piroplasmidea," in *Protozoology*, New York, William Wood, 1926, v. 2, pp. 988–1039). He recognized a suborder of pear-shaped blood parasites, *Piroplasmidea*, within Leuckart's class of Sporozoa. Accordingly, Shilling and Meyer (1930) accepted the designations *Piroplasma* and "piro- plasmoses" for these parasites and their respective animal diseases (C. Schilling and K.F. Meyer, "Piroplasmosen," in W. Kolle and A. von Wassermann, *Handbuch der Pathogenen Mikro-*

organismen, 3rd ed., Jena, Fischer, 1930, v. 8, pp. 1–94). However, in 1960, G. Dinulescu and M. Babes (the diplomat son, Mircea, of Victor Babes) published a one-sided summary of the historical data relating to classification and terminology of the genus *Babesia,* and to priority of discovery (G. Dinulescu and M. Babes, "Sur la Priorité de la Découverte des Babesies. Classification et Terminologie, "*Annales de Parasitologie Humain et Comparée* 35, 1960, 747–754). In 1964, the Committee on Taxonomic Problems, set up by the American Society of Protozoologists, published another classification of the Protozoa which included the *Babesidae* family (B.M. Honigsberg, W. Balamuth, J.D. Corliss, and N.D. Levine, "A Revised Classification of the Phylum Protozoa," *Journal of Protozoology* 11, 1964, 7–20). In 1968, Riek approved the superfamily designation *Babesioidea* (R.F. Riek, "Babesiosis," in D. Weinman and M. Ristic, *Infectious Blood Diseases of Man and Animals,* New York, Academic Press, 1968, v. 2, pp. 219–268).

40. Theobald Smith, Bibliography No. 64.
41. A. Theiler, "East Coast Fever (Due to Piroplasma parvum [n. sp.]) 1," *Journal of the Royal Army Medical Corps* 3 (1904): 599–620.
42. Theobald Smith, Bibliography No. 65.
43. P.C.G. Garnham, J. Donnelly, H. Hoagstrall, C.C. Kennedy, and G.A. Waltin, "Human Babesiosis in Ireland: Further Observations and the Medical Significance of This Infection," *British Medical Journal* 4 (1969): 768–770, where it was observed that "Few places in the world are free of piroplasms."
44. W. Stahl, R. Jackson, G. Turek, and H.A. Gaafar, "Babesiosis: Malaria Mimic," *American Journal of Medical Technology* 44 (1978): 572–574.
45. Theobald Smith, Diary, December 10, 12, 18, 1892.
46. Theobald Smith, Bibliography No. 70.
47. M.A. James, M.G. Levey, and M. Ristic, "Isolation and Partial Characterization of Culture-Derived Soluble *Babesia bovis* Antigens," *Infection and Immunity* 31 (1981): 358–361; R.D. Amith, M.A. James, M. Ristic, M. Aikawa, and C.A. Vega y Munguia, "Bovine Babesisis: Protection of Cattle with Culture-Derived Soluble *Babesia bovis* Antigens," *Science* 212 (April 17, 1981): 335–338.
48. Theobald Smith, Bibliography No. 41.
49. Theobald Smith, Diary, September 28, 1889.
50. Theobald Smith, Diary, July 19, 1990.
51. David Fairchild to Lilian Egleston Smith, December 16, 1934.
52. David Fairchild, *The World Was My Garden. Travels of a Plant Explorer* (New York, Charles Scribner, 1938), p. 24.
53. Theobald Smith, Bibliography No. 41.
54. E.W. Dennis, "The Life-Cycle of *Babesia bigemina* (Smith and Kilbourne) of Texas Cattle-Fever in the Tick *Margaropus annulatus* (Say)," *University of California Publications in Zoology* 36 (1932): 263–298.
55. R.F. Riek, "Babesiosis."
56. Theobald Smith, Diary, June 3, 1892.
57. Theobald Smith to Simon H. Gage, June 6, 1892.
58. Theobald Smith, Diary, June 29, 1892.
59. Theobald Smith, Diary, September 25, 1892.
60. Theobald Smith, Diary, November 10, 1892.
61. Theobald Smith, Bibliography No. 65.

62. Theobald Smith, Diary, March 27, 1893.

63. Cooper Curtice, Manuscript copy of letter, apparently sent ca. 1921 to U.G. Houck, Cooper Curtice Papers, Library of Congress.

64. Simon H. Gage to Theobald Smith, April 3, 1893.

65. George W. Corner, *Anatomist at Large* (New York, Basic Books, 1958), p. 14.

66. Daniel E. Salmon, Letter of Transmittal to Hon. J.M. Rusk, Secretary, U.S. Department of Agriculture, February 6, 1893, in U.S. Bureau of Animal Industry, *Investigations into the Nature, Causation, and Prevention of Texas or Southern Cattle Fever* (Washington, 1893), pp. 7–8.

67. Daniel E. Salmon, "Investigation of Southern Cattle Fever," U.S. Department of Agriculture, *Special Report, U.S. Department of Agriculture for 1879 and 1880.*

68. Theobald Smith to Cooper Curtice, April 29, 1903, Cooper Curtice Papers, Library of Congress.

69. Cooper Curtice to Theobald Smith, May 1, 1903, Cooper Curtice Papers, Library of Congress.

70. Austin Peters to Hom. James Wilson, Secretary, U.S. Department of Agriculture, April 13, 1903, Cooper Curtice Papers, Library of Congress.

71. H.H. Brighman, Acting Secretary, U.S. Department of Agriculture, to A. Peters, April 21, 1903, Cooper Curtice Papers, Library of congress.

72. Theobald Smith to Simon H. Gage, December 21, 1933.

73. Daniel E. Salmon, "Some Examples of the Development of Knowledge Concerning Animal Diseases," U.S. Bureau of Animal Industry, *Sixteenth Annual Report of the Bureau of Animal Industry for 1899* (Washington, 1900), pp. 53–101.

74. Daniel E. Salmon, Cooper Curtice, *et. al.,* "Discussion" (following papers on Texas fever, presented at the Atlantic City meeting, 1901, *Proceedings of the Veterinary Medical Association* (1903): 249–271.

75. Theobald Smith to Simon H. Gage, December 21, 1933.

76. F.L. Kilborne to Hubert Schmidt, March 3, 1936.

77. Hubert Schmidt to F.L. Kilborne, February 11, 1936.

78. Hu. Schuck, *et al., Nobel, the Man and His Prizes* (Amsterdam, Elsevier, 1962), pp. 188–189.

79. Daniel E. Salmon, Cooper Curtice, *et. al.,* "Discussion" (following papers on Texas fever, presented at the Atlantic City meeting of the American Veterinary Medical Association, 1901).

80. Cooper Curtice, Manuscript copy of letter, apparently sent ca. 1921 to U.G. Houck.

81. Cooper Curtice, "The Biology of the Cattle Tick," *Journal of Comparative Medicine and Veterinary Archives* 12 (1891): 313–319; "About Cattle Ticks," *Journal of Comparative Medicine and Veterinary Archives* 13 (1892): 1–7.

82. Cooper Curtice, Manuscript of Autobiographical Notes, ca. 1935, Cooper Curtice Papers, Library of Congress.

83. "Minutes of 150th Meeting," *Proceedings of the Biological Society of Washington* 5 (November 30, 1899): xxii.

84. Cooper Curtice, "The Biology of the Cattle Tick."

85. Cooper Curtice to Theobald Smith, May 1, 1903, Cooper Curtice Papers, Library of Congress.

86. Theobald Smith to Cooper Curtice, May 4, 1903, Cooper Curtice Papers, Library of Congress.

87. Cooper Curtice to the Hon. J. Sterling Morton, March 20, 1893, Cooper Curtice Papers, Library of Congress.

88. Theobald Smith to Simon H. Gage, December 7, 1894.

89. Theobald Smith to Simon H. Gage, December 22, 1896.

90. Theobald Smith to Simon H. Gage, December 21, 1933.

91. Cooper Curtice, Manuscript copy of letter, apparently sent ca. 1921 to U.G. Houck.

92. W.A. Hagen to M.S. Ferguson, September 16, 1957.

93. Theobald Smith to Simon H. Gage, December 7, 1894.

94. Paul de Kruif, "Theobald Smith, Ticks and Texas Fever," in *Microbe Hunters* (New York, Harcourt, Brace and Company, 1926), pp. 234–251.

95. Paul de Kruif to Theobald Smith, November 10 and 16, 1926.

96. Mrs. Maria Kilborne Flaherty to the author, September 12, October 7, and October 27, 1969.

97. Theobald Smith, Bibliography No. 66

98. Harvey Cushing, *The Life of Sir William Osler* (Oxford, Clarendon Press, 1925), v. 1, p. 382.

99. William Osler, "The Practical Value of Laveran's Discoveries," *The Medical News* 67 (1895): 561–564.

100. V.A. Nogaard, "Dipping Cattle for Destruction of Ticks," U.S. Bureau of Animal Industry, *12th and 13th Annual Reports of the Bureau of Animal Industry for 1895–96* (Washington, 1897), pp. 109–118; "In Memoriam. Cooper Curtice, 1856–1939," *Journal of Parasitology* 25 (1939): 517–520.

Chapter 7:

1. See Chapter 3, pp. 51–54.

2. C.E.A. Winslow, *The Life of Hermann M. Biggs.*

3. E.L. Trudeau, *An Autobiography* (Philadelphia, Lea & Febiger, 1916), pp. 173–191, 209–216.

4. L.S. Cutter, "Theobald Smith and His Contributions to Science," *Journal of the American Veterinary Medical Association* 90 (March 1939): 245–255.

5. Robert Koch, "Die Aetiologie der Tuberkolose," *Mittheilungen aus dem Kaiserlichen Gesundheitsamt* 2 (1884): 1–88. The quotations and paginations are cited from Stanley Boyd's translation, reproduced as "The Etiology of Tuberculosis," in *Microparasites in Disease. Selected Essays* (London, New Sydenham Society, 1886), pp. 67–201; also reprinted in *Medical Classics* 2 (1938): 821–880.

6. Editorial: "The Report of the Royal Commission on Tuberculosis," *The Lancet* 1 (April 27, 1895): 1074–1076.

7. J. Law, "International Veterinary Congress," in U.S. Bureau of Animal Industry, *First Annual Report of the Bureau of Animal Industry for 1884*, pp. 321–370; "Tuberculosis in Animals," pp. 350–366, 369–370.

8. G.S. Woodhead, "Tuberculosis and Tabes Mesenterica," *The Lancet* 2 (July 14, 1888): 51–54 (condensed).

9. "Congress for the Study of Tuberculosis. Held at Paris, July 25–31, 1888," *Medical Record*

34 (August 25, September 1, 1888): 217–220, 249–252; Editorial: "The Paris Congress on Tuberculosis, 1888," *The Lancet* 1 (September 1, 1888): 425.

10. Annotation: "The prophylaxis of tuberculosis," *The Lancet* 2 (August 10, 1889): 282.

11. Annotations: "Congress for the Study of Tuberculosis," *The Lancet* 2 (May 9, 1891): 1059; "The Tuberculosis Congress," *The Lancet* 2 (August 22, 1891): 463–464.

12. "Report of a Departmental Committee on Tuberculosis in the United Kingdom," *Practitioner* 41 (December 1888): 466–471.

13. Annotation: "Tuberculosis in Cattle and in Man," *The Lancet* 1 (March 31, 1888): 638–639.

14. "Diseased Meat in Glasgow," *British Medical Journal* (April 27, 1899: 979; "Tuberculous Meat: Judicial Inquiry at Glasgow," *British Medical Journal* 1 (June 29, 1889): 1478.

15. "The Report of the Royal Commission on Tuberculosis," *The Lancet* 1 (April 27, 1895): 1074–1076.

16. Theobald Smith, Diary, January 11, 1890.

17. Theobald Smith, Bibliography No. 41.

18. "Seventh International Congress of Hygiene and Demography, Held in London, Aug. 10–17, 1891," *The Lancet* 2 (August 15, 1891): 349–387.

19. R. Koch, "Ueber bakteriologische Forschung," *Verhandlungen des X. internationalen Kongresses* (Berlin, 1890), v. 1, pp. 35–47. Translated as "Address on Bacteriological Research," *British Medical Journal* 2 (August 16, 1890): 380–383.

20. R. Koch, "Weitere Mittheilungen über ein Heilmittel gegen Tuberkulose," *Deutsche Medizinische Wochenschrift* 16 (November 16, 1890): 1029–1032. Translated as "A further communication on a remedy for tuberculosis," and published as a special supplement to *British Medical Journal* 2 (November 15, 1890); also, *British Medical Journal* 2 (November 22, 1890): 1193–1195.

21. Ibid.

22. John Shaw Billings to Robert Koch, June 20, 1891, Billings Papers, New York Public Library.

23. E.L. Trudeau, *An Autobiography.*

24. Editorial: "Koch's Discovery," *Medical News* (December 6, 1890): 608.

25. R. Koch, "Fortsetzung der Mittheilungen über ein Heilmittel gegen Tuberkulose," *Deutsche Medizinische Wochenschrift* 17 (January 15, 1891): 101. Translated as "A Further Communication on a Remedy for Tuberculosis," *British Medical Journal* 2 (January 17, 1891): 125–127; and abstracted as "The Composition and Preparation of Prof. Koch's Fluid," *The Lancet* 2 (January 17, 1891): 168–169.

26. *Die Wirksamkeit des Koch'schen Heilmittels gegen Tuberculose. Amtliche Berichte der Kliniken, Polykliniken, und Pathologisch-anatomischen Institute der Preussischen Universitäten* (Berlin, Julius Springer, 1891). See also Editorial: "Official Reports on Koch's Treatment," *British Medical Journal* 1 (March 14, 1891): 593–594; and Editorial, *The Lancet* 1 (March 21, 1891): 671–672.

27. Correspondence: "The Twentieth Surgical Congress, Held at Berlin," *The Lancet* 1 (April 11, 1891): 850–851.

28. A. Buchholtz, *Ernst von Bergmann* (Leipzig, F.C.W. Vogel, 1911), pp. 454–456. In the fourth edition (1925) of this work, von Bergmann's speech of welcome to Koch was given in full on pp. 447–455.

29. Paul Ehrlich, "Recent Experiences in the Treatment of Tuberculosis (with Special Refer-

ence to Pulmonary Consumption) by Koch's Method," *The Lancet* 2 (October 24, 1891): 917–920 (abstracted and translated by T.W. Hime).

30. E. Nocard and E. Roux, "Sur la Culture du Bacille de la Tuberculose," *Annales de l'Institut Pasteur* (1887): 19–29.

31. Theobald Smith, Diary, December 10, 11, 14, 28, 1890; January 18, 1891.

32. F.E. Leupps to Theobald Smith, December 18, 1890.

33. Theobald Smith, Bibliography No. 48.

34. John Shaw Billings to Robert Koch, June 20, 1891.

35. Theobald Smith, Bibliography No. 55.

36. Theobald Smith, Bibliography No. 72.

37. W. Gutmann, "Versuche an Tuberculösen Rindern mit dem Koch'schen Mittel," *Berliner Thierärztliche Wochenschrift* 7 (Janaury 8, 1891): 12–13, from *Baltische Wochenschrift für Landwirthschaft,* 1890, No. 51. See also Berlin Correspondent, "Discussion upon Koch's Treatment at the Berlin Medical Societies," *The Lancet* 1 (January 3, 1891): 62–63.

38. B. Bang, "The Diagnostic Value of Tuberculin and Its Employment in Combating Bovine Tuberculosis," *Veterinary Journal and Annals of Comparative Pathology* 39 (1894): 389–394. See also "The Application of Tuberculin in the Suppression of Bovine Tuberculosis," *Massachusetts Agricultural Experiment Station Bulletin No. 41* (Amherst, 1896).

39. A. Eber, "Versuche mit Tuberculinum Kochii bei Rindern zu Diag- nostischen Zwecken. Zusammenfassendes Referat," *Centralblatt für Bakteriologie* 11 (March 9, 1892): 283–288.

40. Special Report, "Tuberculosis in Cattle," *Medical News* 60 (March 26, 1892): 358–362. See also P.F. Clark, *Pioneer Microbiologists of America* (Madison, Wisconsin, 1961), pp. 216, 129.

41. E.C. Schroeder, "Further Experimental Observations on the Presence of Tubercle Bacilli in the Milk of Cows," in U.S. Bureau of Animal Industry *Bulletin No. 7* (Washington, 1894), pp. 75–87.

42. Theobald Smith, Bibliography No. 90.

43. Theobald Smith, Bibliography No. 89.

44. Theobald Smith, Diary, October 20–26, 1893.

45. Theobald Smith, Bibliography No. 92.

46. Theobald Smith, Bibliography No. 78.

47. Theobald Smith to Simon H. Gage, February 25, 1894.

48. Theobald Smith, Bibliography No. 94.

49. Daniel E. Salmon, "Tuberculosis," in Section on the Bureau of Animal Industry in U.S. Department of Agriculture, *Report of the Secretary of Agriculture for 1893* (Washington, 1894), pp. 130–132.

50. A.W. Clement, "Report of the Tuberculosis Committee," *Journal of Comparative Medicine and Veterinary Archives* 14 (December 1893): 380–396.

51. Daniel E. Salmon, "Tuberculosis," in U.S. Department of Agriculture, *Report of the Secretary of Agriculture for 1893.*

52. U.S. Department of Agriculture, *Report of the Secretary of Agriculture for Fiscal Year Ending June 30, 1894* (Washington, 1895), pp. 32–33.

53. B.D. Davis and M.R. Olmsted, "The Sad Fate of Premature Legislation Eradicating Bovine Tuberculosis in Massachusetts," *Harvard Medical Alumni Bulletin* 44 (1970): 18–19.

54. Theobald Smith, Bibliography No. 78.

55. Ibid.

56. Theobald Smith, Bibliography No. 79.

57. B.D. Davis and M.R. Olmsted, "The Sad Fate of Premature Legislation Eradicating Bovine Tuberculosis in Massachusetts."

58. Daniel E. Salmon, "The Work in Regard to Tuberculosis," in Section on the Bureau of Animal Industry, U.S. Department of Agriculture, *Report of the Secretary of Agriculture for Fiscal Year Ending June 30, 1894* (Washington, 1895), p. 111.

59. Theobald Smith, Bibliography No. 89.

60. Theobald Smith, Bibliography No. 91.

61. Theobald Smith, Bibliography No. 92.

62. E.A. de Schweinitz, "The Pasteurization and Sterilization of Milk," in *U.S. Department of Agriculture Yearbook for 1894* (Washington, 1895), 331–356.

63. Theobald Smith, Bibliography No. 92.

64. K.A. Jensen, "Bovine Tuberculosis in Man and Cattle," *Advances in the Control of Zoonoses*, Monograph 19 (Geneva, World Health Organization, 1953).

65. E.L. Trudeau, "Some Cultures of the Tubercle Bacillus Illustrating Variations in Its Mode of Growth and Pathogenic Properties," *Transactions of the Association of American Physicians* 5 (1890): 183–184.

66. Theobald Smith, Bibliography No. 109.

67. Theobald Smith to Simon H. Gage, September 12, 1894.

68. Theobald Smith, Bibliography No. 26.

69. Theobald Smith, Bibliography No. 54.

70. Theobald Smith, Bibliography No. 67.

71. F. Bolton, *London Water Supply* (London, W. Clowes & Sons Ltd., 1884); P. Frankland and [Mrs.] P. Frankland, *Micro-organisms in Water. Their Significance, Identification and Removal* (London, Longmans Green & Co., 1894).

72. Theobald Smith, Diary, January 17, February 14, 16, 17, 21 and 23, 1891.

73. Theobald Smith, Diary, June 25, 29 and 30; July 4 and 5, 1891.

74. Theobald Smith to Lilian Egleston Smith, July 3, 1891 (and Theobald Smith, Diary, July 2, 1891).

75. Theobald Smith, Bibliography No. 57.

76. Theobald Smith, Bibliography No. 18.

77. C.C. Brown, "Fourth Report on Mohawk and Hudson Rivers," in New York State Board of Health, *13th Annual Report for the Year 1892*. (Albany, New York, 1893), pp. 680–726.

78. Theobald Smith, Bibliography No. 43.

79. Theobald Smith, Bibliography No. 75.

80. C.C. Brown, "Fourth Report on Mohawk and Hudson Rivers."

81. Theobald Smith, Bibliography No. 75.

82. Theobald Smith, Bibliography No. 43.

83. Theobald Smith, Bibliography No. 75.

84. Theobald Smith, Bibliography No. 43.

85. Theobald Smith, Bibliography No. 126.

86. "Report of Committee on Standard Methods of Water Analysis to the Laboratory Section of the American Public Health Association," *Journal of Infectious Diseases*, Supplement No. 1 (May 1905): 1–13.

87. Hans Zinsser, "Theobald Smith, 1859–1934," *National Academy of Sciences Biographical Memoirs, No. 12*, 17 (1936): 261–303.

88. Theobald Smith, Bibliography No. 68.
89. Theobald Smith, Bibliography No. 43.
90. Theobald Smith, Bibliography No. 44.
91. Theobald Smith, Bibliography No. 58.
92. Theobald Smith, Bibliography No. 68.
93. Theobald Smith to John S. Billings, April 5, 1894.
94. G.W. Fuller, "The Differentiation of the Bacillus of Typhoid Fever," *Public Documents of Massachusetts, State Board of Health No. 34* (Boston, 1892): 637–644. Also in *Boston Medical and Surgical Journal* 172 (September 1, 1892): 205–207.
95. G.W. Fuller to Theobald Smith, March 9, 1893.
96. Theobald Smith, Bibliography No. 96.
97. Theobald Smith, Bibliography No. 95.
98. E.F. Smith, "Relation of Sugars to the Growths of Bacteria," *The American Naturalist* 50 (January, 1896): 66–67.
99. Theobald Smith, Bibliography No. 79.
100. Theobald Smith to John S. Billings, April 5, 1894.
101. G.M. Kober, "Presentation of the George M. Kober Medal to Dr. Theobald Smith," *Transactions of the Association of American Physicians* 41 (1926): xxxi-xxxii.
102. Theobald Smith, Bibliography No. 32.
103. Theobald Smith, Bibliography No. 76.
104. Theobald Smith to Simon H. Gage, October 2, 1892. In his text, *Principles of Sanitary Science and the Public Health* (1902), William T. Sedgwick discussed Smith's equation under a section headed "Vital Resistance and Susceptibility." Expressing M as MNV, Sedgwick modified the equation to D ? ____ , where N was the number of R micro-organisms involved, V their virulence, and M their "specific character." He admitted that R, the vital resistance of the host, could not be resolved "into any component elements." The first version of Smith's address on mixed cultures was published, early in 1894, in abstract form only. An expanded form, with modified title, was presented at the Annual Meeting of the Association of American Physicians at the end of May 1894, and published in their *Transactions,* late in the same year (Theobald Smith, Bibliography Nos. 76 and 77).
105. Theobald Smith, Bibliography No. 76.
106. Simon H. Gage to Theobald Smith, August 28, 1893.
107. Theobald Smith to Simon H. Gage, September 23, 1893.
108. Theobald Smith, Bibliography No. 68.
109. Theobald Smith, Bibliography No. 75.
110. Printed "Programme of the Quarter-Centennial Celebration of the Opening of Cornell University (1868–1893), Friday, Saturday, and Sunday, October 6th, 7th, and 8th," preserved in Theobald Smith's Scrapbook No. 1.
111. Simon H. Gage to Theobald Smith, August 28, 1893.
112. "The Wilder Quarter-Century Book," *The Cornell Era,* October 9, 1893, pp. 18–20.
113. Ibid.
114. J.G. Schurman to Theobald Smith, October 18, 1893. The Festschrift to Wilder is fully cited in Theobald Smith, Bibliography No. 69.
115. Theobald Smith to Simon H. Gage, July 22, 1894.
116. Theobald Smith, Bibliography No. 99. Also, Nos. 100 and 103.

117.   Theobald Smith, Bibliography No. 115.

118.   Theobald Smith, Bibliography No. 109.

119.   Theobald Smith, Experimental Notes, headed "Abortion & Milk, 1894."

120.   K.F. Meyer, "Medical Research and Public Health," typescript of interviews in 1961 and
       1962 by Edna T. Daniel, Regional Oral History, Bancroft Library, University of Califor-
       nia, Berkeley, p. 71.

121.   Theobald Smith to Simon H. Gage, September 2, 1890.

122.   Ibid.

123.   Theobald Smith to Simon H. Gage, March 27, 1891.

124.   Theobald Smith to Simon H. Gage, September 12, 1894.

125.   Ibid.

126.   Theobald Smith to Simon H. Gage, March 14, 1897.

127.   Simon H. Gage to Theobald Smith, March 24, 1897.

128.   Theobald Smith to Simon H. Gage, September 2, 1890.

129.   Theobald Smith, Diary, February 18, 1892; Banquet Card, dated February 23, 1892, in
       Scrapbook No. 1.

130.   Banquet Card, February 23, 1892.

131.   George L. Burr to Theobald Smith, June 19, 1893, in Theobald Smith, Scrapbook No. 1.

132.   Theobald Smith to Simon H. Gage, June 6, 1892.

133.   James Law, "Unsuspected Poisoning by Sterilized Meat and Milk of Tuberculous Cows,"
       Journal of Comparative Medicine and Veterinary Archives 15 (1894): 101–108.

134.   Theobald Smith to Simon H. Gage, February 26, 1894.

135.   Theobald Smith to Simon H. Gage, May 24, 1894.

136.   Theobald Smith to Simon H. Gage, July 4, 1894.

137.   Theobald Smith to Simon H. Gage, January 2, 1895.

138.   H.P. Walcott to Theobald Smith, January 7, 1895.

139.   Theobald Smith to Simon H. Gage, January 7, 1895.

140.   Theobald Smith to Simon H. Gage, January 11, 1895.

141.   Theobald Smith to Simon H. Gage, January 20, 1895.

142.   Theobald Smith, Diary, January 28 to February 1, 1895.

143.   Theobald Smith to Simon H. Gage, February 17, 1895.

144.   Theobald Smith to the Hon. J. Sterling Morton, Secretary of Agriculture, April 18,
       1895.

145.   J. Sterling Morton to Theobald Smith, April 20, 1895.

146.   Theobald Smith, Diary, April 4, 1895.

147.   Theobald Smith, Bibliography No. 97.

148.   Theobald Smith, Diary, April 30, 1895.

149.   Theobald Smith, Diary, May 4–8, 1895.

Chapter 8:

1.   P.P.E. Roux and A.L. Martin, "Contributions à l'Etude de la Diphtérie (Serum-
     Thérapie)," *Annales de l'Institut Pasteur* 8 (1894): 609–639; also, P.P.E. Roux, A.L. Martin
     and A. Chaillon, "Trois Cents Cas de Diphtérie Traités par la Serum Antidiphtérique,"
     Annales de l'Institut Pasteur 8 (1894): 640–661. The former paper appears in English
     translation as "Contribution to the Study of Serum-Therapy in Diphtheria," *Albany Medi-
     cal Annals* 16 (January 1893): 1–20. A graphic account of Roux's report and its reception

at Budapest appears in V.C. Vaughan, *A Doctor's Memories* (Indianapolis, Bobbs-Merrill Company [1926]), pp. 153–154.

2. H.C. Ernst, "The Preparation of the Antitoxin of Diphtheria," *Transactions of the Association of American Physicians* 10 (1898): 299–311.

3. Harvard Corporation Records, v. 12 (1873–1880), Minutes of October 29, 1874 and March 29, 1875.

4. F.H. Storer to C.W. Eliot, November 20, 1894, Eliot Papers, Harvard University Archives.

5. See Claire Douglas, *Translate This Darkness, The Life of Christiana Morgan* (New York, Simon & Schuster [1993]).

6. Theobald Smith to Lilian Egleston Smith, May 19, 1895.

7. Ibid.

8. Ibid.

9. Theobald Smith to Lilian Egleston Smith, May 31, 1895.

10. Ibid.

11. Theobald Smith to Lilian Egleston Smith, June 2, 1895.

12. Theobald Smith to Simon H. Gage, August 29, 1895.

13. Theobald Smith, Diary, November 18, 1895.

14. Theobald Smith to F.H. Storer, November 26, 1895.

15. Lilian Egleston Smith to Theobald Smith, June 4, 1895.

16. Theobald Smith to Lilian Egleston Smith, May 19, 1895.

17. Theobald Smith to Lilian Egleston Smith, May 31, 1895.

18. Theobald Smith to Lilian Egleston Smith, June 2, 1895.

19. Lilian Egleston Smith to Theobald Smith, June 4, 1895.

20. Theobald Smith to Lilian Egleston Smith, June 2, 1895.

21. Theobald Smith, Diary, June 20–30, 1895.

22. Theobald Smith, Diary, July 18, 1895.

23. Theobald Smith, Diary, July 21, August 9 and 19, 1895.

24. Theobald Smith, Diary, August 24, 1895.

25. Rev. W. Egleston to Theobald Smith, September 2, 1895.

26. Theobald Smith, Diary, October 1, 1895.

27. Theobald Smith, Diary, November 19, 1895.

28. V.A. Moore, "Veterinary Education and Service at Cornell University, 1896–1929," *Cornell Veterinarian* 19 (April 1929): 199–243.

29. Simon H. Gage to Theobald Smith, May 19, 1895.

30. Lilian Egleston Smith to Theobald Smith, May 23, 1895.

31. Lilian Egleston Smith to Theobald Smith, May 26, 1895.

32. Theobald Smith to Simon H. Gage, August 29, 1895.

33. Theobald Smith to Simon H. Gage, August 10, 1895.

34. Theobald Smith to Simon H. Gage, December 22, 1895.

35. Theobald Smith to Simon H. Gage, January 12, 1896.

36. Simon H. Gage to Theobald Smith, February 23, 1896.

37. Theobald Smith to Simon H. Gage, January 26, 1896.

38. Simon H. Gage to Theobald Smith, April 4, 1896.

39. Theobald Smith to Simon H. Gage, April 9, 1896

40. Theobald Smith to Simon H. Gage, December 22, 1896.

41. C.W. Eliot to Theobald Smith, April 21, 1896.

42. C.W. Eliot to C.F. Fabyan, April 3 and 18, 1896, Harard Medical Archives in The Francis A. Countway Library of Medicine.

43. Theobald Smith, Diary, July 18, 19 and 20, 1896.

44. C.W. Eliot to Theobald Smith, April 25, 1896.

45. Harvard University, *President's Annual Report, 1895–96* (Cambridge, 1896), pp. 24–28.

46. Theobald Smith to Simon H. Gage, April 9, 1896.

47. Theobald Smith to Simon H. Gage, March 14, 1897.

48. Harvard University, *President's Annual Report, 1897–98* (Cambridge, 1898), pp. 37–39.

49. Harvard University, *President's Annual Report, 1898–99* (Cambridge, 1899), pp. 24 and 28.

50. Theobald Smith, Bibliography No. 132.

51. Harvard University, *President's Annual Report, 1900–01* (Cambridge, 1901), p. 26.

52. Treasurer's Office, Harvard University, to Theobald Smith, March 11, 1897.

53. F.W. Storer to C.W. Eliot, August 6, 1896, Harvard University Archives.

54. Theobald Smith to Lilian Egleston Smith, August 21, 1896.

55. Theobald Smith to Simon H. Gage, July 6, 1896.

56. Theobald Smith to Lilian Egleston Smith, August 21, 1896.

57. Theobald Smith to Lilian Egleston Smith, August 23-September 3, 1896 (mailed from London).

58. Theobald Smith to Lilian Egleston Smith, September 3–4, 1896 (mailed from Cologne).

59. Theobald Smith to Lilian Egleston Smith, September 6–15, 1896 (mailed from Munich).

60. Ludwig Pfeiffer, "Die Neueren, seit 1887 Genommen Versuche zur Reinzüchtung des Vaccinecontagiums," *Zeitschrift für Hygiene und Infektionskrankheiten* 23 (1896): 306–321.

61. Theobald Smith to Lilian Egleston Smith, September 16–18, 1896 (mailed from Weimar).

62. Theobald Smith to Lilian Egleston Smith, September 19–28, 1896 (mailed from Berlin).

63. H.A. Johne, "Ein Eigenthumlicher Fall von Tuberkolosis beim Rind," *Deutsche Zeitschrift für Tiermedizin* 21 (1895): 438–454.

64. E.L. Stubbs, "Langdon Frothingham (1866–1935)," *Pathologia Veterinaria* 3 (1966): 565–567.

65. Theobald Smith to Lilian Egleston Smith, September 28-October 1, 1896 (mailed from Berlin).

66. Theobald Smith to Lilian Egleston Smith, October 2–6 and 7–9 (both mailed from Antwerp).

67. Koch favored his disciple G. Gaffky for Dunbar's position, but was mollified when his own technical advice was sought and largely followed. To cope with the tremendous increase in bacteriological tests of water supplies during and after the cholera outbreak, the Health Department arranged emergency accommodation in the same building as a cookery school. When Koch came to inspect the establishment, he was furious to find the words "Koch-Institut" over the entrance. (Personal statement to the author by Carl Giles Prausnitz, 1961).

68. Theobald Smith, "Account of the S. S. 'Westerland'," October 9–20, 1896.

69. Theobald Smith to Simon H. Gage, October 6, 1896.

70. Lilian Egleston Smith to Theresia Kexel Schmitt, September 17, 1896.

71. Theobald Smith to Lilian Egleston Smith, September 28-October 1, 1896.

72. Theobald Smith, Scrapbook No. 2.
73. Theobald Smith to Simon H. Gage, April 10, 1897.
74. Theobald Smith to Simon H. Gage, May 10, 1897.
75. Theobald Smith to Simon H. Gage, April 10, 1897.
76. Theobald Smith to Simon H. Gage, May 10, 1897.
77. Theobald Smith to Simon H. Gage, May 22, 1898.
78. Philip Smith, Personal reminiscences narrated to the author.
79. Ibid.
80. C.W. Eliot to Theobald Smith, November 19, 1898.
81. C.W. Eliot to Theobald Smith, May 25, 1901.
82. Theobald Smith, Monthly account book and occasional diary, January 1, 1898 to March 31, 1900.
83. Philip Smith, Personal reminiscences narrated to the author.
84. Ibid.
85. Theobald Smith, Monthly account book and occasional diary, March 1, 1901 to May 31, 1902.
86. Theobald Smith to Simon H. Gage, February 19, 1899.
87. Theobald Smith, Monthly account book and occasional diary, April 1, 1900 to February 28, 1901.
88. Philip Smith, Personal reminiscences narrated to the author.
89. Theobald Smith, Diary, January 6 and 7, 1899.
90. Theobald Smith, Diary, January 29, 1899.
91. Theobald Smith, Diary, February 3, 1899.
92. Theobald Smith to Simon H. Gage, February 19, 1899.
93. Theobald Smith, Diary, May 8, 1899.
94. Theobald Smith, Monthly account book and occasional diary, June 1, 1902 to December 31, 1908.
95. Philip Smith, Personal reminiscences narrated to the author.
96. Theobald Smith, Monthly account book and occasional diary, January 1, 1899 to March 31, 1900.

Chapter 9:

1. Theobald Smith to N.W. Mitchell and S.W. Abbott, December 6 and 9, 1895, from Theobald Smith's "Copybook," Massachusetts Department of Health Laboratories.
2. Theobald Smith, Bibliography No. 147.
3. C.W. Eliot to F.H. Storer, undated, but written June 1 or 2, 1898.
4. F.H. Storer to C.W. Eliot, June 4, 1898.
5. Theobald Smith, Bibliography No. 178.
6. Geoffrey Edsall, "The Massachusetts Antitoxin and Vaccine Laboratory," typescript, 5 pp.
7. Theobald Smith, Bibliography No. 117.
8. Theobald Smith, Bibliography No. 108.
9. Theobald Smith, Bibliography Nos. 133 and 135.
10. Massachusetts State Board of Health, *Annual Reports,* 1901, 1902, and its *Report upon the Production, Distribution and Use of Dephtheria Antitoxin for the Year Ended March 31, 1902,* Public Document No. 34 (Boston, 1902), pp. 438–507.

11. C.W. Eliot, *Animal Experimentation, a Series of Statements Indicating Its Value to Biological and Medical Sciences* (Boston, 1902), pp. 1–3.

12. Lilian Egleston Smith to Theobald Smith, May 11, 1890. The biography Lilian referred to in her letter was probably *Alice, Princess of Great Britain, Grand Dutchess of Hesse. Letters to Her Majesty the Queen. With a Memoir of H.R.H. Princess Christian* (London, John Murray, 1885).

13. Paul Ehrlich, "Die Wertbemessung des Diphteriaheilsorums und Deren Theoretische Grundlagen," *Klinische Jarhbuch* 4 (1897): 299–326.

14. Paul Ehrlich, "Ueber die Constitution des Diphtheriegiftes," *Deutsche Medizinische Wochenschrift* 24 (1898): 597–700.

15. C.E. Dolman, "Paul Ehrlich and William Bulloch. Correspondence and a Friendship (1896–1914)," *Clio Medica* 3 (1868): 65–84.

16. Theobald Smith, Bibliography No. 140.

17. Theobald Smith, Bibliography No. 151.

18. Theobald Smith, Diary, March 6, 1903.

19. "ANTI-TOXIN. Journal Man Sees It Made in Laboratorires of the Bussey Institute," *Boston Sunday Journal,* April 26, 1896.

20. C.W. Eliot, *Animal Experimentaiton, a Series of Statements Indicating Its Value to Biological and Medical Science.*

21. Theobald Smith, Diary, July 24, 1902.

22. Theobald Smith, Diary, March 9, 1905.

23. Theobald Smith, Bibliography Nos. 158 and 178.

24. Editorial: "The Production of Vaccine Lymph," *Boston Medical and Surgical Journal* 146 (January 2, 1902): 22–25.

25. B.M. Phelps, "Boards of Health and the Manufacture of Vaccine Virus and Antitoxins," *Boston Medical and Surgical Journal* 146 (January 23, 1902): 99.

26. For additional background and details, see B.G. Rosenkrantz, *Public Health and the State, Changing Views in Massachusetts, 1842–1936* (Cambridge, Mass., Harvard University Press, 1972), pp. 124–125.

27. Theobald Smith, Bibliography No. 151.

28. Massachusetts State Board of Health, *Annual Reports,* 1901 and 1902, and its *Report upon the Production, Distribution and Use of Diphtheria Antitoxin for the Year Ended March 31, 1902.*

29. Theobald Smith, Bibliography No. 117.

30. Theobald Smith, Bibliography No. 149.

31. Theobald Smith to Simon Flexner, April 1, 1903.

32. Flexner and Smith were both members of the Board of Directors of the recently constituted Rockefeller Institute for Medical Research. Smith had rejected already the offered directorship of the Institute. Flexner, second choice for the post, had accepted.

33. Theobald Smith, Bibliography Nos. 152 and 155.

34. H.H. Gillette, "History of the Diagnostic Laboratory," typescript prepared for the Massachusetts Department of Public Health in 1952, but apparently not published.

35. Massachusetts State Board of Health, *Annual Reports, 1899–1900,* v. 32, pp. 727–729.

36. Theobald Smith, Bibliography Nos. 145 and 148.

37. Theobald Smith, "Proposed Plan of Work for a Department of Comparative Pathology," undated handwritten draft, with addendum of 1898, in "History of the Department of

Comparative Medicine and Tropical Medicine," Harvard Medical Archives in The Francis A. Countway Library of Medicine.

38. Theobald Smith, final version of the preceding, entitled "Proposed Scope of Work in Comparative Pathology," with accompanying letter to President Eliot dated April 30, 1899. Harvard University Archives.

39. Theobald Smith, Bibliography No. 105.

40. Louis Pasteur, "Melanges Scientifiques et Litteraires," *Oeuvres* 7 (1922–1923): 211–221. From a Speech made at Lyon in March 1891.

41. Theobald Smith, Bibliography No. 114.

42. Theobald Smith to Dr. B. Arthur Hughes, January 7, 1905.

43. Theobald Smith to Simon H. Gage, December 22, 1896.

44. E.E. Tyzzer, "Theobald Smith, July 31, 1859 - December 10, 1934," *New England Journal of Medicine* 212 (January 24, 1935): 168–171.

45. Theobald Smith to Simon H. Gage, May 25, 1899.

46. Ibid.

47. Theobald Smith, Bibliography No. 105.

48. George Cheyne Shattuck, Personal interview with the author at the Harvard Medical School on October 25, 1965. Shattuck's father had been Professor of Medicine in Theobald's time and thought very highly of Smith and his work.

49. Theobald Smith, Bibliography No. 142.

50. Notice of copyright is preserved in Smith's Scrapbook No. 2.

51. H.J. Conn, "Professor Herbert William Conn and the Founding of the Society," *Bacteriological Reviews* 12 (1948): 275–296.

52. Theobald Smith, Bibliography No. 137.

53. C-E.A. Winslow, "The First Forty Years of the Society of American Bacteriologists," *Science* 91 (February 9, 1940): 125–129.

54. C.E. Dolman, "Theobald Smith and His Presidential Address to the Society of American Bacteriologists, Philadelphia, December 29, 1903," *ASM News* 47 (1981): 231–235.

55. Esmond R. Long, *History of the American Association of Pathologists and Bacteriologists,* supplement to the *American Journal of Pathology* 77 (1974), No. 1 (Durham, N.C., 1974).

56. Esmond R. Long, *History of the American Society for Experimental Pathology: A Record of Its Annual Meetings with Brief Biographical Sketches of Its Authors* ([Bethesda, Md.], American Society of Experimental Pathology, 1972).

57. B. Cohen, *Chronicles of the Society of American Bacteriologists, 1899–1950* (Baltimore, 1950).

58. Theobald Smith to the Secretary on Fellowships and Memberships of the American Public Health Association, May 11, 1931.

59. Theobald Smith, Bibliography No. 126.

60. Theobald Smith, Diary, October 21 and 22, 1900.

61. Theobald Smith, Bibliography No. 141.

62. Theobald Smith to the Secretary on Fellowships and Memberships of the American Public Health Association, May 11, 1931.

63. E.H. Storer to C.W. Eliot, April 21, 1897, Eliot Papers, Harvard University Archives.

64. M. Fabyan, "History of the Department of Comparative Pathology and Tropical Medicine," Harvard Medical Archives in The Francis A. Countway Library of Medicine.

65. H.P. Walcott, "Memorials to Arthur Tracy Cabot, M.D. I," *Boston Medical and Surgical Journal* 168 (March 20, 1913): 409–412.

66. A.T. Cabot to Theobald Smith, March 20, 1899. In M. Fabyan, "History of the Department of Comparative Pathology and Tropical Medicine."

67. M. Fabyan, "History of the Department of Comparative Pathology and Tropical Medicine."

68. Theobald Smith to N.W. Mitchell and S.W. Abbott, December 6 and 9, 1895.

69. Theobald Smith, Bibliography Nos. 158 and 178.

Chapter 10:

1. George Derby, "The Prevention of Disease," Massachusetts State Board of Health, *Annual Report for 1869* (Boston, 1870), pp. 42–57.

2. Eleanor J. MacDonald, "A History of the Massachusetts Department of Public Health," *The Commonhealth* 23 (1936): 83–124.

3. B.D. Davis and Margaret R. Olmstead, "The Sad Fate of Premature Legislation Eliminating Bovine Tuberculosis in Massachusetts."

4. Theobald Smith, Bibliography No. 177.

5. Theobald Smith, Bibliography No. 176

6. Theobald Smith, Bibliography No. 113.

7. Massachusetts Legislature, *Letter-Report to the Tuberculosis Committee* (Boston, 1897). Massachusetts Legislative Documents, House No. 1341. The testimony of F.S. Billings appears on pp. 26–40, and that of C.R. Wood on pp. 41–49.

8. Theobald Smith, Bibliography No. 121.

9. Theobald Smith to Simon H. Gage, May 22, 1898.

10. Theobald Smith, typescript document, "Proposed Scope of Work in Comparative Pathology," with accompanying letter to President C.W. Eliot, April 30, 1899, Harvard University Archives.

11. Austin Peters and Theobald Smith became firm friends. Peters was a helpful colleague and staunch champion. His official positions gave him weight in veterinary and legislative circles. He also served as consulting veterinarian to the Massachusetts Society for Promoting Agriculture, which assisted Smith's later researches on tuberculosis.

12. J.A. Myers and J.H. Steele, *Bovine Tuberculosis Control in Man and Animals* (St. Louis, W.H. Green, Inc., 1909).

13. Harvard University, *President's Report for 1896–7* (Cambridge, 1897), p. 28.

14. Theobald Smith, Bibliography No. 109.

15. Theobald Smith, Bibliography No. 123.

16. Theobald Smith, Bibliography No. 190.

17. Theobald Smith, Bibliography No. 137.

18. K. Vagadez, "Experimentelle Prüfung der Virulenz von Tuberkelbacillen," *Zeitschrift für Hygiene und Infectiouskrankheiten* 28 (1898): 276–320.

19. Theobald Smith, Bibliography No. 129.

20. Theobald Smith, Bibliography No. 127.

21. Theobald Smith, Bibliography No. 131.

22. Theobald Smith, Bibliography No. 127.

23. Theobald Smith, Bibliography No. 146.

24. "The Tuberculosis Congress: First and Second General Meetings, July 22nd and 23rd," *British Medical Journal* 2 (July 27, 1901): 203–206.

25. Harvey Cushing, *Life of Sir William Osler,* v. 1, pp. 559–561.

26. Robert Koch, "Die Bekämpfung der Tuberkulose unter Berücksightigung der Erfahrungen, Welche bei der Erfolgreichen Bekämpfung Anderer Infektionskrankheiten Gemacht Sind," *Deutsche Medizinische Wochenschrift* 27 (August 15, 1901), pp. 549–554. Also in Koch's *Gesammelte Werke* (Leipzig, Georg Thieme, 1912), v. 1, pp. 566–577; translated version, "The Fight against Tuberculosis in the Light of the Experience That Has Been Gained in the Successful Combat of Other Infectious Diseases," *British Medical Journal* 2 (July 27, 1901): 189–193.

27. British Congress on Tuberculosis, July 22–26, 1901, *Transactions,* v. 3, pp. 603–604.

28. M.P. Ravenel, "The Comparative Virulence of the Tubercle Bacillus from Human and Bovine Strains," *Transactions of the British Congress on Tuberculosis,* July 22–26, 1901, v. 3, pp. 553–581. Also, *Lancet* 2 (1901): 349–356, 443–448.

29. D.B. Bang, "Some Experiments on the Temperature Necessary for Killing Tubercle Bacilli in Milk," *Transactions of the British Congress on Tuberculosis,* v. 3, pp. 592–601.

30. Headline, *Boston Post,* July 31, 1901. The article was about the British Congress on Tuberculosis, which convened at London on July 22 and 23, 1901. A copy is preserved in Smith's Scrapbook No. 2.

31. *Boston Journal,* August 4, 1901, preserved in Scrapbook No. 2.

32. *Brooklyn Eagle,* August 11, 1901, preserved in Scrapbook No. 2.

33. E.G. Janeway to Theobald Smith, November 22, 1901.

34. Theobald Smith, Bibliography No. 146.

35. Robert Koch, "Ubertragbarkeit der Rindertuberkulose auf der Menschen," *Deutsche Medizinische Wochenschrift* 28 (1902): 857–862. Also in Koch's *Gesammelte Werke,* v. 1, pp. 578–590; English translation, "The Transference of Bovine Tuberculosis to Man," *British Medical Journal* 2 (December 20, 1902): 1885–1889.

36. Theobald Smith, Bibliography No. 146.

37. Theobald Smith, Bibliography No. 123.

38. Theobald Smith, Bibliography No. 146.

39. Theobald Smith to Simon H. Gage, May 10, 1897.

40. Theobald Smith to Simon H. Gage, November 13, 1898.

41. K. Vagadez, "Experimentelle Prüfung der Virulenz von Tuberkelbacillen."

42. M.P. Ravenel, "The Comparative Virulence of the Tubercle Bacillus from Human and Bovine Sources."

43. Theobald Smith, Bibliography No. 153.

44. Theobald Smith, Bibliography No. 198.

45. Theobald Smith, Bibliography No. 160.

46. Theobald Smith, Bibliography No. 168.

47. Theobald Smith, Bibliography No. 183.

48. Ibid.

49. Editorials, "Human and Bovine Tuberculosis," *British Medical Journal* 1 (July 4, 1904): 1326–1327, and "The Relations of Human to Bovine Tuberculosis," *Lancet* 1 (June 4, 1904): 1580. See also, "Report of the Royal Commission upon Human and Animal Tuberculosis," *Boston Medical and Surgical Journal* 150 (June 23, 1904): 683–684.

50. Robert Koch, "The Relations of Human and Bovine Tuberculosis, *Journal of the American Medical Association* 51 (October 10, 1908): 1256–1258. For "Conference *in Camara* on Human and Bovine Tuberculosis," see pp. 1262–1268.

51. *Topley and Wilson's Principles of Bacteriology, Virology and Immunity,* 6th edition, edited by Sir Graham Wilson and Sir Ashley Miles (London, Edward Arnold, 1975), v. 2 (Chapter 58), p. 1726.

52. Theobald Smith, Bibliography No. 190.

53. P.A. Lewis, "Tuberculous Cervical Adenitis. A Study of Tubercle Bacilli Cultivated from Fifteen Consequetive Cases," *Journal of Experimental Medicine* 12 (January, 1910): 82–104.

54. M. Fabyan, "The Bovine Type of Bacillus Associated with Three Cases of Tuberculosis in Man," *Archives of Internal Medicine* 6 (July, 1910): 19–23.

55. Alfreda Withington, *My Eyes Have Seen.*

56. W.H. Park and G. Krumwiede, Jr., "The Relative Importance of the Bovine and Human Types of Tubercle Bacilli in the Different Forms of Human Tuberculosis," *Journal of Medical Research* 23 (1910): 205–368.

57. "Final Report of the Royal Commission on Tuberculosis," *British Medical Journal* 2 (July 15, 1911): 122–125; Editorial, "The Report of the Tuberculosis Commission," *British Medical Journal* 2 (July 22, 1911): 180–181. Also, "The Royal Commission on Human and Animal Tuberculosis. Appendix by A.S. Griffith. Vol I. 'Investigation of Viruses Obtained from Cases of Human Tuberculosis Other Than Lupus;' Vol. II. 'Investigation of Viruses Obtained from Cases of Lupus'," *Lancet* 2 (September 23, 1911): 904–908. See also, "The Second Bovine Tuberculosis Report," *Boston Medical and Surgical Journal* 165 (August 10, 1911): 221–222.

58. H. Kossel, A. Weber, and Heuss, "Vergleichende Untersuchungen über Tuberkelbazillen Verschiedener Herkunft," *Tuberkulose Arbeiten den Kaiserlichen Gesundheitsamte* 1 (1904): 1–80; 3 (1905): 1–109; A. Weber and M. Taute, "Weitere Untersuchungen über Tuberkelbazillen Verschiedener Herkunft mit Besonderer Berücksichtigung der Primären Darm- und Mesenterialdrüsen Tuberkulose," *Tuberkulose Arbeiten den Kaiserlichen Gesundsamte* 6 (1907): 15–76.

59. Theobald Smith, Bibliography No. 123.

60. B. Lange, "The Role Played by Bovine Tubercle Bacilli in Human Tuberculosis," *British Medical Journal* 2 (September 10, 1932): 503–506.

61. A.S. Griffith, "Observations on the Bovine Tubercle Bacilli in Human Tuberculosis," *British Medical Journal* 2 (September 10, 1932): 501–503.

62. J.A. Myers and J.H. Steele, *Bovine Tuberculosis Control in Man and Animals.*

63. *Final Report of the Royal Commission on Tuberculosis.*

64. H.M. Biggs, "The Administrative Control of Tuberculosis," *Report of the Henry Phipps Institute for the Study, Treatment and Prevention of Tuberculosis* 1 (1905): 189–193; also, *Medical News* 84 (February 20, 1914): 337–345.

65. Theobald Smith, Bibliography No. 221.

66. Theobald Smith, Bibliography No. 306.

67. C.E. Dolman, "Smith, Theobald (1859–1934)," *Dictionary of Scientific Biography* (New York, Charles Scribner's Sons, 1975), v. 12, pp. 480–486.

68. C.E. Dolman, "Koch, Heinrich Hermann Robert (1843–1910)," *Dictionary of Scientific Biography,* v. 7 (1973), pp. 420–435.

69. F. Neufeld, "Die Typenfrage in der Baketeriologie," *Zentralblatt für Bakteriologie, Parasitenkunde und Infektionskrankheiten Originale* 122 (1931): 104–111.

70. Theobald Smith to Simon Flexner, December 17, 1931.

71. B. Lange, "The Role Played by Bovine Tubercle Bacilli in Human Tuberculosis."

72. A.S. Griffith, "Observations on the Bovine Tubercle Bacillus in Human Tuberculosis."

73. Theobald Smith to Simon H. Gage, November 13, 1898.

74. Theobald Smith, Bibliography No. 146.

75. Theobald Smith, Bibliography No. 306.

Chapter 11:

1. C.L.A. Laveran, *Du Paludisme et de Son Hématozaire* (Paris, 1891); *Traité de Paludisme* (Paris, Masson & Cic, 1898).

2. C.L.A. Laveran, *Paludism* (London, New Sydenham Society, 1893), this being a translation by J.W. Martin of the foregoing.

3. W.T. Councilman, "Certain Elements Found in the Blood in Cases of Malarial Fever," *Transactions of the Association of American Physicians* (1886): 89–95; Discussion, pp. 96–97.

4. W. Osler, "An Address on the Hemotozoa of Malaria," *Transactions of the Pathological Society of Philadelphia*, 13 (1887): 255–276; also in *British Medical Journal*, 1 (1887): 556–562.

5. William Osler to Joseph Leidy, Jr., November 29, 1890. In Harvey Cushing, *The Life of Sir William Osler*, v. 2, pp. 337–338.

6. A.F.A. King, "Insects and Disease—Mosquitoes and Malaria," *Popular Science Monthly* 23 (1883): 644–658.

7. W.S. Thayer and J. Hewetson, *The Malarial Fevers of Baltimore* (Baltimore, 1895). Reprinted from *The Johns Hopkins Hospital Reports* 5 (1895): 3–218.

8. Theobald Smith to Simon H. Gage, August 31, 1884.

9. Theobald Smith, Bibliography No. 154.

10. "Malaria," Massachusetts State Board of Health, *Annual Reports, 1896–97*, pp. 700–704 (Public Document No. 34).

11. Theobald Smith, Diary, September 26, 1895.

12. Theobald Smith to Dr. Leonard D. White, October 12, 1895.

13. Theobald Smith to Leonard D. White, April 25, 1896.

14. Theobald Smith to Leonard D. White, May 14, 1896.

15. Theobald Smith to Leonard D. White, June 30, 1896.

16. Theobald Smith to Leonard D. White, April 9, 1897.

17. The printed form is preserved in Theobald Smith, Scrapbook No. 2, p. 5.

18. In contrast to Smith's laconic diary entries at the time of his Texas Fever discoveries, Ross was moved to compose at Secunderabad in August 1897 the following stanzas for his long poem *In Exile:* This day relenting God / Hath placed within my hand / A wondrous thing; and God / be praised. At His Command, / Seeking His secret deed / with tears and toiling breath, / I find thy cunning seeds, O million-murdering Death. / I know this little thing / A myriad men will save. / O Death, where is thy sting, Thy victory, O Grave! Many years later, John Masefield, the poet laureate, referred to this as "the only poem I ever read which kept me awake half through the night. It is a wonderful work." This is recounted in Ronald Ross's *Memoirs* (London, John Murray, 1923).

19. P. Manson to R. Ross, June 21, 1895.

20. P. Manson to R. Ross, February 7, 1898.

21. W.G. MacCallum, "On the Flagellated Form of the Malarial Parasite," *Lancet* 2 (November 13, 1897): 1740–1741.

22. R. Ross to M. Fabyan, January 4, 1915.

23. R. Ross to Theobald Smith, May 6, 1931.

24. Ross's thirty-year unsuccessful campaign to obtain monetary rewards from Britain and her institutions for solving the "great malaria problem" are described by Eli Chernin, "Sir Ronald Ross, Malaria, and the Rewards of Research," *Medical History* 32, No. 2 (April 1988): 119–141.

25. Theobald Smith, Bibliography, No. 143.

26. Theobald Smith, "Autobiographical Sketch sent to A.W. Milne, Secretary, Liverpool School of Tropical Medicine, 1907."

27. "Malaria," Massachusetts State Board of Health, *Annual Reports, 1896–97.*

28. Theobald Smith, Bibliography No. 143.

29. Theobald Smith, Bibliography No. 136.

30. Lilian Egleston Smith to Theobald Smith, July 9, 1903.

31. Theobald Smith, Bibliography No. 146.

32. Eleanor J. MacDonald, "A History of the Massachusetts Department of Health."

33. Theobald Smith, Diary, June 13, 1902.

34. Theobald Smith, Bibliography No. 156.

35. R.H. Dana to Theobald Smith, September 29, 1904.

36. L.O. Howard, *History of Applied Entomology* (Washington, D.C., 1930). Smithsonian Miscellaneous Collections, No. 84.

37. Ronald Moss, *Memoirs.*

38. Ibid.

39. Theobald Smith, Bibliography No. 306.

40. E.B. McKinley, "Theobald Smith," *Science* 62 (December 20, 1935): 575–586.

41. Theobald Smith, "Autobiographical Sketch sent to A.W. Milne, Secretary, Liverpool School of Tropical Medicine, 1907."

42. Theobald Smith to Simon H. Gage, October 6, 1897.

43. Theobald Smith, Bibliography No. 110.

44. Theobald Smith, Bibliography No. 111.

45. Theobald Smith, Bibliography No. 106.

46. Theobald Smith, Bibliography No. 107.

47. G.A. Soper, "The Epidemic of Typhoid Fever at Ithaca, N.Y.," *Journal of the New England Waterworks Association* 18 (1904): 431–461.

48. Theobald Smith, Bibliography No. 157.

49. Ibid.

50. Theobald Smith, Bibliography No. 188.

51. *Boston Post,* August 29, 1909, in Theobald Smith, Scrapbook No. 3.

Chapter 12:

1. G.W. Corner, *A History of the Rockefeller Institute, 1901–1953.*

2. R.M. Hawthorne, Jr., "Christian Archibald Herter, M.D. (1865–1910)," *Perspectives in Biology and Medicine* 18 (1974): 24–39.

3. W.H. Welch to C.A. Herter, March 31, 1901, Welch Papers, McChesney Archives, Johns Hopkins Medical School.

4. W.H. Welch to Theobald Smith, May 5, 1901.

5. Theobald Smith to Simon H. Gage, June 10, 1901.

6. Ibid.

7. G.W. Corner, *A History of the Rockefeller Institute, 1901–1953.*

8. Theobald Smith to Simon Flexner, June 26, 1904.

9. W.W. Oliver, *The Man Who Lived for Tomorrow. A Biography of William Hallock Park, M.D.* (New York, Dutton & Co., Inc., 1941).

10. W.H. Park and L.E. Holt, "Infant Feeding. Report upon the Results with Different Kinds of Pure and Impure Milk in Infant Feeding in Tenement Houses and Institutions in New York City. A Clinical and Bacteriological Study," *Archives of Pediatrics* 20 (December 1903): 881–909.

11. W.H. Welch to C.A. Herter, January 13, 1902.

12. Ibid.

13. Theobald Smith to W.H. Welch, February 11, 1902.

14. Ibid.

15. W.H. Welch to Theobald Smith, March 4, 1902.

16. L.F. Barker to Simon Flexner, March 5, 1902.

17. G.W. Corner, *A History of the Rockefeller Institute, 1901–1953.*

18. J.T. Flexner, *An American Odyssey. The Story of Helen Thomas and Simon Flexner* (Boston, Little, Brown & Co., 1984).

19. Memorandum, S. Flexner to W.H. Welch, April 8, 1902.

20. Simon Flexner to C.A. Herter, January 6, 1902.

21. C.A. Herter to Theobald Smith, date unascertained, but probably late September 1902.

22. Theobald Smith to C.A. Herter, September 30, 1902.

23. Theobald Smith to C.A. Herter, February 13, 1903.

24. C.A. Herter, *The Influence of Pasteur On Medical Science* (New York, Dodd, Mead & Co., 1904).

25. C.A. Herter to Theobald Smith, March 8, 1903.

26. C.A. Herter to Theobald Smith, December 28, 1903.

27. R.M. Hawthorne, Jr., "Christian Archibald Herter, M.D. (1865–1910)."

28. C.A. Herter to S. Flexner, July 1, 1907.

29. R.M. Hawthorne, Jr., "Christian Archibald Herter, M.D. (1865–1910)."

30. W.H. Welch to Susan Herter, December 6, 1910.

31. Jacques Loeb to Susan Herter, December 6, 1910.

32. Theobald Smith to G.F. Fabyan, March, 1903.

33. Theobald Smith, Scrapbook No. 2.

34. Lilian Egleston Smith to Theobald Smith, July 9, 1903.

35. Lilian Egleston Smith to Theobald Smith, July 16, 1903.

36. Lilian Egleston Smith to Theobald Smith, August 6, 1903.

Chapter 13:

1. Theobald Smith, Diary and Monthly Account Book, September 1903.

2. Theobald Smith, Diary and Monthly Account Book, October 1903.

3. E.J. Cohn, "The Unviersity and the Biooolgical Laboratories of the State of Massachusetts. A Short History," *Harvard Medical Alumni Bulletin* 24 (April 1950): 75–79.

4. Theobald Smith to President C.W. Eliot, August 27, 1904.
5. Theobald Smith to Simon Flexner, March 31, 1904.
6. Theobald Smith, Bibliography No. 158.
7. Theobald Smith, Bibliography No. 178.
8. Theobald Smith to Charles McCarthy, December 22, 1904.
9. Theobald Smith, Bibliography No. 149.
10. Theobald Smith to J.H. Huddleston, January 7, 1905.
11. Theobald Smith to Dr. [T.M.] Rotch, November 30, 1904.
12. Theobald Smith, Bibliography Nos. 97, 104, 108, 112.
13. Paul Ehrlich, "Die Werttemessung des Diphtherieheilserums und Deren Theoretischen Grundlagen."
14. Paul Ehrlich to Theobald Smith, undated, but written in late 1897.
15. Paul Ehrlich to Theobald Smith, January 3, 1898.
16. Theobald Smith to Paul Ehrlich, February 7, 1898, in the stylograph copybook of the Massachusetts State Department of Health Laboratories.
17. Theobald Smith, Bibliography No. 125.
18. Paul Ehrlich, "Ueber die Constitution des Diphtheriegiftes," *Deutsche Medizinische Wochenschrift* 24 (1898): 597–600.
19. Paul Ehrlich to Theobald Smith, December 2, 1898, Ehrlich Copybook, Series I, Book 2, pp. 144–146, Wellcome Historical Medical Library, London; Paul Ehrlich to Theobald Smith, undated, but written in May, 1899, also in Book 2 of Ehrlich's copybooks in the Wellcome Historical Medical Library.
20. Paul Ehrlich, "On Immunity with Special Reference to Cell Life," *Proceedings of the Royal Society of Medicine* 66 (1900): 424–448. This was delivered as the Society's Croonian Lecture.
21. Paul Ehrlich to Theobald Smith, November 15, 1898, Ehrlich Copybook, Series I, Book 2, p. 68. 22. Theobald Smith, *Parasitism and Disease,* p. 110 (Bibliography No. 307).
23. Theobald Smith, Bibliography No. 135.
24. Theobald Smith, Bibliography No. 140.
25. Theobald Smith, Bibliography Nos. 164 and 182.
26. Paul Ehrlich to Theobald Smith, November 18, 1902, Ehrlich Copybook, Series V, Book IX, pp. 300–305.
27. Paul Ehrlich to Theobald Smith, October 15, 1902.
28. Paul Ehrlich to Theobald Smith, November 18, 1902.
29. Paul Ehrlich to Theobald Smith, April 16, 1903, Ehrlich Copybook, Series V, Book XI, p. 123.
30. Theobald Smith, Bibliography No. 140.
31. Paul Ehrlich to Theobald Smith, May 11, 1903, Ehrlich Copybook, Series V, Book XI, pp. 246–248.
32. B. Heymann, "Zur Geschichte der Seitenketten Theorie Paul Ehrlichs," *Klinische Wochenschrift* 7 (1928): 1257–1260, 1305–1309.
33. M. Gruber, "Neue Früchte der Ehrlichschen Toxinlehre," *Wiener Klinische Wochenschrift* 16 (1903): 791–793.
34. Paul Ehrlich, "Toxin und Antitoxin. Entgegung auf den Neuesten Angriff Grubers," *Münchener Medizinische Wochenschrift* 1 (1903): 1428–1432, 1465–1469.
35. C.E. Dolman, "Paul Ehrlich and Willian Bulloch; A Correspondence and Friendship."

36. S. Arrhenius and T. Madsen, "Anwendung der Physikalischer Chemie auf das Studium der Toxine und Antitoxine," *Zeitschrift für Physikalischen Chemie* 44 (1903): 7–62.

37. Paul Ehrlich to Theobald Smith, November 30, 1903.

38. Sir Robert Muir, "Paul Ehrlich, 1854–1915," *Journal of Pathology and Bacteriology* 20 (1915): 349–360.

39. T. Madsen, "La Constitution de la Poison Diphtérique," *Centralblatt für Bakteriologie* 34, I. Abteilung (1903): 630–641.

40. Paul Ehrlich to Theobald Smith, November 12, 1903.

41. Paul Ehrlich to Theobald Smith, November 30, 1903.

42. Paul Ehrlich, I. "The Mutual Relations between Toxin and Antitoxin." II. Physical Chemistry v. Biology in the Doctrines of Immunity." III. "Cytotoxins and Cytotoxic Immunity." *Boston Medical and Surgical Journal* 150 (1904): 443–445, 445–448, 448–450 (translated and abstracted); "The Herter Lectures," reprinted in *The Collected Papers of Paul Ehrlich*, edited by F. Himmelwait and Sir Henry Dale (London, Pergamon Press, 1956), v. 2, pp. 410–413, 414–418, 419–422.

43. E.R. Long, *History of the American Association of Pathologists and Bacteriologists*.

44. M. Marquardt, *Paul Ehrlich* (London, Heinemann, 1949).

45. V.C. Vaughan, *A Doctor's Memories*, pp. 137–138.

46. Paul Ehrlich to Theobald Smith, May 19, 1904, Ehrlich Copybook, Series V, Book XIII, pp. 362–364.

47. H.W. Nernst, "Ueber die Anwendbarkeit der Gesetze des Chemische Gleichgewichts auf Gemische von Toxin und Antitoxin," *Zeitschrift für Elektrochemie* 10 (1904): 377–380.

48. M. Marquardt, *Paul Ehrlich*.

49. C.E. Dolman, "A Fiftieth Anniversary Commemorative Tribute to Paul Ehrlich, with Two Letters to American Friends," *Clio Medica* 1 (1966): 223–234.

50. Christian Herter to Theobald Smith, June 9, 1904.

51. T. Madsen and L. Walbum, "Toxines et Antitoxines. De la Ricine et de l'Antiricine," *Centralblatt für Bakteriologie* 56, I. Abteilung (1904): 242–256.

52. Paul Ehrlich to Theobald Smith, June 9, 1904, Ehrlich Copybook, Series V, Book XIII, pp. 460–462.

53. Paul Ehrlich to Theobald Smith, October 22, 1904.

54. Theobald Smith to Paul Ehrlich, November 2, 1904 (translated from German).

55. Theobald Smith, Bibliography No. 164.

56. Ibid.

57. E. Wernicke, "Ueber die Vererbung der Künstlich Erzeugten Diphtherie-Immunität bei Meerschweinchen," in *Festschrift zur 100 Jährigen Stiftungsfeier des Friedrich Wilhelms Institut* (Berlin, 1895), pp. 525–535.

58. Paul Ehrlich, "Ueber Immunität durch Vererbung und Säugung," *Zeitschrift für Hygiene und Infektionskrankheiten* 12 (1892): 183–203.

59. Theobald Smith, Bibliography No. 182.

60. Theobald Smith, Bibliography No. 191.

61. Ibid.

62. Theobald Smith, Bibliography No. 202.

63. E. von Behring, "Ueber ein Neues Diphtherieschutzmitten," *Deutsche Medizinische Wochenschrift* 29 (1913): 873–876.

64. C.E. Dolman, "A Fiftieth Anniversary Commemorative Tribute to Paul Ehrlich, with

Two Letters to American friends." The controversies aroused by Ehrlich's pioneering studies and proclamations on the mechanisms of toxin-antitoxin reactions have settled into a concept derived from three main sources, of which the predominant component is Ehrlich's hypothesis that diphtheria toxin forms a *chemical* union with its specific anti-toxin. The current view accepts Bordet's postulate that antigen and antibody do not unite in fixed proportions, and also adopts the assumptions of Arrhenius and Madsen that the antigen-antibody complex may be dissociable. See *Topley and Wilson's Principles of Bacteriology, Virology and Immunity,* 6th ed., v. 1 (Chapter 7), p. 254.

65. B. Heymann, "Zur Geschichte der Seitenketten Theorie Paul Ehrlichs."

66. Paul Ehrlich to Theobald Smith, July 29, 1905, Ehrlich Copybook, Series V, Book XVII, pp. 468–470.

67. R. Otto, "Das Theobald Smithsche Phanomen der Serum-Ueberempfindlichkeit," *Von Leuthold-Gedenkschrift* 1 (1906): 153–172.

68. P. Portier and C. Richet, "De l'Action Anaphylactique de Certains Venins," *Comptes Rendus de le Société de Biologie* 54 (1902): 170–172.

69. M.J. Rosenau and J.F. Anderson, *A Study of the Cause of Sudden Death Following the Injection of Horse Serum* (Washington, 1906), Hygenic Laboratory Bulletin No. 29.

70. M.J. Rosenau and J.F. Anderson, *I. Maternal Transmission of Immunity to Diphtheria Toxine. II. Maternal Transmission of Immunity to Diphtheria Toxine and Hypersusceptibility to Horse in the Same Animal* (Washington, 1906), Hygenic Laboratory Bulletin No. 30.

71. M.J. Rosenau and J.F. Anderson, "Hypersusceptibility," *Journal of the American Medical Association* 47 (1906): 1007–1010.

72. Sir Henry H. Dale to F.B. Bang, March 7, 1957.

73. Simon Flexner, The Pathologic Changes Caused by Certain Toxalbumens," *Medical News* 63 (1894): 116–124.

74. P.A. Lewis, "The Induced Susceptibility of the Guinea-Pig to the Toxic Action of the Blood Serum of the Horse," *Journal of Experimental Medicine* 10 (1909): 1–29.

75. Paul Ehrlich to Theobald Smith, February 12, 1910.

76. The allusion to "generous aid" is to a research grant of $10,000 allegedly made by John D. Rockefeller, Sr. as a personal gift to Ehrlich. The details are fuzzy, but Theobald Smith's part in the transaction would have been confined to approval of a proposal before the Board of Directors. The sponsors of the idea were probably Herter, Flexner, Welch, and John D. Rockefeller, Jr. See C.E. Dolman, "A Fiftieth Anniversary Commemorative to Paul Ehrlich, with Two Letters to American Friends."

77. Paul Ehrlich to Theobald Smith, February 12, 1910.

78. Theobald Smith to Paul Ehrlich, March 17, 1910.

79. Paul Ehrlich to Theobald Smith, March 30, 1910.

80. Ibid.

81. C.E. Dolman, "Ehrlich, Paul," in *Dictionary of Scientific Biography.*

82. Theobald Smith to Simon Flexner, March 31, 1904.

83. Theobald Smith, Bibliography No. 125.

84. Theobald Smith, Bibliography No. 306.

85. Theobald Smith, Bibliography No. 161.

86. *New York Tribune,* September 2, 1904; the article is preserved in Theobald Smith's Scrap-book No. 2, p. 71.

87. Theobald Smith, Bibliography No. 162.
88. Theobald Smith, Bibliography No. 165.
89. Theobald Smith, Bibliography No. 172.

Chapter 14:

1. F.C. Shattuck and J.L. Bremer, "The Medical School," in S.E. Morison, editor, *The Development of Harvard University since the Inauguration of President Eliot, 1869–1929* (Cambridge, Mass., Harvard University Press, 1930), 555–594; K.M. Ludmerer, "Reform at Harvard Medical School, 1869–1909," *Bulletin of the History of Medicine* 55 (1981): 343–379. For Harvard's pivotal role in helping reform American medical education, see Ludmerer's *Learning to Heal; the Development of American Medical Education* (New York, Basic Books, 1985).

2. Printed letter from "The Sons of Harvard" to President C.W. Eliot, March 20, 1904, Theobald Smith, Scrapbook No. 2, p. 53.

3. "The Harvard Medical School in 1788–89; Translated by D. Heald from 'Mémoires de Pierre de Sales la Terrière et de Ses Traverses' (1812)," *Boston Medical and Surgical Journal* 162 (April 21, 1910): 517–524. See also H.K. Beecher and M.D. Altschule, *Medicine at Harvard, the First 300 Years* (Hanover, N.H., The University Press of New England, 1977).

4. K.M. Ludmerer, "Reform at Harvard Medical School, 1869–1909;" Beecher and Altschule, *Medicine at Harvard; the First 300 Years.*

5. Editorial: "J.P. Morgan's Gift to Harvard University," *Boston Medical and Surgical Journal* 145 (July 4, 1901): 23–24.

6. F.C. Shattuck and J.L. Bremer, "The Medical School."

7. Editorial: Mr. John D. Rockefeller's Gift to Harvard University," *Boston Medical and Surgical Journal* 146 (February 6, 1902): 150.

8. J.C. Warren to G.F. Fabyan, undated, but probably early March 1902.

9. "The New Harvard Medical School Buildings," in *The Harvard Medical School, 1782–1906* (Cambridge, Mass., Harvard University Press, 1906), pp. 185–193.

10. "The New Harvard Medical School," *Harvard Graduates' Magazine* 14 (June 1906): 1–36.

11. Editorial: "Expansion of Harvard Unviersity Medical School," *Boston Medical and Surgical Journal* 146 (March 20, 1902): 135–136.

12. Theobald Smith, Monthly Account Book and Diary, June 7, 1906.

13. Theobald Smith, Monthly Account Book and Diary, June 6, 1906.

14. Theobald Smith, Monthly Account Book and Diary, March 15, 1904.

15. Theobald Smith, Monthly Account Book and Diary, June 10–15, 1906.

16. Theobald Smith, Monthly Account Book and Diary, Summary for month, July, 1906.

17. Theobald Smith, Day Card, September 25, 1906.

18. F.C. Shattuck, "Medical Education and the Clinics," in *Dedication of the New Buildings of the Harvard Medical School, September 25 and 26, 1906* (Boston, Harvard University Faculty of Medicine, 1906), pp. 12–16.

19. C.W. Eliot, "The Future of Medicine," in *Dedication of the New Buildings at the Harvard Medical School, September 25 and 26, 1906.*

20. W.H. Welch, "The Unity of the Medical Sciences," in *Dedication of the New Buildings at the Harvard Medical School, September 25 and 26, 1906.*

21. Theobald Smith, Monthly Account Book and Diary, September 30, 1906.

22. Theobald Smith to Simon H. Gage, December 13, 1907.

23. J.G. Hart, Secretary, Faculty of Arts and Sciences, Harvard University, to Theobald Smith, December 17, 1908.

24. L. Colebrook, *Almroth Wright, Provocative Doctor and Thinker* (London, Heinemann, 1954).

25. A.E. Wright to W.H. Welch, February 6, 1906.

26. Sir Almroth E. Wright, "The Opsonic Theory," *Canadian Practitioner and Review* 31 (November 1906): 605–620.

27. W.H. Welch to C.A. Herter, October 15, 1906.

28. Theobald Smith, Monthly Account Book and Diary, January 14, 1906.

29. Theobald Smith, Bibliography No. 177.

30. L. Colebrook, *Almoth Wright, Preventive Doctor and Thinker.*

31. Theobald Smith, Bibliography No. 196.

32. Theobald Smith, Bibliography No. 177.

33. Theobald Smith, Bibliography No. 208.

34. Theobald Smith, Bibliography No. 250.

35. Sir Almroth E. Wright, "On the Need for Abandoning Much in Immunology That Has Been Regarded as Assured," *Proceedings of the Royal Society of Medicine* 35 (January, 1942): 161–185.

36. Theobald Smith to C.W. Eliot, November 2, 1906.

37. George F. Fabyan to the President and Fellows of Harvard College, June 12, 1906.

38. Theobald Smith to C.W. Eliot, July 8, 1906.

39. C.W. Eliot to Theobald Smith, July 13, 1906.

40. Theobald Smith to C.W. Eliot, November 13, 1906.

41. C.W. Eliot to Theobald Smith, November 13, 1906, Theobald Smith, Scrapbook No. 2, p. 77.

42. Theobald Smith to C.W. Eliot, mistakenly dated September 31, 1906, but written probably on July 31, 1906.

43. F.H. Storer to C.W. Eliot, May 13, 1906.

44. Theobald Smith, Monthly Account Book and Diary, October 22 and 31, 1906.

45. Theobald Smith, Day Card, August 4, 1906.

46. F.H. Storer to Jerome D. Greene (President Eliot's secretary), May 26, 1906.

47. F.H. Storer to C.W. Eliot, February 17, 1907.

48. F.H. Storer to C.W. Eliot, February 24, 1907.

49. F.H. Storer to C.W. Eliot, April 23, 1907.

50. I.W. Bailey, Professor Emeritus of Forestry, Harvard University, personal interview with C.E. Dolman at the Harvard Herbarium, October 25, 1965.

51. W.H. Wheeler, "The Bussey Institution, 1871–1929," in S.E. Morison, editor, *The Development of Harvard University, 1849–1929*, Chapter XXI, pp. 508–517.

52. P.K. Russo, "The State Laboratory Institute," *Commonhealth* 3 (1974): 3–5; K.F. Girard, "A Tribute to Theobald Smith, M.D.," *Commonhealth* 4 (1975): 14–17.

Chapter 15:

1. Donald MacMillan, "A History of the Struggle to Abate Air Pollution from Copper Smelters of the Far West, 1885–1933," Ph.D. dissertation, University of Montana, 1973. Dr. MacMillan's dissertation was recently edited and published posthumously as *Smoke*

Wars: Anaconda Copper, Montana Air Polution and the Courts, 1890–1924 (Helena, Montana, Montana Historical Society, 2000).

2. *Inter-Mountain,* Butte, May 19, 1909.

3. *Inter-Mountain,* Butte, September 10, 1906.

4. "Anaconda II," *Fortune* 14 (December 1936): 82–95, 225–226, 228, 230, 232; "Anaconda II," *Fortune* 15 (January 1937): 75–77.

5. *Inter-Mountain,* Butte, May 19, 1909.

6. *Inter-Mountain,* Butte, January 22 and 23, 1906.

7. D. McEachern to Theobald Smith, February 20, 1906.

8. W.B. Wherry to Theobald Smith, February 27, 1906.

9. D. McEachern to Theobald Smith, March 7, 1906.

10. Theobald Smith to D. McEachern, March 14, 1906.

11. E.F. Mathewson to Theobald Smith, March 7, 1906.

12. "Autopsied three horses (#20-#22) in the barn near the open door," Theobald Smith, Monthly Account Book and Diary, April 9, 1906.

13. Theobald Smith, Monthly Account Book and Diary, special insert, March 21-April 17, 1906; also, Day Cards, April 18–21, 1906.

14. Theobald Smith to C.W. Eliot, April 23, 1906.

15. "Official Race Program, Butte Fair and Racing Association, Aug. 21 to Sept. 8, 1906," Theobald Smith, Scrapbook No. 2.

16. Theobald Smith, Monthly Account Book and Diary, September 3, 1906.

17. Theobald Smith to C.W. Eliot, September 7, 1906.

18. *Inter-Mountain,* Butte, November 20, 1906.

19. *Inter-Mountain,* Butte, November 21, 1906.

20. *Inter-Mountain,* Butte, November 20–23, 1906.

21. *Inter-Mountain,* Butte, November 24, 1906.

22. Theobald Smith to C.W. Eliot, November 28, 1906.

23. Theobald Smith to V.A. Moore, January 21, 1905.

24. Theobald Smith to Lilian Egleston Smith, December 18, 1906.

25. Theobald Smith, Monthly Account Book and Diary, January 1907.

26. Theobald Smith, Monthly Account Book and Diary, December 18–23, 1906.

27. *Inter-Mountain,* Butte, December 19 and 20, 1906.

28. *Inter-Mountain,* Butte, December 21, 1906.

29. *Inter-Mountain,* Butte, December 28, 29 and 31, 1906.

30. *Inter-Mountain,* Butte, January 8, 1907.

31. *Inter-Mountain,* Butte, January 1, 1907.

32. *Inter-Mountain,* Butte, January 5, 1907.

33. O.H.V. Stalheim, "Daniel Elmer Salmon, the National Veterinary College, and Veterinary Education," *Journal of the American Veterinary Association* 182 (January 1983): 32–36.

34. Theobald Smith to C.W. Eliot, February 27, 1907.

35. Theodore Roosevelt, *Letters, Edited by E.E. Morison* (Cambridge, Mass., Harvard University Press, 1952). Letters to Attorney General C.J. Bonaparte, December 9, 1908 and February 18, 1908, v. 6, pp. 1417–1418, 1527.

36. Theobald Smith to C.W. Eliot, March 10, 1907.

37. *Inter-Mountain,* Butte, October 5, 1907.
38. Theobald Smith to C.F. Kelley, June 7 and 11, 1910.
39. Theobald Smith to C.F. Kelley, June 25, 1910.

Chapter 16:
1. Theobald Smith, Bibliography No. 306.
2. Editorial. "Annual Report of Harvard University, 1905–1906," *Boston Medical and Surgical Journal* 156 (April 11, 1907): 478–480.
3. Theobald Smith, Scrapbook No. 3.
4. Editorial. "Annual Report of Harvard University, 1907–1908," *Boston Medical and Surgical Journal* 160 (April 1, 1909): 417–419.
5. Miscellany. "Harvard Public Medical Lectures for 1911," *Boston Medical and Surgical Journal* 163 (December 29, 1910): 1009.
6. Theobald Smith, Monthly Account and Diary, March 31, 1909.
7. Editorial. "Prof. Theobald Smith's Lowell Institute Lectures," *Boston Medical and Surgical Journal* 160 (April 22, 1909): 522.
8. Theobald Smith, Scrapbook No. 3.
9. Theobald Smith, Bibliography Nos. 194 and 195.
10. Theobald Smith, Bibliography No. 192.
11. C.W. Eliot to Theobald Smith, May 29, 1908.
12. Theobald Smith to C.W. Eliot, June 1, 1908.
13. C.W. Eliot to Theobald Smith, June 2, 1908.
14. Theobald Smith to C.W. Eliot, August 17, 1904.
15. Theobald Smith, Day Card, November 19, 1907.
16. C.W. Eliot to Theobald Smith, November 7, 1904.
17. Theobald Smith, Monthly Account Book and Diary, June 30, 1905.
18. C.W. Eliot to Theobald Smith, July 28, 1908.
19. C.W. Eliot to Theobald Smith, August 26, 1908.
20. C.W. Eliot, "Remarks Made at the 170th Anniversary of the Massachusetts Medical Society," *Boston Medical and Surgical Journal* 138 (June 16, 1898): 570.
21. C.W. Eliot to Theobald Smith, July 9, 1907. "Dr. G——" was Charles Montraville Green.
22. Theobald Smith to C.W. Eliot, July 13, 1907.
23. C.W. Eliot to Theobald Smith, July 15, 1907.
24. Editorial. "Annual Report of Harvard University, 1906–07," *Boston Medical and Surgical Journal* 158 (April 23, 1908): 558–560.
25. H.P. Walcott to C.W. Eliot, September 18, 1908.
26. Theobald Smith to C.W. Eliot, May 4, 1909.
27. Lilian Egleston Smith to Theobald Smith, December 15, 1907.
28. E.L. Trudeau, "An Experimental Study of Preventive Inoculation in Tuberculosis," *Medical Record* 38 (November 22, 1890): 563–568.
29. E.L. Trudeau, "Eye Tuberculosis and Anti-Tubercular Inoculation in the Rabbit," *Transactions of the Association of American Physicians* 8 (1893): 112; discussion, pp. 113–116.
30. E.L. Trudeau, "Remarks on Artificial Immunity in Tuberculosis," *British Medical Journal* 2 (December 25, 1897): 1849–1850.
31. E. von Behring, F. Römer and W.G. Ruppel, "Tuberkulose," *Beiträge zur Experimentelle Therapie* 5 (1902): paged as a separate publication, xviii, 28 pp.

32. L. Pearson and G.H. Gilliland, "Some Experiments upon the Immunization of Cattle against Tuberculosis," *Journal of Comparative Medicine and Veterinary Archives* 21 (November 1902): 673–688.

33. Simon Flexner, "Immunization from Tuberculosis," *Philadelphia Medical Journal* 11 (February 14, 1903): 284–285.

34. Daniel E. Salmon, "Immunization from Tuberculosis," *Philadelphia Medical Journal* 11 (June 13, 1903): 966–970.

35. D.E. Salmon to Simon Flexner, July 14, 1903.

36. Theobald Smith, Bibliography No. 177.

37. H. Noguchi, "A Method for the Cultivation of Pathogenic Treponema Pallidum (Spirochaete Pallida)," *Journal of Experimental Medicine* 14 (1911): 99–108.

38. Theobald Smith, Bibliography No. 168.

39. Theobald Smith, Bibliography No. 177.

40. Theobald Smith, Monthly Account Book and Diary, November 26, 1904.

41. V.Y. Bowditch, *Life and Correspondence of Henry Ingersoll Bowditch* (Cambridge, Mass., Riverside Press, 1902), pp. 217–231.

42. Theobald Smith, Bibliography No. 177.

43. Theobald Smith, Bibliography No. 187.

44. Theobald Smith, Bibliography No. 185.

45. C.W. Eliot to Theobald Smith, July 12, 1908.

46. Theobald Smith to C.W. Eliot, July 14, 1908.

47. Theobald Smith, Bibliography Nos. 203, 223.

48. Simon Flexner to Theobald Smith (telegrams), April 9, 1908, Theobald Smith, Scrapbook No. 3.

49. Robert Koch, Dinner Speech at Waldorf Astoria Hotel, New York, April 11, 1908.

50. "A Dinner to Dr. Robert Koch," *New York Medical Journal* 87 (April 18, 1908): 748–749.

51. Robert Koch, "The Relations of Human and Bovine Tuberculosis," *Journal of the American Medical Association* 51 (October 10, 1908): 1256–1258, followed by "Conference in Camera on Human and Bovine Tuberculosis," pp. 1262–1268.

52. G. Pannwitz, "Koch's Standpunkt in der Frage nach den Beziehungen zwischen Menschen und Kindertuberkulose beim Tuberkulose-Kongress in Washington 1908," *Berliner Klinische Wochenschrift* 45 (November 2, 1908): pp. 2001–2003; discussion, pp. 2003–2006.

53. Theobald Smith, Bibliography No. 230.

54. Theobald Smith, Bibliography No. 305.

55. Theobald Smith, Bibliography Nos. 272 and 273.

56. Theobald Smith, Bibliography No. 272.

57. Theobald Smith, Bibliography No. 273.

58. C.J. Hatfield to Theobald Smith, March 11, 1932.

Chapter 17:

1. Medical Notes. "Prof. Theobald Smith Honored," *Boston Medical and Surgical Journal* 158 (April 12, 1908): 461.

2. Editorial. "The Work of the Cancer Commission of Harvard University," *Boston Medical and Surgical Journal* 162 (April 28, 1910): 579.

3. M. Fabyan, "History of the Department of Comparative Pathology and Tropical Medicine," p. 73.

4. Editorial. "A Department of Tropical Medicine," *Boston Medical and Surgical Journal* 159 (August 13, 1908): 218.

5. A.L. Lowell, "Inaugural Address, October 6, 1909," in S.E. Morison, *The Development of Harvard University,* pp. lxxix-lxxxviii; also in *Harvard Graduates' Magazine* 18 (1909): 211–223.

6. C.W. Eliot, *President's Annual Report of Harvard College, 1904–1905,* p. 52.

7. F.L. Higgingon, "Notice to Subscribers. The Charles W. Eliot Fund, April 28, 1909," in Theobald Smith, Scrapbook No. 3, p. 17.

8. "Official Notice of Appointment," January 11, 1909, in Theobald Smith, Scrapbook No. 3, p. 19.

9. "Provisional Programme, Darwin Commemoration, University of Cambridge, January 30, 1909," in Theobald Smith, Scrapbook No. 3, p. 20.

10. *Final List of Delegates and Other Guests Invited by the University* (Cambridge, Cambridge University Press, June 19, 1909), in Theobald Smith, Scrapbook No. 3, p. 21.

11. Theobald Smith, Monthly Account Book and Diary, June 1910.

12. Theobald Smith, "Address to the Graduating Class, Girls Latin School," June 24, 1910, Transcript, Theobald Smith, Scrapbook No. 3, p. 42.

13. Theobald Smith, Day Card, January 1910. Karl Landsteiner and Erwin Popper had recently, for the first time, transmitted the disease to monkeys, a significant step in the scientific study of poliomyelitis (See Chapter 19, Note 36).

14. "Announcement. Evening Meeting of American Academy of Arts and Sciences, Boston, October 12, 1910," Theobald Smith, Scrapbook No. 3, p. 34.

15. "Dinner Menu and Progam. Celebration of the One Thousandth Meeting, American Academy of Arts and Sciences, University Club, Boston, December 14, 1910," Theobald Smith, Scrapbook No. 3, p. 49.

16. J. O'Sullivan, M.D., City of New York Law Department, to Theobald Smith, July 21, 1911, Theobald Smith, Scrapbook No. 3, p. 64.

17. J.J. Abel to Theobald Smith, April 1, 1907.

18. Theobald Smith to E.J. James, April 9, 1907.

19. Theobald Smith, Scrapbook No. 2, p. 87.

20. Theobald Smith, Day Card, December 28, 1907.

21. University of Illinois, "Proceedings of the Board of Trustees," June 24, 1909, pp. 195–197.

22. Ibid.

23. H.S. Grindley to Theobald Smith, June 10, 1910.

24. E.J. James to Theobald Smith, April 26, 1913.

25. H.S. Grindley, T. Mojonnier and H.C. Porter, *Studies of the Effects of Different Methods of Cooking upon the Thoroughness and Ease of Digestion at the University of Illinois* (Washington, D.C., 1907), *U.S. Department of Agriculture Bulletin No. 193.*

26. Theobald Smith, Bibliography Nos. 121, 193, 215.

27. Theobald Smith, Day Card, January 6, 1911.

28. "Appointment of Professor Theobald Smith to the Referee Board of Consulting Scientific Experts," *American Food Journal* (March 15, 1911): 21, in Theobald Smith, Scrapbook No. 3, p. 52.

29. I. Remsen to Theobald Smith, August 5, 1911, Theobald Smith, Scrapbook No. 3, p. 58.
30. I. Remsen to Mrs. C. Herter, August 5, 1911.
31. Theobald Smith, Bibliography No. 210.
32. Acting Secretary, U.S. Department of Agriculture to Theobald Smith, February 26, 1914.
33. I. Remsen to Theobald Smith, April 10, 1915.

Chapter 18:

1. A.L. Lowell to Theobald Smith, January 6, 1911, Theobald Smith, Scrapbook No. 3, p. 55.
2. Theobald Smith, Day Card, March 13, 1910.
3. Theobald Smith to A.L. Lowell, January 9, 1911.
4. Theobald Smith to A.L. Lowell, January 25, 1911.
5. Jerome G. Greene to Theobald Smith, January 28, 1911.
6. A.L. Lowell to Theobald Smith, March 24, 1911.
7. Theobald Smith to A.L. Lowell, March 26, 1911.
8. Charles S. Minot to Theobald Smith, March 28, 1911.
9. Francis G. Peabody to Theobald Smith, March 31, 1911.
10. Theobald Smith to Francis G. Peabody, April 1, 1911.
11. Carl Flügge to Theobald Smith, May 24, 1911 (translated from German).
12. Theobald Smith to A.L. Lowell, June 14, 1911.
13. Theobald Smith to Carl Flügge, July 15, 1911 (translated from German).
14. H. Uhthuff to Theobald Smith, August 8, 1911 (translated from German).
15. Philip H. Smith to Theobald Smith, August 1, 1911, Theobald Smith, Scrapbook No. 3, p. 64.
16. Theobald Smith, Day Card, December 10–18, 1911.
17. "Die Antrittsvorlesung des Neuen Austauchprofessors," *Berliner Tageblatt* (Abendsausgabe), January 13, 1912; with translated excerpt in *New York Tribune,* February 1, 1912, Theobald Smith, Scrapbook No. 4, pp. 4, 6.
18. "Parasitismus und Krankheit. Antrittsvorlesung des Austauchprofessors Dr. Theobald Smith," *Vossiche Zeitung,* Berlin, January 13, 1912.
19. Theobald Smith, Bibliography No. 205.
20. Berlin Universität, *Studienplan für Mediziner* (Berlin, 1912), Theobald Smith, Scrapbook No. 4, p. 27.
21. Theobald Smith, Diary, March 7, 1912.
22. Theobald Smith, Bibliography No. 204.
23. M. Fabyan, "A Contribution to the Pathogenesis of B. Abortus Bang. II," *Journal of Medical Research* 26 (July 1912): 441–487.
24. "Anglo American Med. Club. Notice of Lecture Meeting on March 9, 1912, at the 'Atlas' Restaurant, Friedrichstrasse 105, Berlin," Theobald Smith, Scrapbook No. 4, p. 33.
25. Abraham Flexner, *Prostitution in Europe* (New York, Century Co., 1914).
26. Abraham Flexner, *I Remember,* pp. 196–197.
27. Kultusminister von Trott zu Solz to Theobald Smith, December 23, 1911.
28. Theobald Smith, Day Card, May 2, 1912.

29. Friedrich Schmidt to Theobald Smith, April 28, 1912.

30. Freie Vereinigung für Mikrobiologie. Provisional Program Appended to a Printed Letter from A. Gärtner, Jena, May 14, 1912, Theobald Smith, Scrapbook No. 4, p. 35.

31. Theobald Smith, Monthly Account Book and Diary, March 26, 1912.

32. Theobald Smith, Day Cards, March 26–30, 1912.

33. *Nachtrag zum Vorlesungsverzeichnis des Hamburgen Kolonialinstitute . . . in das Sommersemester 1912* (Hamburg, 1912), Theobald Smith, Scrapbook No. 4, p. 37.

34. Theobald Smith, Day Cards, June 13–14, 19–20, 1912.

35. Theobald Smith to Simon Flexner, March 4, 1913.

36. Simon Flexner to Theobald Smith, March 8, 1913.

37. W.P. Dunbar, "Investigations into the Question of Bubonic Plague and Assistance in Furthering the Same in India," typescript, November 26, 1912.

38. Theobald Smith, Bibliography No. 210.

39. Theobald Smith, Day Cards, April 15–22, 1912.

40. Hugo Münsterberg to Theobald Smith, April 18, 1911.

41. A.L. Lowell to D.J. Hill (American Ambassador to Germany), April 29, 1911.

42. "Berlin Court Fixes the Social Status of American Exchange Professors," *New York Tribune,* Berlin, February 17, 1912, Theobald Smith, Scrapbook No. 4, p. 6.

43. Dr. Dorothea Smith Farr, personal conversations with C.E. Dolman, February 14–16, 1965.

44. Theobald Smith, Day Card, February 7, 1912.

45. K.O. Bertling to Theobald Smith, December 29, 1911, Theobald Smith, Scrapbook No. 4, p. 22.

46. "Order of Speaking and Menu, Ninth Anniversary Banquet, American Association of Commerce and Trade in Berlin," January 15, 1912, Theobald Smith, Scrapbook No. 4, p. 29.

47. Theobald Smith, "Washington's Birthday, February 22, 1912," Celebration Address to American Colony in Berlin, Zoological Garden Restaurant, the original, much-corrected manuscript of this address is preserved in Theobald Smith's Scrapbook No. 4, p. 18.

48. Calender of the American Church in Berlin, March 3, 1912, Theobald Smith, Scrapbook No. 4, p. 36.

49. Theobald Smith, "Remarks at Farewell Dinner," May 18, 1912, Manuscript in German, Theobald Smith, Scrapbook No. 4, p. 32.

50. "The Final Lecture of the Exchange Professor," *Berliner Tageblatt* (morning edition), June 26, 1912 (translated from German), Theobald Smith, Scrapbook No. 4, p. 55.

51. G.T. Sch., "Professor Theobald Smith on America and Germany. The Difference between American and German Professors and Students," *Berliner Tageblatt,* June 29, 1912 (translated from German), Theobald Smith, Scrapbook No. 4, p. 55.

52. Heslop & Co., Ladies' Tailors, Oxford St., London, "Bill for 3 Ladies' Costumes and a Coat, £18–3–6, August 9, 1912, Lilian Egleston Smith's Address Book.

53. Theobald Smith, Day Cards, August 11–14, 16–19, 1912.

54. C.S. Minot to Theobald Smith, February 16, 1912.

55. C.S. Minot to Theobald Smith, October 10, 1912.

56. Theobald Smith, Day Card, November 23, 1914.

57. K.G. Bertling to Theobald Smith, August 20, 1912 (translated from German).

58. Friedrich Schmidt to Theobald Smith, November 14, 1912 (translated from German).

59. C. Flügge to Theobald Smith, March 16, 1913 (translated from German).

Chapter 19:

1. Theobald Smith to Simon Flexner, September 27, 1912.
2. Theobald Smith, Bibliography No. 207.
3. Theobald Smith, Day Card, November 22, 1912.
4. M.C. Hall to Theobald Smith, January 17, 1913, Theobald Smith, Scrapbook No. 3, p. 76.
5. Theobald Smith, Day Card, April 28, 1914.
6. Theobald Smith, Day Card, March 4, 1914.
7. J.A. Curran, *Founders of the Harvard School of Public Health, with Biographical Notes, 1909–1946* (New York, Josiah Macy Jr. Foundation, 1970).
8. Theobald Smith, Day Cards, December 15, 16 and 17, 1912.
9. Editorial. "The Department of Preventative Medicine and Hygiene and the New Degree of Doctor of Public Health," *Boston Medical and Surgical Journal* 166 (June 13, 1912): 866–867.
10. J.A. Curran, *Founders of the Harvard School of Public Health, with Biographical Notes, 1909–1946.*
11. Ibid, pp. 258–259.
12. "Farewell to Professor Theobald Smith," *New York Tribune,* Berlin, June 24, 1912, of which a clipping is in Theobald Smith's Scrapbook No. 4, p. 40.
13. A.L. Lowell to Theobald Smith, December 23, 1912.
14. Mrs. Elizabeth Putnam to Theobald Smith, December 19, 1912.
15. Theobald Smith, Day Card, December 3, 1912.
16. Theobald Smith, Bibliography No. 204.
17. Ibid.
18. M. Fabyan, "A Contribution to the Pathogenesis of B. Abortus Bang. II."
19. M. Fabyan, "The Persistence of B. Abortus Bang in the Tissues of Inoculated Animals," *Journal of Medical Research* 28 (May 1913): 81–83.
20. M. Fabyan, "A Note on the Presence of B. Abortus in Cow's Milk," *Journal of Medical Research* 28 (May 1913): 85–89.
21. Theobald Smith, Day Card, December 16, 1913.
22. Ibid.
23. Theobald Smith, Bibliography No. 212.
24. Theobald Smith, Monthly Account Book and Diary, November 18, 1913.
25. J.P. McGowan, "Some Observations on a Laboratory Epidemic, Principally among Dogs and Cats, in Which the Animal Effected Presented the Symptoms of the Disease Called 'Distemper'," *Journal of Pathology and Bacteriology* 15 (1911): 372–420.
26. P.P. Laidlaw and G.N. Dunkin, "Studies in Dog Distemper; Immunization of Dogs," *Journal of Comparative Pathology & Therapeutics* 41 (1928): 209–227.
27. Theobald Smith, Day Card, May 22, 1913.
28. Theobald Smith, Day Card, May 28, 1913.
29. Theobald Smith, Bibliography No. 216.
30. R.C. Lancefield, "A Serological Differentiation of Human and Other Groups of Hemolytic Streptococci," *Journal of Experimental Medicine* 61 (1933): 335–349.

31. Theobald Smith, Day Card, January 9, 1910.
32. S. Flexner and P.A. Lewis, "The Transmission of Acute Poliomyelitis to Monkeys," *Journal of the American Medical Association* 53 (November 13, 1909): 1639.
33. Theobald Smith, Day Card, June 17, 1914.
34. Carl TenBroeck (with Introductory Note by Theobald Smith), "Experiments to Determine if Paralyzed Domestic Animals and Those Associated with Cases of Infantile Paralysis May Transmit the Disease," *Monthly Bulletin of the Board of Health of Massachusetts* 28 (1914): 315–334.
35. Ibid.
36. Karl Landsteiner and E. Popper, "Uebertragung der Poliomyelitis Acuta und Affen," *Zeitschrift für Immunitätsforschung und Experimentelle Therapie Originale* 2 (1909): 377–390.
37. Theobald Smith, Bibliography No. 134.
38. S. Flexner and H. Noguchi, "Experiments on the Cultivation of the Virus of Poliomyelitis. Fifteenth Note," *Journal of the American Medical Association* 60 (February 1, 1913): 362.
39. Theobald Smith, Day Card, August 10, 1913.
40. I. Plesset, *Noguchi and His Patrons* (London, Associated University Presses, 1980), pp. 136–141.
41. H. Noguchi, "Contribution to the Cultivation of the Parasite of Rabies," *Journal of Experimental Medicine* 18 (1913): 314–316.
42. Theobald Smith, Day Card, October 27, 1912.
43. Theobald Smith, Day Card, December 6, 1913.
44. Theobald Smith, Day Card, June 12, 1913.
45. Theobald Smith, Day Card, November 8, 1913.
46. C. Curtice, "Foul Typhoid," *Rhode Island Agricultural Experiment Station Bulletin No. 87* (Providence, E.L. Freeman and Son, 1902), pp. 3–10.
47. Theobald Smith, Bibliography No. 217.
48. Theobald Smith, Bibliography No. 218.
49. Theobald Smith, Bibliography No. 219.
50. For instance, *ASM News* for August 1989, was recently mailed to the thousands of current members of the American Society of Microbiologists—a society directly descended from the Society of American Bacteriologists, which Theobald Smith helped to found ninety years before. It contained as a 500 gm. supplement the Program for the Twenty-ninth Interscience Conference on Antimicrobial Agents and Chemotherapy, sponsored by the Society. This program documented 113 sessions and 1,361 presentations. Over 4,430 participants had registered, and there were more than 150 exhibiting companies. In addition, a supporting array of technicians and helpers of various grades carried on in their home laboratories behind this frenzy of gossip and torrent of time-rationed reports.
51. Simon Flexner's natural leadership and organizational talents made him eventually Director of the whole Institute, including the Hospital and the Animal Pathology Department. His initial appointment as a Scientific Director and Director of the Laboratories dated from 1901. Only in 1924, according to Corner's *History of the Rockefeller Institute, 1901–1953* (p. 154), was he formally declared Director of the whole Institute.
52. S.A. Knopf, *A History of the National Tuberculosis Association* (Philadelphia, 1922).
53. Theobald Smith, Bibliography No. 103.
54. Theobald Smith, Bibliography No. 99.

55. L.J. Cole and P.B. Bradley, *Blackhead in Turkeys. A Study in Avian Coccidiosis* (Providence, E.L. Freeman Co. [1910]), pp. 139–271, *Rhode Island Experiment Station Bulletin No. 141*.

56. Theobald Smith, Bibliography No. 197.

57. Theobald Smith, Bibliography No. 148, 149.

58. Theobald Smith, Bibliography No. 197.

59. Theobald Smith, Monthly Account Book and Diary, May 13, 1913.

60. Theobald Smith, Bibliography No. 224.

61. S. Flexner, "J.J. Hill and Dept. of Animal Pathology," Flexner Reminiscences ("Diaries"), Chocorua, New Hampshire, July 17, 1932.

62. Rockefeller Institute for Medical Research, Excerpts from Minutes of the Executive Committee and of the Board of Scientific Directors, headed, "Facts Relating to the Establishment of the Princeton Dept.," October 22, 1913, to April 18, 1914 (Minutes of Executive Committee, October 22, 1913).

63. Paul Ehrlich to Simon Flexner, October 2, 1913 (in German).

64. Theobald Smith to Simon Flexner, October 26, 1913.

65. Simon Flexner to Theobald Smith, October 30, 1913.

66. G.W. Corner, *A History of the Rockefeller Institute, 1901–1953*.

67. Rockefeller Institute for Medical Research, Excerpt from the Minutes of the Executive Commitee, November 12, 1913.

68. Theobald Smith to T.M. Prudden, undated, but written near the end of December 1913.

69. Rockefeller Institute for Medical Research, Excerpt from Minutes of the Board of Scientific Director, January 10, 1914.

70. Theobald Smith, Day Cards, January 19 and February 2, 1914.

71. Rockefeller Institute for Medical Research, Excerpt from Minutes of the Executive Committee, February 5, 1914.

72. Rockefeller Institute for Medical Research, Excerpt from Minutes of the Executive Committee, March 11, 1914.

73. Rockefeller Institute for Medical Research, Excerpt from Minutes of the Executive Committee, March 20, 1914.

74. S. Flexner and J.J. Flexner, *William Henry Welch and the Heroic Age of American Medicine*, p. 295.

75. Rockefeller Institute for Medical Research, Excerpt from Minutes of the Executive Committee, April 1, 1914.

76. Theobald Smith, Day Card, March 31, 1914.

77. Theobald Smith to Simon Flexner, March 31, 1914.

78. Theobald Smith to Simon Flexner, April 1, 1914.

79. S. Flexner to Theobald Smith, March 30, 1914.

80. Theobald Smith, Day Card, May 28, 1914.

81. S. Flexner to Theobald Smith, April 3, 1914.

82. Theobald Smith, Day Card, April 4, 1914.

83. Theobald Smith to Simon Flexner, April 6, 1914.

84. Theobald Smith, Day Card, April 6, 1914.

85. Theobald Smith, Day Card, April 9, 1914.

86. Rockefeller Institute for Medical Research, Excerpt from Minutes of the Executive Committee, April 9, 1914.

87. Theobald Smith, Day Card, April 14, 1914.
88. S. Flexner and J.J. Flexner, *William Henry Welch and the Heroic Age of American Medicine.*
89. Theobald Smith to A.L. Lowell, April 14, 1914.
90. C. Dunham to A.L. Lowell, April 18, 1914.
91. A.L. Lowell to C. Dunham, April 21, 1914.
92. C.W. Eliot to Theobald Smith, April 15, 1914.
93. Theobald Smith to A.L. Lowell, April 22, 1914.
94. Rockefeller Institute for Medical Research, Excerpt from Minutes of the Board of Scientific Directors, April 18, 1914.
95. Ibid.
96. "The Railroaders," in *The Old West* (New York, Time-Life Books, 1973), pp. 221–224.
97. Theobald Smith to Simon Flexner, May 4, 1914.
98. Theobald Smith, Day Card, May 18, 1914.
99. Theobald Smith, Day Cards, May 14–16, 1914.
100. S. Flexner to Theobald Smith, May 20, 1914.
101. P., T. M., "Professor Theobald Smith and a New Outlook in Animal Pathology," *Science* 39 (May 22, 1914): 751–754.
102. "Appointment of Dr. Smith at the Rockefeller Institute," *Boston Medical and Surgical Journal* 170 (May 28, 1914): 848.
103. Theobald Smith to H.P. Walcott, July 2, 1914.
104. M.W. Richardson, Secretary of the Massachusetts State Board of Health, to Theobald Smith, July 11, 1914, Theobald Smith, Scrapbook No. 5, p. 33.
105. Theobald Smith to Simon H. Gage, April 6, 1915.
106. Theobald Smith to Simon H. Gage, August 24, 1915.
107. Theobald Smith to Simon H. Gage, December 24, 1914.
108. Theobald Smith to Simon H. Gage, August 24, 1915.
109. Ibid.

Chapter 20:
1. R.J. Hendrick, "American Contributions to Medical Science," *Harper's Monthly Magazine* 129 (June 1914): 25–32.
2. J. Middlteon, "A Great American Scientist," *The World's Work* (July 1914): 299–302.
3. Theobald Smith, Scrapbook No. 5, p. 9.
4. Theobald Smith, Day Card, March 23, 1914.
5. Theobald Smith, Day Card, June 4, 1914.
6. Theobald Smith, Day Card, July 10, 1914.
7. Theobald Smith to A. Calmette, November 25, 1913.
8. I.J. Paderewski, *Concerto in A Minor for Pianoforte and Orchestra, Op. 17,* Eighteenth Concert Programme, Boston Symphony Orchestra, March 14, 1914. Theobald Smith, Scrapbook No. 5, p. 4.
9. National Academy of Sciences, Program, Annual Meeting, April 21–23, 1914. Theobald Smith, Scrapbook No. 5, p. 10.
10. Theobald Smith, Bibliography No. 220.
11. Theobald Smith, Bibliography No. 306.
12. Abraham Flexner to Lilian Egleston Smith, February 11, 1935.
13. Theobald Smith, Bibliography No. 220.

14. Theobald Smith, Day Card, October 20, 1914.

15. J.J. Sugg, Letter to the Editor, covering A.F. Coca's "'Gestation and Birth' of the *Journal of Immunology* by the Accoucheur," *AAI Newsletter* (October 1985): 2–4.

16. G. Esdall, "What is Immunology?", *Journal of Immunology* 17 (1951): 167–172.

17. Theobald Smith, Bibliography No. 15.

18. Theobald Smith, Bibliography No. 155.

19. R. Otto, "Das Theobald Smithsche Phänomen der Serum-Ueberempfindlichkeit."

20. Theobald Smith, Bibliography No. 182.

21. Theobald Smith, Bibliography No. 191.

22. Theobald Smith, Bibliography No. 253.

23. Theobald Smith, Bibliography No. 177.

24. Theobald Smith, Bibliography No. 196.

25. Theobald Smith, Bibliography No. 208.

26. Theobald Smith, Bibliography No. 227.

27. Theobald Smith, Bibliography No. 250.

28. "Report 97–894. House Appropriations Committee," *AAI Newsletter* (March 1983).

29. Marshal Fabyan, "History of the Department of Comparative Pathology" and "Miscellaneous Notes on Complimentary Dinner to Theobald Smith," Harvard Medical Archives in The Francis A. Countway Library of Medicine.

30. Lilian Egleston Smith to Marshal Fabyan, March 17, 1915.

31. Theobald Smith, Day Card, June 2, 1915.

32. Excerpts from typescript collection of speeches made at a Complimentary Dinner to Theobald Smith, Harvard Club, Boston, June 2, 1915, in "Miscellaneous Notes on Complimentary Dinner to Theobald Smith" (Note 29).

33. Bela Pratt to Theobald Smith, August 8, 1915 and January 26, 1916.

34. See Chapter 11, p. 212.

35. Paul Ehrlich (through Marshal Fabyan) to Theobald Smith, March 9, 1915 (translated from German).

36. William Osler to Marshal Fabyan, January 4, 1915.

37. Editorial. "The Harvard Expeditionary Unit," *Boston Medical and Surgical Journal* 172 (March 18, 1915): 419–420.

38. Excerpts from typescript collection of speeches made at a Complimentary Dinner to Theobald Smith, Harvard Club, Boston, June 2, 1915.

39. "Complimentary Dinner to Dr. Theobald Smith," *Boston Medical and Surgical Journal* 82, No. 23 (June 10, 1915): 873.

40. Theobald Smith, Monthly Account Book and Diary, June 2, 1915.

41. Marshal Fabyan and H.P. Aitken, "Thanks to You, Theobald Smith," Theobald Smith, Scrapbook No. 5, p. 52. For further details, see Eli Chernin, "A Unique Tribute to Theobald Smith, 1915," *Review of Infectious Diseases* 9, no. 3 (May-June 1987): 625–635.

42. W.S. Halsted to Marshal Fabyan, June 14, 1915.

43. William Osler to Marshal Fabyan, June 22, 1915.

44. William Noyes to Marshal Fabyan, June 3, 1915.

45. J.P. Van Derveer to Marshal Fabyan, June 10, 1915.

46. H. Lee Higginson to Francis Wright Fabyan, June 3, 1915.

47. George Fabyan to A.L. Lowell, June 17, 1915.

48. A.L. Lowell to George Fabyan, July 1, 1915.

49. George Fabyan to A.L. Lowell, July 7, 1915.

50. A.L. Lowell to George Fabyan, July 13, 1915.

51. George Fabyan to A.L. Lowell, July 15, 1915.

52. A.L. Lowell to George Fabyan, July 21, 1915.

53. Theobald Smith, Day Card, August 16 and 17, 1915.

54. Theobald Smith, Bibliography No. 224.

55. Theobald Smith to Simon H. Gage, August 24, 1915.

56. Program, Radcliffe College Commencement, Sanders Theatre, June 23, 1915, Theobald Smith, Scrapbook No. 5, p. 43.

57. "Resignation [Prof. Theobald Smith]," *Harvard University Gazette* 10 (May 15, 1915): 3.

58. Theobald Smith, Day Cards, August 16 and 17, 1915.

59. Philip Smith, Personal communication to Claude E. Dolman.

60. G.H. Palmer, "Münsterberg," in S.E. Morison, editor, *Development of Harvard University, 1869–1929* (Cambridge, Mass., Harvard University Press, 1939), pp. 17–19.

61. Mrs. Theobald Smith, X-ray, right shoulder and arm, October 12, 1915, Theobald Smith, Scrapbook, No. 5, p. 57.

62. Simon Flexner to Theobald Smith, July 16, 1913.

63. Theobald Smith to Simon Flexner, July 26, 1913.

64. Theobald Smith, Day Card, September 16, 1913.

65. Theobald Smith, Day Card, October 15, 1913.

66. Theobald Smith, Bibliography No. 216.

67. Philip Smith, Personal communication to Claude E. Dolman.

68. Theobald Smith to Simon H. Gage, December 24, 1914.

69. Theobald Smith, Day Cards, December 12 and 13, 1914.

Chapter 21:

1. G.W. Corner, *A History of the Rockefeller Institute, 1901–1953,* p. 131.

2. Theobald Smith to Simon Flexner, June 8, 1915.

3. Simon Flexner to Theobald Smith, April 7, 1915.

4. E.G. Conklin to Theobald Smith, June 5, 1914.

5. Simon Flexner to Theobald Smith, June 24, 1915.

6. Simon Flexner, Autobiographical Notes, July 19, 1927. Cited in J.T. Flexner, *An American Saga,* p. 421.

7. J.T. Flexner, *An American Saga,* p. 443.

8. Peyton Rous, Personal communication to the author, October 1, 1968.

9. G.W. Corner, *A History of the Rockefeller Institute, 1901–1953,* p. 160.

10. J.T. Flexner, *An American Saga,* pp. 427–428.

11. Simon Flexner, Diary, May 2, 1928, "Noguchi's illness and death."

12. Simon Flexner, "The Pathologic Changes Caused by Certain Toxalbumins—an Experimental Study," *Transactions of the Pathological Society of Philadelphia* 17 (1896): 212–231.

13. Simon Flexner to Carl TenBroeck, May 14, 1935.

14. J.T. Flexner, *An American Saga,* p. 420.

15. G.W. Corner, *A History of the Rockefeller Institute, 1901–1953,* p. 513.

16. Henry James, Jr., *Charles W. Eliot* (Cambridge, Mass., The Riverside Press, 1930), 2 vols.

17. Peyton Rous, Personal communication to the author, October 1, 1968.

18. Henry James, Jr., to Theobald Smith, June 18, 1913.

19. Theobald Smith to Henry James, Jr., June 19, 1913.

20. Henry James, Jr., to Theobald Smith, April 9, 1914.

21. Ibid.

22. Theobald Smith, Day Card, April 20, 1914.

23. Theobald Smith, Day Card, April 21, 1914.

24. National Academy of Sciences, Program, Annual Meeting, Washington, D.C., April 21–23, 1914, Theobald Smith, Scrapbook No. 5, p. 10.

25. Theobald Smith, Day Card, June 14, 1914.

26. Henry James, Jr., to Theobald Smith (telegram and letter), June 27, 1914.

27. Theobald Smith to Henry James, Jr. (telegram and letter), June 29, 1914.

28. Messrs. Shepley, Rutan and Coolidge, "An Estimate of the Cost of Improvements at the Farm, Rockefeller Institute," undated, but undertaken between April and July, 1914.

29. Henry James, Jr., to Theobald Smith, June 27, 1914.

30. Henry James, Jr., to Theobald Smith, June 29, 1914.

31. Henry James, Jr., to Theobald Smith, July 7, 1914.

32. Theobald Smith to Henry James, Jr., July 8, 1914.

33. Henry James, Jr., to Theobald Smith, October 5, 1914.

34. Theobald Smith to Simon Flexner, April 6, 1914.

35. Theobald Smith, Day Card, May 24, 1914.

36. Editorial. "A Revolutionary Bill," *Boston Transcript,* May 14, 1914, Theobald Smith, Scrapbook No. 5, p. 19.

37. Simon Flexner to Lilian Egleston Smith, May 28, 1914.

38. Simon Flexner, Autobiographical Notes, July 19, 1927.

39. G.W. Corner, *A History of the Rockefeller Institute, 1901–1953,* pp. 132–133.

40. J.D. Greene to Simon Flexner (telegram), February 25, 1915.

41. "The New Rockefeller Institute for Medical Research and Adjacent Properties," *Princeton Press,* April 17, 1915, p. 11.

42. Theobald Smith to Simon Flexner, November 12, 1915.

43. Simon Flexner to Theobald Smith, November 16, 1914.

44. Theobald Smith to Simon Flexner, November 17, 1914.

45. George Fabyan to A.L. Lowell (telegram), January 11, 1915.

46. Theobald Smith to Simon Flexner, January 14, 1915.

47. Theobald Smith to George Fabyan, January 18, 1915.

48. Editorial. "Famous Harvard Medical Expert Called to Save Illinois Herds," *Chicago Herald,* January 12, 1915, Theobald Smith, Scrapbook No. 5, p. 36.

49. Editorial. "Harvard Savant Presents Plan to End Plague," *Chicago Herald,* February 4, 1915, Theobald Smith, Scrapbook No. 5, p. 37.

50. Ibid.

51. Theobald Smith, Day Card, February 12, 1915.

52. Theobald Smith, Bibliography No. 150.

53. F. Loeffler and P. Frosch, "Berichte der Kommission zur Entforschung der Maul und Kleuenseuche bei dem Institut für Infektionskrankheiten in Berlin," *Zentralblatt für Baktriologie* 23, Abt. I (1898): 371–391.

54. Editorial. "Abolish the 'Horse Doctor'," *The Country Gentleman,* March 6, 1915, Theobald Smith, Scrapbook No. 5, p. 38.

55. Theobald Smith, Bibliography No. 221.

56. Editorial. "The Obstinate Farmer," New York *Evening Globe,* March 13, 1915.

57. Editorial. "Senator Wilson's Son," New York *Globe,* March 30, 1915.

58. *Boston Transcript,* April 10, 1915.

59. E.B. Smith to Theobald Smith, March 18, 1915.

60. E.G. Conklin to Theobald Smith, May 30, 1914.

61. Theobald Smith, Day Card, June 26, 1915.

62. Theobald Smith to E.G. Conklin, July 5, 1915.

63. E.G. Conklin to Theobald Smith, July 10, 1915.

64. Theobald Smith to E.G. Conklin, August 13, 1915.

65. Theobald Smith to E.G. Conklin, August 27, 1915.

Chapter 22:

1. Theobald Smith, Day Card, November 13, 1915.

2. Editorial. "A Step Forward," *The Princeton Pictorial Review* 4 (March 4, 1916): 200.

3. Simon Flexner, "The Rockefeller Institute for Medical Research. The Department of Animal Pathology," *The Princeton Pictorial Review* 4 (March 4, 1916): 202.

4. Lilian Egleston Smith to Theobald Smith, July 4, 1914.

5. Theobald Smith to Simon Flexner, March 4, 1913.

6. Theobald Smith to Simon Flexner, August 24, 1914.

7. Theobald Smith to Simon Flexner, May 10, 1915.

8. Theobald Smith to Simon Flexner, May 18, 1915.

9. Theobald Smith, Day Cards, November 18 and December 15, 1915 and February 2, 1916.

10. Theobald Smith to Simon Flexner, January 4, 1918.

11. Simon Flexner to Theobald Smith, May 4, 1914.

12. Simon Flexner to Theobald Smith, May 6, 1914.

13. Theobald Smith to Simon Flexner, April 21, 1915.

14. Simon Flexner to Theobald Smith, April 26, 1915.

15. Theobald Smith to Simon Flexner, April 27, 1915.

16. Theobald Smith to Henry James, Jr., March 29, 1916.

17. Theobald Smith to Henry James, Jr., August 9, 1916.

18. Theobald Smith to Henry James, Jr., November 29, 1916.

19. Theobald Smith to Simon Flexner, February 2, 1917.

20. Theobald Smith to Simon Flexner, March 26, 1917.

21. Rhoda Erdmann, "Cytological Observations on the Behavior of Chicken Bone Marrow in Plasma Medium," *American Journal of Anatomy* 22 (1917): 73–125.

22. Theobald Smith to Rhoda Erdmann, June 29, 1917.

23. Simon Flexner to Theobald Smith, July 6, 1917.

24. Lilian Egleston Smith to Theobald Smith, June 28, 1917.

25. Theobald Smith to Henry James, Jr., May 9, 1914.

26. Henry James, Jr., to Theobald Smith, May 15, 1914.

27. Henry James, Jr., to Theobald Smith, July 7, 1914.

28. Theobald Smith to Henry James, Jr., October 25, 1914.

29. Theobald Smith to Simon Flexner, November 12, 1914.

30. F.C. Winkler to Theobald Smith, January 2, 1915.

31. Theobald Smith to F.C. Winkler, January 4, 1915.

32. Theobald Smith to R.B. Little, January 4, 1915.
33. Theobald Smith to R.B. Little, January 7, 1915.
34. Theobald Smith to Henry James, Jr., April 23, 1915.
35. Theobald Smith, Day Card, June 30, 1916.
36. Theobald Smith, Day Cards, July 3–5, 1916.
37. Theobald Smith to Henry James, Jr., August 9, 1916.
38. Theobald Smith to Simon Flexner, December 1, 1917.
39. Theobald Smith to Simon Flexner, November 5, 1919.
40. Theobald Smith, "Memorandum to Director and Executive Committee, Rockefeller Institute for Medical Research Hog Cholera Research Program," April 1915.
41. Theobald Smith, "Memorandum to Board of Trustees, Rockefeller Institute for Medical Research Hog Cholera Research Program," December 23, 1915.
42. Henry James, Jr., to Theobald Smith, December 28, 1915.
43. Theobald Smith, Day Cards, February 7 and March 20, 1916.
44. Theobald Smith to Simon Flexner, March 22, 1916.
45. Henry James, Jr., to Theobald Smith, July 13, 1916.
46. J.J. Hill to H.M. Biggs, January 20, 1914.
47. Theobald Smith, Day Card, November 29, 1915.
48. Carnegie Institute, Invitation from Trustees to Attend Celebration of the Twentieth Founder's Day, Theobald Smith, Scrapbook No. 5.
49. Theobald Smith, "The Topography of Pneumonic Lesions in Certain Mammals," typed Notice of Staff Meeting, Rockefeller Institute for Medical Research, April 28, 1916, Theobald Smith, Scrapbook No. 5, p. 73.
50. Seating List, Harvey Society's Supper Party at Sherry's Honoring William Henry Welch, November 29, 1915, Theobald Smith, Scrapbook No. 5, p. 75.
51. W. H. Welch, "Medical Education in the United States," *Harvey Lectures (1915–16),* pp. 366–382.
52. S. Flexner and J.F. Flexner, *William Henry Welch and the Heroic Age of American Medicine,* p. 336.
53. Theobald Smith, Bibliography No. 227.
54. Congress of American Physicians, Program, 10th Triennial Session, Theobald Smith, Scrapbook No. 5, p. 76.
55. Lectures on the Herter Foundation, Ninth Course, 1916, Theobald Smith, Scrapbook No. 5, p. 96.
56. Theobald Smith, Bibliography No. 307.
57. Theobald Smith, Bibliography No. 230. See also Theobald Smith, Scrapbook No. 5, p. 79, for formal announcement.
58. Theobald Smith, Monthly Accounts for May 1916 and January 1917.
59. Simon H. Gage to Theobald Smith, May 16, 1916.
60. Theobald Smith, Bibliography No. 226.
61. "Professor Gage's Response," in *The Gage Memorial; a Report of the Exercises in Connection with the Presentation of the Fund for the Simon H. Gage Fellowship in Animal Biology to Cornell University* (Ithaca, N.Y., Cornell University, 1916), p. 21.
62. Simon H. Gage to Theobald Smith, October 28, 1915.
63. Theobald Smith, Day Card, April 20, 1916.
64. Theobald Smith, Day Card, May 31, 1916.

65. Theobald Smith, Bibliography No. 228.
66. Theobald Smith, Bibliography Nos. 228 and 229.
67. Theobald Smith, Day Card, November 15, 1916.
68. R.B. Little, Personal interview with the author, February 1965.
69. N. Shaw, "Memoir of Theobald Smith," and letter to Philip H. Smith, November 30, 1939.
70. Ibid.
71. Ibid.
72. Theobald Smith, Day Cards, April 8 and 9, 1916.
73. Theobald Smith to Secretary, Yale Corporation, June 21, 1916, Theobald Smith, Scrapbook No. 5, p. 84.
74. N. Shaw, "Memoir of Theobald Smith," and letter to Philip H. Smith, November 30, 1939.
75. Theobald Smith, Day Card, June 19, 1916.
76. N. Shaw, "Memoir of Theobald Smith," and letter to Philip H. Smith, November 30, 1939.
77. Ibid.
78. T.M. Prudden to Henry James, Jr., October 28, 1918. Reproduced in Lillian T. Prudden, ed., *Biographical Sketches and Letters of T. Mitchell Prudden,* p. 169.
79. N. Shaw, "Memoir of Theobald Smith," and letter to Philip H. Smith, November 30, 1939.
80. Theobald Smith, Day Card, September 13, 1916.
81. Theobald Smith to Henry James, Jr., December 13, 1916.
82. Peyton Rous, Personal interview with the author, October 1, 1968.
83. Theobald Smith to Henry James, Jr., April 20, 1916.
84. Henry James, Jr., to Theobald Smith, April 25, 1916.
85. Henry James, Jr., to Starr J. Murphy, August 9, 1916.
86. Theobald Smith, Bibliography No. 231.
87. Theobald Smith, Day Cards, September 25 to October 3, 1917.
88. Theobald Smith to Simon H. Gage, January 13, 1918.
89. Simon Flexner to T.M. Prudden, September 5, 1918.
90. T.M. Prudden to Henry James, Jr., October 28, 1918.
91. Theobald Smith, Day Card, February 7, 1918.

Chapter 23:
1. I. Fisher to Theobald Smith, May 10, 1917.
2. Circular letter from Lella Faya Secor, Secretary, Emergency Peace Federation, February 8, 1917.
3. Theobald Smith to the Hon. J. Fralinghaysen, March 31, 1917.
4. Theobald Smith to G. Geffky, October 7, 1914 (in German).
5. Theobald Smith to H. Kossel, October 5, 1914.
6. H. Kossel to Theobald Smith, November 1, 1914.
7. D. Weber to Theobald Smith, December 28, 1914.
8. F. Schmidt to Theobald Smith, August 24, 1914.
9. Theobald Smith to F. Schmidt, October 18, 1914 (in German).

10. Lilian Egleston Smith to Theobald Smith, June 26, 1916.

11. Lilian Egleston Smith to Theobald Smith, July 12, 1916.

12. Lilian Egleston Smith to Theobald Smith, June 28, 1917.

13. Rev. E. Cummings to Theobald Smith, December 24, 1919.

14. Adjutant General's Office to Theobald Smith, October 7, 1908; signed by John E. Wright, Secretary of War, and countersigned by President Theodore Roosevelt.

15. Commission of Theobald Smith as Major, Medical Section, U.S. Army Officer Reserve Corps., from Secretary of War, to rank from April 11, 1915.

16. Association of Military Surgeons to Major Theobald Smith, notifying him of election to active membership, to date from January 1, 1921; signed by Captain F.L. Pleadwell, U.S.N. and Colonel J.R. Church, September 3, 1921.

17. Adjutant General, U.S. Army to Major Theobald Smith, March 29, 1923.

18. Jacques Loeb, "Biology and War," *Science* 45 (January 26, 1917): pp. 73–77.

19. Simon Flexner to Theobald Smith, September 16, 1918.

20. T.M. Prudden to Henry James, Jr., October 28, 1918.

21. W.H. Welch to Simon Flexner (telegrams), June 10 and 12, 1917.

22. E.W. Smillie, Personal interview with the author, October 15–16, 1966.

23. C.G. Bull and I.W. Pritchett, "Identity of the Toxins of Different Strains of *Bacillus Welchii* and Factors Influencing Their Production *in Virto,*" *Journal of Experimental Medicine* 26 (1917): 867–883.

24. W.H. Welch and G.H.F. Nuttall, "A Gas-Producing Bacillus (*Bacillus Aerogenes Capsulatus, Nov. spec.*) Capable of Rapid Development in the Blood Vessels after Death," *Johns Hopkins Hospital Bulletin* 3 (1892): 81–91.

25. Theobald Smith to Simon Flexner, February 26, 1917.

26. W.F. Nicholson, Admiralty, London, to Secretary, Rockefeller Institute for Medical Research, New York, September 1, 1919.

27. Simon Flexner, Diary, July 21, 1938, "Carrel."

28. Simon Flexner to T.M. Prudden, April 4, 1919.

29. A. Carrel and G. Dehelly, *The Treatment of Infected Wounds* (New York, Hoebner, 1916).

30. A.D. Bevan to W.H. Welch, October 25, 1917.

31. Simon Flexner to W.H. Welch, undated, but about the end of October 1917.

32. Simon Flexner, Diary, July 21, 1938, "Carrel."

33. Theobald Smith, Day Card, Janaury 17, 1920.

34. Theobald Smith to Simon Flexner, October 5, 1919.

35. T.M. Prudden to Simon Flexner, undated, but about December 1919.

36. Alexis Carrel and C.A. Lindbergh, *The Culture of Organs* (New York, Hoebner, 1938).

37. Alexis Carrel, *Man the Unknown* (New York, Harper & Bros., 1935).

38. G.W. Corner, *A History of the Rockefeller Institute, 1901–1953,* pp. 227–229.

39. Simon Flexner, Diary, June 21, 1938, "Carrel."

40. J.T. Durkin, *Hope for Our Time—Alexis Carrel on Men and Society* (New York, Harper & Row, 1965), p. 130.

41. Editorial. "Carrel the Unknown," *Washington Post,* September 14, 1944.

42. Simon Flexner to T.M. Prudden, September 5, 1918.

43. T.M. Prudden to Simon Flexner, October 20, 1918.

44. Simon Flexner to T.M. Prudden, September 5, 1918.

45. T.M. Prudden to Simon Flexner, October 20, 1918.
46. Simon Flexner to T.M. Prudden, February 7, 1919.
47. E.W. Smillie, Personal interview with the author, October 15–16, 1966.
48. Ibid.
49. Ibid.
50. Ibid.
51. Ibid.
52. TenBroeck always spelled his name as one word, with a capital B in the middle. Theobald Smith split the name into "Ten" and "Broeck," and Flexner followed suit. The one-word spelling has been adapted here, except where it appears in quotation, where it is left as written.
53. Carl TenBroeck to Theobald Smith, October 26, 1918.
54. Simon Flexner and J.T. Flexner, *William Henry Welch and the Heroic Age of American Medicine*, pp. 397–415.
55. Carl TenBroeck to Theobald Smith, November 15, 1920.
56. Carl TenBroeck to Theobald Smith, January 25, 1921.
57. Carl TenBroeck to Theobald Smith, August 28, 1921.
58. Carl TenBroeck to Theobald Smith, January 25, 1921.
59. Theobald Smith to Carl TenBroeck, July 19, 1921.
60. Simon Flexner and J.T. Flexner, *William Henry Welch and the Heroic Age of American Medicine*, pp. 397–415.
61. Whether an official invitation to Theobald Smith was ever under consideration is not clear. If so, the proposal could have been vetoed by Simon Flexner, or by John D. Rockefeller, Jr., himself, who still awaited an invitation to visit the new department near Princeton.
62. Carl TenBroeck to Theobald Smith, October 2, 1921.
63. Theobald Smith to Simon H. Gage, August 24, 1915.
64. Theobald Smith to Simon H. Gage, April 8, 1918.
65. Lilian Egleston Smith to Theobald Smith, July 12, 1916.
66. Theobald Smith, Day Card, July 14, 1917.
67. Lilian Egleston Smith to Theobald Smith, July 5–8, 1917.
68. Theobald Smith, Day Cards, April 13–16, 1918; Theobald Smith, Diary, April 15, 16 and 21, 1918.
69. Theobald Smith, Diary, May 28 and June 12, 1918.
70. Theobald Smith, Diary, September 11, 1918.
71. Theobald Smith, Day Card, July 20, 1918.
72. Philip H. Smith, Personal communications to the author during various interviews, June 1966 to March 1977.
73. Ibid.
74. Theobald Smith, Day Card, March 29, 1920.
75. Theobald Smith, Day Card, January 3, 1922.
76. T.M. Prudden to Simon Flexner, August 21, 1920.
77. Lilian Egleston Smith to Theobald Smith, June 28, 1916.
78. Theobald Smith, Day Card, March 26, 1919.
79. Theobald Smith, Day Card, May 16, 1922.

80. Theobald Smith, Day Card, October 13, 1922.

81. Theobald Smith, Notes for letter to Secretary, Harvard Corporation, undated but written about May 20, 1920, Theobald Smith, Scrapbook No. 6, p. 28.

82. Theobald Smith, Day Card, February 3, 1920.

83. Theobald Smith, Day Card, December 3, 1920.

84. Theobald Smith, Day Card, October 14, 1922.

85. Theobald Smith, Day Card, November 9, 1922.

86. Theobald Smith, Day Card, May 13, 1922.

87. Theobald Smith to Simon H. Gage, April 8, 1918.

88. Theobald Smith to Simon H. Gage, March 24, 1918.

89. John D. Rockefeller, Jr., to Simon Flexner, September 26, 1919.

90. Theobald Smith to Simon Flexner, October 5, 1919.

91. Theobald Smith, Day Card, May 16, 1923.

92. Simon Flexner to Theobald Smith, December 9, 1919.

93. Theobald Smith, Bibliography No. 244.

Chapter 24:

1. Theobald Smith, Bibliography Nos. 225, 228, 229.

2. Theobald Smith, Bibliography Nos. 226, 227, 230, 231.

3. Theobald Smith to Simon Flexner, January 4, 1918.

4. Simon Flexner to Theobald Smith, February 15, 1919.

5. Theobald Smith to Simon Flexner, February 17, 1919.

6. Simon Flexner to Theobald Smith, September 8, 1919.

7. Simon Flexner to T.M. Prudden, September 28, 1920.

8. Theobald Smith to Simon Flexner, September 10, 1919.

9. Theobald Smith to T.M. Prudden, January 13, 1920.

10. Ibid.

11. Simon Flexner to T.M. Prudden, November 4, 1920.

12. T.M. Prudden to Theobald Smith, November 18, 1920.

13. Theobald Smith to T.M. Prudden, November 22, 1920.

14. Theobald Smith, Bibliography Nos. 240, 241, 242.

15. Simon Flexner to William H. Welch, January 26, 1921.

16. J.F. Huddleson to Simon Flexner, September 5, 1919.

17. Theobald Smith to Simon Flexner, January 4, 1918.

18. Karl F. Meyer, "Medical Research and Public Health."

19. Theobald Smith to Simon Flexner, June 20, 1921.

20. Simon Flexner to Theobald Smith, June 27, 1921.

21. Karl F. Meyer, "Medical Research and Public Health."

22. Simon Flexner to William H. Welch, January 5, 1922.

23. Theobald Smith recorded on his Day Card of January 20, 1922 that he and Lilian went with the Howes, where he saw "many old friends." Smith's scrapbook for the immediate postwar period shows the extent to which he relieved his gloominess by concerts featuring such performers as Fritz Kreisler and Pablo Casals. Musical programs went into his scrapbooks even more frequently than notices of honorary degrees, special lectureships, and other distinctions. His Scrapbook No. 5 contains, on p. 92, an elaborate engraved in-

vitation card and an 8-page program of a song receital by Reinhold Warlich that he and Lilian co-hosted with the Simon Frasers, the Rufus Coles, and Henry James, followed by supper at the Cosmopolitan Club, with invitations going to the Rockefeller Institute staff and their spouses. The program provided the words of Warlich's songs in French, German and Russian, together with English translations.

24. Simon Flexner to William H. Welch, January 5, 1922.
25. Simon Flexner to A. Schuster, August 23, 1919.
26. Theobald Smith, Day Card, December 15, 1919.
27. Theobald Smith, Bibliography No. 227.
28. About two years after his Washington engagement, Smith declined the presidency of the Eleventh Triennial Congress due to meet in 1919. Exactly three years after the Tenth Congress symposium, he was notified by the Secretary of the American Association of Immunologists, Dr. Arthur F. Coca, that he had been elected to "active membership" in the Association. This notice was sent several years after Theobald Smith supposedly reported to Coca "Immunology is dead." (Theobald Smith to A.F. Coca, May 10, 1922. The unlikelihood of his earlier claim is discussed in Chapter 20.)
29. Theobald Smith, Bibliography No. 230.
30. Theobald Smith, Day Card, June 7 and 8, 1917.
31. Theobald Smith, Bibliography No. 231.
32. Ibid.
33. Theobald Smith, Bibliography No. 220.
34. Theobald Smith to William H. Welch, February 27, 1921.
35. Theobald Smith to Charles W. Eliot, December 31, 1920.
36. Theobald Smith, Day Card, October 20, 1920.
37. "Announcement and Description of M. Douglas Flattery Prize, Harvard University," Theobald Smith, Scrapbook No. 5.
38. F.W. Hunnewell, Secretary, President's Office, Harvard University, to Theobald Smith, , Theobald Smith, Scrapbook No. 5.
39. Theobald Smith to F.W. Hunnewell, pencilled draft, Theobald Smith Scrapbook No. 5.
40. A.L. Lowell to Theobald Smith, Card of acknowledgement of gift to the Harvard Endowment Fund, Theobald Smith, Scrapbook No. 5.
41. Theobald Smith, Day Cards, September 21–29, 1920.
42. Theobald Smith, Bibliography No. 244.
43. Charles W. Eliot to Theobald Smith, December 27, 1920.
44. Theobald Smith to Charles W. Eliot, December 27, 1920.
45. Theobald Smith, Day Card, June 10, 1921.
46. Theobald Smith, Bibliography No. 249.
47. David Fairchild to Theobald Smith, August 5, 1921.
48. T.M. Prudden to Theobald Smith, October 3, 1921.
49. T.M. Prudden to Theobald Smith, December 7, 1921.
50. J.G. Wilson to Theobald Smith, March 18, 1920, Theobald Smith, Scrapbook No. 5, p. 16.
51. Theobald Smith to J.G. Wilson, March 22, 1920, Theobald Smith, Scrapbook No. 5, p. 26.
52. Theobald Smith, Bibliography No. 250.
53. Theobald Smith, Day Cards, October 20, 21 and 22, 1921.

54. Walt Whitman, "The Song of the Open Road."

55. T.M. Prudden to Theobald Smith, March 29, 1922.

56. Theobald Smith, Day Card, January 22, 1916.

57. Theobald Smith, Day Card, April 1, 1915.

58. T.M. Prudden to Theobald Smith, June 3, 1918.

59. Theobald Smith to T.M. Prudden, June 4, 1918.

60. Theobald Smith, "Report on a Proposed Cooperation between the Department of Animal Pathology and the Walker-Gordon Laboratories Company in the Prosecution of Research in Bovine Pathology and Dairy Sanitation," November 9, 1920.

61. Simon Flexner to T.M. Prudden, November 5, 1920.

62. Theobald Smith, Day Card, April 4, 1921.

63. Theobald Smith to Simon Flexner, November 10, 1919.

64. Theobald Smith, Bibliography No. 234.

65. Theobald Smith, Bibliography No. 237.

66. Theobald Smith, Bibliography No. 256.

67. Great Britain, Board of Agriculture and Fisheries, Committee to Inquire on Epizootic Abortion. "*Report of the Departmental Committee Appointed . . . to Enquire on Epizootic Abortion.* (London, H.M. Stationery Office [1909–10]). Appendix to pt. I, Epizootic Abortion in Cattle, 1909; Appendix to pt. III, Abortion in Sheep, 1913. Both appendices by Sir J. MacFadyean and Sir Stewart Stockman (London, Printed for H.M. Stationery Office by Eyre and Spottiswoode, 1909, 1913).

68. Theobald Smith, Bibliography No. 234.

69. Theobald Smith, Bibliography No. 236.

70. Theobald Smith, Bibliography No. 238.

71. Theobald Smith, Bibliography No. 247.

72. Theobald Smith, Bibliography No. 235.

73. Theobald Smith, Bibliography No. 238.

74. Theobald Smith, Bibliography No. 239.

75. Theobald Smith, Bibliography No. 262.

76. Theobald Smith, Bibliography No. 247.

77. Theobald Smith, Day Card, January 22, 1921.

78. Theobald Smith, Bibliography Nos. 240, 241, 242.

79. Theobald Smith, Bibliography Nos. 233, 248, 251.

80. C.E. Dolman, D.E. Kerr, H. Chang, and A.R. Shearer, "Two Cases of Ratbite Fever due to *Streptobacillus moniliformis*," *Canadian Journal of Experimental Medicine* 1951, 42:228–241.

81. R.B. Little and M.L. Orcutt, "The Transmission of Agglutinins for *Bacillus abortus* from cow to calf in the colostrum," *Journal of Experimental Medicine* 35 (1921): 161–171.

82. Theobald Smith, Bibliography No. 253.

83. Theobald Smith, Bibliography No. 254.

84. Theobald Smith, Bibliography No. 257.

85. Theobald Smith, Bibliography No. 259.

86. Theobald Smith, Bibliography No. 255.

87. Theobald Smith, Bibliography No. 258.

88. Theobald Smith, "Suggestions concerning Directions of Growth of the Department of Animal Pathology in the Near Future," 1923. Typescript, 15 pp.

Chapter 25:

1. J. Lorain Smith to Theobald Smith, July 5, 1923.
2. Theobald Smith to J. Lorain Smith, July 23, 1923.
3. J. Lorain Smith to Theobald Smith, August 14, 1923.
4. Theobald Smith, Day Card, November 23, 1923.
5. Theobald Smith, Day Card, November 24, 1923.
6. Theobald Smith, Day Card, November 26, 1923.
7. Theobald Smith, Day Card, November 27, 1923.
8. Theobald Smith, Bibliography No. 261.
9. J. Lorain Smith to Theobald Smith, November 16, 1923.
10. Theobald Smith, Day Card, November 29, 1923.
11. Theobald Smith, Bibliography No. 260.
12. Ibid.
13. Sir Robert Philip to Theobald Smith, February 7, 1924.
14. Sir Robert Philip to Theobald Smith, December 8, 1923. Theobald Smith, President of the National Tuberculosis Association, gave his address, entitled "Remarks on the Co-operation of Science and Practice in Tuberculosis" at the opening of the Fifth Conference of the International Union Against Tuberculosis, Washington, D.C., September 30, 1926.
15. Dean of Medicine Sidney Smith to Theobald Smith, June 8, 1934.
16. Theobald Smith, Day Card, December 18, 1923.
17. Theobald Smith, Day Card, October 18, 1924.
18. T.M. Prudden to Theobald Smith, November 16, 1893.
19. T.M. Prudden to Theobald Smith, September 1, 1918.
20. T.M. Prudden to Theobald Smith, January 27, 1919.
21. T.M. Prudden to Theobald Smith, March 25, 1919.
22. T.M. Prudden to Theobald Smith, July 29, 1919.
23. T.M. Prudden to Theobald Smith, October 21, 1920.
24. T.M. Prudden to Theobald Smith, June 10, 1922.
25. T.M. Prudden to Theobald Smith, March 1, 1923.
26. Theobald Smith, Day Card, April 12, 1924.
27. John D. Rockefeller, Jr., to T.M. Prudden, May 1923, quoted from Lillian E. Prudden, ed., *Sketches and Letters of T. Mitchell Prudden, M.D.*, p. 170.
28. Theobald Smith, Bibliogaphy No. 264.
29. Theobald Smith, Bibliogaphy No. 265.
30. Theobald Smith, Bibliogaphy No. 267.
31. Theobald Smith, Bibliogaphy No. 266.
32. Theobald Smith, Diary, July 1, 1925.
33. Theobald Smith, Day Cards, September 28–29, 1925.
34. Theobald Smith, Day Cards, November 19–21, 1925.
35. Theobald Smith, Bibliography No. 273
36. Theobald Smith, Diary, Day Card, October 4, 1926.
37. Theobald Smith, Bibliography No. 272.
38. Elizabeth M. O'Hern, "Alice Evans and the Brucellosis Story," *Annali Sclavo; Rivista di Microbiologia e di Immunologia* 19, no. 1 (January-February 1977): 12–19. This is preceeded by a brief summary which contains a bibliography of Evans's publications.

39. Alice C. Evans, "Further Studies on Bacterium Abortus and Related Bacteria. II. A Comparison of Bacterium Abortus with Bacterium Bronchiosepticus and with the Organism Which Causes Malta Fever," *Journal of Infectious Diseases* 22 (1918): 580–593.

40. Theobald Smith, Bibliogaphy No. 204.

41. Theobald Smith, Bibliogaphy No. 238.

42. Theobald Smith, Bibliogaphy No. 269.

43. Theobald Smith, Bibliogaphy No. 270.

44. Theobald Smith, Bibliogaphy No. 284.

45. Theobald Smith, Bibliogaphy No. 288.

46. Theobald Smith, Bibliogaphy No. 269.

47. Theobald Smith, Bibliogaphy No. 289.

48. Theobald Smith, Bibliogaphy Nos. 262, 270.

49. Theobald Smith, Bibliogaphy No. 290.

50. Theobald Smith, Bibliogaphy No. 304.

51. As examples of this type of correspondence in Smith's preserved papers, the following two letters can be cited as somewhat typical examples: Theobald Smith to B.S. Oppenheim (of the Mt. Sinai Hospital in New York City), November 30, 1931; Theobald Smith to G.D. Morrison (of the newspaper *New Orleans States*), November 10, 1931.

52. In addition to the article on Evans cited in note 38, Elizabeth O'Hern wrote the biography of Alice Evans in *Notable American Women: The Modern Period* (Cambridge, Mass.: Harvard University Press, 1980), pp. 19–21. The information cited here comes from "Alice Evans and the Brucellosis Story," pp. 17–18.

53. Eli Chernin, "Paul de Kruif's *Microbe Hunters* and an Outraged Ronald Ross," *Reviews of Infectious Diseases* 10, no. 3 (May-June 1988): 661–667.

54. Tom Rivers, *Reflections of a Life in Medicine and Science, an Oral History Memoir Prepared by Saul Benison* (Cambridge, Mass., M.I.T. Press [1967]), pp. 180–181.

55. Paul de Kruif, *The Sweeping Wind, a Memoir* (New York, Harcourt, Brace & World [1962]), p. 27.

56. Ibid, p. 55.

57. Tom Rivers, *Reflections of a Life in Medicine and Science,* p. 181.

58. Paul de Kruif, *Microbe Hunters,* Chapter VIII.

59. Eli Chernin, "Paul de Kruif's *Microbe Hunters* and an Outraged Ronald Ross."

60. Theobald Smith to Simon Flexner, December 1, 1931.

61. Simon Flexner to Theobald Smith, December 11, 1931.

62. Theobald Smith to Simon Flexner, July 31, 1926.

63. Theobald Smith, Bibliogaphy No. 274.

64. Theobald Smith, Bibliogaphy No. 275.

65. Theobald Smith, Bibliogaphy No. 276.

66. Theobald Smith, Bibliogaphy No. 265.

67. Theobald Smith, Bibliogaphy No. 280.

68. Theobald Smith, Bibliogaphy No. 281.

69. Theobald Smith, Bibliogaphy No. 282.

70. Theobald Smith, Bibliogaphy No. 285.

71. Theobald Smith, Bibliogaphy No. 277.

72. Theobald Smith, Day Card, April 1, 1927.

73. Theobald Smith, Bibliogaphy No. 278.

74. Theobald Smith, Bibliogaphy No. 279.
75. Theobald Smith to Simon Flexner, January 19, 1927.
76. Theobald Smith, Bibliogaphy No. 286.
77. Theobald Smith, Bibliogaphy No. 291.

Chapter 26:
1. Much of the information appearing here was published previously in Claude E. Dolman's "Hideyo Noguchi (1876–1928): His Final Effort in West Africa," *Clio Medica* 12, nos. 2–3 (June-September 1977): 131–145.
2. Quoted from Simon Flexner's "Diary," which was irregularly kept. Ten entries about Noguchi appeared between May 22, 1928 and July 12, 1931.
3. Ibid.
4. The classical publication on the subject, "Experimental Transmission of Yellow Fever to Laboratory Animals," by Adrian Stokes, J.H. Bauer and N.P. Hudson, appeared in the *American Journal of Tropical Medicine* 8 (1928): 103–164.
5. Theobald Smith, Bibliography No. 287.
6. Gustav Eckstein to Theobald Smith, March 3, 1929.
7. Theobald Smith to Gustav Eckstein, March 5, 1929.
8. Gustav Eckstein to Theobald Smith, March 27, 1929.
9. Gustav Eckstein, *Noguchi* (New York, Harper and Brothers, 1931).
10. Tom Rivers, *Reflections of a Life in Medicine and Science,* pp. 95–96.
11. Ibid., pp. 96–97.
12. Claude E. Dolman, "Noguchi (Seisaki), Hideyo," *Dictionary of Scientific Biography* (New York, Charles Scribner's Sons [1974]), pp. 141–145.
13. P.A. Lewis to Theobald Smith, May 14, 1921.
14. P.A. Lewis to Simon Flexner, January 20, 1923; P.A. Lewis to Theobald Smith, January 24, 1923; Simon Flexner to Theobald Smith, January 26, 1923; P.A. Lewis to Theobald Smith, January 27, 1923; P.A. Lewis to Theobald Smith, January 28, 1923; P.A. Lewis to Theobald Smith, January 29, 1923.
15. P.A. Lewis to Theobald Smith, July 11 and 21, 1923.
16. P.A. Lewis to Theobald Smith, August 20, 1925.
17. Simon Flexner to P.A. Lewis, December 4, 1925.
18. Simon Flexner to Theobald Smith, December 21, 1925.
19. Simon Flexner to P.A. Lewis, August 1, 1927.
20. Simon Flexner to Theobald Smith, September 12, 1927.
21. Simon Flexner to P.A. Lewis, September 22, 1927.
22. Simon Flexner to Theobald Smith, January 27, 1928.
23. Theobald Smith to Simon Flexner, February 28, 1928.
24. Simon Flexner to P.A. Lewis, April 27, 1928.
25. Simon Flexner to Theobald Smith, June 18, 1928.
26. Simon Flexner to Theobald Smith, June 20, 1928.
27. Simon Flexner to Theobald Smith, June 22, 1928.
28. Simon Flexner to Theobald Smith, June 30, 1928.
29. F.F. Russell to Simon Flexner, October 26, 1928.
30. Simon Flexner to F.F. Russell, October 29, 1928.
31. F.F. Russell to Theobald Smith, October 30, 1928.

32. P.A. Lewis to Theobald Smith, February 1, 1929.
33. Theobald Smith to P.A. Lewis, February 19, 1929.
34. P.A. Lewis to Simon Flexner, April 12, 1929.
35. Simon Flexner to Theobald Smith, June 30, 1929.
36. Simon Flexner to Theobald Smith, July 1, 1929.
37. Simon Flexner, "Paul Adin Lewis," *Science* n.s. 70 (August 9, 1929): 133–134.
38. Simon Flexner to Theobald Smith, July 27, 1929.
39. John Auer and Paul A. Lewis, "The Physiology of the Immediate Reaction of Anaphylaxis in the Guinea-Pig," *Journal of Experimental Medicine* 12 (1910): 151–175.
40. Simon Flexner and Paul A. Lewis, "Experimental Poliomyelitis in Monkeys: Active Immunization and Passive Serum Protection," *Journal of the American Medical Association* 54 (1910): 1780–1782.
41. Theobald Smith to Simon Flexner, July 31, 1926.
42. Simon Flexner to Theobald Smith, August 6, 1926.
43. Simon Flexner to Theobald Smith, November 23, 1926.
44. Theobald Smith to Simon Flexner, December 31, 1926.
45. Carl TenBroeck to Theobald Smith, January 14, 1927.
46. Western Union Cablegram, undated; in a letter to Smith of February 27, Flexner reported that in accordance with their telephone conversation they had sent such a cablegram to TenBroeck.
47. Theobald Smith to Simon Flexner, July 29, 1927.
48. Simon Flexner to Abraham Flexner, September 21, 1927.
49. Abraham Flexner to Carl TenBroeck, September 30, 1927.
50. Simon Flexner to Theobald Smith, January 25, 1928.
51. Theobald Smith to Simon Flexner, January 26, 1928.
52. Theobald Smith to Simon Flexner, September 22, 1928.
53. Theobald Smith to Simon Flexner, November 29, 1928.
54. Theobald Smith to Simon Flexner, December 12, 1928.
55. Simon Flexner to Theobald Smith, January 28, 1929.
56. Simon Flexner to Theobald Smith, April 29, 1929.
57. Charles Rupert Stockard (1879–1939) was one of America's outstanding biological scientists of the twentieth century. While he did not succeed Theobald Smith as Director of the Institute's Department of Animal Pathology, he did succeed him as President of the Institute's Board of Scientific Directors upon Smith's death in 1935.
58. Theobald Smith to Simon Flexner, April 30, 1929.
59. Theobald Smith to Simon Flexner, May 27, 1929.
60. Theobald Smith to Simon Flexner, May 28, 1929.
61. Simon Flexner to Theobald Smith, May 29, 1929.
62. Simon Flexner to Theobald Smith, June 6, 1929.
63. Theobald Smith to Simon Flexner, June 27, 1929.
64. Simon Flexner to Theobald Smith, June 28, 1929.
65. Theobald Smith, Day Card, July 1, 1929.
66. Theobald Smith, Day Card, July 8, 1929.
67. Simon Flexner to Theobald Smith, July 27, 1929.
68. Simon Flexner to Theobald Smith, July 30, 1929.
69. Theobald Smith, Day Cards, October 5 and 7, 1929.

70. Theobald Smith, Day Card, November 7, 1929.

71. Theobald Smith, Day Card, November 8, 1929.

72. Theobald Smith, Day Cards, November 9 and 10, 1929.

73. Theobald Smith, Day Cards, November 18 and 19, 1929.

74. Theobald Smith, Day Cards, November 23 and 26, 1929.

75. Theobald Smith, Day Card, December 19, 1929.

76. Simon Flexner to Theobald Smith, September 25, 1929.

77. Theobald Smith to Simon Flexner, September 27, 1929.

78. Simon Flexner to Theobald Smith, December 16, 1929.

79. Theobald Smith to Simon Flexner, December 24, 1929.

80. Simon Flexner to Theobald Smith, January 6, 1930.

81. Simon Flexner to Theobald Smith, February 3, 1930.

82. "The London Correspondent of the Journal of the American Medical Association. . . ." *Science* n.s. 71 (January 31, 1930): 122.

83. "Memorial to Manson," *Journal of the American Medical Association* 95, no. 5 (February 2, 1930): 351.

84. Smith was referring here to Dr. George C. Low of the London School of Tropical Medicine, who, with his colleague Dr. Luigi Sambon, in 1900 carried out under the auspices of the Colonial Office a series of experiments to test the truth of the mosquito theory of malaria by a practical application. Living for six months in the heart of the swamps in the Romana Compagna, near Ostia, a notoriously malarious region of Italy, and enclosing themselves in a mosquito-proof hut from an hour before sunset until an hour after sunrise each day so as to avoid being bit by mosquitos, which were believed to feed only at night, they survived infection entirely without the aid of quinine or other drugs. During the day, when mosquitos did not bite, they occupied themselves by collecting animal and insect life, including mosquitos, and making observations on the anopheles and their larvae. Further confirmation of the theory was afforded by the report of similar success by a team sent by the Liverpool school to the most malarious spots of Nigeria, where its members maintained their immunity through the careful use of mosquito nets at night. See the *British Medical Journal* 2 (1900): 847–848, 1266, 1679–1682, and *Nature* 62 (1900): 230, 531. In a connected experiment carried on by Dr. Manson, infected anopheles mosquitos were sent by Prof. Bastianelli in Rome to London where Manson allowed them to bite a volunteer (his son), who developed malaria fifteen days later and was cured by quinine. See the *British Medical Journal* 2 (1900): 949–951.

85. Theobald Smith to Simon Flexner, February 7, 1930.

86. Simon Flexner to Theobald Smith, February 10, 1930.

87. Theobald Smith to Simon Flexner, February 12, 1930.

88. Simon Flexner to Theobald Smith, April 1, 1930.

89. Simon Flexner to Theobald Smith, April 10, 1930.

90. Theobald Smith to Simon Flexner, April 16, 1930.

91. Theobald Smith's diary records that he did begin sitting for his portrait on May 1 (two sessions) and that he visited Borie again on May 2, 13, 14, 21, 24, 27, and June 2, 9 and 14. Born in Paris in 1877, and completing his education in Munich, Borie came to Philadelphia before 1910 and specialized in portrait painting. He died in 1934 at the age of fifty-seven, not long after completing Smith's portrait.

92. Theobald Smith to Simon Flexner, September 10, 1929.

93. Simon Flexner to Theobald Smith, October 16, 1929.
94. Theobald Smith, Bibliography Nos. 293, 294, 295.
95. Theobald Smith, Bibliography No. 253.
96. Theobald Smith, Bibliography No. 266.
97. Theobald Smith, Bibliography No. 297.
98. Theobald Smith to Simon Flexner, April 29, 1930.
99. Theobald Smith, Day Cards, May 5–8, 1930.
100. Theobald Smith to Simon Flexner, May 23, 1930.
101. Theobald Smith, Day Cards, May 16, June 2 and June 29, 1930.
102. Marshal Fabyan to Theobald Smith, September 19, 1930.
103. Marshal Fabyan to Theobald Smith, January 12, 1931.
104. Simon Flexner to Theobald Smith, February 14, 1930.
105. Theobald Smith to Simon Flexner, February 16, 1930.
106. Theobald Smith, Bibliography No. 301.
107. Theobald Smith, Bibliography No. 302.
108. Theobald Smith, Day Cards, October 17 and 18, 1930.
109. Howard T. Krasner to Theobald Smith, April 28, 1930.
110. Homer N.C. Iver to Theobald Smith, September 23, 1930.
111. Milton J. Rosenau to Theobald Smith, April 24, 1931.
112. Theobald Smith to Simon Flexner, January 27, 1931.
113. Simon Flexner to Theobald Smith, January 31, 1931.
114. Theobald Smith to Simon Flexner, February 1, 1931.
115. Simon Flexner to Theobald Smith, February 3, 1931.
116. E.B. McKinley to Frederick P. Gay, January 8, 1930; Frederick P. Gay to Theobald Smith, January 14, 1930.
117. Theobald Smith to Frederick P. Gay, January 20, 1930.
118. Frederick P. Gay to Theobald Smith, January 21, 1930.
119. E.B. McKinley to Theobald Smith, January 27, 1930.
120. Theobald Smith to E.B. McKinley, February 10, 1931.
121. Theobald Smith to E.B. McKinley, February 11, 1931; E.B. McKinley to Theobald Smith, February 17, 1931.
122. Theobald Smith, Day Cards, January 30–31, February 3, February 27–March 3, 1931.
123. Theobald Smith, Day Cards, March 12–30, 1931.
124. E.B. McKinley to Theobald Smith, April 8, 1931.

Chapter 27:

1. Theobald Smith, Bibliography No. 299.
2. Theobald Smith, Day Cards, April 16–19, 1931.
3. Theobald Smith, Day Cards, May 18–21, 1931.
4. Theobald Smith, Day Cards, June 8-September 26, 1931.
5. Flexner reported to Smith in a letter of April 30, 1930, written after Smith had declined his invitation to represent the Institute at the various European congresses during the coming summer due, in part, to the need to vacate the Director's quarters, that he had spoken to E.B. Smith about deferring leasing the house until autumn and that they would not begin altering it before then, allowing Theobald and Lilian to remain at Larkfields longer. An exchange of several other letters on this subject followed.

6. These notes are referred to in the very first endnote in this book, Note 1 of Chapter I.

7. Simon Flexner, Diary, November 18, 1931.

8. Peyton Rous, Personal communication to the author, October 1, 1968.

9. Simon Flexner, Diary Notes, November 18, 1931.

10. "Speeches. Testimonial Dinner Given to Dr. Theobald Smith on the Occasion of the Opening of 'the Theobald Smith House' at the Rockefeller Institute, Princeton, N.J. November 30, 1931." Typescript, 32 pp. A number of copies were bound for distribution to honorees and guests, and copies exist on thin typewriter paper as well.

11. Ibid., pp. 27–31.

12. Simon Flexner to Theobald Smith, August 7, 1931.

13. Theobald Smith to Simon Flexner, August 12, 1931.

14. Mark Wyman Richardson (brother of the late Harvard Professor of Surgery Maurice Howe Richardson), received the Harvard M.D. degree in 1894 and served as Secretary of the Massachusetts State Board of Health from 1909 to 1914, during Smith's last years in Boston. He wrote on bacteriology and immunology and on the epidemiology of poliomyelitis.

15. Simon Flexner to Theobald Smith, August 13, 1931.

16. Simon Flexner to Theobald Smith, August 14, 1931.

17. Theobald Smith to Simon Flexner, September 10, 1931.

18. Theobald Smith to Simon Flexner, September 15, 1931.

19. Simon Flexner to Theobald Smith, September 11, 1931.

20. Ellsworth Huntington, "The Matamek Conference on Biological Cycles, 1931," *Science* 74 (September 4, 1931): 229–235.

21. Theobald Smith to Leslie T. Webster, November 16, 1931. Webster's paper, "Experimental Epidemiology," subsequently appeared in *Science* 75 (April 29, 1932): 445–452, and in *Medicine* 11 (September 1932): 321–344.

22. Simon Flexner to Theobald Smith, November 22, 1931.

23. Simon Flexner to Theobald Smith, December 16, 1931.

24. Fred Neufeld, "Die Typenfrage in der Bakteriologie."

25. See pp. 204–205.

26. Theobald Smith, Bibliography No. 300.

27. Simon Flexner to Theobald Smith, February 24, 1932.

28. Theobald Smith to Simon Flexner, February 25, 1932.

29. Simon Flexner to Theobald Smith, February 24, 1932, a letter totally dissimilar from the one cited in Note 27. This was devoted solely to a program to be put on at the Institute in New York on the semi-centennial of the tubercle bacillus discovery. In it, Flexner told that he would cable Neufeld to speak if such a program was possible.

30. Simon Flexner to Theobald Smith, February 26, 1932.

31. Theobald Smith, Day Card, March 8, 1932.

32. Theobald Smith, Day Card, March 14, 1932.

33. Theoald Smith, Bibliography No. 303.

34. Theobald Smith, Day Card, March 24, 1932.

35. C.M. Wenyon to Theobald Smith, April 1, 1932.

36. Simon Flexner to Theobald Smith, May 29, 1932.

37. Theobald Smith to Simon Flexner, June 1, 1932.

38. Theobald Smith, Day Card, May 11–14, 1932.

39. Lord Rayleigh (Foreign Secretary) to Theobald Smith, June 3, 1932.

40. For Cannon's experience, see Elin L. Wolfe, A. Clifford Barger and Saul Benison, *Walter B. Cannon, Science and Society* (Boston, Boston Medical Library in The Francis A. Countway Library of Medicine; Distributed by the Harvard University Press, 2000), pp. 290–291.

41. Theobald Smith, Day Cards, September 19–22, 1932.

42. There is a folder in the Theobald Smith Papers marked "Battle Road House" which contains correspondence and other matters relating to the construction of the house; Theobald's diary entries can be found in the file for the years 1930–1932 under dates cited.

43. Theobald Smith to Simon Flexner, October 27, 1932.

44. Theobald Smith, Day Cards, January 3–10, 1933.

45. Theobald Smith, Day Cards, January 13–14, 18, 1933.

46. Theobald Smith, Day Cards, March 3–21, 1933.

47. Theobald Smith, Day Cards, April 5–7, May 6, 1933.

48. Theobald Smith, Bibliography No. 305.

49. Theobald Smith, Day Cards, April 18–19, 1933.

50. Theobald Smith to Simon Flexner, August 23, 1933.

51. Theobald Smith, Day Cards, May 31-October 9, 1933.

52. The letter from Dale about the Copley Medal was dated November 2, 1933. Dale expressed the hope that Smith could attend the Society's November 30th meeting to receive it. On November 15, Smith sent his regrets that circumstances prevented his indulgence in that pleasure, and the medal was later delivered to the American Embassy in London for transmittal to him.

53. Theobald Smith, Day Cards, October 28-December 31, 1933.

54. Theobald Smith, Day Cards, January 3-June 30, 1934.

55. Simon Flexner to Theobald Smith, July 3, 1934.

56. The biography of Welch, completed by Flexner with the help of his son James, was, of course, *William Henry Welch and the Heroic Age of American Medicine*.

57. Theobald Smith, Bibliography No. 307.

58. Theobald Smith to Simon Flexner, December 22, 1933.

59. Simon Flexner to Theobald Smith, December 27, 1933.

60. Simon Flexner to Theobald Smith, July 28, 1934.

61. William Bulloch, *The History of Bacteriology* (London, Oxford University Press, 1938).

62. William Bulloch, "Theobald Smith," *Journal of Pathology and Bacteriology* 30 (1935): 634.

63. Theobald Smith, Day Cards, June 29-October 5, 1934.

64. Theobald Smith, Day Cards, October 6–27, 1934.

65. Simon Flexner, Diary, November 18, 1934.

66. Theobald Smith, Day Card, November 18, 1934.

67. Simon Flexner, Diary, November 20, 1934.

68. Ibid.

69. Simon Flexner, Diary, December 13, 1934.

70. Ibid.

71. Simon Flexner, Diary, December 25, 1934.

72. Lilian Egleston Smith to Mr. and Mrs. Edric B. Smith, December 21, 1934.

73. Edric B. Smith to Lilian Egleston Smith, January 28, 1935.

74. Simon Flexner, Diary, January 1935.

75. In addition to his important blackhead work, Ernest Tyzzer is remembered today for having been among the first to do research on human leucocyte antigens—HLA—and on the heredity of mouse cancer as well as being the first to recognize inclusion bodies in varicella. See Clarence Cook Little and Ernest Edward Tyzzer, "Further Experimental Studies on the Inheritance of Susceptibility to a Transplantable Tumor, Carcinoma (J.W.A.) of the Japanese Walzing Mouse," *Journal of Medical Research* 33 (1916): 393–427; E.E. Tyzzer, "A Study of Heredity in Relation to the Development of Tumors in Mice," *Journal of Medical Research* 17 (1907–08): 199–211; and E.E. Tyzzer, "The Histology of the Skin Lesions in Varicella," *Journal of Medical Research* 14 (1905–06): 361–392.

76. E.E. Tyzzer to the Senate of the Caroline Medico-Chirurgical Institute, Stockholm, January 11, 1921; a copy is in the Harvard Medical Archives, Countway Library.

77. Howard T. Karsner to Theobald Smith, October 20, 1922.

78. Theobald Smith to Howard T. Karsner, October 23, 1922.

79. Peyton Rous to the Nobel Committee for Physiology and Medicine, January 5, 1925.

80. Peyton Rous to Carl TenBroeck, October 26, 1931.

81. Carl TenBroeck to Peyton Rous, October 27, 1931.

82. A.W. Meyer to Simon Gage, October 4, 1935.

83. Frederick B. Bang to the Nobel Prize Committee, November 17, 1958.

84. Nils K. Ståhle for the Nobel Foundation to Frederick B. Bang, November 26, 1958.

85. Tom Rivers, *Reflections on a Life in Medicine and Science,* pp. 86–87.

86. Ibid., pp. 146–147.

87. Simon Flexner, Diary, December 13, 1934.

88. Simon Flexner, Diary, December 14, 1934.

89. Charles Stockard, "Theobald Smith," *Science* 80 (December 21, 1934): 569–580.

90. William Bulloch, "Theobald Smith," p. 621.

INDEX

INDEX